ANNALS OF THE NEW YORK ACADEMY OF SCIENCES

Volume 485

BIOREGULATORY FUNCTIONS OF THROMBIN

ANNALS OF THE NEW YORK ACADEMY OF SCIENCES
Volume 485

BIOREGULATORY FUNCTIONS OF THROMBIN

Edited by Daniel A. Walz, John W. Fenton II,
and Marc A. Shuman

The New York Academy of Sciences
New York, New York
1986

Cover photo: *Electron micrograph of a pulmonary vessel in a dog following thrombin infusion; neutrophils and platelets are found associated with fibrin. A neutrophil is observed forming a phagocytic vacuole engulfing fibrin fibrils, indicating active phagocytosis of fibrin by neutrophils.* *See p. 298.*

Library of Congress Cataloging-in-Publication Data

Bioregulatory functions of thrombin.

(Annals of the New York Academy of Sciences, ISSN 0077-8923; v. 485)
"This volume is the result of a conference entitled Conference on Bioregulatory Functions of Thrombin, held in New York City on February 5-7, 1986, by the New York Academy of Sciences"—Contents p.
Includes bibliographies and index.
1. Thrombin—Congresses. I. Walz, Daniel A. II. Fenton, John W. III. Shuman, Marc A. IV. Conference on Bioregulatory Functions of Thrombin (1986 : New York, N.Y.) V. New York Academy of Sciences. VI. Series. [DNLM: 1. Thrombin—congresses. W1 AN 626YL v.485 / WH 310 B6156 1986]
Q11.N5 vol. 485 500 s 86-33321
[QP93.5] [612'.115]
ISBN 0-89766-365-9
ISBN 0-89766-366-7 (pbk.)

PCP
Printed in the United States of America
ISBN 0-89766-365-9 (cloth)
ISBN 0-89766-366-7 (paper)
ISSN 0077-8923

ANNALS OF THE NEW YORK ACADEMY OF SCIENCES

Volume 485
December 29, 1986

BIOREGULATORY FUNCTIONS OF THROMBIN[a]

Editors and Conference Organizers
DANIEL A. WALZ, JOHN W. FENTON II, AND MARC A. SHUMAN

CONTENTS

[a]This volume is the result of a conference entitled Conference on Bioregulatory Functions of Thrombin, held in New York City on February 5-7, 1986, by the New York Academy of Sciences.

Part III. Cellular Events Mediated by Thrombin

Part IV. Poster Papers

Financial assistance was received from:

- AMERICAN HEART ASSOCIATION, COUNCIL ON THROMBOSIS
- ARMOUR PHARMACEUTICAL COMPANY
- ARMY MEDICAL RESEARCH AND DEVELOPMENT COMMAND
- LILLY RESEARCH LABORATORIES
- McNEIL PHARMACEUTICAL
- OFFICE OF NAVAL RESEARCH (GRANT NO 0014-85-G-0137)
- PENTAPHARM LTD
- PFIZER CENTRAL RESEARCH
- SEARLE RESEARCH AND DEVELOPMENT
- SYNTEX RESEARCH
- THE UPJOHN COMPANY

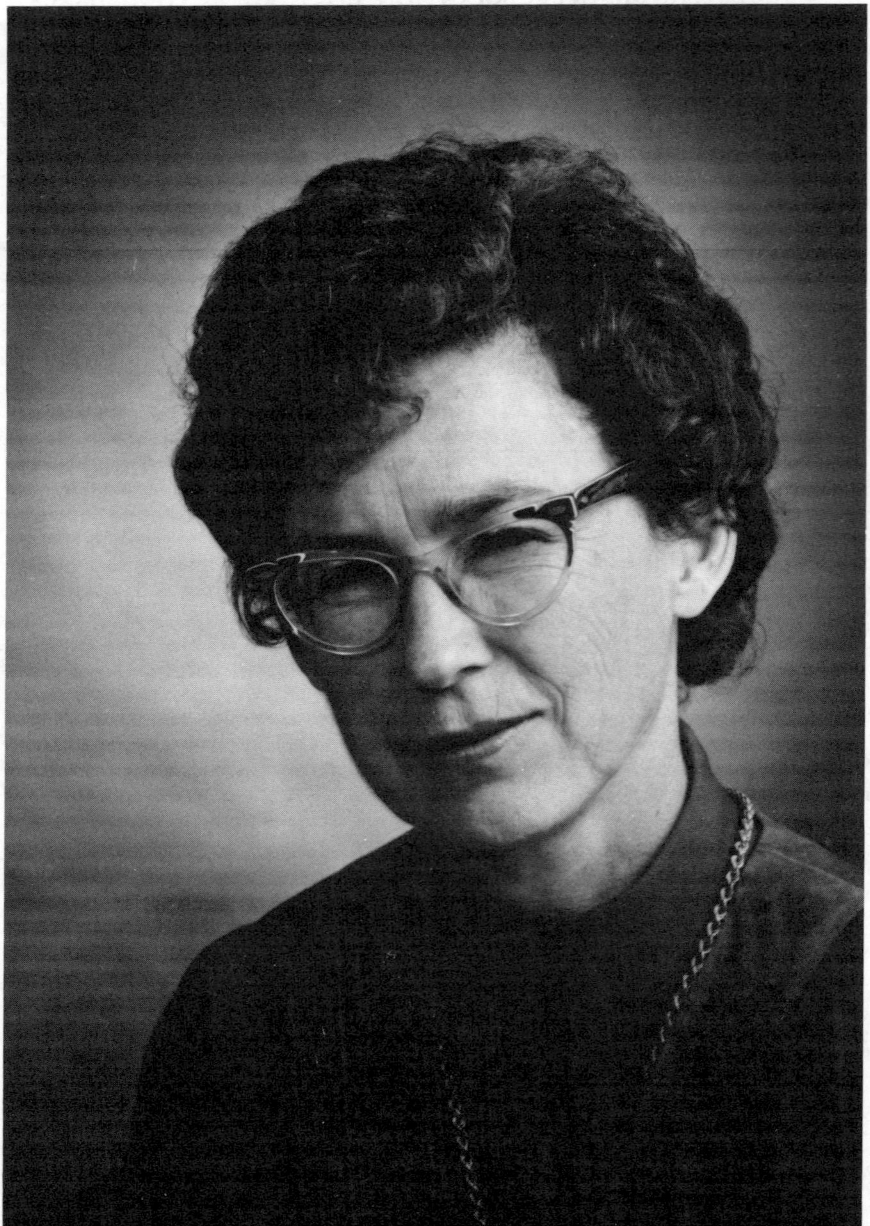

Marion I. Barnhart
1921-1985

In Memoriam

Marion I. Barnhart

DANIEL A. WALZ

Department of Physiology
School of Medicine
Wayne State University
Detroit, Michigan 48201

Marion Barnhart was scheduled to be a speaker at the Conference on Bioregulatory Functions of Thrombin, and it was both a personal and professional loss to learn of her death on December 23, 1985. Marion Barnhart was an internationally recognized research scientist who contributed numerous and important observations in the fields of cellular physiology, blood coagulation and thrombosis, platelet vessel wall interactions, and other aspects of hematology research. During her 34-year career in Wayne State University's Department of Physiology, she served as an invaluable faculty member, adviser to graduate students, and teacher of medical students. She inspired and encouraged everyone through her enthusiasm and energetic approach to life. The recollection of her authorship of 150 scientific papers, book chapters, and instructional monographs emphasizes the diversity of her interests. She served on numerous editorial boards, National Institutes of Health advisory and scientific committees, as well as state and local organization committees. Marion Barnhart was often the spark that kept things moving.

At the time of her death, Marion was the Director of the Academic Program in Transfusion Medicine, Director of the Bargman Laboratory for Cell and Molecular Research, and a Professor in Physiology at Wayne State University. She was the program director for a multidisciplinary training program in Experimental Hematology at Wayne State University. In addition, she was the chairperson of the Blood Diseases and Resources/Hemostasis Advisory Committee of the National Institutes of Health.

Marion Barnhart was vitally involved in many research and educational programs at Wayne State University, and her death leaves a void that will be impossible to fill. She had looked forward with her typical enthusiasm to participating in this conference on thrombin, and her absence is our collective loss.

Introduction

JOHN W. FENTON II

Wadsworth Center for Laboratories and Research
School of Public Health Sciences
New York State Department of Health
Albany, New York 12201

MARC SHUMAN

Department of Medicine
Cancer Research Institute
University of California Medical Center
San Francisco, California 94143

DANIEL A. WALZ

Department of Physiology
School of Medicine
Wayne State University
Detroit, Michigan 48201

Thrombin has central bioregulatory functions in hemostasis.[1] Some 30 years ago, thrombin was shown to function as a highly selective proteolytic enzyme in the clotting of fibrinogen solutions.[2] It was also found to be an esterolytically active enzyme,[3] and relative to this activity, its clotting activity could be differentially lost by chemical modification[4] or by autoproteolytic degradation.[5] More recently, thrombin has also been demonstrated to function nonenzymically, or hormonally, in the stimulation of specific cellular activities. Both enzymic and nonenzymic mechanisms are required for the initiation of fibroblast proliferation.[7]

The development of our understanding of thrombin functions has paralleled our understanding of its structure, which in turn has depended on the availability of methods and material. Bovine thrombin became available in large amounts through advances made at Wayne State University,[8] and human thrombin by members of the same group who had moved to Albany.[9,10] The amino acid sequence of bovine prothrombin was determined in Denmark,[11] that of human prothrombin by contributions from three groups.[12–14] The genes for the two prothrombins were subsequently sequenced in Seattle.[15,16] Although crystals of bovine thrombin were grown more than a decade ago,[17] the crystallographic structure is not yet available. Three-dimensional models have been deduced for the thrombin B chain based on its homology with chymotrypsin.[18] In addition to the catalytic site, the enzymic form with high clotting activity (α-thrombin) has an important exosite involved in fibrin(ogen) interactions and other biological activities.[19]

The biological effects of thrombin comprise those on the plasma proteins (*e.g.*, fibrinogen; coagulation factors V, VIII, and XIII; and protein C), and the blood cellular components (*e.g.*, platelets and leukocytes) and vascular tissues (*e.g.*, endothelium and smooth muscle). Thrombin generation is believed to occur, predominantly, on cell surfaces.[20] Prior to clot formation, low levels of thrombin activate factors V and VIII and stimulate platelets.[21] As the process proceeds in whole blood, most of the prothrombin is consumed, but serum thrombin concentrations remain at only approximately 10% of that which would be generated following complete activation

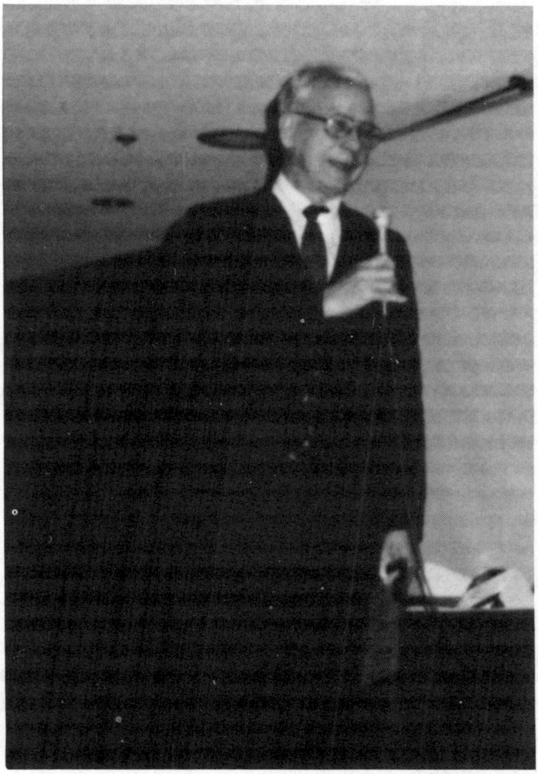

JOHN M. BUCHANAN

of the zymogen.[22] Such thrombin concentrations correspond to sublethal doses that cause maximal contraction of aortic smooth muscles.[23]

A large portion of the thrombin generated in blood is believed to be incorporated into the fibrin clot, where it remains until disruption of the clot.[24] Thus, thrombin can be partitioned within the clot and can potentially emerge from the protected environment of cell-to-clot surfaces, where it may also mediate nonclotting functions. Because thrombin is a potent mitogenic substance, such functions might include the stimulation of cell growth in the wound-healing process.[25] It is in this regard that we have chosen to honor Dr. John M. Buchanan at this conference for his leadership in the discovery of the induction of cell proliferation by thrombin. This discovery opened the way for many other investigators to probe the cellular aspects of the bioregulatory functions of thrombin.

We thank various members of the New York Academy of Sciences and especially our scientific advisory committee, Dr. Greenberg, Dr. Messite, and Dr. Strand. In particular, we wish to single out the efforts of Ellen A. Marks and Albert Capozzelli, whose patience and experience in convening such a gathering of scientists made our organizing efforts all the easier. We are grateful to those organizations and corporations who made financial contributions to help underwrite the expenses of this conference. We thank Ethicon Inc. for funding the award to Dr. Buchanan.

REFERENCES

1. Walz, D. A. & L. E. McCoy, Eds. 1981. Ann. N.Y. Acad. Sci. **370**.
2. Lorand, L. 1951. Nature (London) **167:** 992-994.
3. Sherry, S. & W. Troll. 1954. J. Biol. Chem. **208:** 95-105.
4. Landaburu, R. & W. H. Seegers. 1959. Can. J. Biochem. Physiol. **37:** 1361-1366.
5. Seegers, W. H., J. Reuterby, G. Murano, L. E. McCoy & B. B. L. Agrawal. 1971. Thromb. Diath. Haemorrh. Suppl. **47:** 325-337.
6. Bar-Shavit, R., A. Kahn, J. W. Fenton II & G. D. Wilner. 1983. J. Cell Biol. **96:** 282-285.
7. Carney, D. H., J. Stiernberg & J. W. Fenton II. 1984. J. Cell. Biochem. **26:** 181-195.
8. Seegers, W. H. 1962. Prothrombin. Harvard University Press. Cambridge, MA.
9. Miller, K. D. & W. H. Copeland. 1965. Exp. Mol. Pathol. **4:** 431-437.
10. Fenton II, J. W., M. J. Fasco, A. B. Stackrow, D. L. Aronson, A. M. Young & J. S. Finlayson. 1977. J. Biol. Chem. **252:** 3587-3598.
11. Magnusson, S., T. E. Petersen, L. Sottrup-Jensen & H. Claeys. 1975. Proteases and Biological Control. Cold Spring Harbor. New York.
12. Butkowski, R. J., J. Elion, M. R. Downing & K. G. Mann. 1977. J. Biol. Chem. **252:** 4942-4957.
13. Thompson, A. R., D. L. Enfield, L. H. Ericsson, M. E. Legaz & J. W. Fenton II. 1977. Arch. Biochem. Biophys. **178:** 356-367.
14. Walz, D. A., D. Hewett-Emmett & W. H. Seegers. 1977. Proc. Natl. Acad. Sci. USA **74:** 1969-1972.
15. Degen, S., R. T. A. MacGillivray & E. W. Davie. 1983. Biochemistry **22:** 2087-2097.
16. MacGillivray, R. T. A. & E. W. Davie. 1984. Biochemistry **23:** 1626-1634.
17. Tsernoglou, D., D. A. Walz, L. E. McCoy & W. H. Seegers. 1974. J. Biol. Chem. **249:** 999.
18. Bing, D. H., R. Laura, D. J. Robinson, B. Furie, B. C. Furie & R. J. Feldman. 1981. Ann. N.Y. Acad. Sci. **370:** 496-510.
19. Fenton II, J. W. 1981. Ann. N.Y. Acad. Sci. **370:** 468-495.
20. Rodgers, G. M. & M. Shuman. 1983. Proc. Natl. Acad. Sci. **80:** 7001-7005.
21. Shuman, M. A., & P. W. Majerus. 1976. J. Clin. Invest. **58:** 1249-1258.
22. Aronson, D. L., L. Stevan, A. P. Ball, B. B. Franza & J. S. Finlayson. 1977. J. Clin. Invest. **60:** 1410-1418.
23. Walz, D. A., G. Anderson, R. E. Ciaglowski, M. Aiken & J. W. Fenton II. 1985. Proc. Soc. Exp. Biol. Med. **80:** 518-526.
24. Seegers, W. H., M. L. Nieft & E. C. Loomis. 1945. Science **100:** 520-521.
25. Chen, L. B., & J. M. Buchanan. 1975. Proc. Natl. Acad. Sci. USA **72:** 131-135.

Thrombin[a]

JOHN W. FENTON II

Wadsworth Center for Laboratories and Research
School of Public Health Sciences
New York State Department of Health
Albany, New York 12201

Department of Physiology
The Albany Medical College of Union University
Albany, New York 12208

Thrombin (EC 3.4.21.5) is the central bioregulatory enzyme in hemostasis.[1–3] Hemostasis is the containment of circulating blood, an adaptation of higher animals in order to supply nutrients and remove wastes from dependent tissue. Thrombin functions at all levels of hemostasis—the fluid or plasma level, the blood cell or cellular level, and the blood vessel or vascular level (FIGURE 1).

Thrombin is generated from its zymogen, prothrombin, through the concerted action of several factors in the blood coagulation pathways.[1,4–6] Unlike most coagulation zymogens (factors), prothrombin circulates in plasma at relatively high concentrations. Like most other plasma proteins, prothrombin is synthesized by the liver but is a vitamin K-dependent protein (as are factors VII, IX, and X, as well as proteins C and S). Vitamin K is required for the post-ribosomal formation of the residues in the NH_2-terminal lead peptide of the zymogen.[7] These are believed to be involved in Ca^{2+} binding and forming salt bridges to phospholipids in prothrombin activation.[4,8]

Following the lead peptide, prothrombin has two homologous "kringle structures" indicative of ancestral gene duplication in the zymogen.[7] These structures are then followed by a connecting peptide segment which forms the thrombin A chain and joins to the much larger B-chain moiety. The thrombin B chain constitutes approximately half of the CO_2H-terminal polypeptide of the zymogen and is homologous with other serine enzymes. The consequences of this assemblage is that the two halves of prothrombin are structurally and functionally unrelated (FIGURE 1 in Reference 6; FIGURE 4 in Reference 9). Whereas the function of the NH_2-terminal moiety is the regulation of thrombin generation (e.g., zymogen biosynthesis, circulation, and activation[1,6]), that of the CO_2H-terminal moiety is to carry out the regulatory functions of the activated zymogen (e.g., clotting of fibrinogen and various other activities in FIGURE 1). Although thrombin is a proteolytic enzyme in the majority of interactions with plasma proteins, it also has nonenzymic or hormone-like activities involving receptor-mediated processes with a variety of cells.[10–15] Thus, a new term is perhaps needed connoting a protein activation product with both enzymic and hormonal bioregulatory activities or either activities. Such a term might be a "proteinoid bioregulant."

In the prothrombinase complex (composed of prothrombin and activated factors X and V, as well as Ca^{2+} and phospholipid[4,8]), prothrombin is cleaved between the

[a]Supported in part by National Institutes of Health Grant HL13160.

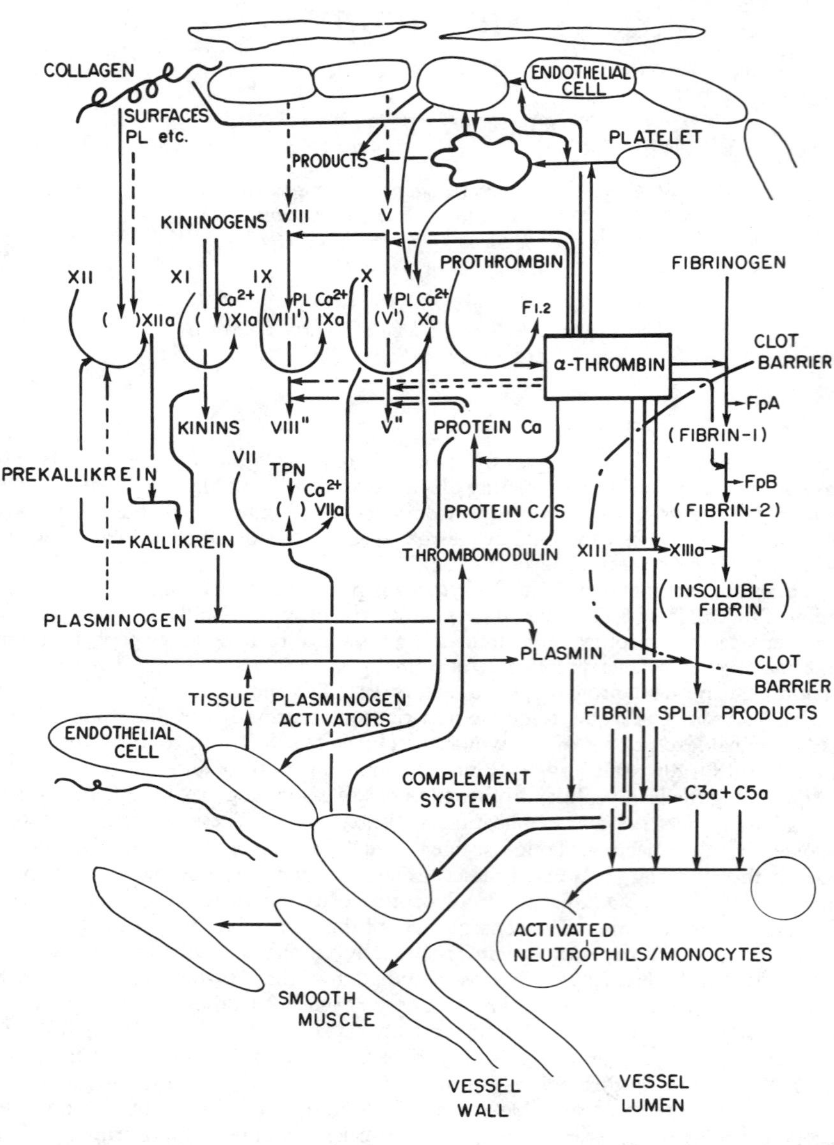

FIGURE 1. The central bioregulatory functions of α-thrombin in hemostasis. Roman numerals are used for coagulation factor zymogens and are followed by "a" for the activated enzymes. Primes and double primes are used respectively for the activated and inactivated forms of factors V and VIII. Other abbreviations used are: F1·2, the prothrombin activation fragment; FpA, fibrinopeptide A; FpB, fibrinopeptide B; PL, phospholipid; and TPN, thromboplastin. The upper left-hand and lower right-hand corners of the figure portray "preclotting" and "postclotting" events, respectively. This figure is further designed to incorporate certain aspects of Figure 1 in Reference 1 and Figure 10 in Reference 76. (Reprinted with permission from Fenton.[2])

propiece (fragment F1·2) and thrombin ("prethrombin 2") moieties followed by a second cleavage generating the disulfide-linked thrombin A and B chains.[4] Despite the fact that activation involves the two proteolytic cleavages, which clearly require enzymic processes, the catalytic turnover of the complex may not be complete, causing "burst" or dose-related thrombin generation. In the preparative activation of thrombin where high concentrations of the enzyme are generated (e.g., >500 units/ml),[16–18] human thrombin autoproteolytically removes a 13-residue NH_2-terminal fragment (F3) from the A chain (FIGURE 1 in Reference 6). However, in the clotting of whole blood, $>80\%$ of the zymogen is activated, but $<10\%$ of the potential enzyme concentration is ever achieved (e.g., 5 to 15 units/ml), presumably due to inclusion of thrombin within fibrin clots.[19,20] The 13-residue fragment remains intact under these conditions and is also believed to do so under physiological conditions.[21]

In contrast to most other plasma serine proteinases (e.g., factor Xa and other coagulation factors,[22] tissue plasminogen activator,[23] plasmin[24]), the propiece and enzyme halves of prothrombin are not joined by a disulfide bridge.[7,24] Thus, thrombin is generated as a free moiety of half the size and with properties independent of its zymogen. Moreover, thrombin is essentially a neutrally charged protein (major pI values 7.2 to 7.6)[17,18] and readily adheres to apolar and negatively charged surfaces.[25] This enables the enzyme to be easily separated from other activation products with cationic exchange resins.[17,26] The propiece fragments (F1 and F2) can be subsequently purified from the nonadhering fraction from such resins, and these fragments appear to be spent activation products with no known biologic activities.[27]

The thrombin A chain is a remnant activation fragment and is attached by a single disulfide bridge to the serine enzyme homologous B chain. Not unexpectedly the A chain is unrelated to the activation peptides of the pancreatic serine proteins.[7,28] These peptides are relatively short and are lost upon cleavage in the activation of these enzymes. Contrastingly, the thrombin A chain is only a small portion of the "extended activation peptide" of prothrombin (fragment F1·2 plus A chain). This extended activation peptide has evolved for regulating thrombin generation and undoubtedly has arisen through gene translocation and duplication processes (see above).

The consequence of the thrombin A chain being attached to the B chain raises questions as to its functions, if any. Clearly, the 13-residue NH_2-terminal fragment (F3) of the human thrombin chain is not required for fibrinogen clotting or other enzymic activities.[17] On the other hand, the A chain is located near the thrombin active site, since it can be labeled by an active-site-directed affinity-labeling reagent with a reactive group on an extended chain.[29] This labeling is further independent of requirements for clotting activity (i.e., the reagent labels human α- and γ-thrombins in the same manner) suggesting the A chain may participate in the formation of active-site regions neighboring the catalytic site (see below) and the arginine side-chain pocket.[28,29]

The thrombin B chain is more closely related to chymotrypsin than any other pancreatic serine proteinase.[28,30–32] When the amino acid sequences of bovine thrombin B chains are aligned with those of bovine chymotrypsin, the greatest homologies occur within peptides forming the β-barrel structures of chymotrypsin and assuming the crystallographic structure of chymotrypsin. Three dimensional models can be generated by computer graphic techniques.[30–32]

When the amino acid sequence of the human B chain is similarly aligned (FIGURE 1 in Reference 3) and the polypeptide chain structure of chymotrypsin is assumed,[33] a first approximation model of human thrombin can be constructed (FIGURE 2). In the center of this model, His-57, Asp-102, and Ser-195 constitute the catalytic site, per se, and Glu-192 is the counter ion at the bottom of the arginine side-chain pocket. The polypeptide substrate groove begins at ~7 o'clock and runs through the catalytic site, where it is believed to drop downward toward 4 o'clock.[3] The former corresponds to the fibrinopeptide side, while the latter to the fibrin side of the Aα cleavage site in fibrinogen.

The active-site groove is predominantly composed of residues with apolar side chains and is lined with those with charged groups.[3] Notably, residues, such as Trp-215 in the fibrinopeptide groove adjacent to the catalytic site, form the apolar binding

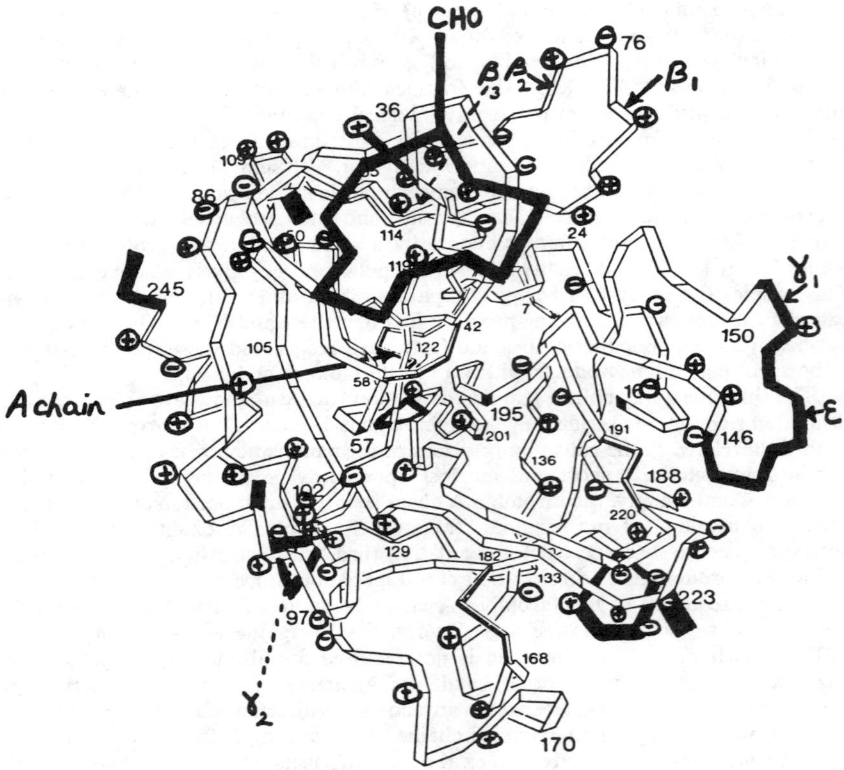

FIGURE 2. A polypeptide chain model of human α-thrombin. The chain structure of α-chymotrypsin[33] is assumed where the disulfide at residues 136 to 201 is removed. Inserted residues of the human thrombin B chain (Figure 1 in Reference 3) are drawn in and represent uncertain configurations. The catalytic site consists of His-57, Asp-102, and Ser-195, as well as adjacent residues. The carbohydrate (CHO) attachment and charged residues (+ or −) are shown. The autoproteolytic or tryptic (β and γ) and elastolytic (ϵ) cleavage sites are also indicated (see text). The A-chain disulfide bridge connects to Cys-122 on the back side of the model.

site.[30,34,35] This site binds proflavin,[34,35] indole derivatives, and other aromatic compounds,[34] and presumptively explains the requirement for apolar residues preceding arginine in chromogenic tripeptide substrates.[36] Furthermore, such substrates have (or can assume) bent structures,[37] such as that caused by proline adjacent to the arginine, as has been found for the majority of known thrombin-susceptible bonds in proteins.[38] These bent configurations, therefore, would agree with kinked active-site groove predicted by the computer graphic B-chain model.[3]

On the other hand, the Aα cleavage site in fibrinogen is perhaps one of the most thrombin-susceptible bonds known but lacks the adjacent proline and other characteristics of most thrombin cleavage sites in proteins.[1,2] This suggests that the fibrinopeptide A chain must assume a unique configuration in order to interact selectively with the enzyme.[39] Since α-thrombin is the enzymic form with high fibrinogen clotting activity and its autoproteolytic or tryptic derivative forms, β- and γ-thrombins, lack clotting activity,[17,18] the conformation of the fibrinopeptide appears not to explain α-thrombin specificity for fibrinogen.[1,2] In these regards, β- and γ-thrombins exhibit kinetic parameters with chromogenic substrates similar to those of α-thrombin, suggesting that their active-site regions associated with the fibrinopeptide groove are largely unaltered.[37,40] On the other hand, certain regions of the active site in γ-thrombin are more constrained than in α-thrombin.[41,42] The reason for the specificity of α-thrombin with fibrinogen must reside elsewhere and presumptively on the fibrin side of the groove.[1,2]

Conformation rearrangements undoubtedly occur with the loss of clotting activity in formation of degradative enzyme forms.[9] Human α-thrombin prepared by thromboplastin activation converts slowly autoproteolytically or is very rapidly converted by tryptic digestion to β- and γ-thrombin forms, where β-thrombin behaves as an intermediate form.[16–18] The cleavage sites β_1, β_2, and γ_1 have been identified for autolyzed material,[43] whereas the β_2 and γ_1 sites have been found for material made by passage through immobilized trypsin.[18] The β_3 and γ_2 sites, on the other hand, have been reported for the autolytic degradation of α-thrombin made by activation with snake venom,[44] and may be due to copurified venom proteinases.[45] The ε cleavage is produced by elastase from either pancreatic[46,47] or neutrophil[48,49] sources and causes a dramatic loss in clotting activity.[46–49] Bovine thrombin has the corresponding tryptic β_2 and pancreatic elastase ε cleavage sites but lacks the γ_1 site.[47] In this regard, the lysine at the γ_1 site in human thrombin is replaced by glutamic acid in bovine thrombin.[18] Like human γ-thrombin, bovine β-thrombin prepared by passage through trypsin immobilized on agarose lacks any significant clotting activity.[37] Thus, cleavage of either the β or γ/ε domain destroys or markedly reduces clotting activity.[49]

When radiolabeled catalytically inactivated α-thrombins (e.g., ^{125}I-*i*-Pr_2P- or ^{125}I-Ph$MeSO_2$-α-thrombins) are incubated with fibrinogen and trace amounts of α-thrombin to initiate clotting, they incorporate into clots like the labeled native enzyme, whereas labeled γ-thrombin and the hirudin complex of labeled α-thrombin do not similarly incorporate.[50] Likewise, catalytically inactivated α-thrombin binds to nonpolymerized fibrin(ogen) immobilized on agarose in the same manner as α-thrombin, while γ-thrombin binds weakly and the hirudin complexes of all thrombin forms do not bind.[51] Furthermore, the NaCl concentrations required to elute various thrombin forms from the fibrin(ogen) resin correlate with those required to elute these forms from the cation exchange resin Amberlite CG-50.[52] The binding of α-thrombin and its derivative forms to heparin immobilized on agarose occurs in a similar manner and such binding is likewise blocked by hirudin.[53] These findings and the elution of α-thrombin from fibrin(ogen) resin with various anionic substances[54] have suggested that α-thrombin has a true exosite (completely independent of the catalytic site) involved in fibrin(ogen) recognition.[1,2]

The β cleavage sites are, notably, in a peptide segment unusually rich in arginines and lysines (FIGURE 2). The γ_1 and ε sites are also in positively charged segments, which in concert with those in preceding segments could form an anionic binding site of major importance.[2,3] If the proper alignment of the catalytic site in α-thrombin and of an anionic binding exosite in the enzyme is required for a prominent negatively charged surface on the substrate, then a double-site mechanism can be envisioned to account for the specificity of α-thrombin.

This hypothesized double-site mechanism is supported by the very high affinity noncovalent binding of hirudin to α-thrombin.[55] Hirudin is a small protein ($M_r \sim 7000$) consisting of an oily disulfide knot followed by a noncleavable Pro-Lys-Pro sequence and a very negatively charged tail.[56] Cleavage of either the disulfide bridges or the tail destroys its inhibitory activity.[57,58] It noncompetitively inhibits human α-thrombin ($K_i \sim 60$ pM) and competitively inhibits γ-thrombin with a 200-fold reduction in binding.[9,59] Thus, hirudin binding appears to involve the apolar binding site, regions neighboring the catalytic site, and the anionic binding exosite.[3]

Hirudin binding also blocks various nonenzymic or hormonal activities of thrombin[10,12,14] but does not block the accessibility of the carbohydrate side chain of thrombin (FIGURE 2) to complex with concanavalin A immobilized on agarose.[53] Partial removal of the carbohydrate side chain[60] does not affect enzymic properties of α-thrombin in blood coagulation[61,62] or the nonenzymic chemotactic response of monocytes,[63] suggesting that this side chain is well removed from the active site. The carbohydrate attachment site, nevertheless, must represent an exposed protein surface for postribosomal carbohydrate synthesis and most likely functions in regulating the circulating half-life of prothrombin.[6,9]

The carbohydrate attachment occurs within the largest insertion peptide found in the thrombin B chain (FIGURE 2). This insertion begins at the three to four exon junction in chymotrypsin[64] and is followed by the most variable segments found among serine proteinases.[3] Preceding the carbohydrate attachment, this insertion contains the unusual Tyr-Pro-Pro-Trp sequence, where the tandem prolines would form a double kink structure, which should place the Tyr-60A and Trp-60D in close proximity to one another. A prominent mound of these and other apolar residues is believed to reside just above the catalytic site.[3,30–32] This mound or bulge caused by the carbohydrate-attachment insertion peptide is further believed to be an important structural feature of the chemotactic domain. However, since the chemotactic domain is contained within an isolated CNBr fragment corresponding to roughly the first third of the B chain,[63] other peptide segments cannot be ignored which are contained within the fragment and are unique to thrombin.[3] Such peptides following the carbohydrate-attachment insertion peptide are unusually rich in arginines and lysines. Furthermore, the β cleavage sites are contained in this peptide segment (FIGURE 2). Since human α- and γ-thrombins are similarly chemotactic[11] and since the β sites are cleaved in γ-thrombin,[9,18,29] the integrity of this peptide segment is not required for chemotactic activity. On the other hand, γ-thrombin does not bind to certain high-affinity receptors, whereas catalytically inactivated forms of α-thrombin (e.g., ^{125}I-*i*-Pr$_2$P-α-thrombin) will bind like α-thrombin to such receptors on platelets[65] and fibroblasts.[66,67] This implies that the arginine/lysine-rich segment is required for this type of receptor binding.

The α-thrombin form has been elegantly shown by Carney and co-workers to stimulate fibroblast receptors by two mechanisms.[11,68] The first can be initiated by catalytically inactivated α-thrombin but not γ-thrombin. This mechanism involves high-affinity receptors requiring occupancy for signal generation and increases cAMP levels. The second can be initiated by γ-thrombin but not by catalytically inactivated α-thrombin. Consequently, this mechanism requires the functional enzyme and presumptively involves a proteolytic cleavage in the activation of phosphoinositide turnover and Ca^{2+} mobilization. Both mechanisms are necessary for initiation of mitogenesis in these cells.

A third mechanism can also be envisioned where high-affinity binding and proteolytic cleavage are coupled. This could involve the initial binding of α-thrombin to a membrane component (receptor-1) other than the neighboring target component (receptor-2). Because binding to the first component would increase the effective concentration of the enzyme and enhance interaction with the second component, this would become an "affinity-enhanced enzymic process." This type of mechanism may be involved in platelet stimulation[69,70] as previously suggested.[1]

The variety of physiological processes stimulated by thrombin make it one of the most interesting bioregulators known. With the exception perhaps of the mammalian erythrocyte, all cell types or tissues examined to date have to varying extents been responsive to thrombin.[1–3] This includes such bizarre examples as stimulation of nerve cells,[71] contraction of smooth muscle tissue,[72] initiation of bone resorption,[73] and enhancement of viral infectivity.[74] The extents to which such biologic activities are of physiological significance or whether thrombin is merely mimicking another bioregulant (e.g., thrombin-like enzyme or hormone-like substance) remains to be determined in many cases.

What is apparent in the multiple functions of α-thrombin in the blood coagulation pathways is that the enzyme in its native or modified forms is not just involved in the clotting process (FIGURE 1). The forming fibrin clot actively incorporates α-thrombin within its interstices where the enzyme is stored and protected from scavaging proteinase inhibitors in plasma.[20,50,75] In the advanced stages of thrombin-induced pulmonary edema and vascular injury, neutrophil sequestering occurs.[76] Notably, the activated neutrophil releases elastase, which can partially degrade fibrin clots and potentially release α-thrombin as well as convert it into the elastase-degraded form lacking clotting activity.[49] Since this form, like γ-thrombin, could retain certain other biological activities, it is a potential candidate for carrying out thrombin-mediated processes in postclotting events. These include the initiation of cellular stimulatory and proliferative processes leading to the recovery of tissue damage in wound healing.[77,78]

ACKNOWLEDGMENTS

I wish to thank many colleagues who have shared information and ideas leading to the formation of my thoughts and understanding of the bioregulatory functions of thrombin. In particular, I am indebted to Dr. Kent D. Miller, who introduced me to the field and taught me the preparation of thrombin. I further thank various persons in my laboratory and persons with whom I have collaborated with over the years. I lastly thank Mary Jane Boulay for her secretarial assistance in preparing the manuscript.

REFERENCES

1. FENTON II, J. W. 1981. Thrombin specificity. Ann. N.Y. Acad. Sci. **370:** 468-495.
2. FENTON II, J. W. 1986. Structural regions and bioregulatory functions of thrombin. *In* Cell Proliferation: Recent Advances. A. L. Boynton & H. L. Leffert, Eds. Vol. II. Academic Press. New York, N.Y. In press.
3. FENTON II, J. W. & D. H. BING. 1986. Thrombin active-site regions. Semin. Thromb. Hemostasis. **12:** 200-208.
4. SUTTIE, J. W. & C. M. JACKSON. 1977. Prothrombin structure, activation, and biosynthesis. Physiol. Rev. **57:** 1-70.

5. Davie, E. W., K. Fujkawa, K. Kurachi & W. Kisiel. 1979. The role of serine proteases in the blood coagulation cascade. Adv. Enzymol. **48:** 277-318.
6. Fenton II, J. W. & B. H. Landis. 1981. Prothrombin and thrombin transformation: bioregulations and functions. *In* Perspectives in Hemostasis. J. Fareed, H. L. Messmore, J. W. Fenton II & K. M. Brinkhous, Eds.: 31-52. Pergamon Press. New York, N.Y.
7. Magnuson, S., T. E. Petersen, L. Sottrup-Jensen & H. Claeys. 1975. Complete primary structure of prothrombin: isolation, structure, and reactivity of ten carboxylated glutamic acid residues and regulation of prothrombin activation by thrombin. *In* Proteases and Biological Control. E. Reich, D. B. Rifkin & E. Shaw, Eds.: 123-149. Cold Spring Harbor Laboratory. Cold Spring Harbor, N.Y.
8. Mann, K. G., M. E. Nesheim, L. S. Hibbard & P. B. Tracy. 1981. The role of factor V in the assembly of the prothrombinase complex. Ann. N.Y. Acad. Sci. **370:** 378-388.
9. Fenton II, J. W., B. H. Landis, D. A. Walz, D. H. Bing, R. D. Feinman, M. P. Zabinski, S. A. Sonder, L. J. Berliner & J. S. Finlayson. 1979. Human thrombin: preparative evaluation, structural properties and enzymic specificity. *In* The Chemistry and Physiology of Human Plasma Proteins. D. H. Bing, Ed.: 151-183. Pergamon Press. New York, N.Y.
10. Bar-Shavit, R., A. Kahn, G. D. Wilner & J. W. Fenton II. 1983. Monocyte chemotaxis: stimulation by specific exosite region in thrombin. Science **220:** 728-731.
11. Carney, D. H., J. Stiernberg & J. W. Fenton II. 1984. Initiation of proliferative events by human α-thrombin requires both receptor binding and enzymic activity. J. Cell Biochem. **26:** 181-195.
12. Bizios, R., L. Lai, J. W. Fenton II, S. A. Sonder & A. B. Malik. 1985. Thrombin induced aggregation of lymphocytes: nonenzymic induction by a hirudin-blocked thrombin exosite. Thromb. Res. **38:** 425-431.
13. Garcia, J. G. N., A. Siflinger-Birnboim, R. Bizios, P. J. Del Vecchio, J. W. Fenton II & A. B. Malik. 1986. Thrombin-induced increases in albumin transport across cultured endothelial monolayers. Am. J. Physiol. **128:** 96-104.
14. Bar-Shavit, R. & G. D. Wilner. 1986. Biological activities of nonenzymatic thrombin: elucidation of a macrophage interactive domain. Semin. Thromb. Hemostasis. **12:** 244-249.
15. Booyse, F. M., R. Bruce, M. Gover & L. C. Casey. 1986. Rapid release and deactivation of plasminogen activators in human endothelial cell cultures in the presence of thrombin and ionophore A23187. Semin. Thromb. Hemostasis **12:** 228-230.
16. Fenton II, J. W., W. P. Campbell, J. C. Harrington & K. D. Miller. 1971. Large-scale preparation and preliminary characterization of human thrombin. Biochem. Biophys. Acta **229:** 26-32.
17. Fenton II, J. W., M. J. Fasco, A. B. Stackrow, D. L. Aronson, A. M. Young & J. S. Finlayson. 1977. Human thrombins. Production, evaluation, and properties of α-thrombin. J. Biol. Chem. **252:** 3587-3598.
18. Fenton II, J. W., B. H. Landis, D. A. Walz & J. S. Finlayson. 1977. Human thrombins. *In* Chemistry and Biology of Thrombin. R. L. Lundblad, J. W. Fenton II & K. G. Mann, Eds.: 43-70. Ann Arbor Science Publishers. Ann Arbor, Mich.
19. Aronson, D. L., L. Stevan, A. P. Ball, B. R. Franza, Jr. & J. S. Finlayson. 1977. Generation of the combined prothrombin activation peptide (F1-2) during the clotting of blood and plasma. J. Clin. Invest. **60:** 1410-1418.
20. Liu, C. Y., H. L. Nossel & K. L. Kaplan. 1979. The binding of thrombin by fibrin. J. Biol. Chem. **254:** 10421-10425.
21. Walz, D. A. & T. R. Brown. 1980. Human prothrombin activation: radioimmunoassay of fragment 3. *In* Vitamin K Metabolism and Vitamin K-Dependent Proteins. J. W. Suttie, Ed.: 116-120. University Park Press. Baltimore, Md.
22. Neurath, H. 1985. Proteolytic enzymes, past and present. Fed. Proc. **44:** 2907-2913.
23. Ny, T., F. Elgh & B. Lund. 1984. The structure of the human tissue-type plasminogen activator genes: correlation of intron and exon structures to functional and structural domains. Proc. Natl. Acad. Sci. USA **81:** 5355-5359.
24. Magnusson, S., L. Sottrup-Jensen, T. E. Petersen, G. Dudek-Wojciechowska & H. Claeys. 1976. Homologous "kringle" structures common to plasminogen and prothrombin. Substrate specificity of enzymes activating prothrombin and plasminogen. *In*

Proteolysis and Physiological Regulation. D. W. Ribbons & K. Brew, Eds. **11:** 203-238. Miami Winter Symposia. Academic Press. New York, N.Y.
25. Wasiewski, W., M. J. Fasco, B. M. Martin, T. C. Detwiler & J. W. Fenton II. 1976. Thrombin adsorption to surfaces and prevention with polyethylene glycol 6,000. Thromb. Res. **8:** 881-886.
26. Miller, K. D. & W. H. Copeland. 1962. Isolation of human thrombin. Proc. Soc. Exp. Biol. Med. **111:** 512-514.
27. Aronson, D. L., A. P. Ball, R. B. Franza, T. E. Hugli & J. W. Fenton II. 1980. Human prothrombin fragments F1($\alpha\beta$) and F2: preparation and characterization of structural and biological properties. Thromb. Res. **20:** 239-253.
28. Magnusson, S. 1971. Thrombin and prothrombin. *In* The Enzymes. P. D. Boyer, Ed. **3:** 227-321. Academic Press. New York, N.Y.
29. Bing, D. H., M. Cory & J. W. Fenton II. 1977. Exo-site affinity labeling of human thrombins. Similar labeling of the A chain and B chain/fragments of clotting α- and nonclotting γ/β-thrombins. J. Biol. Chem. **252:** 8027-8034.
30. Bing, D. H., R. Laura, D. J. Robinson, B. C. Furie & R. J. Feldman. 1981. A computer-generated three-dimensional model of the B chain of bovine α-thrombin. Ann. N.Y. Acad. Sci. **370:** 496-510.
31. Furie, B., D. H. Bing, R. J. Feldman, D. J. Robison, J. P. Burnier & B. C. Furie. 1982. Computer-generated models of blood coagulation factor Xa, factor IXa, and thrombin based upon structural homology with other serine proteinases. J. Biol. Chem. **257:** 3875-3882.
32. Bing, D. H., R. J. Feldmann & J. W. Fenton II. 1986. Structure-functioning relationships of thrombin based on the computer-generated three-dimensional model of the B chain of bovine thrombin. Ann. N.Y. Acad. Sci. This volume.
33. Birktoft, J. J. & D. M. Blow. 1972. Structure of crystalline α-chymotrypsin. V. The atomic structure of tosyl-α-chymotrypsin at 20 resolution. J. Mol. Biol. **68:** 187-240.
34. Berliner, L. J. & Y. Y. L. Shen. 1977. Physical evidence for an apolar binding site near the catalytic center of human α-thrombin. Biochemistry **16:** 4622-4626.
35. Sonder, S. A. & J. W. Fenton II. 1984. Proflavin binding within the fibrinopeptide groove adjacent to the catalytic site of human α-thrombin. Biochemistry **23:** 1818-1823.
36. Claeson, G., L. Aurell, G. Karlson & P. Friberger. 1977. Substrate structure and activity relationships. *In* New Methods for the Analysis of Coagulation Using Chromogenic Substrates. I. Witt, Ed.: 39-54. Walter de Gruyter. Berlin, FRG.
37. Sonder, S. A. & J. W. Fenton II. 1986. Thrombin specificity with tripeptide substrates. Comparison of human and bovine thrombins with and without fibrinogen clotting activities. Clin. Chem. **32:** 934-937.
38. Chang, J-Y. 1985. Thrombin specificity. Requirement for apolar amino acid adjacent to the thrombin cleavage site of polypeptide substrate. Eur. J. Biochem. **151:** 217-224.
39. Marsh, H. C., Jr., Y. C. Meinwald, T. W. Thannhauser & H. A. Scheraga. 1983. Mechanism of action of thrombin on fibrinogen. Kinetic evidence for involvement of aspartic acid at position P_{10}. Biochemistry **22:** 4170-4174.
40. Lottenberg, R., J. A. Hall, J. W. Fenton II & C. M. Jackson. 1982. The action of thrombin on peptide *p*-nitroanilide substrates: hydrolysis of Tos-Gly-Pro-Arg-pNA and *D*-Phe-Pip-Arg-pNA by human α and γ and bovine α and β-thrombins. Thromb. Res. **28:** 313-332.
41. Berliner, L. J., R. S. Bauer, T-L. Chang, J. W. Fenton & Y. Y. L. Shen. 1981. Active-site topography of human coagulant (α) and noncoagulant (β/γ) thrombins. Biochemistry **20:** 1831-1837.
42. Villanueva, G. B. 1981. Conformational differences between high clotting human α-thrombin and nonclotting γ-thrombin. Biochemistry **20:** 6519-6525.
43. Chang, J-Y. Personal communication.
44. Boissel, J-P., N. Lebonniec, M-J. Rabiet, D. Labie & J. Elion. 1984. Covalent structures of β and γ autolytic derivatives of human α-thrombin. J. Biol. Chem. **259:** 5691-5697.
45. Landis, B. H. Personal communication.
46. Karvabata, S., T. V. Morita, S. Iwanaga & H. Igaraski. 1985. Staphylocoagulase-binding region in human prothrombin. J. Biochem. **97:** 325-331.

47. WALZ, D. A., T. A. OLSON, S. A. SONDER & J. W. FENTON II. Unpublished data.
48. WALZ, D. A. & M. S. BROWER. Personal communication.
49. BROWER, M. S., K. E. GARRY & J. W. FENTON II. 1986. Proteolysis of human α-thrombin by human neutrophil elastase results in decreased fibrinogen clotting and platelet-stimulatory activity. Ann. N.Y. Acad. Sci. This volume.
50. WILNER, G. D., M. P. DANITZ, M. S. MUDD, K-H. HSIEH & J. W. FENTON II. 1981. Selective immobilization of α-thrombin by surface-bound fibrin. J. Lab. Clin. Med. **97:** 403-411.
51. FENTON II, J. W., M. P. ZABINSKI, K. HSIEH & G. D. WILNER. 1981. Thrombin non-covalent-protein binding and fibrin(ogen) recognition. Thromb. Haemost. **46:** 177.
52. OLSON, T. A., M. P. ZABINSKI & J. W. FENTON II. Unpublished data.
53. OLSON, T. A., S. A. SONDER, G. D. WILNER & J. W. FENTON II. 1986. Heparin binding in proximity to the catalytic site of human α-thrombin. Ann. N.Y. Acad. Sci. This volume.
54. BERLINER, L. J., Y. SUGAWARA & J. W. FENTON II. 1985. Human α-thrombin binding to non-polymerized fibrin-sepharose: evidence for an anionic binding region. Biochemistry **24:** 7005-7009.
55. WALSMANN, P. & F. MARKWARDT. 1981. Biochemische und parmakologische aspeckte de thrombininhibitors hirudin. Die Parmazie **36:** 653-660.
56. DODT, J., H-P. MULLER, V. SEEMULLER & J-Y. CHANG. 1984. The complete amino acid sequence of hirudin, a thrombin specific inhibitor. FEBS Lett. **165:** 180-183.
57. BAGDY, D., E. BARBAS, L. GRAF, T. E. PETERSEN & S. MAGERUSSON. 1976. Hirudin. Methods Enzymol. **45:** 669-678.
58. CHANG, J-Y. 1984. The functional domain of hirudin, a thrombin-specific inhibitor. FEBS Lett. **164:** 307-313.
59. LANDIS, B. H., M. P. ZABINSKI, G. J. M. LAFLEUR, D. H. BING & J. W. FENTON II. 1978. Human α- and γ-thrombin differential inhibition with hirudin. Fed. Proc. **37:** 1445.
60. NILSON, B., MCD. K. HORNE III & H. R. GRALNICK. 1983. The carbohydrate of human thrombin: structural analysis of glycoprotein oligosaccharides by mass spectrometry. Arch. Biochem. Biophys. **224:** 127-133.
61. HORNE, MCD. K., III & H. R. GRALNICK. 1984. The oligosaccharide of human thrombin: investigations of functional significance. Blood **63:** 188-194.
62. ROSENFELD, L. & I. DANISHEFSKY. 1984. Effects of enzymic deglycosylation on the biological activities of human thrombin and antithrombin. Arch. Biochem. Biophys. **229:** 359-367.
63. BAR-SHAVIT, R., A. KAHN, M. S. MUDD, G. D. WILNER, K. G. MANN & J. W. FENTON II. 1984. Localization of a chemotactic domain in human thrombin. Biochemistry **23:** 397-400.
64. BELL, G. I., C. QUINTO, M. QUIROGA, P. VELENZUELA, C. S. CRAIK & W. J. RUTTR. 1984. Isolation and sequence of a rat chymotrypsin B gene. J. Biol. Chem. **259:** 14265-14270.
65. TOLLEFSEN, D. M., J. R. FEAGLER & P. M. MAJERUS. 1974. The binding of thrombin to the surface of human platelets. J. Biol. Chem. **249:** 2646-2651.
66. GLENN, K. C., D. H. CARNEY, J. W. FENTON II & D. D. CUNNINGHAM. 1980. Thrombin-active site regions required for fibroblast receptor binding and initiation of cell division. J. Biol. Chem. **255:** 6609-6616.
67. PERDUE, J. F., W. LUBENSKYI, E. KIVITY & J. W. FENTON II. 1981. Characterization of human α-thrombin binding on cultured avian and mammalian cells. *In* Plasma and Cellular Modulatory Proteins. D. H. Bing & R. A. Rosenbaumd, Eds.: 109-123. Center for Blood Research. Boston, Mass.
68. CARNEY, D. H., G. J. HERBOSA, J. STIERNBERG, J. S. BERGMAN, E. A. GORDON, D. SCOTT & J. W. FENTON II. 1986. Double signal hypothesis for thrombin initiation of cell proliferation. Semin. Thromb. Hemostasis **12:** 231-240.
69. MCGOWAN, E. B. & T. C. DETWILER. 1986. Modified platelet responses to thrombin. Evidence for two types of receptors or coupling mechanisms. J. Biol. Chem. **261:** 739-746.
70. TAKAMATSU, J., MCD. K. HORNE III & H. R. GRALNICK. 1986. Identification of the

thrombin receptor on human platelets by chemical cross linking. J. Clin. Invest. **77:** 362-368.
71. Snider, R. M., M. McKinney, C. Forray & E. Richelson. 1984. Neurotransmitter receptors mediate cyclic GMP formation by involvement of arachidonic acid and lipoxygenase. Proc. Natl. Acad. Sci. USA **81:** 3905-3909.
72. Walz, D. A., G. F. Anderson, R. E. Ciaglowski, M. Aiken & J. W. Fenton II. 1985. Thrombin-elicited contractile responses of aortic smooth muscle. Proc. Soc. Exp. Biol. Med. **180:** 518-526.
73. Gustafson, G. T. & U. Lerner. 1983. Thrombin, a stimulator of bone resorption. Biosci. Rep. **3:** 255-261.
74. Dubovi, E. J., J. D. Geratz & R. R. Tidwell. 1983. Enhancement of respiratory syncytial virus-induced cytopathology by trypsin, thrombin, and plasmin. Infect. Immun. **40:** 351-358.
75. Francis, C. W., R. E. Markham, Jr., G. H. Barlow, T. M. Florack, D. M. Dobrzynski & V. J. Marder. 1983. Thrombin activity of fibrin thrombi and soluble plasmic derivatives. J. Lab. Clin. Med. **102:** 220-230.
76. Malik, A. B. 1983. Pulmonary micro-embolism. Physiol. Rev. **63:** 1114-1207.
77. Chen, L. B. & J. M. Buchanan. 1975. Mitogenic activity of blood components. I. Thrombin and prothrombin. Proc. Natl. Acad. Sci. USA **72:** 131-135.
78. Buchanan, J. M., L. B. Chen & B. R. Zetter. 1976. Protease-related effects in normal and transformed cells. *In* Cancer Enzymology. J. Schultz & F. Ahmad, Eds. **12:** 1-24. Miami Winter Symposia. Academic Press. New York, N.Y.

Proteolytic Derivatives of Thrombin[a]

JACQUES ELION,[b] JEAN-PAUL BOISSEL,[b]
BERNARD LE BONNIEC,[b] ANNIE BEZEAUD,[b]
MARTINE JANDROT-PERRUS,[c] MARIE-JOSÈPHE RABIET,[b]
AND MARIE-CLAUDE GUILLIN[c]

[b]*Laboratoire de Biochimie B*
[c]*Laboratoire de Recherche sur l'Hémostase et la Thrombose*
Faculté Xavier Bichat
75018, Paris, France

INTRODUCTION

Native α-thrombin, the end product of the clotting factor activation cascade, is a serine protease which not only catalyzes the conversion of fibrinogen into fibrin, but also clearly plays a central regulatory role in hemostasis by interacting with a wide variety of plasmatic and cellular components.[1,2] Its catalytic mechanism seems rather similar to that of other serine proteases and like trypsin, thrombin cleaves preferentially peptide bonds involving the carboxyl group of basic amino acids, yet with a marked preference for arginine residues.[3,4] Because of the number of its macromolecular substrates, thrombin cannot be considered a uniquely specific enzyme. However, unlike the pancreatic serine proteases, it exhibits for each given substrate a remarkably narrow specificity by cleaving only a very limited number of peptide bonds. Attempts to establish the molecular bases of thrombin specificity have generated a great deal of research in the past years. Its amino acid sequence has been determined in both the bovine[5] and human[6] species allowing comparisons with the other members of the serine protease family.[5,7] Systematic mapping of the active site[1,8,9] and construction of computer-generated spatial models[10] have also provided a great deal of information. However, although thrombin has been crystallized,[11,12] its exact three-dimensional structure, which would probably generate more definite elements, still remains to be elucidated. Limited proteolysis of thrombin gives rise to at least two definite derivative forms referred to as β- and γ-thrombins.[13–16] In sharp contrast to a mostly preserved catalytic activity on small synthetic and some proteic substrates, these derivatives exhibit dramatic alterations in activity toward some other specific macromolecular substrates including fibrinogen. Although no physiological relevance has been demonstrated to date for these proteolytic derivatives, because of these remarkable features they have been extensively used as models in the general effort to define the structure-function relationship in the thrombin molecule. It is the purpose of this

[a]This work was supported by Grants from the Centre National de la Recherche Scientifique (Génie Biomédical 81), from the Institut National de la Santé et de la Recherche Médicale (CRL 81-5-022 and 84-5-007), and from the Faculté Xavier Bichat, Université Paris VII. B.L.B. was a recipient of a fellowship from the Ministère de la Recherche et de l'Industrie.

paper to describe results we have obtained concerning the preparation and the structural characterization of the proteolytic derivatives of human thrombin as well as some aspects of their function and to compare them to the data of the literature.

PREPARATION OF PROTEOLYTIC DERIVATIVES OF THROMBIN

Proteolytic derivatives of human thrombin can be obtained by limited proteolysis by trypsin or by autolysis at alkaline pH in the presence of a high concentration of monovalent cations.[16,17] Treatment of thrombin with other trypsin-like enzymes such as plasmin or factor Xa has also been reported to give rise to similar derivatives.[16]

Typically, autolysis of human α-thrombin can be carried out at room temperature in sterile vials at a concentration of 60 to 100 nmol/ml in 20 mM Tris, 0.5 M NaCl, pH 9.0.[10] Under such conditions, clotting activity decreases rapidly; 50% is lost in the first 20 hr and virtually all the activity is lost by 180 hr (FIGURE 1A). Amidolytic activity measured on H-D-Phe-Pip-Arg-*p*NA, however, decreases much more slowly and 65% of the activity still remains after 180 hr of incubation. By contrast, α-thrombin at the same concentration is perfectly stable for the same period of time in 0.3 M NaCl at pH 6.2 to 6.7. Increasing the temperature of incubation and the thrombin or NaCl concentration accelerates autolysis but makes more difficult the isolation of the intermediate form, β-thrombin.

The proteolytic fragmentation of α-thrombin can be followed by sodium dodecyl sulfate (SDS)-polyacrylamide gel electrophoresis (FIGURE 1B). In the absence of a reducing agent, α-thrombin corresponds to a single band with a molecular weight of 35.6 kDa. Four bands of lower molecular weights appear during autolysis. The 25- and 13-kDa bands are the first to be formed. They are the consequence of the α to β conversion in which cleavage of the thrombin B chain gives rise to two fragments, B1 with an apparent molecular weight of 13 kDa and B2. This last fragment and the A chain, to which it is covalently bound by a disulfide bridge (B2-A), correspond to the 25-kDa band. At later stages of autolysis, the 25-kDa species is replaced by the two 12- and 10-kDa bands resulting from the further fragmentation in γ-thrombin of B2-A into B3-A (11 kDa) and B4 (13 kDa). Limited proteolysis of α-thrombin by trypsin gives rise to a similar fragmentation pattern. The fact that proteolytic cleavages occur in a sequential manner suggests that the α to β conversion alters the conformation of native thrombin exposing new sites to proteolytic attack, hence leading to the production of γ-thrombin.

Preparative separation of the autolytic derivatives of human thrombin can be achieved by ion exchange chromatography on Biorex 70. A 1 × 38-cm column is equilibrated at 4°C in 0.15 M NaCl, pH 8.0 and a flow rate of 80 ml/hr is maintained. Gamma- and β-thrombins are eluted sequentially by raising the ionic strength to 0.30 M NaCl and the remaining undegraded α-thrombin can be eluted at 0.75 M NaCl. FIGURE 2A shows such a separation performed after 80 hr of autolysis and FIGURE 2B the analysis of the different fractions by SDS-polyacrylamide gel electrophoresis.

Human α-thrombin can also be satisfactorily prepared by controlled passage through a trypsin-Sepharose column.[16]

Proteolytic derivatives of bovine thrombin can be obtained after activation of crude prothrombin in 25% trisodium citrate, pH 7.2, followed by repeated sulfopropyl-Sephadex chromatography.[19]

The existence of multiple forms of porcine thrombin has also been reported.[20]

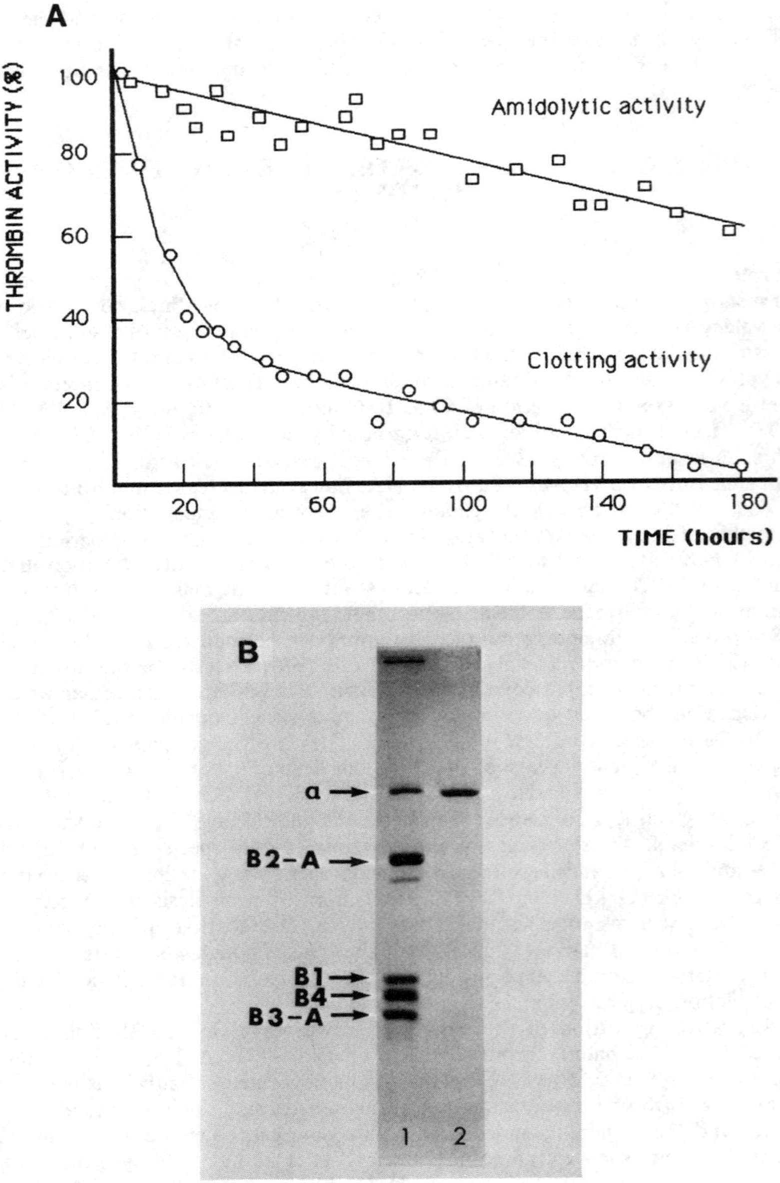

FIGURE 1. Autolytic degradation of human α-thrombin. **(A)** Thrombin activity as measured on fibrinogen (○) and on H-D-Phe-Pip-Arg-*p*NA (□). Thrombin autolysis was carried out under the conditions described in the text. **(B)** SDS-polyacrylamide gel electrophoresis of (1) the autolytic products after 100 hr of incubation and (2) the starting material (α-thrombin). Polyacrylamide gels were run in the absence of reducing agent. The polyacrylamide concentration was 15% and the acrylamide/bisacrylamide ratio was 30/1.

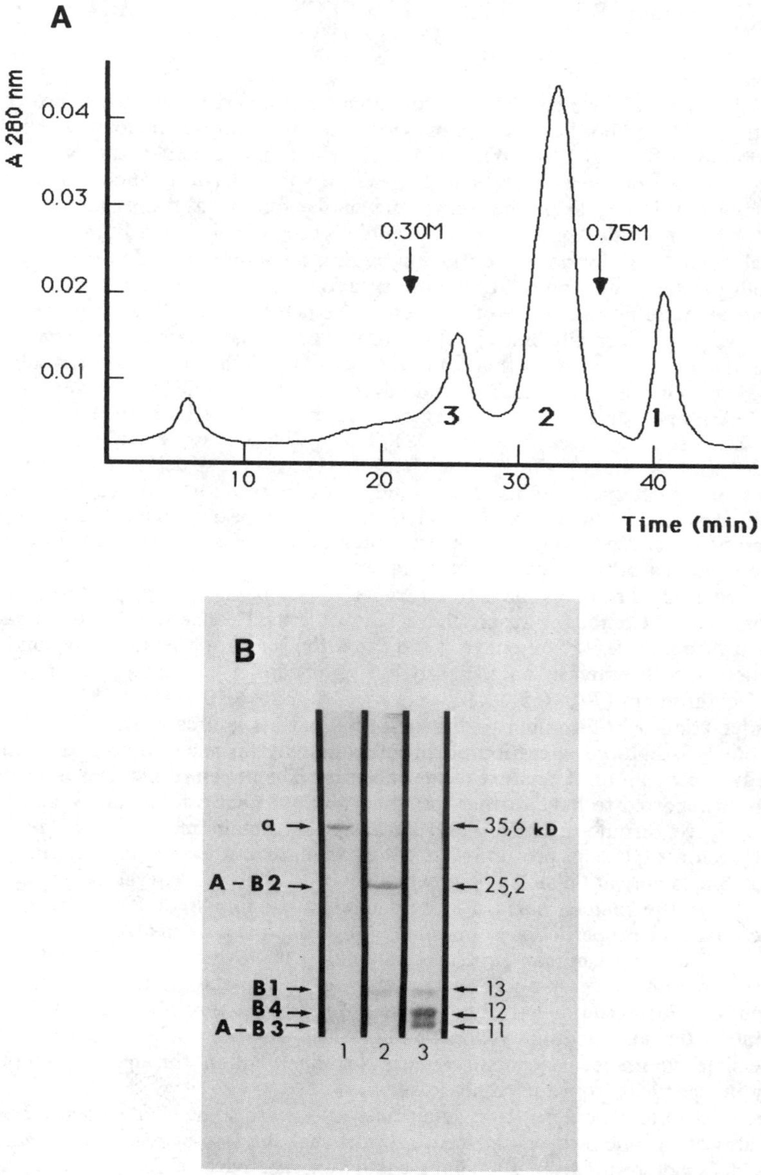

FIGURE 2. Chromatographic separation of the autolytic derivatives of human thrombin. **(A)** Chromatographic profile of an autolytic mixture after 80 hr of incubation. Chromatography on Biorex 70 was performed as described in the text. Arrows indicate stepwise changes in the NaCl concentration of the eluting buffer. Peaks 1, 2, and 3 correspond to α-, β- and γ-thrombins, respectively. **(B)** SDS-polyacrylamide gel electrophoresis of the purified products, carried out as stated in the caption for FIGURE 1. Lanes, 1, 2, and 3 correspond to peaks 1, 2, and 3 on the chromatogram.

FUNCTIONAL PROPERTIES OF PROTEOLYTIC DERIVATIVES OF THROMBIN

Published results concerning the functional characterization of the proteolytic derivatives of thrombin have been mostly obtained by using the major final products of degradation, namely, β-thrombin in the bovine species and γ-thrombin in the human. Because of the extreme similarity in structure between human and bovine β-thrombins, it is very likely that they share similar functional properties. As already mentioned, proteolytic degradation of thrombin is accompanied by a dramatic decrease in its ability to clot fibrinogen contrasting with a moderate alteration of the activity on small synthetic substrates. Active-site titration using *p*-nitrophenyl *p*′-guanidinobenzoate shows a normal value of one active site per molecule. The serine residue of the catalytic triad normally binds [^{14}C]diisopropyl fluorophosphate. Esterolytic activity measured with benzoyl-Arg-ethyl ester or tosyl-Arg-methyl ester is essentially unchanged.[16,19] The slight decrease in amidolytic activity on anilide substrates such as benzoyl-Arg-*p*NA or H-D-Phe-Pip-Arg-*p*NA is the result of both an increase in K_m and a decrease in k_{cat} (see Reference 21). These results favor a slight alteration of both the primary binding site and the charge relay system. A decrease of the nucleophilicity of the catalytic-site histidine as judged by its reaction with tosyl-Lys-CH_2Cl has been reported.[22] Studies on the catalytic mechanism of trypsin[23] indicate that such an alteration is indeed likely to decrease amide or anilide hydrolysis, but to have no effect on the hydrolysis of ester substrates.

Proteolyzed thrombins have been reported to be normally inhibited by α_2-macroglobulin.[9] Conflicting results have been described concerning their interaction with antithrombin III.[24,25] We have found[26] that the second-order rate constant of the inhibition of γ-thrombin is only slightly but significantly reduced when compared to that of α-thrombin ($7 \pm 0.5 \times 10^3$ versus $11 \pm 1.7 \times 10^3$ M^{-1} sec^{-1}, $p < 0.02$). The interaction of γ-thrombin with hirudin in contrast is drastically altered.[16]

Proteolysis-induced alteration of thrombin activity on macromolecular substrates is highly dependent on the nature of the substrate. The nonclotting forms of thrombin have been reported to have further lost their ability to activate factors V and VIII[16] and to cleave thrombospondin.[27] By contrast, they retain most of their reactivity toward factor XIII[28] and prothrombin.[29] We found, like others,[30] that the capacity of γ-thrombin to activate platelets is greatly reduced, whereas cleavage of glycoprotein V (GPV) at the platelet surface is only moderately impaired. Recently, we have characterized the properties of γ-thrombin in regard to the protein C/thrombomodulin system.[26] The rate of human protein C activation by γ-thrombin in the absence of thrombomodulin is very much decreased when compared to that obtained with α-thrombin. Furthermore, γ-thrombin fails to displace α-thrombin from its complex with rabbit thrombomodulin. It has therefore lost the ability of α-thrombin to form a reversible equimolecular complex with thrombomodulin through an interaction totally independent from the catalytic site.[31]

Because proteolytic derivatives retain activity toward some of the macromolecular substrates of thrombin, it would seem a priori that the loss of reactivity toward the others does not result from the slight change of reactivity of the catalytic and/or primary binding sites but rather to the alteration or even loss of specific recognition sites remote from the catalytic site itself. It has been reported that γ-thrombin fails to bind fibrinogen or fibrin monomers, or to incorporate in fibrin clots.[16] In the bovine system, however, it has more recently been shown that fibrinogen behaves as a competitive inhibitor in the hydrolysis of H-D-Phe-Pip-Arg-*p*NA by β-thrombin with a K_i identical to that found for α-thrombin.[22] This indicates that the fibrinogen binding site is not affected in bovine β-thrombin and that the loss of clotting activity could be related solely to changes in reactivity of the active-site histidine. Further work is required to extend these conclusions to the human derivative and most obviously to the other macromolecular substrates toward which activity is lost in the proteolyzed thrombins.

STRUCTURE OF THE PROTEOLYTIC DERIVATIVES

To elucidate the exact nature of the proteic material lost in the proteolytic derivatives of human thrombin, we purified[18] the constitutive peptide chains of reduced and carbamidomethylated β- and γ-thrombins by a combination of gel filtration and reverse-phase high-performance liquid chromatography (HPLC). Their amino acid composition was determined by standard procedures. NH_2-terminal sequences were obtained by manual DABITC Edman degradation[32] and the DABTH derivatives independently identified by both thin-layer chromatography (TLC) and HPLC. Amino acids liberated by carboxypeptidase B and/or Y digestion were converted to DABTC derivatives prior to independent analysis by TLC and HPLC and used to establish COOH-terminal sequences. Our results are summarized in FIGURE 3. Autolysis only affects the B chain since native human α-thrombin and its two β and γ derivatives have identical A chains. The α to β conversion results from two cleavages at Arg-62 and -73 in the B chain giving rise to the B1 chain extending from residues 1 to 62 and the B2 chain from residues 74 to 259. Confirmation of these cleavages comes from the isolation of an intact 11-residue peptide extending from residues 63 to 73 after 72 hr of autolysis. The B1 chain contains one of the residues of the catalytic triad, His-43, and the carbohydrate chain linked to Asn-53. These results confirm that, as mentioned above, the B1 chain is not covalently bound to the rest of the derivative molecule; the B2 chain on the contrary is bound to the A chain by the disulfide bond involving Cys-119. Beta to γ conversion results from at least two additional cleavages at Arg-123 and Lys-154 subdividing the B2 chain into B3 and B4 chains. It is likely that several cleavages occur in the 124 to 154 region since we were unable to isolate an intact peptide containing this region of the molecule. In γ-thrombin therefore, there is only one covalent interchain linkage, namely, the disulfide bond between the B3 and A chains. The three residues of the catalytic site, His-43, Asp-99, and Ser-205, are located on three different and noncovalently bound peptide chains, respectively B1, B3, and B4. Our results are in agreement with the minimal cleavages previously reported for the autolytic degradation of human thrombin. The covalent structures of the β and γ human autolytic derivatives are schematized in FIGURE 3 in comparison to that of α-thrombin.

The noncovalent association of the constitutive peptide chains in γ-thrombin is most probably responsible for the decreased stability of the molecule.[33,34] γ-Thrombin has been elegantly used as a model to study the folding of multichain proteins.[35]

From our results it is also possible to determine the exact molecular weights of the constitutive peptide chains of the proteolytic derivatives of human thrombin (TABLE 1). It is to be noted that most probably because of the presence of the carbohydrate moiety, the B1 chain has an abnormally low electrophoretic mobility which does not correspond to its actual molecular weight. Despite the difference in mass between β- and γ-thrombins, it is not possible to separate these two derivatives either by conventional gel filtration or by high-performance gel permeation.

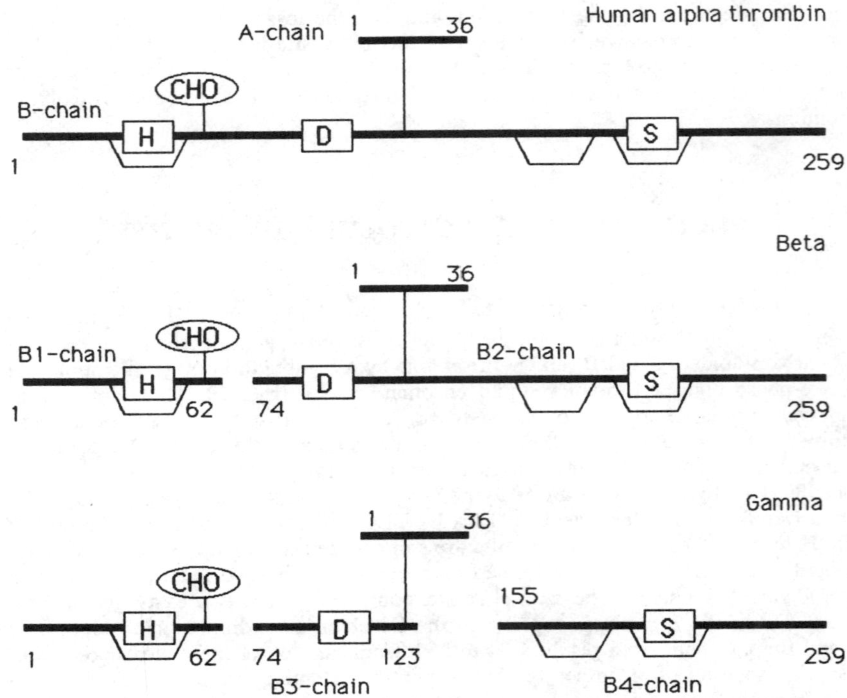

FIGURE 3. Structures of native human α-thrombin and of its β and γ autolytic derivatives. Numbering of the residues is that of human thrombin A and B chains, respectively. In the B chain, H, D, and S correspond to the catalytic site residues, His-43, Asp-97, and Ser-205. CHO indicates the carbohydrate moiety linked to Asn-53. Thrombin contains four disulfide bridges which are schematized in the figure, one between the A and B chains and three in the B chain.

Comparison with the reported structural events of the bovine thrombin proteolytic degradation reveals several differences.[36] First the A chain is affected by the proteolytic process in the bovine system only. The human A chain is 13 residues shorter on the NH_2-terminal side, due to a Pro-Arg-(−1)-Thr-1 sequence in human prothrombin (versus Glu-Lys-Thr in bovine thrombin) which is cleaved off by thrombin during human prothrombin activation. Proteolytic degradation of bovine thrombin results in cleavages at Lys-(−1) and Lys-17 in the A chain. Despite an identical amino acid sequence surrounding Lys-17 in the two species, we did not observe autolytic cleavage at this site in the human system. The A chain of human derivatives is therefore homologous to its bovine counterpart on the NH_2-terminal end, but 19 residues longer on the COOH-terminal end. Autolytic cleavages in the B chain are also different in the two species. In human β-thrombin, the region extending from residues 63 to 73 is cleaved off, as compared to residues 66 to 73 in the bovine B chain, even though the sequence surrounding Arg-62 (human cleavage site) and Lys-65 (bovine cleavage site) is strictly identical in both species. In the bovine system, β-thrombin is the major final product of proteolytic degradation. Although the existence of a γ form has been reported, available quantities of this derivative have been insufficient to date to clearly establish its covalent structure. This is a remarkable difference from the human system in which β-thrombin is a somewhat labile intermediate and γ-thrombin is the final proteolytic product. Therefore, despite an 84% degree of identity between human and bovine thrombins, during the proteolytic process, only one cleavage (at Arg-73) is identical between the two species. It might be worth mentioning, however, that the region cleaved off in human γ-thrombin contains the highest incidence of substitutions between the two species (38.7 versus 14.7% for the entire B chain).

From sequence comparisons of thrombin with the pancreatic serine proteases,[7,10] speculations have been made concerning the direct or indirect involvement of the observed insertions of peptide material (loops, as defined in Reference 7) in the formation of specific recognition sites for thrombin macromolecular substrates. One of them (loop A) is the COOH-terminal portion of the A chain which is no longer present in bovine β-thrombin. However, it is conserved in the human derivatives and therefore its loss in itself cannot account for the altered activity of the bovine proteolytic derivative. One other major insertion (loop B) is the peptide region containing the carbohydrate moiety at Asn-53 in the B chain. It might be of interest to note that the loss of clotting activity seems to be related solely to the excision of the 63-73 peptide (or 66-73 in bovine thrombin) located in the proximity of this loop.

A computer-generated model of the three-dimensional structure of thrombin[10] indicates, as for all serine proteases, a two β barrel structure, each barrel formed by six extended β structures. In this model, the autolytic 63-73 peptide is located in the NH_2-terminal barrel between the D and E extended β structures (FIGURE 4). Its deletion in the proteolytic derivatives could severely affect the structure of this molecular domain which contains two residues of the catalytic triad (His-43 and Asp-99). If this were the case, it could represent the molecular basis for the reduced reactivity of His-43 and/or indicate that structural integrity of the NH_2-terminal barrel is essential for the recognition of some of the thrombin macromolecular substrates. The region of the peptide chain lost during the β to γ conversion affects the interdomain region. Cleavage in the homologous region of chymotrypsin does not affect its activity. The two generated fragments, however, unlike in γ-thrombin, remain covalently linked by a disulfide bridge.[37] From the lack of apparent major functional

TABLE 1. Molecular Weights of the Human Thrombin Derivatives[a]

	Peptide Molecular Weight	Total Molecular Weight
α-Thrombin	33,659	35,600
β-Thrombin	32,924	34,300
γ-Thrombin	29,152	31,100
Thrombin A chain	4,091	4,091
B chain	29,568	31,500
B1 chain	7,058	9,000
B2 chain	21,145	21,145
B3 chain	6,080	6,080
B4 chain	11,923	11,923

[a]Peptide molecular weights are calculated from the amino acid sequence data (References 6 and 18) and the total molecular weights assuming a 8.2% carbohydrate content in prothrombin and a symmetrical three-chain distribution.

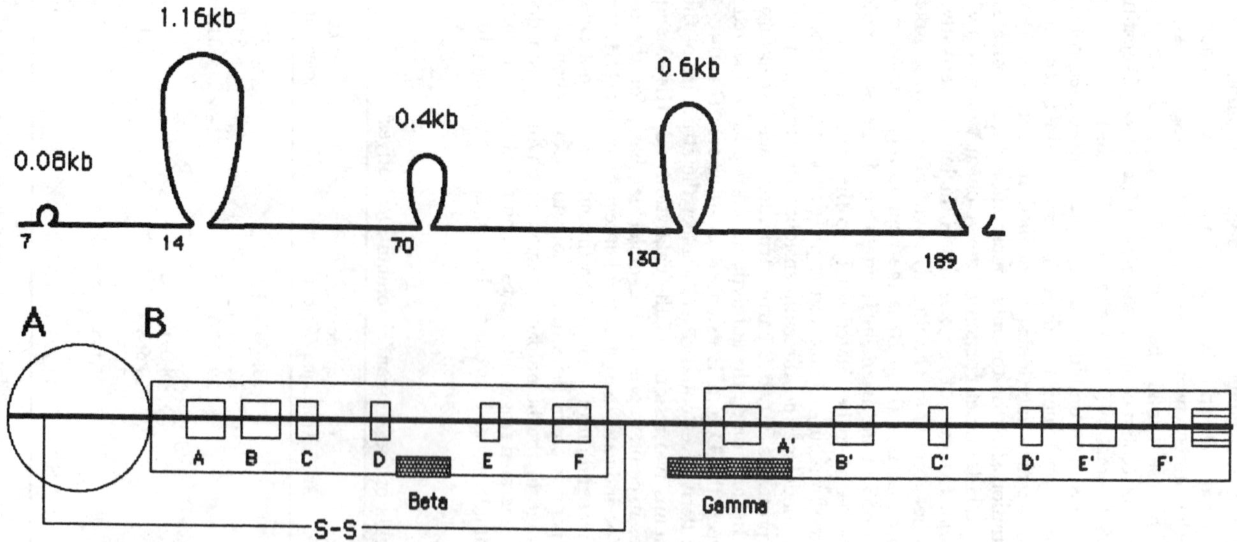

FIGURE 4. Comparison of the structure of thrombin and that of the region of the prothrombin gene corresponding to the NH_2-terminal part of thrombin. In the lower part of the figure, the structure of thrombin is schematized. The A chain is represented by a circle and the B chain by two rectangles corresponding to the two β barrels. In each barrel, the six regions of extended β structure are represented: A to F in the NH_2-terminal barrel and A′ to F′ in the COOH-terminal barrel. Shaded areas correspond to the regions of the peptide chain cleaved off upon autolysis. The upper part of the figure represents the structure of the region of the prothrombin gene corresponding to the NH_2-terminal part of thrombin. Introns are represented as loops and their respective sizes are given in kilobases (kb). The other numbers indicate residues in the A and B chains at which the exon/intron junctions occur. The structure of the region of the prothrombin gene corresponding to the COOH-terminal part of thrombin has not been published to date.

differences between bovine β- and human γ-thrombins, it could be hypothesized that a similar situation exists for thrombin, although the loss of peptide material is much more extensive than in chymotrypsin and includes the whole A′ extended β structure of the COOH-terminal barrel.

Finally, because of the proposed relation between exons and functional domains in proteins,[38] and the structure of the prothrombin gene now being established,[39] it might be of interest to realize that the 0.4- and 0.6 kilobase (kb) introns of the genomic DNA are located in the regions cleaved off during proteolysis (FIGURE 4). The position of the 0.6-kb intron actually corresponds to the hinge region between the two β barrels of the thrombin molecule.

The demonstration that the COOH-terminal part of the thrombin A chain does not participate in fibrinogen recognition and some insights on the role of His-43 in the catalytic triad, are direct consequences of the studies performed with the proteolytic derivatives. It is likely, as more data accumulate, that such studies will provide an appreciable contribution to the general attempt to define the precise molecular mechanisms of thrombin function.

REFERENCES

1. FENTON, J. W. 1981. Ann. N.Y. Acad. Sci. **370:** 468-495.
2. MANN, K. G. & R. L. LUNDBLAD. 1982. *In* Hemostasis and Thrombosis, Basic Principles and Clinical Practice. R. W. Colman, J. Hirsch, V. J. Mard & E. W. Salzman, Eds.: 112-126. J. B. Lippincott Co. Philadelphia, Pa.
3. DOWNING, M. R., J. ELION, R. J. BUTKOWSKI & K. G. MANN. 1978. *In* Recent Progress in Blood Coagulation and Thrombosis Research. Bibliotheca Haematologica, pp. 39-53. Karger Verlag. Basel, Switzerland.
4. CHANG, J. Y. 1985. Eur. J. Biochem. **151:** 217-224.
5. MAGNUSSON, S., T. E. PETERSON, L. SOTTRUP-JENSEN & H. CLAEYS. 1974. *In* Proteases and Biological Control. E. Reich & D. B. Rifkin, Eds.: 123-149. Cold Spring Harbor Editor. Cold Spring Harbor, N.Y.
6. BUTKOWSKI, R. J., J. ELION, M. R. DOWNING & K. G. MANN. 1977. J. Biol. Chem. **252:** 4942-4957.
7. ELION, J., M. R. DOWNING, R. J. BUTKOWSKI & K. G. MANN. 1977. *In* Chemistry and Biology of Thrombin. R. L. Lunblad, J. W. Fenton & K. G. Mann, Eds.: 97-111. Ann Arbor Science Publisher. Ann Arbor, Mich.
8. SHERAGA, H. A. 1977. *In* Chemistry and Biology of Thrombin. R. L. Lunblad, J. W. Fenton & K. G. Mann, Eds.: 145-158. Ann Arbor Science Publisher. Ann Arbor, Mich.
9. BERLINER, L. J. 1984. Mol. Cell. Biochem. **61:** 159-172.
10. FURIE, B., D. H. BING, R. J. FELDMANN, D. J. ROBINSON, J. P. BURNIER & B. C. FURIE. 1982. J. Biol. Chem. **257:** 3875-3882.
11. TSERNOGLOU, D., D. A. WALZ, L. E. MCCOY & W. H. SEEGERS. 1974. J. Biol. Chem. **249:** 999.
12. MCKAY, D. B., L. M. KAY & R. M. STROUD. 1977. *In* Chemistry and Biology of Thrombin. R. L. LUNBLAD, J. W. FENTON & K. G. MANN, Eds.: 113-121. Ann Arbor Science Publisher. Ann Arbor, Mich.
13. SEEGERS, W. H., L. MCCOY, R. K. KIPFER & G. MURANO. 1968. Arch. Biochem. Biophys. **128:** 194-201.
14. MANN, K. G., R. YIP, C. M. HELDEBRANT & D. A. FASS. 1973. J. Biol. Chem. **248:** 1868-1875.
15. WORKMAN, E. F., JR. & R. L. LUNDBLAD. 1980. *In* CRC Handbook Series in Clinical Laboratory Science, Vol. III. Section I: Hematology. R. M. Schmidt, Ed.: 149-169. CRC Press. Boca Raton, Fla.

16. FENTON, J. W., B. H. LANDIS, D. A. WALZ & J. S. FINLAYSON. 1977. *In* Chemistry and Biology of Thrombin. R. L. Lunblad, J. W. Fenton & K. G. Mann, Eds.: 43-70. Ann Arbor Science Publisher. Ann Arbor, Mich.
17. FENTON, J. W., M. J. FASCO, A. B. STOCKROW, D. L. ARONSON, A. M. YOUNG & J. S. FINLAYSON. 1977. J. Biol. Chem. **252:** 3587-3598.
18. BOISSEL, J. P., B. LE BONNIEC, M. J. RABIET, D. LABIE & J. ELION. 1984. J. Biol. Chem. **259:** 5691-5697.
19. WORKMAN, E. F., JR., L. C. UHTEG, H. S. KINGDON & R. L. LUNBLAD. 1977. *In* Chemistry and Biology of Thrombin. R. L. Lunblad, J. W. Fenton & K. G. Mann, Eds.: 23-42. Ann Arbor Science Publisher. Ann Arbor, Mich.
20. ROSSI, A. & J. R. GIGLIO. 1974. Can. J. Biochem. **52:** 336-344.
21. LOTTENBERG, R., J. A. HALL, J. W. FENTON & C. M. JACKSON. 1982. Thromb. Res. **28:** 313-332.
22. LUNDBLAD, R. L., M. E. NEISHEIM, D. L. STRAIGHT, S. SAILOR, J. BOWIE, J. W. BENZANO, J. D. ROBERTS & K. G. MANN. 1984. J. Biol. Chem. **259:** 6991-6995.
23. ELROD, J. P., J. L. HOGG, D. M. QUINN, J. S. VENKATASUBBAN & R. L. SCHOWEN. 1980. J. Am. Chem. Soc. **102:** 3917-3922.
24. CHANG, T. L., R. D. FEINMAN, B. H. LANDIS & J. W. FENTON. 1979. Biochemistry **18:** 113-119.
25. MACHOVICH, R., A. BORSODI, G. BLASKO & S. A. ORAKZAI. 1977. Biochem. J. **167:** 393-398.
26. BEZEAUD, A., M. H. DENNINGER & M. C. GUILLIN. 1985. Eur. J. Biochem. **153:** 491-496.
27. TAKAHASHI, K., M. AIKEN, J. W. FENTON & D. A. WALZ. 1984. Biochem. J. **224:** 673-676.
28. LORAND, L. & R. B. CREDO. 1977. *In* Chemistry and Biology of Thrombin. R. L. Lunblad, J. W. Fenton & K. G. Mann, Eds.: 311-323. Ann Arbor Science Publisher. Ann Arbor, Mich.
29. SEEGERS, W. H., H. I. HASSOUNA, D. HEWETT-EMETT, D. A. WALZ & T. J. ANDARY. 1975. Semin. Thromb. Hemostasis **1:** 211-283.
30. CHARO, I. F., R. D. FEINMAN & T. C. DETWILER. 1977. J. Clin. Invest. **60:** 866-873.
31. ESMON, N. L., W. G. OWEN & C. T. ESMON. 1982. J. Biol. Chem. **257:** 859-864.
32. CHANG, J. Y. 1981. Biochem. J. **199:** 557-564.
33. BAUER, R. S., T. L. CHANG & L. J. BERLINER. 1980. J. Biol. Chem. **255:** 5900-5903.
34. CHANG, T. L., R. S. BAUER & L. J. BERLINER. 1980. J. Biol. Chem. **255:** 5904-5906.
35. VILLANUEVA, G. B. 1981. Biochemistry **20:** 6519-6525.
36. LUNDBLAD, R. L., C. M. NOYES, K. G. MANN & H. S. KINGDON. 1979. J. Biol. Chem. **254:** 8524-8528.
37. MELOUN, B., I. KLUH, V. KOSTKA, L. MORAVECK, Z. PRUSIK, J. VANECEK, B. KEIL & F. SORM. 1966. Biochim. Biophys. Acta **130:** 543-546.
38. GILBERT, W. 1978. Nature **271:** 501.
39. FRIEZNER-DEGEN, S. J., R. T. A. MC GILLIVRAY & E. W. DAVIE. 1983. Biochemistry **22:** 2087-2097.

Difference in Enzymatic Properties between "Staphylothrombin" and Free α-Thrombin[a]

SHUN-ICHIRO KAWABATA,[b] TAKASHI MORITA,[b]
TOSHIYUKI MIYATA,[b] SHIGENORI KAIDA,[b]
HIDEO IGARASHI,[c] AND SADAAKI IWANAGA[b]

[b]*Department of Biology*
Faculty of Science
Kyushu University 33
Fukuoka 812, Japan

[c]*Department of Microbiology*
Tokyo Metropolitan Research Laboratory of Public Health
Tokyo 160, Japan

Human prothrombin forms an equimolar complex with staphylocoagulase, a bacterial nonenzymatic protein.[1,2] The resulting molecular complex, termed "staphylothrombin," has the ability to form a fibrin clot, like α-thrombin.[3,4] This staphylocoagulase-mediated activation of prothrombin does not involve any proteolytic cleavage along the polypeptide chain of the prothrombin molecule.[5-7] Thus, it differs entirely from the mechanism of prothrombin activation by factor Xa and snake venom procoagulant, as shown in FIGURE 1. Our objective in the present study is to elucidate how active zymogen is formed by the interaction between prothrombin and staphylocoagulase. We discuss in this paper the difference in enzymatic properties between staphylothrombin and free α-thrombin, and also the covalent structure of the active fragment derived from staphylocoagulase.

ENZYMATIC PROPERTIES OF STAPHYLOTHROMBIN[d]

Staphylocoagulase was purified from culture filtrates of *Staphylococcus aureus* strain 213 as described in previous papers.[9,10] The isolated staphylocoagulase gave a single band corresponding to a molecular weight of 64,000 on sodium dodecyl sulfate-polyacrylamide gel electrophoresis (SDS-PAGE) (for experimental details see references 7,8,11-13).

[a]This work was supported by a Grant-in-Aid for Scientific Research from the Ministry of Education, Science and Culture of Japan.

[d]See references 7 and 8.

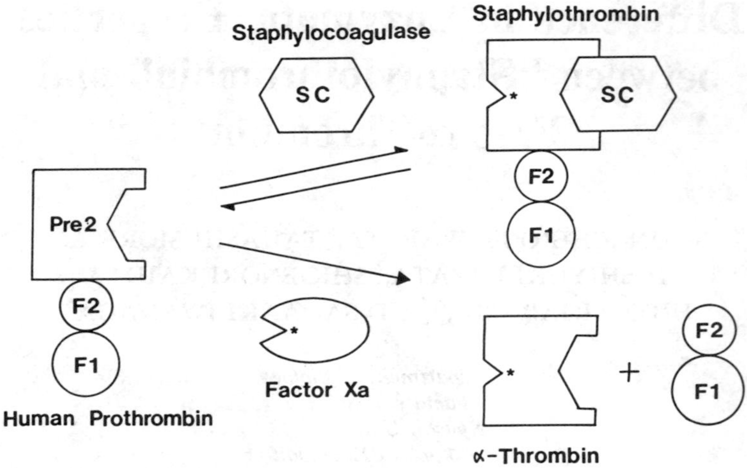

FIGURE 1. Activation of human prothrombin by factor Xa and staphylocoagulase. Pre2, F1, and F2 show prethrombin domains, prethrombin 2, fragment 1, and fragment 2, respectively.

TABLE 1 shows the enzymatic properties of staphylothrombin and α-thrombin. The fibrinogen clotting activity of staphylothrombin was 20% of that of α-thrombin. Staphylothrombin also activated protein C and factor XIII like α-thrombin. However, the staphylothrombin activity was not inhibited at all by antithrombin III and hirudin. Synthetic inhibitors, diisopropyl fluorophosphate (DFP) and benzamidine, inhibited the amidase activity of staphylothrombin. In order to determine whether DFP is incorporated into prothrombin or staphylocoagulase after the complex formation, human prothrombin and prethrombin 1 were incubated, separately, with staphylocoagulase at 25°C for 1 hr in the presence of tritiated DFP, and the mixtures were subjected to SDS-PAGE. The results are shown in FIGURE 2. Lanes 1 and 2 are prothrombin and prethrombin 1, respectively. Lanes 3 and 4 are the complexes of prothrombin + staphylocoagulase and prethrombin 1 + staphylocoagulase, respectively. Asterisks denote fluorograms of the corresponding SDS-PAGE. From the data

TABLE 1. Enzymatic Properties of Staphylothrombin and Human α-Thrombin

	Staphylothrombin	α-Thrombin
Clotting activity (NIH units/mg)	250-300	2500
(NIH units/nmol)	20	100
Activator activity		
Factor XIII	+	+
Effect of inhibitor		
Antithrombin III-heparin	Not inhibited	Inhibited
Hirudin	Not inhibited	Inhibited
DFP	Inhibited	Inhibited
Benzamidine (K_i, M)	1.2×10^{-4}	1.0×10^{-4}

of lanes 3 and 3*, the staphylothrombin activity was not completely inhibited by DFP under the conditions used. Thus, a part of prothrombin was transformed into prethrombin 1, and DFP was incorporated into these two precursors. However, no tritiated DFP was incorporated into staphylocoagulase. As to the prethrombin 1 + staphylocoagulase complex (lanes 4 and 4*), only prethrombin 1 was labeled. These results indicate that a DFP-sensitive active site is formed in the prothrombin part but not in the staphylocoagulase molecule. Moreover, there was no cleavage of the peptide linkage between A and B chains constituting the α-thrombin molecule.

TABLE 2 shows the steady-state kinetic parameters of staphylothrombin, staphyloprethrombin 1, and α-thrombin. The K_m and k_{cat} values were determined by measuring the initial rate at pH 8.0 and 37°C, using synthetic peptide substrates. The values obtained on active-site titration for both staphylothrombin and staphyloprethrombin 1 with *p*-nitrophenyl *p*′-guanidinobenzoate·HCl (NPGB) were essentially

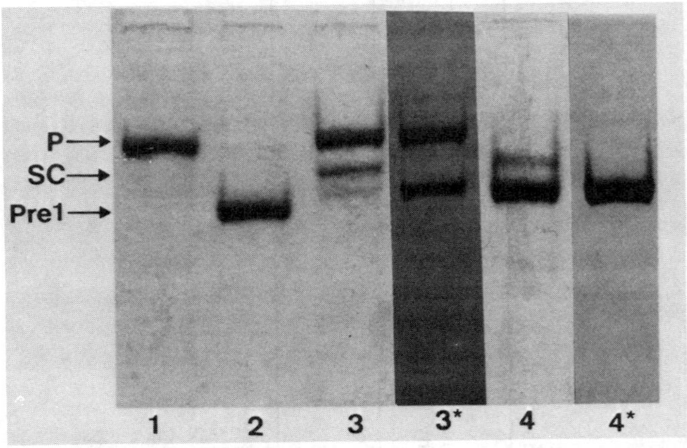

FIGURE 2. Incorporation of [^{3}H]DFP into the active complex. Lane 1, human prothrombin; lane 2, human prethrombin 1; lane 3, a mixture of human prothrombin and staphylocoagulase; lane 3*, a fluorogram of lane 3; lane 4, a mixture of human prethrombin 1 and staphylocoagulase; lane 4*, a fluorogram of lane 4.

the same as that for α-thrombin, thus indicating that one residue of active site per one molecule was formed in both complexes. The rates of acylation were very fast for all enzymes, since the immediate burst of *p*-nitrophenol was observed within 5 sec. The clotting activities of staphylothrombin and staphyloprethrombin 1 were approximately one-seventh of that of α-thrombin. The K_m values of staphyloprethrombin 1 were somewhat larger than those of α-thrombin. The k_{cat} values of staphyloprethrombin 1 were about a half of those of α-thrombin. FIGURE 3 shows the pH profiles of α-thrombin and staphyloprethrombin 1 obtained using Boc-Val-Pro-Arg-MCA (MCA = 4-methylcoumaryl-7-amide) as substrate. As expected, α-thrombin showed a bell-shaped profile with an optimum at around pH 8.5. However, the pH profile of staphyloprethrombin 1 differed significantly from that of α-thrombin especially at alkaline pH, and the maximum was found at pH 10.2. At the higher pH of 10.5 the activity rapidly decreased, showing that the complex might be dissociated or denatured at this pH.

TABLE 2. Enzymatic Properties of Staphylothrombin, Staphyloprethrombin 1, and α-Thrombin

Enzyme	Active-Site Titration (%)	Clotting Activity (NIH units/nmol)	Boc-Val-Pro-Arg-MCA[a]			S-2238[a]		
			K_m (μM)	k_{cat} (sec^{-1})	k_{cat}/K_m (sec^{-1} μM^{-1})	K_m (μM)	k_{cat} (sec^{-1})	k_{cat}/K_m (sec^{-1} μM^{-1})
Staphylothrombin	95 ± 2	14	—[b]	—	—	—	—	—
Staphyloprethrombin 1	81 ± 8	12	28	54	1.9	18	115	6.4
α-Thrombin	95 ± 3	97	21	105	5	7.9	197	25

[a] The K_m and k_{cat} values were determined by measuring the initial rate at pH 8.0 and at 37°C. Substrate concentrations of Boc-Val-Pro-Arg-MCA or H-D-Phe-Pip-Arg-*p*NA (S-2238) ranged from 7 to 70 μM or 2.2 to 22 μM, respectively.

[b] Since staphylothrombin digests autocatalytically the NH_2-terminal portion of human prothrombin,[7] a competition with the synthetic substrate will occur. Thus, its kinetic parameters for these synthetic substrates have not been estimated.

All the results mentioned above suggest that the microenvironments of the active sites are not identical for staphylothrombin and free α-thrombin. Possibly, complex formation blocks access to the substrate binding site located near the active site of α-thrombin due to steric hindrance.

THE PROCOAGULANT- AND PROTHROMBIN-BINDING DOMAIN DERIVED FROM STAPHYLOCOAGULASE[e]

Our recent studies demonstrate that chymotryptic digestion of staphylocoagulase under controlled conditions yields mainly three large fragments, of 43, 30, and 20

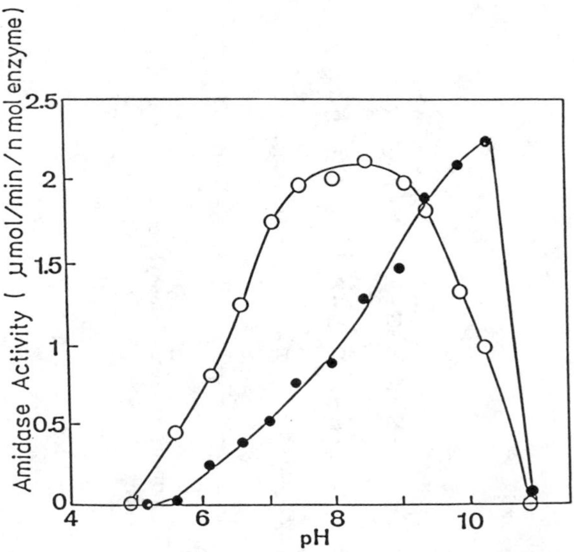

FIGURE 3. Effect of pH on the amidase activities of staphyloprethrombin 1 and α-thrombin. Staphylocoagulase (100 μg/ml) was incubated with human prethrombin 1 (25 μg/ml) for 5 min at 0°C. Then, 20-μl aliquots were added to 600 μl of Britton-Robinson's buffer, and the activity was measured at 37°C using Boc-Val-Pro-Arg-MCA as substrate. The amidase activity of human α-thrombin alone was also measured over the same pH range. ●, staphyloprethrombin 1; ○, α-thrombin.

kDa, all of which give a single band on SDS-PAGE.[12] To align these fragments in the staphylocoagulase molecule, their NH_2-terminal sequences were first determined. The NH_2-terminal sequence of the 43-kDa fragment up to the 22nd amino acid corresponded to the NH_2-terminal sequence established for intact staphylocoagulase, as shown in FIGURE 4. On the other hand, the NH_2-terminal sequence of the 30-kDa fragment up to the 15th amino acid was the same as that of the 20-kDa fragment.

[e] See reference 12.

```
                    1                 10                  20                  30
Staphylocoagulase   I-V-T-K-D-Y-S-K-E-S-R-V-N-E-K-S-K-K-G-A-T-V-S-D-Y-Y-Y-W-K-I-

43-kDa Fragment     I-V-T-K-D-Y-S-K-E-S-R-V-N-E-K-S-K-K-G-A-T-V-

30-kDa Fragment     Q-F-N-K-E-V-K-E-I-E-H-K-N-V-D-L-K-Q-F-D-K-D-G-E-D-K-A-T-K-E-

20-kDa Fragment     Q-F-N-K-E-V-K-E-I-E-H-K-N-V-D-
```

FIGURE 4. NH_2-terminal sequence of staphylocoagulase and its chymotryptic fragments.

Moreover, the COOH-terminal-Val-Ala-Leu sequence of the 43-kDa fragment determined by carboxypeptidase Y digestion, was consistent with that of the 30-kDa fragment, indicating that the 43-kDa fragment must be located in the NH_2-terminal portion of the intact molecule, and that it must include the entire sequence constituting the 30-kDa fragment. FIGURE 5 shows the amino acid compositions of these isolated fragments. The composition of the intact staphylocoagulase is also shown for comparison. The overall compositions were very similar to one another, with a high content of lysine, aspartic acid, and glutamic acid together constituting nearly 50% of the total residues in each of the fragments.

TABLE 3 shows the kinetic parameters of the complex formed between chymotryptic fragment and prethrombin 1. The clotting activity of the 43-kDa fragment complex was almost equivalent to that of the intact staphylocoagulase complex, and one active site per complex was titrated by NPGB. The k_{cat} over K_m value of the 43-kDa fragment complex for fluorogenic substrate was three times higher than that of the intact complex, and this value was comparable to that of α-thrombin, indicating that the 43-kDa fragment retains the full functional activity. On the other hand, the 30-kDa fragment complex showed no detectable clotting activity. The amidase parameter of the 30-kDa fragment complex was reduced to only 0.5% of that of the intact complex. The 30-kDa fragment complex also had one active site per complex. The esterase activities of the complexes were also examined by using *N*-α-tosyl-L-arginine methylester (TAME) as a substrate. As shown in TABLE 4, the prethrombin 1-43-kDa fragment complex exhibited the highest esterase activity, which was two times higher than that of α-thrombin. As to the 20-kDa fragment complex, clotting, amidase, and esterase activities were not detectable. However, the 20-kDa fragment had the ability to bind to a bovine prothrombin-Sepharose column.

The rate of incorporation of DFP into the complexes was determined at 1 mM DFP by following the time course of inactivation of the amidase activity.[12] The prethrombin 1-43-kDa fragment complex was most reactive to DFP. The apparent first-order rate constants of inactivation were 0.3, 1.4, and 0.015 min^{-1} for the intact staphylocoagulase complex, the 43-kDa fragment complex, and the 30-kDa fragment complex, respectively. Thus, the inactivation rate of the prethrombin 1-30-kDa fragment complex was 20-fold slower than that of the intact complex. Several synthetic peptides of arginine chloromethyl ketone are known to selectively inhibit the α-thrombin activity.[15] We have undertaken the study of the inhibition of active complexes by peptidyl chloromethyl ketone, D-Phe-Pro-Arg-CH_2Cl, which is the most potent synthetic inhibitor of α-thrombin.[16] The kinetic study was performed by monitoring the progress of inhibition in the presence of Boc-Val-Pro-Arg-MCA with the method of Walker *et al.*[17] The amidase activities of the complexes were inhibited more effectively than that of α-thrombin, even in the case of the prethrombin 1-30-kDa fragment complex (TABLE 5). However, the inhibition constant (K_i) and the first-order rate constant (k_i) for the prethrombin 1-30-kDa fragment complex were considerably higher than those of other complexes. These results suggest that there is some difference either in the state of amino acid residues associated with the catalytic triad, or the substrate binding site between the prethrombin 1-staphylocoagulase complex and the prethrombin 1-30-kDa fragment complex.

TABLE 6 shows the apparent dissociation constant of the complex formed between chymotryptic fragment and prothrombin. The concentration of the complex was calculated from the specific activity and the data were analyzed by a Scatchard plot. Intact staphylocoagulase formed a tight complex with an apparent K_d of 0.46 nM. The 43-kDa fragment bound to prothrombin with a K_d of 1.7 nM, which is comparable to that of the intact complex. The 30-kDa fragment complex gave a K_d of 120 nM, indicating a much weaker interaction of this fragment with prothrombin. In all cases,

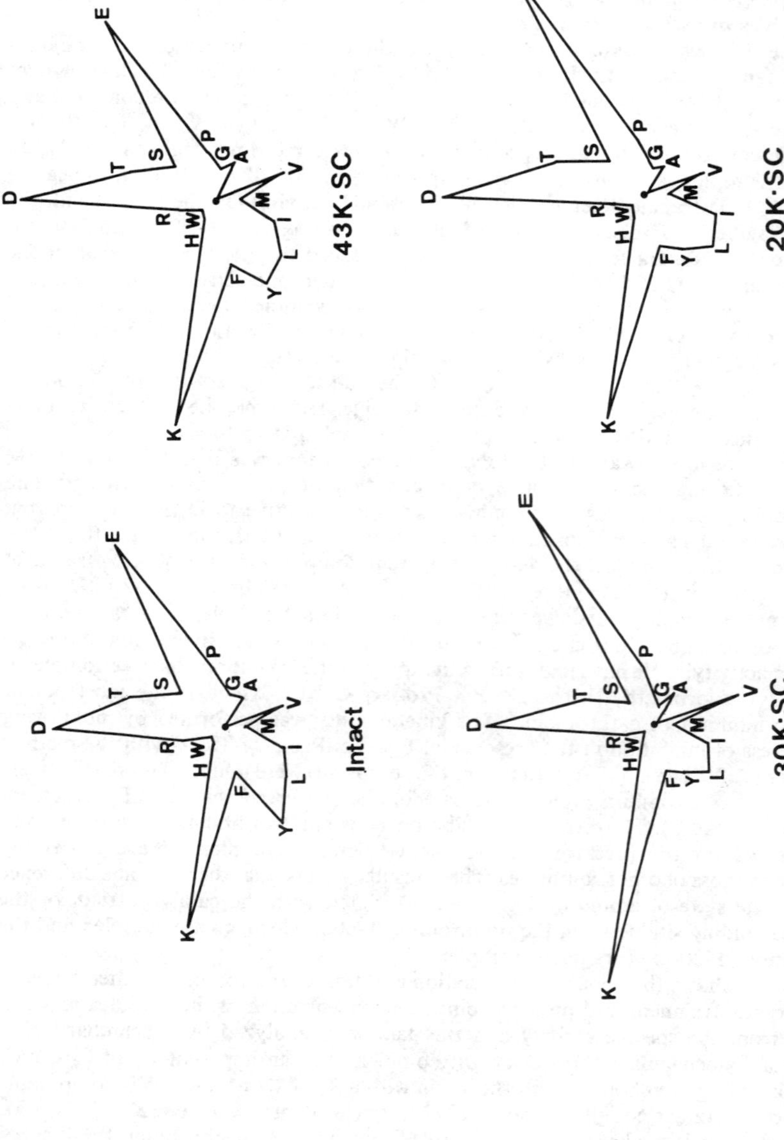

FIGURE 5. Amino acid compositions of intact staphylocoagulase and the isolated fragments.

TABLE 3. Kinetic Parameters of the Complex Formed between Chymotryptic Fragment and Human Prethrombin 1 (Pre1)

Complex	Active-Site Titration (mol NPGB/mol complex)	Clotting Activity (NIH units/nmol)	Boc-Val-Pro-Arg-MCA		
			K_m (μM)	k_{cat} (sec^{-1})	k_{cat}/K_m (sec^{-1} μM^{-1})
Pre1-staphylocoagulase	0.81 ± 0.08	18	22	48	2.2
Pre1-43-kDa fragment	0.90 ± 0.09	19	15	90	6.0
Pre1-30-kDa fragment	0.93 ± 0.12	ND[a]	138	1.6	0.01
Human α-thrombin	0.95 ± 0.03	97	22	121	5.5

[a]Not detectable.

TABLE 4. TAME-Esterase Activity of the Molecular Complex[a]

Complex	Esterase Activity (mol/min/mol enzyme)
Pre1-staphylocoagulase	240
Pre1-43-kDa fragment	351
Pre1-30-kDa fragment	22
Pre1-20-kDa fragment	0
Human α-thrombin	158

[a]The assay was performed at 25°C at pH 8.0. Calculations were based on the molar absorption difference of 740 cm^{-1} M^{-1} at 247 nm.

the stoichiometry was between 1.0 and 1.2. These results indicate that of the three fragments, the 43-kDa fragment has almost the same prothrombin activator activity as that of the parent molecule. For this reason, we next determined the covalent structure of the functionally active 43-kDa fragment.

FIGURE 6 shows the whole sequence of the 43-kDa fragment. It consists of 324 residues with the NH_2-terminal isoleucine and the COOH-terminal leucine. As staphylocoagulase lacks half-cystine, this represents the complete covalent structure. The calculated molecular weight based on the whole sequence is 38,098. The most notable aspect of the overall amino acid composition on the basis of this sequence is the high content of Asp (28 residues), Asn (22), Glu (35), Gln (9), and Lys (52). The sum of these residues accounts for more than 45% of the total residues. Moreover, there are some unusual features in the amino acid sequence. One is the uneven distribution of certain residues in the sequence: most of the tyrosine residues are found in the NH_2-terminal half, while the proline residues are mainly distributed in the COOH-terminal half of the molecule. Another unique feature is the frequent repetitions, found along the whole sequence, of the various kinds of dipeptides: for instance, Lys-Lys is repeated 7 times, Lys-Glu 10 times, and Thr-Lys 7 times.

We compared the structure of the 43-kDa fragment with that of streptokinase established recently by Jackson and Tang.[14] However, it did not reveal any obvious sequence homologies. Moreover, there was no sequence homology with the structures of serine proteases including trypsin, chymotrypsin, and elastase.

FIGURE 7 shows a gross structure of staphylocoagulase and alignments of its chymotryptic fragments. As we mentioned before, the 43-kDa fragment displayed high ability for binding with human prothrombin (K_d = 1.7 nM), as well as the intact staphylocoagulase (K_d = 0.49 nM), and the enzyme activities of its complex with prothrombin did not differ significantly from those of the intact protein complex. On

TABLE 5. Parameters for Inactivation of the Complexes by Peptidyl Chloromethyl Ketone, D-Phe-Pro-Arg-CH_2Cl

Complex	K_i (nM)	k_i (min^{-1})	k_i/K_i (min^{-1} nM^{-1})
Pre1-staphylocoagulase	1.5	1.3	0.87
Pre1-43-kDa fragment	0.7	1.8	2.6
Pre1-30-kDa fragment	28	11.8	0.42
Human α-thrombin	27	4.5	0.17

the other hand, the molecular complex of 30-kDa fragment with prothrombin showed only a very weak clotting activity, although it still exhibited the binding ability with prothrombin (K_d = 120 nM). These results suggest that the prothrombin-binding site is located in the COOH-terminal portion, which includes the entire structure of the 30-kDa fragment, and that the functional region of staphylocoagulase for activating prothrombin is localized in the NH_2-terminal half of the molecule. Further studies on the identification of functional residues from these regions in staphylocoagulase activity are now under way.

SUMMARY

Bacterial protein, staphylocoagulase, binds stoichiometrically to human prothrombin resulting in a coagulant complex, staphylothrombin. The enzymatic properties of staphylothrombin differ from those of α-thrombin in their substrate specificities toward natural and synthetic substrates, in addition to their interaction with protease inhibitors. In order to obtain information about the region of staphylocoagulase that

TABLE 6. Dissociation Constant of the Complex Formed between Staphylocoagulase or Chymotryptic Fragment and Human Prothrombin (HP)

Interaction	K_d (M)	Stoichiometry
HP + staphylocoagulase	4.6×10^{-10}	1.1
HP + 43-kDa fragment	1.7×10^{-9}	1.2
HP + 30-kDa fragment	1.2×10^{-7}	1.0

interacts with human prothrombin, staphylocoagulase was cleaved by α-chymotrypsin. This limited α-chymotryptic cleavage of staphylocoagulase yielded three large fragments, fragments of 43, 30, and 20 kDa. The 43-kDa fragment exhibited a high affinity for human prothrombin (K_d = 1.7 nM), which is comparable to the affinity observed using intact staphylocoagulase (K_d = 0.46 nM). A complex of the 43-kDa fragment and prothrombin possessed both clotting and amidase activities essentially identical to those observed in a complex of intact staphylocoagulase and prothrombin. The 30-kDa fragment exhibited weaker affinity for prothrombin (K_d = 120 nM). While a complex of this fragment and prothrombin did not exhibit clotting activity, it nonetheless possessed a weak amidase activity. The 20-kDa fragment was found only to bind to prothrombin. The NH_2-terminal sequence analyses of these fragments revealed that the 43-kDa fragment constitutes the NH_2-terminal portion of staphylocoagulase, and contains the 30-kDa and 20-kDa fragments. It is therefore concluded that the functional region of staphylocoagulase for binding and activation of prothrombin is localized in the NH_2-terminal region of the intact protein.

The 43-kDa fragment contains 324 amino acids with a molecular weight of 38,098. The 43-kDa fragment has an unusual amino acid composition based on the sequence, in which the sum of Asp (28 residues), Asn (22), Glu (35), Gln (9), and Lys (52)

```
                                          20                                        40
  1  I V T K D Y S K E S R V N E K S K K G A T V S D Y Y Y W K I I D S L E A Q F T G

                                          60                                        80
 41  A I D L L E N Y K Y G D P I Y K E A K D R L M T R V L G E D Q Y L L K K K I D E

                                          100                                       120
 81  Y E L Y K K W Y K S S N K N T N M L T F H K Y N L Y N L T M N E Y N D I F N S L

                                          140                                       160
121  K D A V Y Q F N K E V K E I E H K N V D L K Q F D K D G E D K A T K E V Y D L V

                                          180                                       200
161  S E I D T L V V T Y Y A D K D Y G E H A K E L R A K L D L I L G D T D N P H K I

                                          220                                       240
201  T N E R I K K E M I D D L N S I I D D F F M E T K Q N R P N S I T K Y D P T K H

                                          260                                       280
241  N F K E K S E N K P N F D K L V E E T K K A V K E A D E S W K N K T V K K Y E E

                                          300                                       320
281  T V T K S P V V K E E K K V E E P Q L P K V G N Q Q E V K T T A G K A E E T T Q

321  P V A L                    Total 324      Mr = 38, 098

     D 28   N 22   T 23   S 14   E 35   Q 9    P 9    G 9    A 14   V 21
     M 5    I 16   L 23   Y 21   F 9    K 52   H 5    W 3    R 6
```

FIGURE 6. Amino acid sequence of the 43-kDa fragment. The 30-kDa and 20-kDa fragments are localized, respectively, in the COOH-terminal regions from Gln-126 to Leu-324 and from Gln-126 to Tyr-278.

residues accounts for more than 45% of the total residues. A comparison of the amino acid sequence of the 43-kDa fragment with that of streptokinase did not reveal any obvious sequence homology. There was also no sequence homology with those of trypsin, α-chymotrypsin, and elastase.

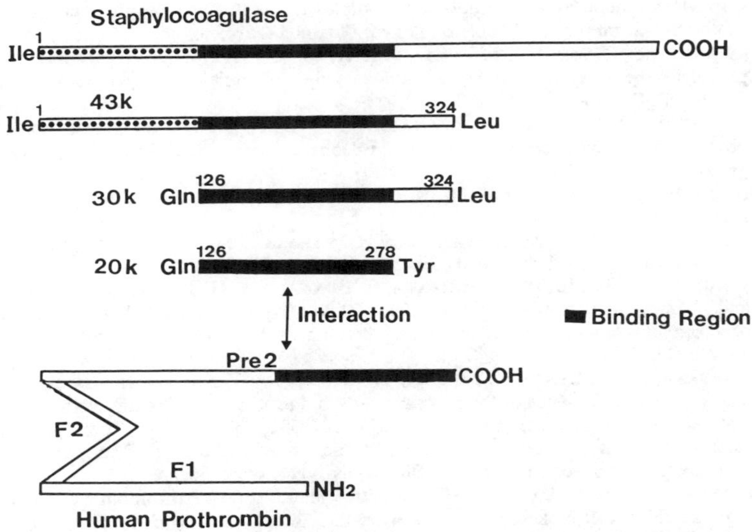

FIGURE 7. Alignments of the fragments of 43, 30, and 20 kDa along the polypeptide chain of staphylocoagulase. Solid area represents the binding region. Dotted area is required for manifestation of the staphylocoagulase activity.

ACKNOWLEDGMENT

We thank Mizumo Akiyoshi for her expert secretarial assistance.

REFERENCES

1. ZAJDEL, M., Z. WEGRZYNOWICZ, J. SAWECKA, J. JELJASZEWICZ & G. PULVERER. 1976. Mechanism of action of staphylocoagulase. *In* Staphylococci and Staphylococcal Disease. J. Jeljaszewicz, Ed.: 546-575. Gustav Fischer Verlag. Stuttgart, FRG.
2. ZAJDEL, M., Z. WEGRZYNOWICZ, J. JELJASZEWICZ & G. PULVERER. 1973. Mechanism of action of staphylocoagulase and clumping factor. *In* Staphylococci and Staphylococcal Infections. J. Jeljaszewicz, Ed.: 364-375. S. Karger. Basel, Switzerland.
3. TAGER, M. & M. C. DRUMMOND. 1965. Staphylocoagulase. Ann N.Y. Acad. Sci. **128:** 92-111.
4. SOULIER, J. P., O. PROÙ & L. HALLÉ. 1970. Further studies on thrombin-coagulase. Thromb. Diath. Haemorrh. (Stuttgart) **23:** 37-49.

5. HEMKER, H. C., B. M. BAS & A. D. MULLER. 1975. Activation of a proenzyme by a stoichiometric reaction with another protein. The reaction between prothrombin and staphylocoagulase. Biochim. Biophys. Acta **379:** 180-188.
6. HENDRIX, H., T. LINDHOUT, K. MERTENS, W. ENGELS & H. C. HEMKER. 1983. Activation of human prothrombin by stoichiometric levels of staphylocoagulase. J. Biol. Chem. **258:** 3637-3644.
7. KAWABATA, S., T. MORITA, S. IWANAGA & H. IGARASHI. 1985. Enzymatic properties of staphylothrombin, an active molecular complex formed between staphylocoagulase and human prothrombin. J. Biochem. (Tokyo) **98:** 1603-1614.
8. KAWABATA, S., T. MORITA, S. IWANAGA & H. IGARASHI. 1985. Difference in enzymatic properties between α-thrombin-staphylocoagulase complex and free α-thrombin. J. Biochem. (Tokyo) **97:** 1073-1078.
9. IGARASHI, H., T. MORITA & S. IWANAGA. 1979. A new method for purification of staphylocoagulase by a bovine prothrombin-Sepharose column. J. Biochem. (Tokyo) **86:** 1615-1618.
10. MORITA, T., H. IGARASHI & S. IWANAGA. 1981. Staphylocoagulase. Methods Enzymol. **80:** 311-319.
11. KAWABATA, S., T. MORITA, S. IWANAGA & H. IGARASHI. 1985. Staphylocoagulase-binding region in human prothrombin. J. Biochem. (Tokyo) **97:** 325-331.
12. KAWABATA, S., T. MORITA, T. MIYATA, S. IWANAGA & H. IGARASHI. 1986. Isolation and characterization of staphylocoagulase chymotryptic fragment. Localization of the procoagulant- and prothrombin-binding domain of this protein. J. Biol. Chem. **261:** 1427-1433.
13. KAWABATA, S., T. MIYATA, T. MORITA, T. MIYATA, S. IWANAGA & H. IGARASHI. 1986. The amino acid sequence of the procoagulant- and prothrombin-binding domain isolated from staphylocoagulase. J. Biol. Chem. **261:** 527-531.
14. JACKSON, K. W. & J. TANG. 1982. Complete amino acid sequence of streptokinase and its homology with serine proteases. Biochemistry **21:** 6620-6625.
15. KETTNER, C. & E. SHAW. 1977. The selective inactivation of thrombin by peptides of arginine chloromethyl ketone. *In* Chemistry and Biology of Thrombin. R. L. Lundbald, J. W. Fenton II, and K. G. Mann, Eds.: 129-143. Ann Arbor Science Publishers Inc. Ann Arbor, Mich.
16. KETTNER, C. & E. SHAW. 1979. D-Phe-Pro-Arg-CH_2Cl—a selective affinity label for thrombin. Thromb. Res. **14:** 969-973.
17. WALKER, B., P. WIKSTROM & E. SHAW. 1985. Evaluation of inhibitor constants and alkylation rates for a series of thrombin affinity labels. Biochem. J. **230:** 645-650.

Mechanisms for Inhibition of the Generation of Thrombin Activity by Sulfated Polysaccharides[a]

F. A. OFOSU, G. J. MODI, J. HIRSH,
M. R. BUCHANAN, AND M. A. BLAJCHMAN

The Canadian Red Cross Society
Blood Transfusion Service
Hamilton, Ontario, Canada
and
Departments of Pathology and Medicine
McMaster University
Hamilton, Ontario, Canada L8N 3Z5

INTRODUCTION

The catalytic action of standard heparin on the antiprotease action of antithrombin III is considered to be the predominant mechanism for its anticoagulant and antithrombotic activities.[1] Heparin has been shown to accelerate the inhibition of several serine proteases of coagulation by antithrombin III.[1–6] Whereas it is possible to estimate the efficiency of heparin in catalyzing protease inhibition by antithrombin III with purified protease-antithrombin III systems,[2–6] the protease-antithrombin III inhibition system most sensitive to catalysis by heparin during plasma coagulation is unknown. Published methods for estimating the relative efficiency of heparin as a catalyst of antithrombin III-mediated inhibition of activated clotting factors utilize conditions that are significantly different from those that obtain during blood coagulation.[2–6] Some reports suggest that the application of results obtained with purified systems may not reflect coagulation in plasma.[7–9]

In recent studies, we found that the inhibition of factor Xa by antithrombin III, even when catalyzed by the octasaccharide fragment of heparin with high affinity to antithrombin III, which has high antifactor Xa activity, was very ineffective in inhibiting the generation of thrombin activity in plasma.[8] By contrast, dermatan sulfate, which only catalyzes thrombin inhibition by heparin cofactor II, was more effective than the octasaccharide fragment of heparin in inhibiting the generation of thrombin activity.[8] The poor effect of the octasaccharide on inhibiting the generation of thrombin activity may be related to the protection afforded factor Xa from inhibition by antithrombin III-heparin when factor Xa is associated with coagulant surfaces.[7,9–12] In addition, it has been demonstrated that relatively little factor Xa (approximately 1

[a] This work was supported in part by Grants-in-Aid from the Stroke and Heart Foundation of Ontario and the Medical Research Council of Canada.

nM) is required for optimal activation of prothrombin and thus the generation of thrombin activity in plasma.[7,8] The concentration of factor Xa generated when factor X is activated by the intrinsic pathway in plasma containing standard heparin and other sulfated polysaccharides exceeds this figure.[8] Support for the concept that catalysis of factor Xa inhibition *per se* was not the activity responsible for the anticoagulant and antithrombotic activities of sulfated polysaccharides has been obtained both *in vitro* and *in vivo*.[8,13–15] Several recent studies show that the catalytic effect of heparin and other sulfated polysaccharides on thrombin inhibition, rather than factor Xa inhibition, is critical to the expression of their anticoagulant and optimal antithrombotic effects.[8,13–16]

There are four possible mechanisms by which inhibition of the generation of thrombin activity can be achieved by sulfated polysaccharides: (1) catalysis of thrombin inhibition by antithrombin III; (2) catalysis of thrombin inhibition by heparin cofactor II; (3) inhibition of either the formation or the activity of prothrombinase complex (*i.e.* direct inhibition of prothrombin activation); and (4) inhibition of the generation of factor Xa activity. Inhibition of the generation factor Xa is unlikely to be important, as it has been shown that sulfated polysaccharides that catalyze factor Xa inhibition, but do not catalyze thrombin inhibition, are not effective inhibitors of the generation of thrombin activity in plasma.[8,13] Such sulfated polysaccharides are also relatively weak antithrombotic agents.[8,13,14,16]

Currently available techniques for estimating anticoagulant effects of sulfated polysaccharides do not permit the delineation of the relative contributions of the first three mechanisms to the inhibition of the generation of thrombin activity. We have designed experiments to assess the contributions of each of the first three mechanisms listed above to the anticoagulant activities of four sulfated polysaccharides. Prothrombin activation was measured after adding [^{125}I]prothrombin to human plasma and initiating coagulation by either the intrinsic or extrinsic pathway. Heparin cofactor activities of the sulfated polysaccharides were determined by estimating enhanced formation of [^{125}I]thrombin complexes with antithrombin III and/or heparin cofactor II. As used here, heparin cofactor activity is defined as the ability of a sulfated polysaccharide to catalyze thrombin inhibition by plasma. D-Phe-L-Pro-L-ArgCH_2Cl (PPACK), a fast and specific chloromethyl ketone inhibitor of thrombin,[17] was added to the plasma in some experiments in order to estimate antithrombin III-independent and heparin cofactor II-independent effects of sulfated polysaccharides on prothrombin activation. The expectation was that PPACK would inhibit the formation of thrombin-antithrombin III and thrombin-heparin cofactor II complexes but not inhibit prothrombin activation in normal plasma. Unexpectedly, PPACK completely inhibited prothrombin activation. This inhibition was reversed by adding thrombin to the plasma prior to the addition of PPACK, suggesting a critical role of trace amounts of thrombin in efficient prothrombin activation in plasma. These observations led us to perform studies to delineate the relative inhibitory effects of various sulfated polysaccharides on the heparin cofactor-dependent and heparin cofactor-independent mechanisms for inhibiting the generation of thrombin activity.

MATERIAL AND METHODS

Material

Human α-thrombin was a generous gift from Dr. John Fenton II, New York Department of Health, Albany, NY. Porcine skin dermatan sulfate (Lot number 64F-

0413) was obtained from Sigma Chemical Co., St. Louis, MO. Heparan sulfate from bovine kidney, (Chondroitinase ABC-treated, lot number S 8402) was obtained from Miles Laboratory, Toronto, Ontario. Porcine mucosal heparin, (specific activity: 145 USP units/mg) was obtained from Diosynth BV, Oss, The Netherlands. Pentosan polysulfate was a gift of Bene-Chemie, Munich, Federal Republic of Germany. Automated partial thromboplastin time reagent was obtained from General Diagnostics, Toronto, Ontario. D-Phe-L-Pro-L-ArgCH_2Cl (PPACK) and dansyl-L-Glu-Gly-L-Arg-CH_2Cl were obtained from Behring-Calbiochem, San Diego, CA. Tissue thromboplastin from human brain was obtained from the National Reference Laboratory, Manchester, England. Human prothrombin was isolated from factor IX concentrates[18] and iodinated by the modified chloramine-T method to a specific activity of 1.0×10^6 dpm/μg.[19]

Methods

Effects of Sulfated Polysaccharides on Prothrombin Activation by the Intrinsic Pathway

Pooled human plasma, anticoagulated with citrate, was prepared as previously described.[7,8] The intrinsic activation of prothrombin in this plasma and the effects of each of the four sulfated polysaccharides on prothrombin activation were performed by modification of procedures previously described for the generation of thrombin activity in plasma.[7,8] In these experiments, the plasma also contained 1-2 μg of [^{125}I]human prothrombin/mL of plasma. The intrinsic activation of prothrombin was terminated by subsampling a 1 volume aliquot of the thrombin generating system into 4 volumes of a 5 mM EDTA buffer.[7,8] In addition to EDTA, the buffer also contained 0.05 M Tris-HCl, 0.15 M NaCl, 1.0×10^{-6} M PPACK, and 1.0×10^{-6} M dansyl-L-Glu-Gly-L-ArgCH_2Cl, pH 7.4. This buffer served to inactivate any free thrombin and factor Xa generated in the plasma. An aliquot of the above mixture was then subjected to SDS-polyacrylamide gel electrophoresis and subsequent autoradiography.[19,20]

In some experiments, human α-thrombin (1.0 NIH units/mL final concentration) was added to the plasma 2 min after the initiation of contact activation, to activate factor VIII and factor V. One min later, the calcium chloride and PPACK (1.0×10^{-6} M final concentration) were added simultaneously to initiate prothrombin activation. In other experiments, the PPACK was added to the plasma for 1 min during contact activation to ensure that no thrombin activity was generated. When added with $CaCl_2$, the final concentration of each sulfated polysaccharide used were one of 0.66, 6.6, or 66.0 μg/mL of plasma. When added with PPACK and $CaCl_2$, the final concentrations of each sulfated polysaccharide used were also 0.66, 6.6, or 66.0 μg/mL. This last set of experimental conditions estimated the heparin-cofactor-independent effects of each sulfated polysaccharide, as no complexes of thrombin with plasma inhibitors were detectable in plasma containing 1.0×10^{-6} M PPACK.

Effect of Sulfated Polysaccharides on Extrinsic Prothrombin Activation

Previously described procedures for quantitating prothrombin activation in plasma initiated by the extrinsic pathway were used to estimate the effects of each of the four sulfated polysaccharides on extrinsic prothrombin activation.[7] The plasma also contained [^{125}I]prothrombin, however, and the activation of prothrombin was terminated as described above. The effects of PPACK on extrinsic prothrombin activation, both in the presence or absence of a sulfated polysaccharide were also determined.

RESULTS

Effect of PPACK on Intrinsic and Extrinsic Prothrombin Activation

The effects of the presence of PPACK on prothrombin activation, initiated by either the intrinsic or extrinsic pathway, are summarized in FIGURE 1. There was no activation of prothrombin, as measured by the formation of prothrombin $F_1 \cdot F_2$, when PPACK was added simultaneously with calcium chloride to plasma. The inhibitory effects of PPACK were completely reversed when thrombin was added to the plasma for 1 min during contact activation, and before PPACK and calcium chloride were added (see below). These results demonstrate the importance of trace amounts of thrombin for the efficient activation of prothrombin by both pathways.

Effects of Sulfated Polysaccharides on Intrinsic Activation of Prothrombin

In preliminary experiments in which thrombin generation was quantitated over 10 min, recalcification of contact-activated plasma resulted in the cleavage of [^{125}I]prothrombin to [^{125}I]thrombin and [^{125}I]prothrombin F_1;$\cdot F_2$. The thrombin, in turn, formed complexes with antithrombin III, heparin cofactor II, and α_2-macroglobulin. Maximum cleavage of prothrombin, with minimum inhibition of the thrombin formed by the above inhibitors, was observed 1 min after recalcification in the absence of a sulfated polysaccharide. Longer incubations after recalcification resulted in greater inhibition of the thrombin.

The effects of the four sulfated polysaccharides on the formation of thrombin, prothrombin $F_1 \cdot F_2$, and complexes of thrombin with its inhibitors in plasma containing one of the four sulfated polysaccharides are shown in FIGURES 2A-2D. The data in FIGURE 2 are those obtained 1 min after recalcification. At this time, greater than 95% of the prothrombin in the control plasma had been cleaved to thrombin and prothrombin $F_1 \cdot F_2$ (lane 2, FIGURES 2A-2D). In plasma containing heparin, the lowest concentrations of heparin completely prevented the activation of prothrombin. Higher concentrations of heparin had no additional effect (FIGURE 2A). Prothrombin activation proceeded normally in plasma containing heparan sulfate (FIGURE 2B). Some of the thrombin formed was inactivated predominantly by antithrombin III. Formation of the thrombin-antithrombin III complex was thus accelerated by heparan sulfate (FIGURE 2B).

Dermatan sulfate enhanced the formation of thrombin-heparin cofactor II complex (FIGURE 2C). In contrast to heparan sulfate, the highest concentration of dermatan sulfate also resulted in the inhibition of prothrombin activation (lane 5, FIGURE 2C). Pentosan polysulfate also appeared to inhibit the intrinsic generation of thrombin activity by the two mechanisms described for dermatan sulfate. The lowest concentration (0.66 μg/mL of plasma) catalyzed the formation of thrombin-heparin cofactor II (FIGURE 2D). No activation of prothrombin could be demonstrated with higher concentrations of pentosan polysulfate (FIGURE 2D).

Effects of Sulfated Polysaccharides on Prothrombin Activation in Plasma Containing Factor VIIIa and Factor Va

The intrinsic activation of prothrombin was also determined in plasma containing factor Va and factor VIIIa, in order to assess the role of the catalysis of thrombin

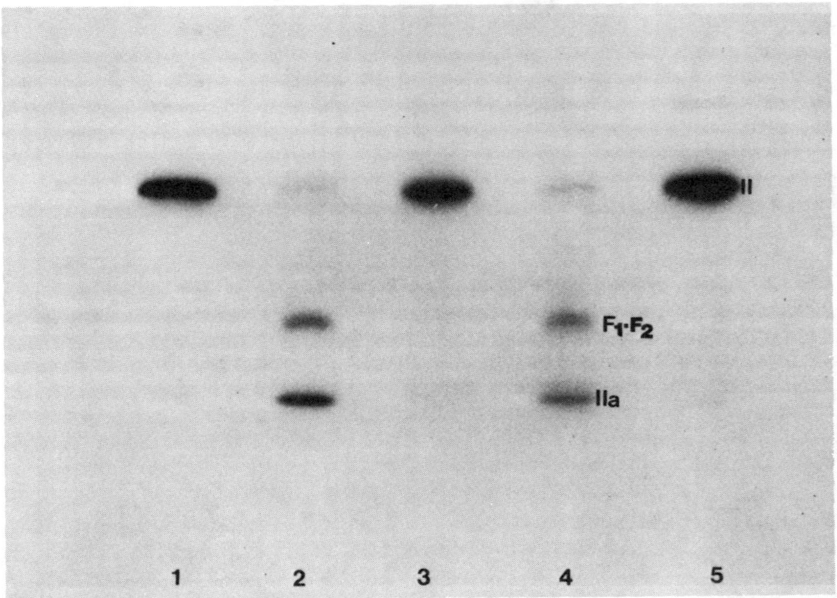

FIGURE 1. The effect of PPACK on the activation of [^{125}I]prothrombin in undiluted human plasma. Prothrombin activation was initiated by either the intrinsic or extrinsic pathway. Lane 1, nonactivated control plasma; lane 2, prothrombin activated by the intrinsic pathway; lane 3, intrinsic activation of prothrombin in plasma containing 1.0×10^{-6} M PPACK; lane 4, prothrombin activated by extrinsic pathway; lane 5, extrinsic pathway activation of prothrombin in plasma containing 1.0×10^{-6} M PPACK. Abbreviations used in FIGURE: $F_1 \cdot F_2$, [^{125}I]prothrombin fragment 1.2; IIa, [^{125}I]thrombin; II, [^{125}I]prothrombin.

inhibition (*i.e.* the heparin cofactor-dependent effects) to the expression of the anticoagulant effects of the four sulfated polysaccharides. As shown in FIGURE 1, the fast and specific inhibitor of thrombin, PPACK, completely inhibited intrinsic and extrinsic prothrombin activation. In the next series of experiments, factor V and factor VIII were activated in the plasma by adding thrombin 2 min after the initiation of contact activation. PPACK and $CaCl_2$ were then added simultaneously 1 min later to the plasma.

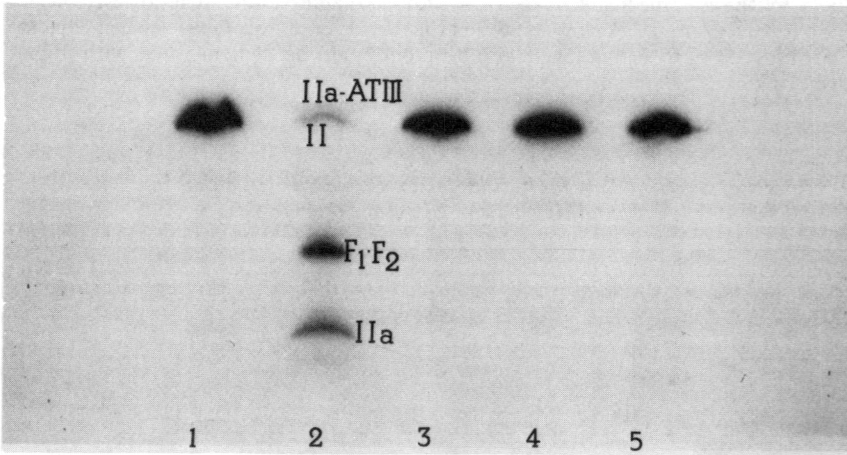

A

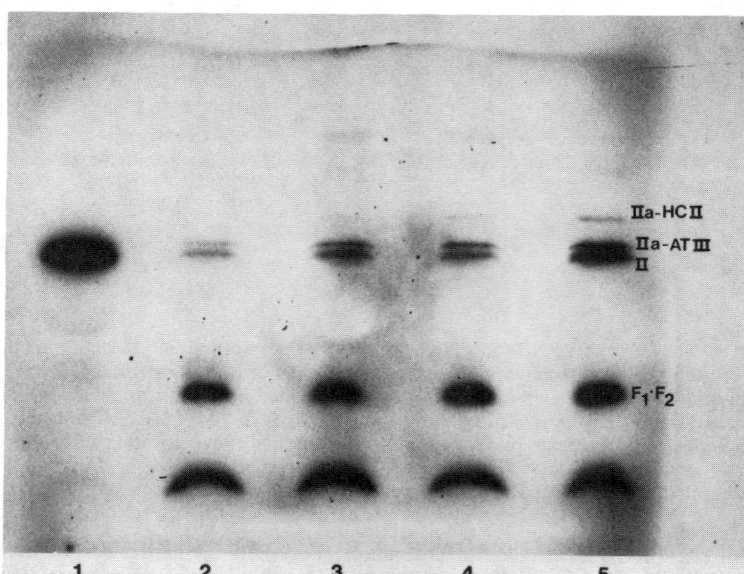

B

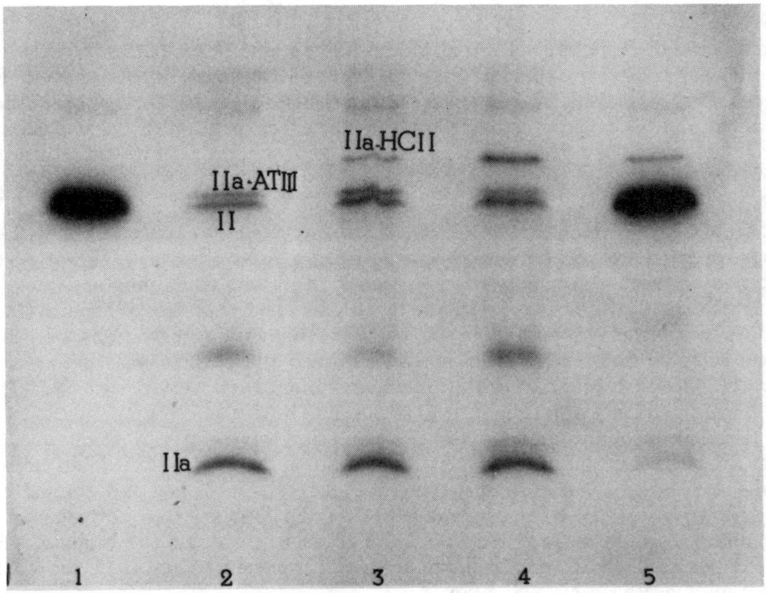

C

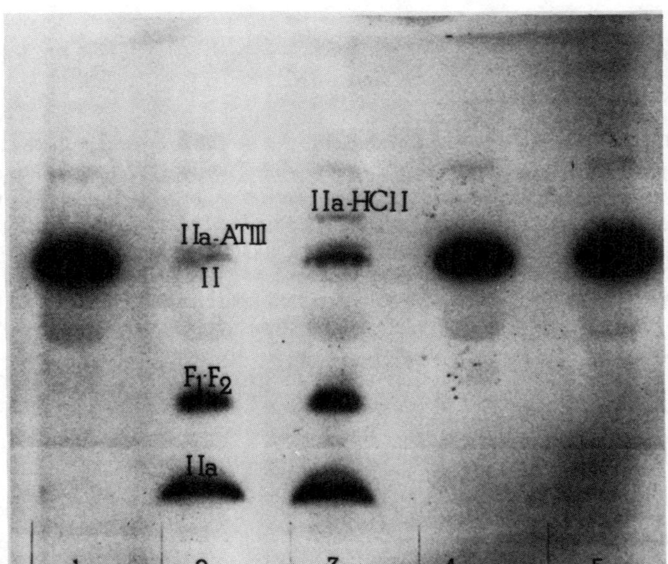

D

FIGURE 2. Effects of heparin (**A**), heparan sulfate (**B**), dermatan sulfate (**C**), or pentosan polysulfate (**D**) on intrinsic pathway activation of [^{125}I]prothrombin in plasma. Lane 1, unactivated plasma; lane 2, contact-activated plasma; lane 3-5, contact-activated plasma containing 0.66, 6.6, and 66 μg of sulfated polysaccharide/mL of plasma. Abbreviations used: IIa-ATIII, [^{125}I]thrombin-antithrombin III complex; IIa-HCII, [^{125}I]thrombin-heparin cofactor II complex; II, [^{125}I]prothrombin.

When PPACK was added simultaneously with $CaCl_2$ to the contact-activated plasma containing factor VIIIa and factor Va, no complexes of thrombin with antithrombin III, heparin cofactor II, or α_2-macroglobulin could be detected in the plasma. The conditions, therefore, made it possible to assess the heparin cofactor-dependent and the heparin cofactor-independent effects of sulfated polysaccharides in normal plasma. The effects of heparin and pentosan polysulfate on prothrombin activation under these conditions are summarized in FIGURE 3.

When thrombin was added to the plasma prior to heparin and calcium chloride to activate factor VIII and factor V, the complete inhibition caused by 0.66 μg/mL of heparin in plasma containing unactivated factor V and factor VIII was reversed. Inhibition of prothrombin activation, however, in plasma containing activated factor VIII and factor V was observed with the two higher concentrations of heparin (FIGURE 3A). As was observed with heparin, only the higher concentrations of pentosan polysulfate inhibited prothrombin activation when the plasma was pretreated with thrombin. More inhibition of prothrombin activation was observed with 66.0 μg than with 6.6 μg pentosan polysulfate/mL of plasma (FIGURE 3B).

The addition of thrombin to the plasma, prior to recalcification, eliminated the ability of dermatan sulfate and heparan sulfate to inhibit prothrombin activation (results not shown). These results, therefore, suggest that a key and common characteristic aspect of the anticoagulant action of the four sulfated polysaccharides is their ability to catalyze thrombin inhibition. If efficient enough, the catalytic effect of sulfated polysaccharides on thrombin inhibition appears to result in the complete inhibition of prothrombin activation.

Effects of Sulfated Polysaccharides on the Extrinsic Pathway of Prothrombin Activation

The effects of the four sulfated polysaccharides on the extrinsic pathway activation of prothrombin are summarized in FIGURE 4A-4D. The data shown are those obtained 30 sec after recalcification, as maximum activation of prothrombin, with minimum inhibition of the thrombin formed, was obtained 30 sec after recalcification. Heparin was the most efficient of the four sulfated polysaccharides in inhibiting prothrombin activation by the extrinsic pathway. In contrast to the intrinsic pathway, complete inhibition of extrinsic prothrombin activation by heparin was demonstrable only with 6.6 and 66.0 μg of heparin/mL of plasma. The lowest concentration of heparin, which completely inhibited prothrombin activation by the intrinsic pathway, did not inhibit extrinsic prothrombin activation but appeared to catalyze the inactivation of the thrombin formed by antithrombin III (FIGURE 4A). The other three sulfated polysaccharides, with the exception of the highest concentration of pentosan polysulfate, did not inhibit prothrombin activation, but catalyzed the inhibition of the thrombin generated. Heparan sulfate primarily catalyzed the formation of thrombin-antithrombin III complex (FIGURE 4B), whereas dermatan sulfate and pentosan polysulfate catalyzed the formation of thrombin-heparin cofactor II complex (FIGURES 4C and D).

DISCUSSION

The anticoagulant effect of heparin has been attributed to its ability to accelerate the inhibition, by antithrombin III, of a variety of serine proteases of blood coagu-

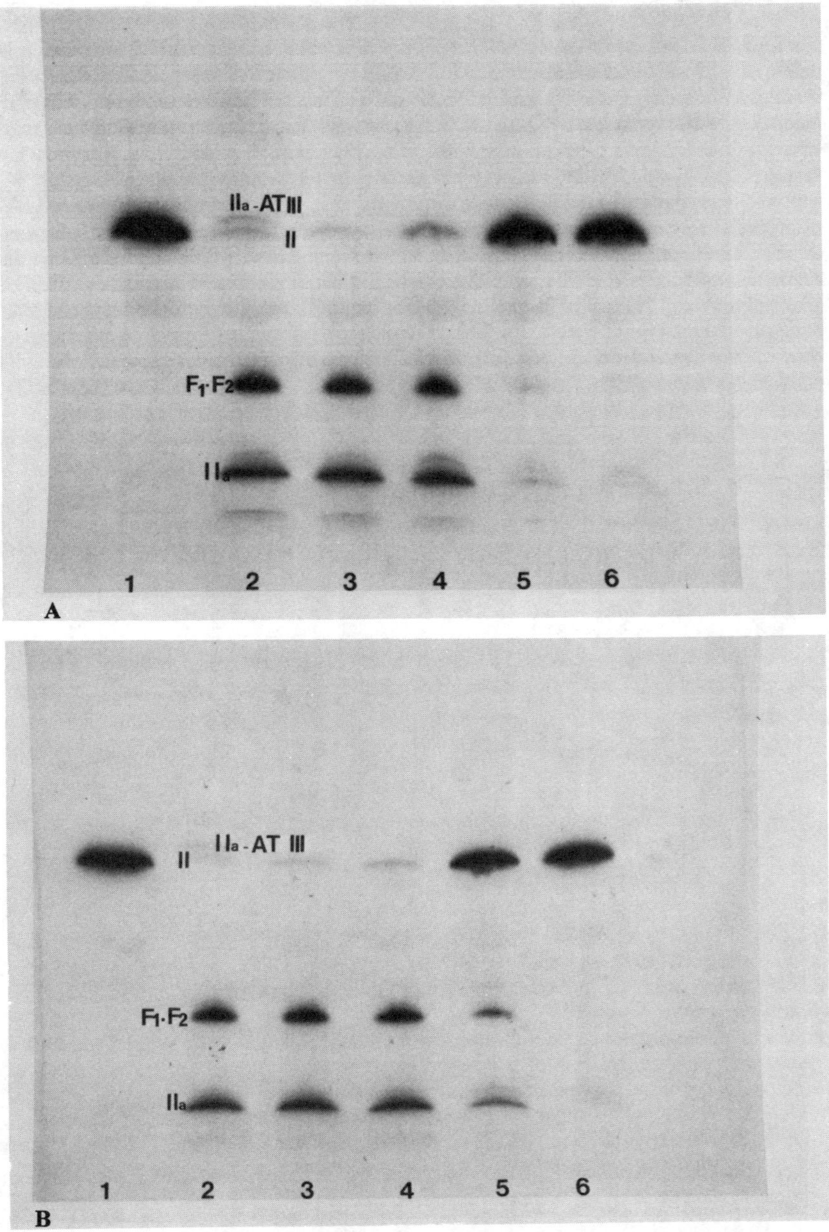

FIGURE 3. Effects of heparin (**A**) and pentosan polysulfate (**B**) on intrinsic pathway activation of plasma containing factor VIIIa and factor Va. Factor VIIIa and factor Va were generated *in situ* by the addition of thrombin to the plasma during contact activation. PPACK, sulphated polysaccharide, and $CaCl_2$ were then added simultaneously 1 min after thrombin addition to initiate prothrombin activation. Lane 1, unactivated plasma; lane 2, contact-activated plasma; lane 3, contact-activated plasma + PPACK; lanes 4-6, contact-activated plasma + PPACK and sulfated polysaccharide of 0.66, 6.6, and 66.0 μg/mL of plasma.

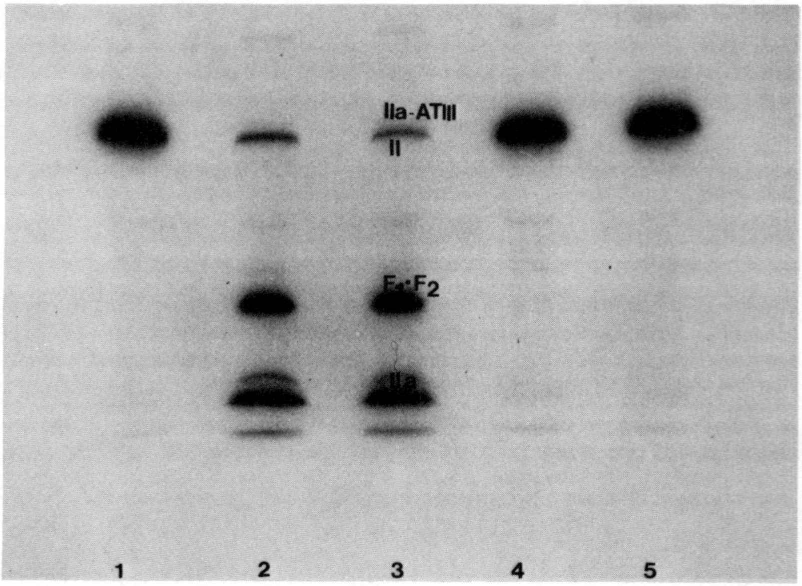
IIa-ATIII
II
F1·F2
IIa
1
2
3
4
5

A

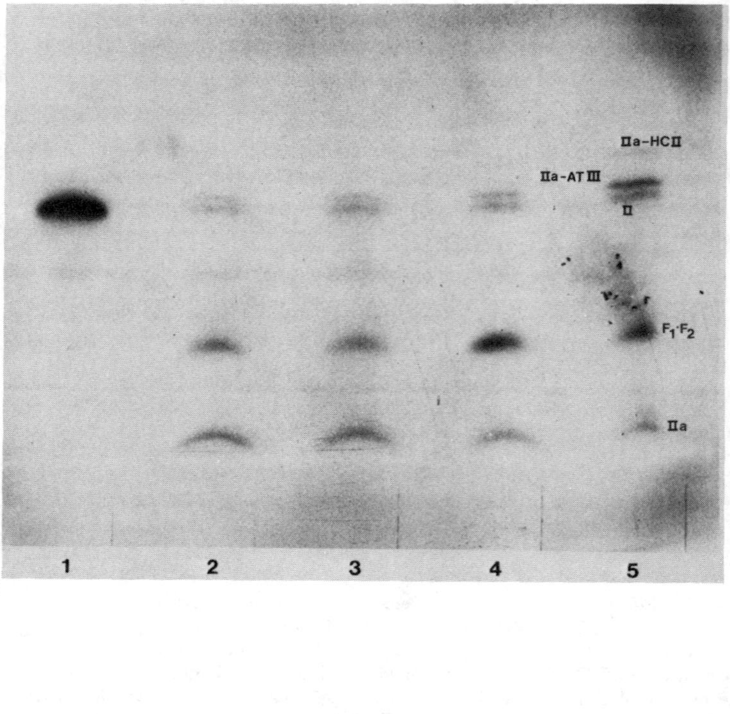
IIa-HCII
IIa-AT III
II
F1·F2
IIa
1
2
3
4
5

B

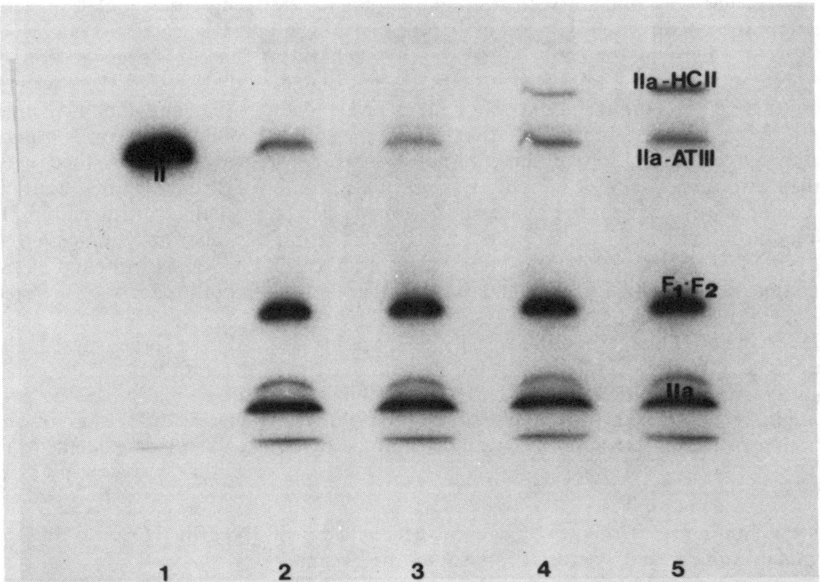

C

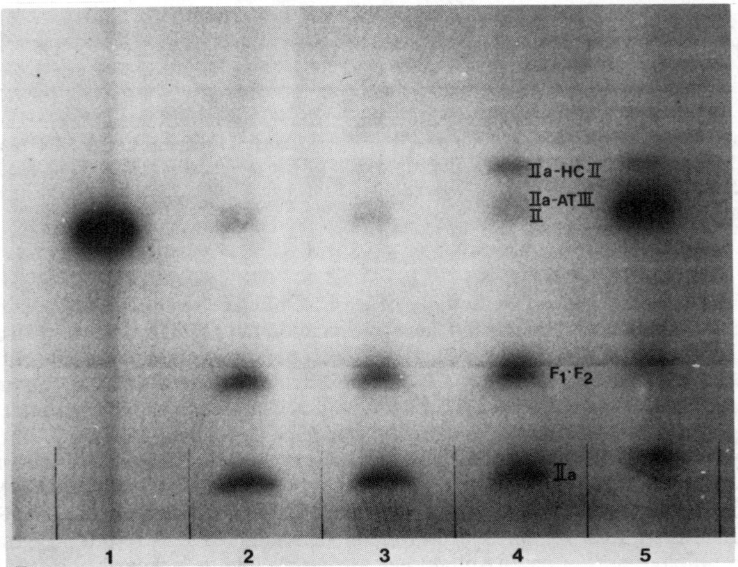

D

FIGURE 4. Effects of heparin (**A**), heparan sulfate (**B**), dermatan sulfate (**C**), and pentosan polysulfate (**D**) on extrinsic pathway activation of [^{125}I]prothrombin in pooled human plasma. Lane 1, unactivated plasma; lane 2, activated plasma with no sulfated polysaccharides; lane 3-5, activated plasma containing 0.66, 6.6, and 66.0 μg of sulfated polysaccharides/mL of plasma.

lation.[1–6] It has been difficult with routine methods for assessing anticoagulant effects, to determine relative sensitivities of various antithrombin III-protease systems to catalysis, by heparin (or other sulfated polysaccharides) during the generation of thrombin activity in plasma. Recent experiments that directly assessed the catalytic effects of heparin on the inhibition of factor XIIa, factor XIa, and factor IXa by antithrombin III indicate that, relative to factor Xa and thrombin, heparin is a poor catalyst for the inhibition of these three enzymes.[21–23] Kinetic data obtained with purified thrombin, factor Xa, factor IXa and antithrombin III, and optimal concentrations of a well characterized heparin fragment, also suggest that antithrombin III inhibits thrombin best.[2] Furthermore, recent reports from our laboratory indicate that catalysis of thrombin inhibition, rather than that of factor Xa, is critical for the expression of the anticoagulant and possibly the antithrombotic effects of sulfated polysaccharides.[8,13]

Heparin can inhibit thrombin activity or thrombin formation in three ways: 1) the catalysis of thrombin inhibition by antithrombin III; 2) the catalysis of thrombin inhibition by heparin cofactor II; and 3) the inhibition of the formation of the prothrombinase complex or the expression of its activity. Whereas inhibition of the formation of the prothrombinase complex may be heparin cofactor-dependent, inhibition of the expression of the activity of prothrombinase complex may occur independently of antithrombin III and heparin cofactor II.[24,25] The present experiments indicate that the four sulfated polysaccharides operate to inhibit the generation of thrombin activity by one or more of these mechanisms. These mechanisms and the relative effectiveness of the four sulfated polysaccharides in acting to inhibit the generation of thrombin activity by these mechanisms are summarized in TABLE 1.

TABLE 1. Summary of the Anticoagulant Mechanisms of Heparin, Heparan Sulfate, Dermatan Sulfate, and Pentosan Polysulfate in Plasma.[a]

Sulfated Polysaccharide	Mechanism I	Mechanism II	Mechanism III
Heparin	1	3	1
Heparan Sulfate	3	5	5
Dermatan Sulfate	5	3	5
Pentosan Polysulfate	4	2	2

[a] Mechanism I represents catalysis of thrombin inhibition by antithrombin III; mechanism II represents catalysis of thrombin inhibition by heparin cofactor II; mechanism III represents direct inhibition of the formation or the expression of the activities of prothrombinase and/or tenase complexes. The numerical indices used are 1 through 5, where 1 indicates strong activity and 5 indicates weak activity.

Heparan sulfate catalyzes the formation of the thrombin-antithrombin III complex but does not significantly inhibit prothrombin activation. Dermatan sulfate catalyzes the formation of the thrombin-heparin cofactor II complex. At the highest dose used, dermatan sulfate also inhibited prothrombin activation. These results suggest that heparan sulfate and dermatan sulfate act as anticoagulants primarily by catalyzing antithrombin III and heparin cofactor II respectively, as has been postulated previously.[20] This was confirmed in experiments in which thrombin was added to the plasma prior to the addition of either heparan sulfate or dermatan sulfate. No inhibition of prothrombin activation was observed under these conditions, suggesting that these two agents did not directly inhibit the expression of the activity of the prothrombinase complex. Similarly, we have previously reported that heparan sulfate and dermatan sulfate fail to inhibit prothrombin activation in plasma immunologically depleted of both antithrombin III and heparin cofactor II.[26]

The specific thrombin inhibitor, PPACK, completely inhibited prothrombin activation by both the intrinsic and extrinsic pathways. The inhibition of prothrombin activation by PPACK thus indicates that the presence of trace quantities of thrombin is essential for efficient activation of prothrombin by both pathways. This has previously been suggested by other investigators.[27–30] The reversal of the inhibitory effect of PPACK by the addition of thrombin, prior to the addition of PPACK, indicates that the activation of factor V and factor VIII by thrombin are necessary for the efficient formation of the prothrombinase complex.

All three concentrations of heparin completely inhibited the intrinsic activation of prothrombin. The inhibition of prothrombin activation by heparin was only partially reversed when thrombin was added to plasma before heparin. If catalysis of inhibition of thrombin was the only effect of heparin, then preactivation of plasma factor VIII and factor V by thrombin addition would completely reverse the inhibition of prothrombin activation by heparin, as was the case with PPACK. The failure to reverse the inhibitory effect of heparin suggests that heparin also inhibits prothrombin activation by additional mechanisms. Heparin appears to directly inhibit either the formation, or the expression of the enzymatic activity of the prothrombinase complex. Similar effects were observed with pentosan polysulfate.

Heparin and pentosan polysulfate thus appear to directly inhibit prothrombin activation by a number of mechanisms. They catalyze the inhibition of the initial trace amounts of thrombin formed by antithrombin III (heparin) or heparin cofactor II (pentosan polysulfate), and so inhibit the formation of the prothrombinase complex by reducing factor V activation by thrombin. Heparin and pentosan polysulphate have an additional effect on prothrombin activation, which is demonstrable in plasma containing factor Va and factor VIIIa. This effect results in the direct inhibition of prothrombin activation. The direct inhibition of prothrombin activation occurs by the inhibition of the formation of the prothrombinase complex or inhibition of the expression of the catalytic activity of the prothrombinase complex. These effects, demonstrable with higher concentrations of heparin and pentosan polysulfate, result from the disruption of the interactions of the constituents of the prothrombinase complex, as well as prothrombin, with coagulant surfaces.[24,25]

The present studies indicate that inhibition of the formation, or the catalytic activity of the prothrombinase complex, is the primary mechanism by which sulfated polysaccharides act as anticoagulants. These studies also indicate that the presence of thrombin activity is critical for efficient prothrombin activation. Thus, the efficient catalysis of the formation of thrombin-inhibitor complexes by sulfated polysaccharides reduces the rate of assembly of the prothrombinase complex and results in the inhibition of prothrombin activation.

SUMMARY

Three mechanisms by which sulfated polysaccharides act as anticoagulants and possibly as antithrombotic agents have been described. These are the two heparin cofactor-dependent mechanisms involving the catalysis of the inhibition of various proteases of coagulation by either antithrombin III or heparin cofactor II. The third is a heparin cofactor-independent mechanism involving the inhibition of formation of prothrombinase and tenase complexes. Four sulfated polysaccharides previously shown to have anticoagulant and antithrombotic effects were assessed to determine which of the three mechanisms operate in the expression of their anticoagulant effects. To do this, [^{125}I]prothrombin was added to undiluted human plasma, and the inhibition of [^{125}I]prothrombin activation, or the catalysis of the formation of thrombin-inhibitor complexes was determined in plasma containing one of the four sulfated polysaccharides. Prothrombin activation was demonstrated by the formation of [^{125}I]prothrombin fragment 1.2 and [^{125}I]thrombin. The effect of the thrombin-specific inhibitor, D-Phe-L-Pro-L-ArgCH$_2$Cl (PPACK), on prothrombin activation was also investigated to determine the role of thrombin-dependent feedback reactions on efficient prothrombin activation. Use of PPACK with sulfated polysaccharides also facilitated estimation of the role of the heparin cofactor-independent effects of sulfated polysaccharides on prothrombin activation. Three concentrations of each of the sulfated polysaccharides were used: 0.66, 6.6, and 66 μg/ml of plasma.

PPACK (1.0×10^{-6}M) completely inhibited both intrinsic and extrinsic prothrombin activation. The inhibition of prothrombin activation caused by PPACK was abolished when thrombin was added to the plasma before PPACK. These observations indicate that the presence of trace thrombin activity is critical for efficient prothrombin activation by both the intrinsic and extrinsic pathways.

All three concentrations of standard heparin completely inhibited the intrinsic activation of prothrombin. This inhibition was only partially abolished when thrombin was added to the plasma before heparin, indicating that heparin inhibits prothrombin activation both by catalyzing the inhibition of thrombin activity and by a heparin cofactor-independent mechanism. Heparan sulfate did not inhibit intrinsic prothrombin activation but catalyzed the inhibition of the thrombin generated by the formation of thrombin-antithrombin III complex. Dermatan sulfate inhibited intrinsic prothrombin activation only at the highest concentration. At the two lower concentrations, dermatan sulfate catalyzed formation of thrombin-heparin cofactor II. Pentosan polysulfate completely inhibited intrinsic prothrombin activation, whereas the lowest concentration only catalyzed the formation of thrombin-heparin cofactor II. Pretreatment of the plasma with thrombin partially abolished the inhibition obtained with pentosan polysulfate and completely abolished inhibition by heparan sulfate and dermatan sulfate. These observations indicate that heparan sulfate and dermatan sulfate primarily catalyzed thrombin inhibition, whereas pentosan polysulfate, like heparin, also inhibited prothrombin activation. The four sulfated polysaccharides had similar effects on the extrinsic activation of prothrombin except that the extrinsic pathway generation of thrombin was less sensitive to the effects of these sulfated polysaccharides. The presence of thrombin activity is thus critical for the efficient activation of prothrombin by both the intrinsic and extrinsic pathways. Furthermore, efficient catalysis of the formation of thrombin-inhibitor complexes by sulfated polysaccharides, which results in the inhibition of thrombin activity, reduces the rate of assembly of the prothrombinase complex and thus results in the inhibition of prothrombin activation.

REFERENCES

1. ROSENBERG, R. D. 1982. Heparin-Antithrombin System. *In* Hemostasis and Thrombosis. Basic Principles and Clinical Practice. R. W. Colman, J. Hirsh, V. J. Marder & E. W. Salzman, Eds.: 962-985. J. B. Lippincott Co. Philadelphia and Toronto.

2. JORDAN, R. E., G. M. OOSTA, W. T. GARDNER & R. D. ROSENBERG. 1980. J. Biol. Chem. **255:** 10081-10090.
3. CERSKUS, A. L., K. J. BIRCHALL, F. A. OFOSU, M. A. BLAJCHMAN & J. HIRSH. 1984. Can. J. Biochem. Cell Biol. **62:** 975-983.
4. ROSENBERG, J. S., P. MCKENNA & R. D. ROSENBERG. 1975. J. Biol. Chem **250:** 883-888.
5. STEAD, N., A. P. KAPLAN & R. D. ROSENBERG. 1976. J. Biol. Chem. **251:** 6481-6488.
6. KURACHI, K., K. FUJIKAWA, G. SCHMIER & E. W. DAVIE. 1976. Biochemistry **15:** 373-377.
7. OFOSU, F. A., A. L. CERSKUS, J. HIRSH, L. M. SMITH, G. J. MODI & M. A. BLAJCHMAN. 1984. Br. J. Haematol. **57:** 229-238.
8. OFOSU, F. A., M. A. BLAJCHMAN, G. J. MODI, L. M. SMITH, M. R. BUCHANAN & J. HIRSH. 1985. Br. J. Haematol. **60:** 695-704.
9. ELLIS, V., M. F. SCULLY & V. V. KAKKAR. 1986. Biochem. J. **233:** 161-165.
10. MARCINIAK, E. 1973. Br. J. Haematol. **24:** 391-400.
11. WALSH, P. N. & R. BIGGS. 1972. Br. J. Haematol. **22:** 743-760.
12. TEITEL, J. M. & R. D. ROSENBERG. 1983. J. Clin. Invest. **71:** 1383-1391.
13. BUCHANAN, M. R., B. BONEU, R. A. OFOSU & J. HIRSH. 1985. Blood **65:** 198-201.
14. BARROWCLIFFE, T. W., R. E. MERTON, S. J. HAVERCROFT, L. THUNBERG, U. LINDHAL & D. P. THOMAS. 1984. Thromb. Res. **34:** 135-133.
15. THOMAS, D. P., R. E. MERTON, T. W. BARROWCLIFFE, L. THUNBERG & U. LINDHAL. 1982. Thromb. Haemostasis **47:** 244-248.
16. OCKELFORD, P. A., C. J. CATER, L. MITCHELL & J. HIRSH. 1982. Thromb. Res. **28:** 401-412.
17. KETTNER, C. & E. SHAW. 1979. Thromb. Res. **14:** 969-973.
18. MODI, C. J., M. A. BLAJCHMAN & F. A. OFOSU. 1984. Thromb. Res. **36:** 537-547.
19. TOLLEFSEN, D. M., D. W. MAJERUS & M. K. BLANK. 1982. J. Biol. Chem. **257:** 2162-2169.
20. OFOSU, F. A., G. J. MODI, J. M. SMITH, A. L. CERSKUS, J. HIRSH & M. A. BLAJCHMAN. 1984. Blood **64:** 742-745.
21. PIXLEY, R. A., M. SCHAPIRA & R. W. COLMAN. 1985. Blood **66:** 198-203.
22. SCOTT, C. F., M. SCHAPIRA & R. W. COLMAN. 1982. Blood **60:** 940-947.
23. MCNEELEY, T. B. & M. J. GRIFFITH. 1985. Blood **65:** 1226-1231.
24. WALKER, F. J. & C. T. ESMON. 1979. Biochim. Biophys. Acta. **585:** 405-451.
25. OFOSU, F. A., M. A. BLAJCHMAN & J. HIRSH. 1980. Thromb. Res. **20:** 391-403.
26. SIE, P., F. A. OFOSU, F. FERNANDEZ, M. R. BUCHANAN, M. PITITOU, B. BONEU. 1986. Br. J. Haem. In Press.
27. NESHEIM, M. E. & K. G. MANN. 1979. J. Biol. Chem. **254:** 1326-1334.
28. ROSING, J., G. TANS, J. W. P. GOVERS-REIMSLAG, R. F. A. ZWAAL & H. C. HEMKER. 1980. J. Biol. Chem. **255:** 274-283.
29. NESHEIM, M. E., C. KETTNER, E. SHAW & K. G. MANN. 1981. J. Biol. Chem. **256:** 6537-6540.
30. NESHEIM, M. E., S. EID, K. G. MANN. 1981. J. Biol. Chem. **256:** 9874-9882.

Congenitally Abnormal Prothrombin and Thrombin[a]

MARIE-CLAUDE GUILLIN, ANNIE BEZEAUD, MARIE-JOSÈPHE RABIET, AND JACQUES ELION

Laboratoire de Recherche sur l'Hémostase et la Thrombose
Laboratoire de Biochimie B
Faculté Xavier Bichat
75018, Paris, France

Isolated prothrombin deficiencies due to inherited qualitative defects are very rare conditions. Fourteen nonrelated families with distinct dysprothrombinemias have been identified to date.[1-14] In each case, an immunoassay has revealed the presence of prothrombin molecules with little or no activity. According to the international nomenclature, most of the prothrombin variants have been designated by the name of the city of birth of the proband. Purification of the abnormal prothrombin has led to the unambiguous characterization of the functional defect of several variants.

In this review, we will briefly summarize the clinical features associated with congenital dysprothrombinemias and will describe in some detail the functional defects that characterize different prothrombin variants studied in our laboratory and in others.

MODE OF INHERITANCE

Congenital dysprothrombinemia has been diagnosed in 52 subjects belonging to 14 families. The defect is inherited as an autosomal trait. Results of family studies have allowed classification of most of the probands according to their respective genotype (TABLE 1). The homozygous form, as would be expected, is very rare and seems to be confirmed so far in only two cases, namely prothrombins Barcelona[2] and Madrid.[8] Probands with prothrombins Brussels,[4] Cardeza,[1] Clamart,[14] and Padua[3] are heterozygotes. Other variants are found in more complex genotypic situations. Probands carrying prothrombins Habana,[12] Metz,[11] and Molise[6] are characterized by a double heterozygosity for abnormal prothrombin and true prothrombin deficiency, with the four possible genetic combinations encountered among the various family members. Probands with prothrombins Quick[15] and San Juan[5] are both compound heterozygotes for two distinct abnormal prothrombins. The low prothrombin antigen level (34% of normal) reported in the patient with prothrombin Quick could reflect

[a] This work was supported by Grants from the Institut National de la Santé et de la Recherche médicale (CRL 78 2 103 1 and 82 50 11) and from the Faculté Xavier Bichat, Université Paris VII.

TABLE 1. Congenital Dysprothrombinemias: Genetic Status

Genetic Status	Prothrombin Variants
Homozygotes	Barcelona, Madrid
Heterozygotes	Brussels, Cardeza Clamart, Padua
Compound heterozygotes for abnormal prothrombin and true hypoprothrombinemia	Habana, Metz, Molise
Compound heterozygotes for two different abnormal prothrombins	Quick, San Juan

a shortened survival of one of the variants or of both of them; such a mechanism has been reported for fibrinogen Philadelphia.[16] The unequal distribution of the two variants present in the plasma San Juan (San Juan I = 75%, San Juan II = 25%) has been tentatively ascribed to differential rates of synthesis or catabolism of the two abnormal proteins.[5]

CLINICAL FEATURES

A mild bleeding syndrome is generally ascribed to congenital dysprothrombinemias (TABLE 2). Excessive bleeding after a trauma or a surgical procedure is frequent (10 probands out of 14) and most often requires blood transfusions.[3–5,7–9,12] Other bleeding manifestations consist mainly of easy bruising and epistaxis.[2,3,6,8,9,12] Meno- and metrorrhagia are frequent[6,8,10,11] and may be severe; they have required transfusions of blood or prothrombin complex concentrates on several occasions in the proband with prothrombin Madrid,[8] and have led to hysterectomy in both twins with prothrombin Gainesville.[10] Hematomas[2,7,12] have been reported, as well as one severe neonatal umbilical bleeding.[12]

A poor correlation is observed between the severity and frequency of bleeding on the one hand, and the level of prothrombin activity on the other. The patient with prothrombin Salakta is asymptomatic, although his prothrombin activity is 15% of normal,[13] whereas patients with higher prothrombin activities such as San Juan[5] and Gainesville[10] are considered abnormal bleeders.

TABLE 2. Congenital Dysprothrombinemias: Bleeding Manifestations

	Frequency (Percent)
Posttrauma or surgery bleeding	79
Easy bruising, epistaxis	43
Meno and metrorrhagias	38
Hematomas	21
No abnormal bleeding	21

DIAGNOSIS

The presence of an abnormal prothrombin is associated with a prolonged prothrombin time (PT) and activated partial thromboplastin time (APTT). APTT, however, is less sensitive than PT for the detection of prothrombin defects. Prothrombin activity (TABLE 3) is decreased when measured by the classical one- or two-stage assays. By contrast, prothrombin antigen measured by the Laurell technique is most often normal.[1-5,8,10,13,14] Yet it has been found decreased to approximately 50% of normal in five probands;[6,7,9,11,12] in all these cases, however, the antigen level is higher than the activity level. Four of these probands have been classified as double heterozygotes, either for an abnormal prothrombin and a true hypoprothrombinemia,[6,11,12] or for two distinct prothrombin variants.[15] A constant feature is the decrease of the activity/antigen ratio below normal values; it ranges from less than 0.10 (Barcelona, Habana, Houston, Madrid, and Quick) to 0.50 (Brussels, Cardeza, and Padua), with intermediate values for Salakta, Metz, San Juan, Molise, and Gainesville (0.15 to 0.35).

Functional assays based on the use of various prothrombin activators are generally employed as tools for a preliminary characterization of the variants prior to purification and extensive study of the abnormal molecule. These activators, which include the prothrombinase complex, various snake venom enzymes and staphylocoagulase, activate prothrombin by different pathways (TABLE 4). The prothrombinase complex consists of factor Xa, calcium ions, negatively charged phospholipids, and factor Va. Factor Xa cleaves human prothrombin at the Arg (271)-Thr and Arg (320)-Ile peptide bonds.[17-20] These cleavages appear to occur in a concerted fashion in the presence of the full prothrombinase complex.[21] Although factor Xa alone will catalyze prothrombin conversion, the other components of the prothrombinase complex enhance the reaction

TABLE 3. Congenital Dysprothrombinemias: Plasma Prothrombin Assay

	Prothrombin Activity (Percent)					Prothrombin
Variant	one-stage	two-stage	TSV[b]	ECV[c]	Staphylo-coagulase	Antigen (percent)
Barcelona	5	12	—	—	100	100
Brussels	35	48	64	—	50	71
Cardeza	—	50	—	100	100	100
Clamart	50	50	48	100	100	100
Gainesville[a]	25	40	20	12	—	72
Habana	1-5	5-10	—	—	40-50	50
Houston	5	10	—	abN	—	52
Madrid	3	10	8	94	—	103
Metz	10	—	—	25	50	50
Molise	12	10	9.5	14	50	36-52
Padua	52	50	32	98	105	100
Quick	—	2	2	2	—	34
Salakta	15	17	—	17	18	100
San Juan	—	20	—	—	80	93

[a] Prothrombin Gainesville is present in both identical twins; the results are similar for the two probands.

[b] TSV: taipan snake venom

[c] ECV: *Echis carinatus* venom

TABLE 4. Mechanism of Action of Various Prothrombin Activators

Activator	Peptide Bonds Cleaved in Prothrombin[a]	Cofactors
Xa	Arg (271)-Thr; Arg (320)-Ile	Phospholipids, Ca^{++} Factor Va
Taipan	Arg (271)-Thr; Arg (320)-Ile	Phospholipids, Ca^{++}
Echis carinatus or *Dispholidus typus* venom	Arg (320)-Ile	None
Staphylocoagulase	None[b]	None

[a] The cleavages that are indicated do not include the cleavages catalyzed by thrombin produced during the activation process.

[b] Staphylocoagulase activates prothrombin by the formation of a complex, unmasking the thrombin active site.

rate by about five orders of magnitude;[22–24] kinetics of prothrombin activation is therefore clearly dependent on the interaction of prothrombin with each of the components of the complex. Incubation of prothrombin with the enzyme present in Taipan snake venom results in the same products as those found upon prothrombinase action, suggesting that the cleaved peptide bonds are identical;[25] the reaction rate is slightly enhanced by phospholipids and calcium, but is not modified by factor Va.[26] Prothrombin-activating enzymes from *Echis carinatus* or *Dispholidus typus* venoms are not dependent on the presence of calcium, phospholipids, or factor Va and are responsible for the cleavage of a unique peptide bond (Arg (320)-Ile) in the prothombin molecule.[27,28] Whatever the activator (prothrombinase, Taipan snake, *Echis carinatus* or *Dispholidus typus* venoms), the scission of the Arg (320)-Ile bond unmasks the thrombin active site, which is then responsible for autocatalytic proteolysis of prothrombin or its derivatives at Arg (155)-Ser, Arg (271)-Thr, and Arg (284)-Thr. Therefore, the final activation products (fragment 1, fragment 2, fragment 3, and thrombin) are identical, although the pathways and intermediate products differ. In contrast to the previously mentioned activators, staphylocoagulase activates prothrombin by way of the formation of an equimolecular complex, and the thrombin active site is unmasked without detectable proteolysis of prothrombin.[29]

The 14 distinct variants identified to date are characterized by a decrease in prothombin activity, measured by the usual one- or two-stage assays employing prothrombinase as the activator. Comparison (TABLE 3) of the results obtained when measuring prothrombin activity in plasma, by using the various activators described above, may identify a priori different types of functional defects. An abnormality of the thrombin active site would be detected whatever activator one used for prothrombin assay, as illustrated by prothrombin Salakta. An impairment of the interaction of prothrombin with the components of the prothrombinase complex would be detected by the usual one- or two-stage assays, whereas assays performed with *Echis carinatus* or *Dispholidus typus* venoms, and with staphylocoagulase, would be normal, as illustrated by prothrombins Barcelona or Madrid. Theoretically, the assay performed with Taipan snake venom should be helpful for the identification of a defect in factor Va binding. One should stress, however, that results of assays performed in whole plasma have to be taken with some caution: the functional activity of prothrombin Metz and Molise has been found to be normal in plasma by the staphylocoagulase assay,[6,11] whereas study of the purified variants has allowed us to demonstrate an abnormality of the thrombin active site.[30,31] The reason for this apparent discrepancy is not clear at this point.

Heterogeneity of the variants is further illustrated by the analysis of their electrophoretic mobility in plasma. Mobility of prothrombins Brussels,[4] Madrid,[8] Metz,[11] Molise,[6] Padua,[3] and Salakta[13] is normal, either in the presence or absence of calcium ions. Electrophoretic migration of prothrombins Barcelona,[2] Habana,[12] Houston,[9] and San Juan[5] is more anodal than normal; the abnormal migration rate of prothrombin San Juan I is apparently related to a defect in calcium binding.[5] An abnormal electrophoretic pattern of prothrombin derivatives in serum has been reported for some variants,[1,3,4,6] suggesting a defect in the prothrombin cleavage pathway.

ISOLATION OF THE VARIANTS

So far, all of the variants have been shown to be adsorbable on barium salts, and conventional prothrombin purification procedures have been used for their isolation.[5,13,14,30–34] An abnormal behavior on ion-exchange chromatography has been reported for some of the variants. Prothrombin San Juan I was less tightly retained to DEAE Sephadex than normal prothrombin, whereas prothrombin Madrid was more tightly bound. By DEAE Sephadex chromatography, prothrombin Barcelona was resolved into two peaks, both of which reacted with antiprothrombin antibodies. The major peak (2/3 of total prothrombin) had a low prothrombin activity, similar to plasma prothrombin activity, and eluted at a slightly higher ionic strength than normal prothrombin, whereas the minor peak eluted ahead of normal prothrombin and was devoid of activity.[32] This unexpected behavior of prothrombin Barcelona on DEAE Sephadex still remains unexplained.

Analysis of purified prothrombin variants by polyacrylamide gel electrophoresis, either in the absence or presence of sodium dodecyl sulfate (SDS), has failed to detect any abnormality, except for prothrombin Barcelona, which appeared to be more negatively charged than normal prothrombin.[32]

FUNCTIONAL CHARACTERIZATION OF THE VARIANTS

Availability of purified prothrombin variants has allowed investigators to precisely determine the functional defect of nine of the variants. On theoretical bases, different types of defects can be considered: 1) impairment of factor Xa-induced cleavages; 2) defect in prothrombin interaction with calcium and/or phospholipids, and/or factor Va; 3) production of an abnormal thrombin molecule. A classification of the prothrombin variants according to these theoretical defects is presented in TABLE 5.

An impairment of factor Xa-induced cleavages has been demonstrated in four variants by SDS polyacrylamide gel electrophoresis analysis of the activation products. It can affect either one of the Arg (271)-Thr or Arg (320)-Ile cleavages.

Prothrombins Barcelona and Madrid are both characterized by a defective cleavage at Arg (271)-Thr.[34,35] Impairment of this cleavage results, in both cases, in the production of high molecular weight intermediates, as illustrated in FIGURE 1 for prothrombin Madrid. These high molecular weight intermediates consist of meizothrombin and meizothrombin-des-F1, and correspond respectively to prothrombin and prethrombin 1 cleaved at the Arg (320)-Ile bond. They are specifically devoid of clotting activity, but their activity towards small peptidic substrates is similar to that of thrombin: this is illustrated by the dissociation between a normal generation of amidolytic activity and a decreased production of clotting activity upon factor Xa activation (FIGURE 2). Although meizothrombin is unable to clot fibrinogen, it is able, however, to interact with some macromolecular substrates, as its conversion to meizothrombin-des-F1 is an autolytic process. Production of meizothrombin and meizothrombin-des-F1 by prothrombins Barcelona and Madrid was the first evidence that Xa-induced cleavage at Arg (320)-Ile was not dependent upon the Xa-induced cleavage at Arg (271)-Thr.

Prothrombins Cardeza and Clamart appear to present with a defective Arg (320)-Ile factor Xa-induced cleavage.[14,36] The production of thrombin activity by prothrombin Clamart upon Xa action was shown to proceed at a two-fold decreased rate, but in contrast with prothrombins Barcelona and Madrid, amidolytic activity production

TABLE 5. Classification of the Prothrombin Variants According to the Functional Defects

1. Impairment of Xa-induced proteolysis
   —at Arg (271)-Thr : Barcelona, Madrid
   —at Arg (320)-Ile : Cardeza, Clamart
2. Defective calcium binding
   San Juan
3. Defective thrombin active site
   Metz, Molise, Quick I, Salakta

paralleled that of clotting activity (FIGURE 2). SDS polyacrylamide gel electrophoresis analysis of the proteolytic pattern in the presence of factor Xa revealed the prolonged persistence of prethrombin 2 in conditions where normal prothrombin is entirely converted into thrombin (FIGURE 3). Similar features characterize prothrombin Cardeza.[14] The mutation, however, is unlikely to affect Arg 320 or Ile 321 because the cleavage rate of this peptide bond by *Echis carinatus* venom is normal both in prothrombins Cardeza and Clamart. Rather, a mutation in the vicinity of the Arg (320)-Ile peptide bond could affect its accessibility to factor Xa.

A defective interaction with the cofactors of the prothrombinase complex has been suggested for prothrombin San Juan I. This variant is thought to have a calcium binding defect,[36] which could be responsible for the observed decreased activation rate by prothrombinase.

An abnormality of the thrombin active site has been demonstrated for prothrombins Metz, Molise, Quick I, and Salakta. In these cases, factor Xa-induced prothrombin proteolysis proceeds normally but gives rise to a thrombin molecule that is abnormal in its catalytic behavior. The enzymatic activity of thrombin Metz,[30] Molise,[31] and Salakta[13,37] is clearly abnormal whatever substrate is used to test it (H-D-Phe-Pip-

Arg-*p*NA, fibrinogen, factor V, protein C, antithrombin III, platelets). This strongly suggests that the molecular defect disturbs the function of the catalytic site itself rather than specific interactions with some macromolecular substrates. Characterization of the enzymatic properties of thrombin Salakta[37] has demonstrated that the quantitative incorporation of [^{3}H]diisopropylfluorophosphate (DFP) by the abnormal molecule is normal, as well as the active site titration with *p*-nitrophenyl *p'*-guanidino benzoate. By contrast, the kinetics of inhibition by DFP and benzamidine are abnormal. These results suggest that the structural defect of thrombin Salakta does not reside in the catalytic triade, but rather disturbs the function of the primary binding site. Thrombin Quick I differs from thrombins Metz, Molise, and Salakta in that its esterolytic and amidolytic activities are not affected.[38] Thrombin Quick I interacts

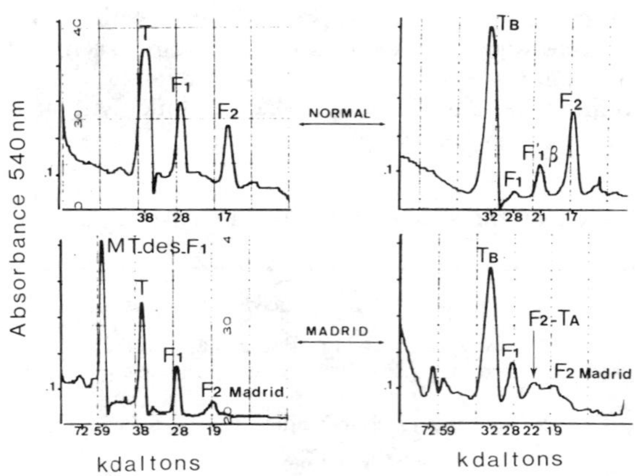

FIGURE 1. SDS gel analysis of prothrombin Madrid activation by factor Xa. Prothrombin (1 mg/ml) was incubated with bovine Xa (10 U/ml) and human brain cephalin (50 μg/ml) in 50 mM NaCl, 10 mM $CaCl_2$, 20 mM Tris, pH 7.5, for 8 hours at 20°C. Aliquots were submitted to electrophoresis in 10% acrylamide gels containing 0.1% SDS, either in nonreduced (left panels) or reduced (right panels) conditions, and the gels were scanned at 540 nm. Prothrombin Madrid yielded a 59 kDa product (MT-des-F1), consisting of two disulfide-linked chains (TB and F2-TA). The abnormal migration rate of F2 Madrid was ascribed to the absence of cleavage at Arg (271)-Thr, F2 Madrid consisting of F2 plus the 13 amino acids peptide F3 still attached to it.[34]

Abbreviations: T:thrombin; F1:fragment; F2:fragment 2; MT-des-F1:meizothrombin-des-fragment 1; TB:thrombin B chain; F'1 β:subfragment β of F1 split at Arg (51)-Thr by thrombin; F2-TA: F2 plus thrombin A chain attached to it.

normally with the inhibitor dansylarginine-*N*-(3-ethyl-1,5-pentanediyl)-amide, whereas its activity towards fibrinogen, prothrombin, platelets, and endothelial cells is abnormal.[38–40] The molecular defect of thrombin Quick I could, therefore, alter primarily its binding to macromolecular substrates. No information is yet available on the functional properties of thrombin Quick II.

Although none of the mutations of the prothrombin variants have to date been identified, availability of such molecules presenting with specific functional defects provides a unique opportunity for the investigation of the structural features that are critical for either the prothrombin activation process or the mechanism of thrombin functions.

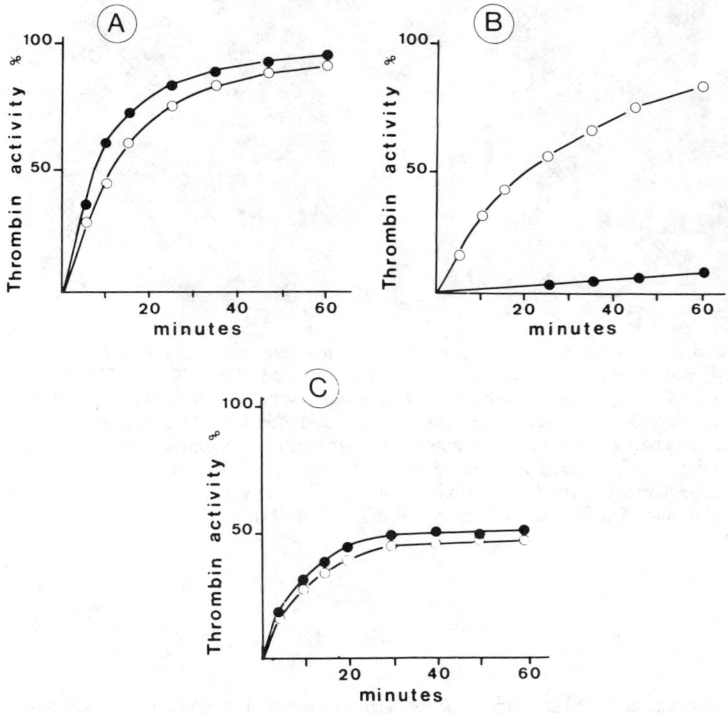

FIGURE 2. Prothrombin Madrid and Clamart activation by factor Xa: production of thrombin-like clotting and amidolytic activities. Prothrombin (10 μg/ml) was incubated with bovine Xa (0.1 U/ml) and human brain cephalin (50 μg/ml) in 50 mM NaCl, 10 mM $CaCl_2$, 20 mM Tris, pH 7.5, at 20°C. At timed intervals, aliquots were assayed for clotting activity using purified human fibrinogen (●——●) and for amidolytic activity using S2238 (○——○). Thrombin-like activity was expressed as per cent maximum thrombin produced by normal prothrombin. Panel A: normal prothrombin; panel B: prothrombin Madrid; panel C: prothrombin Clamart.

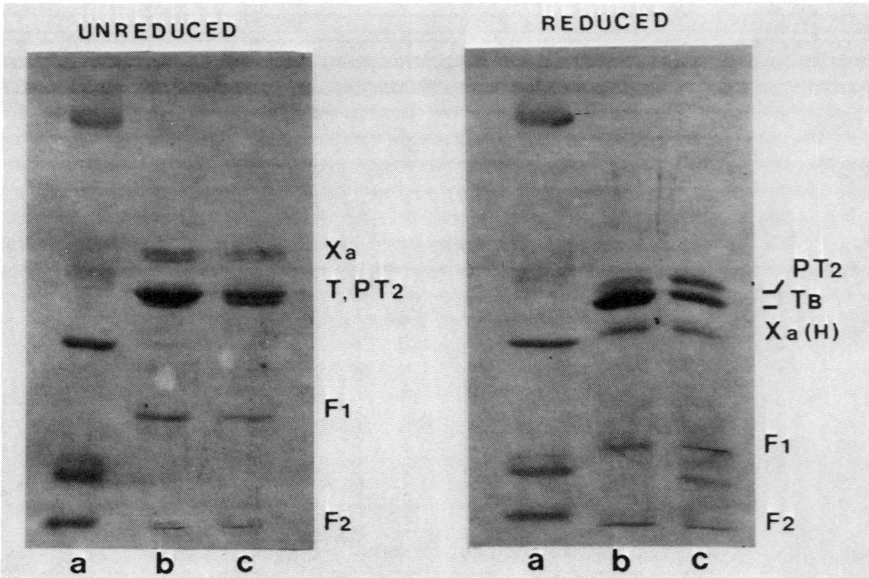

FIGURE 3. SDS gel analysis of prothrombin Clamart activation by factor Xa. Prothrombin (0.28 μM) was incubated with Xa (200 U/ml) in 150 mM NaCl, 10 mM $CaCl_2$, 20 mM Tris, pH 7.4. After 24 hours incubation at 20°C, aliquots were submitted to SDS slab gel electrophoresis in 10% acrylamide, before and after disulfide bonds reduction. Prothrombin Clamart yielded equal amounts of PT2 and T, whereas normal prothrombin was almost entirely converted to T. Lane a: mixture of standard markers of molecular weight 67,000, 30,000, 20,000, and 12,000. Lane b: Xa-activated normal prothrombin. Lance c: Xa-activated prothrombin Clamart.

Abbreviations: T:thrombin; PT2:prethrombin 2; Xa(H):Xa heavy chain; F1:fragment 1; F2:fragment 2.

REFERENCES

1. Shapiro, S. S., J. Martinez & R. R. Holburn. 1969. J. Clin. Invest. **48:** 2251-2259.
2. Josso, F., J. Monasterio de Sanchez, J. M. Lavergne, D. Menache & J. P. Soulier. 1971. Blood **38:** 9-16.
3. Girolami, A., G. Bareggi, A. Brunetti & A. Sticchi. 1974. J. Lab. Clin. Med. **84:** 654-666.
4. Kahn, M. J. P. & A. Govaerts. 1974. Thromb. Res. **5:** 141-156.
5. Shapiro, S. S. 1975. *In* Prothrombin and Related Factors. H. C. Hemker & J. J. Veltkamp, Eds.: 205-212. Leiden University Press. Leiden, the Netherlands.
6. Girolami, A., S. Coccheri, G. Palaretti, M. Poggi, A. Burul & G. Cappellato. 1978. Blood **52:** 115-125.
7. Owen, C. A., R. A. Henriksen, F. C. McDuffie & K. G. Mann. 1978. Mayo Clin. Proc. **53:** 29-33.
8. Bezeaud, A., M. C. Guillin, F. Olmeda, M. Quintana & G. Gomez. 1979. Thromb. Res. **16:** 47-58.
9. Weinger, R. S., C. Rudy, J. L. Moake, J. D. Olson & P. L. Cimo. 1980. Blood **55:** 811-816.
10. Smith, L. G., L. A. H. Coone & C. S. Kitchens. 1981. Am. J. Hematol. **11:** 223-231.
11. Josso, F., Y. Rio & S. Beguin. 1982. Haemostasis **12:** 309-316.

12. Rubio, R., D. Almagro, A. Cruz & J. F. Corral. 1983. Br. J. Haematol. **54:** 553-560.
13. Bezeaud, A., L. Drouet, C. Soria & M. C. Guillin. 1984. Thromb. Res. **34:** 507-518.
14. Huisse, M. G., M. Dreyfus & M. C. Guillin. 1985. Thromb. Haemost. **54:** 274. (Abstract.)
15. Henriksen, R. A. & W. G. Owen. 1981. Thromb. Haemost. **46:** 121. (Abstract.)
16. Martinez, J., R. R. Holburn, S. S. Shapiro & A. J. Erslev. 1974. J. Clin. Invest. **53:** 600-611.
17. Heldebrant, C. M. & K. G. Mann. 1973. J. Biol. Chem. **248:** 3642-3652.
18. Heldebrant, C. M., R. J. Butkowski, S. P. Bajaj & K. G. Mann. 1973. J. Biol. Chem. **248:** 7149-7163.
19. Esmon, C. T. & C. M. Jackson. 1974. J. Biol. Chem. **249:** 7782-7790.
20. Owen, W. G., C. T. Esmon & C. M. Jackson. 1974. J. Biol. Chem. **249:** 594-605.
21. Nesheim, M. E. & K. G. Mann. 1983. J. Biol. Chem. **258:** 5386-5391.
22. Miletich, J. P., C. M. Jackson & P. W. Majerus. 1978. J. Biol. Chem. **253:** 6908-6916.
23. Nesheim, M. E., J. B. Taswell & K. G. Mann. 1979. J. Biol. Chem. **254:** 10952-10962.
24. Rosing, J., G. Tans, J. W. P. Govers-Riemslag, R. F. A. Zwaal & H. C. Hemker. 1980. J. Biol. Chem. **255:** 274-283.
25. Owen, W. G. & C. M. Jackson. 1974. Thromb. Res. **3:** 705-714.
26. Pirkle, H., M. McIntosh, I. Theodor & S. Vernon. 1972. Thromb. Res. **1:** 559-568.
27. Morita, T., S. Iwanaga & T. Suzuki. 1976. J. Biochem. **79:** 1089-1108.
28. Guillin, M. C., A. Bezeaud & D. Menache. 1978. Biochim. Biophys. Acta **537:** 160-168.
29. Hendrix, H., T. Lindhout, K. Mertens, W. Engels & H. C. Hemker. 1983. J. Biol. Chem. **258:** 3637-3644.
30. Rabiet, M. J., M. Jandrot-Perrus, J. P. Boissel, J. Elion & F. Josso. 1984. Blood **63:** 927-934.
31. Rabiet, M. J. 1985. Thromb. Haemost. **54:** 273. (Abstract.)
32. Benarous, R., J. M. Lavergne, D. Labie & F. Josso. 1974. Biochem. Biophys. Res. Commun. **60:** 976-982.
33. Rabiet, M. J., R. Benarous, D. Labie & F. Josso. 1978. FEBS Lett. **87:** 132-134.
34. Guillin, M. C. & A. Bezeaud. 1981. Ann. N.Y. Acad. Sci. **370:** 414-425.
35. Rabiet, M. J., J. Elion, R. Benarous, D. Labie & F. Josso. 1979. Biochim. Biophys. Acta **584:** 66-75.
36. Shapiro, S. S. & S. McCord. 1978. Prog. Hemostasis Thromb. **4:** 177-209.
37. Bezeaud, A., M. Jandrot-Perrus & M. C. Guillin. 1985. Blood **665**(Suppl. 1): 1207. (Abstract.)
38. Henriksen, R. A., W. G. Owen, M. E. Nesheim & K. G. Mann. 1980. J. Clin. Invest. **66:** 934-940.
39. Henriksen, R. A. & A. F. A. Brotherton. 1983. J. Biol. Chem. **258:** 13717-13721.
40. Henriksen, R. A. & W. G. Owen. 1985. Thromb. Haemostasis **54:** 1553. (Abstract.)

The Prothrombin Gene and Serine Proteinase Evolution

SANDRA J. FRIEZNER DEGEN[a]
AND EARL W. DAVIE[b]

[a]*Children's Hospital Research Foundation and the University of Cincinnati Medical School Cincinnati, Ohio 45229*

[b]*Department of Biochemistry University of Washington Seattle, Washington 98195*

The structure of human prothrombin has been well defined. Mature human prothrombin, the form found circulating in the blood, is a single chain glycoprotein with a molecular weight of 72,000; it contains 579 amino acids and 8% carbohydrate.[1-3] The amino acid sequence of human and bovine prothrombin have been determined by amino acid sequencing procedures[4-8] and deduced from the DNA sequence of cDNA clones coding for both the human and bovine protein.[2,9] The amino acid sequence for the human protein is shown in FIGURE 1. The apparent carbohydrate attachment sites are at Asn 78, 100, and 373 (see FIGURE 1). Vitamin K is required for the biosynthesis of this protein and is involved in the carboxylation of the first ten glutamic acid residues and their conversion to γ-carboxyglutamic acid (GLA).[4,10-12] Immediately following the GLA region are two homologous domains called kringles.[4] These domains contain approximately 80 amino acids linked together by three disulfide bonds. Kringle structures are highly conserved and have been implicated as domains involved in interactions with other proteins;[13] for example, the second kringle of prothrombin appears to be involved in the binding of the protein to its cofactor, factor V.[14] The carboxyl terminal region of prothrombin contains the catalytic region, which is homologous to trypsin, as well as all other serine proteases.[15]

In order to gain further information on the location of the intervening sequences in the gene for prothrombin and the relationship of the introns with the structural domains of the protein and, also to investigate the regulation and expression of prothrombin, we have isolated and characterized the gene for human prothrombin using recombinant DNA techniques.

ISOLATION OF THE HUMAN PROTHROMBIN GENE

An almost full-length cDNA coding for human prothrombin has been previously isolated and found to code for 36 amino acids of the leader sequence, 579 amino acids of the mature protein, a stop codon of TAG and the complete 3′ noncoding region of 97 base pairs (bp).[2] This cDNA was used to screen genomic DNA libraries prepared

-43 -35 -30 -20
Met Ala Arg Val Arg Gly Leu Gln Leu Pro Gly Cys Leu Ala Leu Ala Ala Leu Cys Ser Leu Val His Ser Gln His Val Phe Leu Ala

-10 -1 1 10
Pro Gln Gln Ala Arg Ser Leu Leu Gln Arg Val Arg Arg Ala Asn Thr Phe Leu GLA GLA Val Arg Lys Gly Asn Leu GLA Arg GLA Cys

20 30 40
Val GLA GLA Thr Cys Ser Tyr GLA GLA Ala Phe GLA Ala Leu GLA Ser Ser Thr Ala Thr Asp Val Phe Trp Ala Lys Tyr Thr Ala Cys

50 60 70
Glu Thr Ala Arg Thr Pro Arg Asp Lys Leu Ala Ala Cys Leu Glu Gly Asn Cys Ala Glu Gly Leu Gly Thr Asn Tyr Arg Gly His Val

80 90 100
Asn Ile Thr Arg Ser Gly Ile Glu Cys Gln Leu Trp Arg Ser Arg Tyr Pro His Lys Pro Glu Ile Asn Ser Thr Thr His Pro Gly Ala

110 120 130
Asp Leu Gln Glu Asn Phe Cys Arg Asn Pro Asp Ser Ser Asn Thr Gly Pro Trp Cys Tyr Thr Thr Asp Pro Thr Val Arg Arg Gln Glu

140 150 160
Cys Ser Ile Pro Val Cys Gly Gln Asp Gln Val Thr Val Ala Met Thr Pro Arg Ser Glu Gly Ser Ser Val Asn Leu Ser Pro Pro Leu

170 180 190
Glu Gln Cys Val Pro Asp Arg Gly Gln Gln Tyr Gln Gly Arg Leu Ala Val Thr Thr His Gly Leu Pro Cys Leu Ala Trp Ala Ser Ala

200 210 220
Gln Ala Lys Ala Leu Ser Lys His Gln Asp Phe Asn Ser Ala Val Gln Leu Val Glu Asn Phe Cys Arg Asn Pro Asp Gly Asp Glu Glu

230 240 250
Gly Val Trp Cys Tyr Val Ala Gly Lys Pro Gly Asp Phe Gly Tyr Cys Asp Leu Asn Tyr Cys Glu Glu Ala Val Glu Glu Glu Thr Gly

260 270 280
Asp Gly Leu Asp Glu Asp Ser Asp Arg Ala Ile Glu Gly Arg Thr Ala Thr Ser Glu Tyr Gln Thr Phe Phe Asn Pro Arg Thr Phe Gly

290 300 310
Ser Gly Glu Ala Asp Cys Gly Leu Arg Pro Leu Phe Glu Lys Lys Ser Leu Glu Asp Lys Thr Glu Arg Glu Leu Leu Glu Ser Tyr Ile

320 330 340
Asp Gly Arg Ile Val Glu Gly Ser Asp Ala Glu Ile Gly Met Ser Pro Trp Gln Val Met Leu Phe Arg Lys Ser Pro Gln Glu Leu Leu

350 360 370
Cys Gly Ala Ser Leu Ile Ser Asp Arg Trp Val Leu Thr Ala Ala His Cys Leu Leu Tyr Pro Pro Trp Asp Lys Asn Phe Thr Glu Asn

380 390 400
Asp Leu Leu Val Arg Ile Gly Lys His Ser Arg Thr Arg Tyr Glu Arg Asn Ile Glu Lys Ile Ser Met Leu Glu Lys Ile Tyr Ile His

410 420 430
Pro Arg Tyr Asn Trp Arg Glu Asn Leu Asp Arg Asp Ile Ala Leu Met Lys Leu Lys Lys Pro Val Ala Phe Ser Asp Tyr Ile His Pro

440 450 460
Val Cys Leu Pro Asp Arg Glu Thr Ala Ala Ser Leu Leu Gln Ala Gly Tyr Lys Gly Arg Val Thr Gly Trp Gly Asn Leu Lys Glu Thr

470 480 490
Trp Thr Ala Asn Val Gly Lys Gly Gln Pro Ser Val Leu Gln Val Val Asn Leu Pro Ile Val Glu Arg Pro Val Cys Lys Asp Ser Thr

500 510 520
Arg Ile Arg Ile Thr Asp Asn Met Phe Cys Ala Gly Tyr Lys Pro Asp Glu Gly Lys Arg Gly Asp Ala Cys Glu Gly Asp Ser Gly Gly

530 540 550
Pro Phe Val Met Lys Ser Pro Phe Asn Asn Arg Trp Tyr Gln Met Gly Ile Val Ser Trp Gly Glu Gly Cys Asp Arg Asp Gly Lys Tyr

560 570 579
Gly Phe Tyr Thr His Val Phe Arg Leu Lys Lys Trp Ile Gln Lys Val Ile Asp Gln Phe Gly Glu

FIGURE 1. The amino acid sequence of human prothrombin as deduced from the sequence of the cDNA and gene. The leader sequence is numbered −43 to −1, whereas the amino acid sequence of the mature protein found circulating in the blood is numbered 1 to 579. Apparent carbohydrate attachment sites are indicated by ◆, and peptide bonds cleaved by factor Xa during the activation of prothrombin to thrombin are indicated by arrows above the sequence. The active site residues histidine, aspartic acid, and serine are amino acid residues 363, 419, and 525, respectively. Open arrows below the sequence indicate the placement of the 13 intervening sequences in the gene with respect to the amino acid sequence. An arrow between two amino acids indicates that in the gene the intervening sequence occurs between the two triplet codons coding for these amino acids, whereas an arrow placed after the first or second letter of the amino acid indicates that the intervening sequence is located after the first or second nucleotide of the triplet codon coding for that amino acid.

from human fetal liver[16] and placental DNA. These libraries contained fragments of approximately 20 kilobases (kb) of human DNA inserted into a lambda bacteriophage vector. Screening of the recombinant phage was performed by the method of Benton and Davis[17] as modified by Woo.[18] Several phage isolates were found that contained portions of the human prothrombin gene. DNA isolated from these clones were mapped with restriction endonucleases followed by southern hybridization analysis.[19] Overlapping fragments, obtained by restriction endonuclease digestion of the recombinant phage, were subcloned into pBR322 and further characterized by DNA sequence analysis.

CHARACTERIZATION OF THE GENE FOR HUMAN PROTHROMBIN

Comparison of the sequence to that determined for the cDNA indicates that the gene is composed of 14 exons and 13 intervening sequences. The intervening sequences range in size from 84 bp to over 8 kb in length. The 5′ and 3′ ends of all intervening sequences agree with the consensus sequence of Mount[20] and have the typical GT-AG recognition sequence for splicing.[21] At least eleven copies of Alu repetitive DNA[22] are contained within the intervening sequences. The role of these sequences within the human prothrombin gene is unknown. The 14 exons range in size from 25 to 315 bp. Present evidence indicates that the gene is approximately 24 kb in length. This is larger than that reported for the gene for bovine prothrombin, which is 15 kb in length and has the same number of intervening sequences.[23]

It is apparent from the sequence of the gene and the cDNA that prothrombin is synthesized with an amino terminal extension of 43 amino acids.[2,9] This leader sequence ends with two arginine residues preceding the amino terminal Ala present in the mature protein (residue 1 in FIGURE 1). Because Arg-Ala is not a typical signal peptidase cleavage site, it is likely that the leader sequence contains a signal and a pro peptide.[24] Pro peptides have also been identified in other plasma proteins,[25–31] but their function is unknown. It is likely that the signal peptidase cleaves somewhere in the middle of the leader sequence. The signal sequence has the typical hydrophobic stretch of amino acids and is removed before secretion from the cell, whereas the pro piece is removed by additional processing in the liver or in blood.

The location of intervening sequences with respect to the amino acid sequence and domain structure of human prothrombin is shown in FIGURES 1 and 2. The first intervening sequence (intron A) occurs at amino acid −17 in the leader sequence. Intervening sequences B (between amino acid residues 37 and 38) and C (at amino acid residue 46) are immediately following the GLA region. Introns D (at amino acid residue 63) and F (at amino acid residue 144) flank the first kringle domain. Intron E (at amino acid residue 98) is present within this domain. The second kringle domain is flanked by intron F and intron G (at amino acid residue 249). Further downstream, the two factor Xa cleavage sites are separated by introns H (at amino acid residue 292) and I (at amino acid residue 334). The remaining intervening sequences separate each of the active site amino acids into individual exons. The exon containing the active site histidine is flanked by introns I and J (at amino acid residue 390), the active site aspartic acid by introns J and K (at amino acid residue 448), and the active site serine by introns L (at amino acid residue 509) and M (between amino acid residues 532 and 533). The entire 3′ noncoding region of the mRNA is present in the last exon and is not interrupted by an intervening sequence. The placement of intervening sequences with respect to the triplet codon they interrupt has been categorized:[32] type 0 intervening sequences interrupt the coding region between two triplet codons, type I occurs after the first nucleotide in the codon, and type II occurs after the second nucleotide in the codon. Intervening sequences of all three types are found in the gene for human prothrombin; there are two of type 0, 7 of type I, and 4 of type II.

COMPARISON OF THE PLACEMENT OF INTERVENING SEQUENCES WITH RESPECT TO DOMAINS IN THE GENES CODING FOR PROTHROMBIN AND OTHER SERINE PROTEASES

It has been proposed that the genes coding for the serine proteases present today are the result of duplication and divergence from a common ancestral gene.[33] Further

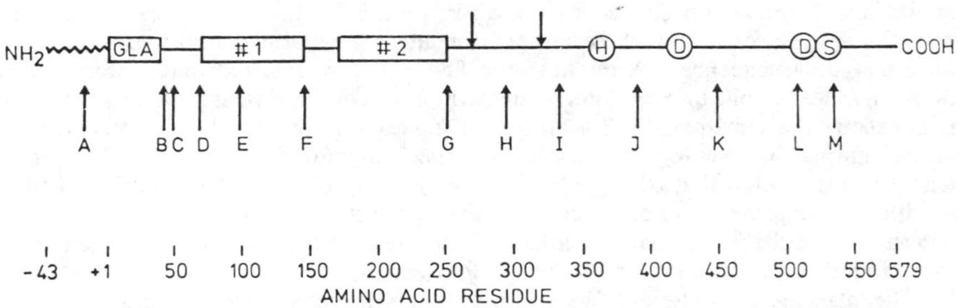

FIGURE 2. Placement of intervening sequences with respect to functional and structural domains in the gene coding for human prothrombin. The protein is represented on the top line with the amino- and carboxyl-terminal ends indicated by NH_2 and COOH, respectively. The leader sequence is represented by ∿∿∿ , the region containing the ten γ-carboxyglutamic acid residues by GLA, and the first and second kringle by #1 and #2. Amino acids in the active site and substrate binding pocket are represented as H (histidine), D (aspartic acid), and S (serine). Factor Xa cleavage sites are indicated by arrows above the protein. Placement of intervening sequences in the gene for human prothrombin are indicated by the lettered arrows below the protein.

diversification has been proposed to occur by recombination of exons from different primodial genes (exon shuffling).[34-36] In this way, proteins having domains in common occur, even if the remainder of the protein is very different. Prothrombin and the other proteins involved in coagulation and fibrinolysis appear to have evolved by these mechanisms.[36] Comparison of the organization of genes for related proteins and analysis of the placement of intervening sequence with respect to functional and structural domains is one way to study how these proteins have evolved.

The organization of the human prothrombin gene reflects the domain structure of the protein (FIGURE 2). The GLA region, second kringle, and each active site amino acid are each in individual exons. The first kringle, although divided into two exons, retains intervening sequences exactly at positions proposed to delineate this domain.

Factor IX and protein C, like prothrombin, contain GLA residues and are zymogens of serine proteases. The organization of the genes for factor IX and protein C have been reported.[29,37] Comparison of the placement of the intervening sequences in these three genes reveals a number of similarities. For example, the intervening sequence present within the signal sequence and the two immediately following the GLA region in prothrombin (intervening sequences A, B, and C in FIGURE 2) are found in similar positions in the genes for factor IX and protein C. The regions spanned by these intervening sequences are highly homologous between these three proteins and, in fact, are the most conserved part of these proteins. The growth factor domains (regions found to be homologous to epidermal growth factor) of factor IX and protein C follow the GLA domain and have no similarity to the kringle domains of prothrombin; the gene structure in these two different domains are not comparable. The placement of intervening sequences with respect to the active site amino acids in these proteins is discussed below.

Plasminogen, factor XII, tissue-plasminogen activator (t-PA), and urokinase (u-PA) are the only other proteins, besides prothrombin, known to contain kringle domains; plasminogen has five,[38] t-PA has two,[31] and u-PA and factor XII both have one.[39,40] The structure of the genes for t-PA and u-PA have been completely elucidated,[41–44] whereas that for plasminogen has been partially characterized.[45] The organization of intervening sequences in the t-PA and u-PA genes are extremely similar over the entire protein. All three kringle domains are separated into two exons with an intervening sequence present near the first and last cysteine that delineate this domain, as well as one internal intervening sequence. This internal intervening sequence is in exactly the same position for all three kringles, but different from the placement of the internal intervening sequence in the first kringle of prothrombin. This agrees with the observation that t-PA and u-PA are more closely related to each other than to other serine proteases. For plasminogen, the gene structure of kringle #4 has been determined, and the internal placement of the intervening sequence is distinct from those found in prothrombin, t-PA, and u-PA.

The placement of the active-site amino acids in separate exons has also been observed in the genes coding for other serine proteases. The three active-site amino acids (His, Asp, and Ser) are in individual exons in t-PA,[41,42] u-PA,[43,44] pancreatic kallikrein,[46] complement factor B,[47] trypsin,[48] chymotrypsin,[49] and elastase,[50] and in many cases the intervening sequences are located in similar positions with respect to these amino acids. In the genes for human factor IX[37] and protein C,[29] only the active site histidine is in an individual exon; the aspartic acid and serine are contained in the same exon.

These observations fit with the proposal that the genes coding for serine proteases evolved from a common ancestor.[33] Assuming that the ancestral gene contained intervening sequences, it seems reasonable to assume that each active site amino acid was present in individual exons. Any differences in number of intervening sequences may be attributed to insertions or deletions occurring throughout evolution, and slight variations in placement may be due to the sliding of intron-exon junctions.[51,52] The situation with regard to kringle domains is interesting. One possibility that accounts for the least number of insertions and/or deletions of intervening sequences could be that the ancestral gene containing the kringle domain coded for a kringle in one exon, as is the case for the second kringle of prothrombin. For prothrombin, this exon duplicated to form two kringle regions followed by random insertion of an intervening sequence in the first kringle domain, whereas for t-PA and u-PA, the random insertion of an intervening sequence occurred before duplication of the kringle domain, resulting in the identical placement of intervening sequences in these kringles. This same placement might also be expected in the gene for factor XII, because the kringle in this protein is most homologous to the kringles in t-PA and u-PA.

SUMMARY

The gene coding for human prothrombin has been isolated from two human genomic DNA libraries using a human prothrombin cDNA. Present evidence indicates that the gene is approximately 24 kb in length with about 90% of the DNA representing intervening sequence. Thirteen intervening sequences were found to interrupt the region coding for the mRNA into 14 exons. These intervening sequences vary greatly in size and contain at least 11 copies of Alu repetitive DNA. The positions where several of the intervening sequences interrupt the coding region appear to separate functional and structural domains of the protein. A similar placement of intervening sequences in genes coding for proteins homologous to prothrombin has been observed and provides additional evidence that these proteins have evolved from a common ancestor.

REFERENCES

1. MANN, K. G. & J. ELION. 1980. *In* CRC Handbook Series in Clinical Laboratory Science, Section I: Hematology. R. M. Schmidt, Ed. Vol. 3: 15-31. CRC Press. Boca Raton, FL.
2. DEGEN, S. J. F., R. T. A. MACGILLIVRAY & E. W. DAVIE. 1983. Biochemistry **22:** 2087-2097.
3. DISCIPIO, R. G., M. A. HERMODSON, S. G. YATES & E. W. DAVIE. 1977. Biochemistry **16:** 698-706.
4. MAGNUSSON, S., T. E. PETERSEN, L. SOTTRUP-JENSEN & H. CLAEYS. 1975. *In* Proteases and Biological Control. E. Reich, D. B. Rifkin & E. Shaw, Eds.: 123-149. Cold Spring Harbor Laboratories. Cold Spring Harbor, NY.
5. BUTKOWSKI, R. J., J. ELION, M. R. DOWNING & K. G. MANN. 1977. J. Biol. Chem. **252:** 4942-4957.
6. THOMPSON, A. R., D. L. ENFIELD, L. H. ERICSSON, M. E. LEGAZ & J. W. FENTON II. 1977. Arch. Biochem. Biophys. **178:** 356-367.
7. WALZ, D. A., D. HEWETT-EMMETT & W. H. SEEGERS. 1977. Proc. Natl. Acad. Sci. USA **74:** 1969-1972.
8. SEEGERS, W. H. 1979. Prog. Chem. Fibrinolysis Thrombolysis **4:** 241-254.
9. MACGILLIVRAY, R. T. A. & E. W. DAVIE. 1984. Biochemistry **23:** 1626-1634.
10. STENFLO, J., P. FERNLUND, W. EGAN & P. ROEPSTORFF. 1974. Proc. Natl. Acad. Sci. USA **71:** 2730-2733.
11. NELSESTUEN, G. L, T. H. ZYTKOVICZ & J. B. HOWARD. 1974. J. Biol. Chem. **249:** 6347-6350.
12. SUTTIE, J. W. 1983. *In* Plasma Protein Secretion by the Liver. H. Glaumann, T. Peters, Jr. & C. Redman, Eds.: 375-403. Academic Press. London.
13. PATTHY, L., M. TREXLER, Z. VALI, L. BANYAI & A. VARADI. 1984. FEBS Lett. **171:** 131-136.
14. ESMON, C. T. & C. M. JACKSON. 1974. J. Biol. Chem. **249:** 7791-7797.
15. ELION, J., M. R. DOWNING, R. J. BUTKOWSKI & K. G. MANN. 1977. *In* Chemistry and Biology of Thrombin. R. L. Lundbland, J. W. Fenton II & K. G. Mann, Eds.: 97-111. Ann Arbor Science Publishers. Ann Arbor, MI.
16. LAWN, R. M., E. F. FRITSCH, R. C. PARKER, G. BLAKE & T. MANIATIS. 1978. Cell **15:** 1157-1174.
17. BENTON, W. D. & R. W. DAVIS. 1977. Science **196:** 181-182.
18. WOO, S. L. C. 1979. Methods Enzymol. **68:** 389-395.
19. SOUTHERN, E. M. 1975. J. Mol. Biol. **98:** 503-517.
20. MOUNT, S. M. 1982. Nucleic Acids Res. **10:** 459-472.
21. BREATHNACH, R., C. BENOIST, K. O'HARE, F. GANNON & P. CHAMBON. 1978. Proc. Natl. Acad. Sci. USA **75:** 4853-4857.

22. SCHMID, C. W. & W. R. JELINEK. 1982. Science **216:** 1065-1070.
23. IRWIN, D. M., K. G. AHERN, G. D. PEARSON & R. T. A. MACGILLIVRAY. 1985. Biochemistry **24:** 6854-6861.
24. BLOBEL, G., P. WALTER, C. N. CHANG, B. M. GOLDMAN, A. H. ERICKSON & R. LINGAPPA. 1979. *In* Secretory Mechanisms. C. R. Hopkin & C. J. Duncan, Eds. Vol. **33:** 9-36. Cambridge University Press. London.
25. PATTERSON, J. E. & D. M. GELLER. 1977. Biochem. Biophysics Res. Commun. **74:** 1220-1226.
26. LAWN, R. M., J. ADELMAN, S. C. BOCK, A. E. FRANKE, C. M. HOUCK, R. C. NAJARIAN, P. H. SEEBURG & K. L. WION. 1981. Nucleic Acids Res. **9:** 6103-6114.
27. KURACHI, K. & E. W. DAVIE. 1982. Proc. Natl. Acad. Sci. USA **79:** 6461-6464.
28. FUNG, M. R., R. M. CAMPBELL & R. T. A. MACGILLIVRAY. 1984. Nucleic Acids Res. **12:** 4481-4492.
29. FOSTER, D. C., S. YOSHITAKE & E. W. DAVIE. 1985. Proc. Natl. Acad. Sci. USA **82:** 4673-4677.
30. BECKMANN, R. J., R. J. SCHMIDT, R. F. SANTERRE, J. PLUTZKY, G. R. CRABTREE & G. L. LONG. 1985. Nucleic Acids Res. **13:** 5233-5247.
31. PENNICA, D., W. F. HOLMES, W. J. KOHR, R. N. HARKINS, G. A. VEHAR, C. A. WARD, W. F. BENNET, E. YELVERTON, P. H. SEEBURG, H. L. HEYNEKER, D. V. GOEDDEL & D. COLLEN. 1983. Nature **301:** 214-221.
32. SHARP, P. A. 1981. Cell **23:** 643-646.
33. KATAYAMA, K., L. H. ERICSSON, D. L. ENFIELD, K. A. WALSH, H. NEURATH, E. W. DAVIE & K. TITANI. 1979. Proc. Natl. Acad. Sci. USA **76:** 4990-4994.
34. GILBERT, W. 1985. Science **228:** 823-824.
35. ROGERS, J. 1985. Nature **315:** 458-459.
36. PATTHY, L. 1985. Cell **41:** 657-663.
37. YOSHITAKE, S., B. G. SCHACH, D. C. FOSTER, E. W. DAVIE & K. KURACHI. 1985. Biochemistry **24:** 3736-3750.
38. SOTTRUP-JENSEN, L., H. CLAEYS, M. ZAJDEL, T. E. PETERSEN & S. MAGNUSSON. 1978. *In* Fibrinolysis and Thrombolysis. T. F. Davidson, R. M. Rowan, M. M. Samama & P. C. Desnoyer, Eds. Vol. **3:** 191-209. Raven Press. New York.
39. GUNZLER, W. A., G. J. STEFFENS, F. OTTING, S-M. A. KIM, E. FRANKUS & L. FLOHE. 1982. Hoppe-Seyler's Z. Physiol. Chem. **363:** 1155-1165.
40. MCMULLEN, B. A. & K. FUJIKAWA. 1985. J. Biol. Chem. **260:** 5328-5341.
41. DEGEN, S. J. F., B. RAJPUT & E. REICH. 1986. J. Biol. Chem. **261:** 6972-6985.
42. NY, T., F. ELGH & B. LUND. 1984. Proc. Natl. Acad. Sci. USA **81:** 5355-5359.
43. NAGAMINE, Y., D. PEARSON, M. S. ALTUS & E. REICH. 1984. Nucleic Acids Res. **12:** 9525-9541.
44. RICCIO, A., G. GRIMALDI, P. VERDE, G. SEBASTIO, S. BOAST & F. BLASI. 1985. Nucleic Acid Res. **13:** 2759-2771.
45. MALINOWSKI, D. P., J. E. SADLER & E. W. DAVIE. 1984. Biochemistry **23:** 4243-4250.
46. MASON, A. J., B. A. EVANS, D. R. COX, J. SHINE & R. I. RICHARDS. 1983. Nature **303:** 300-307.
47. CAMPBELL, R. D. & R. R. PORTER. 1983. Proc. Natl. Acad. Sci. USA **80:** 4464-4468.
48. CRAIK, C. S., Q-L. CHOO, G. H. SWIFT, C. QUINTO, R. J. MACDONALD & R. J. RUTTER. 1984. J. Biol. Chem. **259:** 14255-14264.
49. BELL, G. I., C. QUINTO, M. QUIROGA, P. VALENZUELA, C. S. CRAIK & R. J. RUTTER. 1984. J. Biol. Chem. **259:** 14265-14270.
50. SWIFT, G. H., C. S. CRAIK, S. J. STARY, C. QUINTO, R. G. LAHAIE, W. J. RUTTER & R. J. MACDONALD. 1984. J. Biol. Chem. **259:** 14271-14278.
51. STONE, E. M., K. N. ROTHBLUM & R. J. SCHWARTZ. 1985. Nature **313:** 498-500.
52. CRAIK, C. S., W. J. RUTTER & R. FLETTERICK. 1983. Science **220:** 1125-1129.

Recombinant Genetic Approaches to Functional Mapping of Thrombin[a]

ROSS T. A. MacGILLIVRAY,[b] DAVID M. IRWIN,[b]
ENRIQUETA R. GUINTO,[b] AND JAMES C. STONE[c]

[b]*Department of Biochemistry*
University of British Columbia
Vancouver, British Columbia V6T 1W5 Canada

[c]*The Jackson Laboratory*
Bar Harbor, Maine 04609

INTRODUCTION

During the final stages of blood coagulation, prothrombin is converted from an inactive zymogen to a serine protease called thrombin. This reaction is catalyzed by factor Xa in the presence of phospholipid, calcium ions, and an accessory protein called factor Va.[1] Thrombin then cleaves the fibrinopeptides A and B from the aminoterminal regions of the α and β chains of fibrinogen, respectively. The resulting fibrin monomers polymerize spontaneously to form the fibrin network that is the basis of the blood clot. These fibrin polymers are further strengthened by the action of factor XIIIa, which introduces covalent cross-links between the γ chains of adjacent fibrin molecules. Factor XIIIa is stored in plasma as an inactive precursor (factor XIII) that is also activated by thrombin (see ref. 2 for a recent review). In addition to its proteolytic effects of fibrinogen and factor XIII, thrombin also activates factor V,[3,4] factor VIII[5] and, in the presence of thrombomodulin, protein C.[6] In each of these cases, the activation involves limited proteolysis of the polypeptide chains by thrombin.

In contrast to many of the other clotting factors, thrombin has other activities that are independent of its proteolytic function. For example, proteolytically inactive thrombin is chemotactic for peripheral blood monocytes and cells belonging to the monocyte/macrophage family.[7–10] In addition, thrombin has mitogenic properties towards fibroblasts[11] and macrophages.[12] The latter growth factor activity is independent of esterolytic activity and has been localized to the "loop B" insertion sequence of the thrombin B chain.[12]

During the past few years, the many naturally occurring mutants of hemoglobin have allowed a detailed investigation of structural/functional relationships in this protein. The paucity, however, of such mutant forms of many proteins has limited this approach. The development of recombinant DNA techniques has introduced a powerful new method to study structural/functional relationships in any protein. Once a complementary DNA (cDNA) or gene coding for a protein has been cloned and characterized, it can be expressed in bacteria, yeast, or eukaryotic cells. By careful

[a] This work has been supported in part by a Grant from the British Columbia Heart Foundation.

selection of the appropriate regulatory sequences, large amounts of the corresponding protein can be expressed and characterized. Specific residues of the protein can then be changed or deleted by *in vitro* mutagenesis (see ref. 13 for a recent review). The effects of these changes on protein function can then be evaluated. In this paper, we discuss the application of *in vitro* mutagenesis approaches to studying the various activities of thrombin.

PROTHROMBIN cDNA CLONES

Several cDNA clones coding for both bovine and human prothrombin have been isolated. Initially, MacGillivray *et al.* used immunoadsorption of bovine liver polysomes to purify bovine prothrombin mRNA.[14,15] The resulting mRNA preparation was sufficiently pure to be used as a hybridization probe to screen a bovine liver cDNA library. Three positives were isolated and DNA sequence analysis showed that pBII3 contained DNA coding for the carboxyterminal 160 amino acid residues of prothrombin in addition to a 3′ untranslated region of 119 base pairs (bp) and a poly(A) tail (FIG. 1).

To isolate cDNA clones coding for the remainder of bovine prothrombin mRNA, a cDNA library was constructed that contained 90,000 independent recombinants containing cDNA inserts that were greater than 1,000 bp in size.[15] When this library was screened by using pBII3 as a hybridization probe, many positive clones were identified.[15] Two of these, pBII102 and pBII111, contained overlapping DNA coding for 5 bp of 5′ untranslated sequence, a leader peptide of 43 amino acids, the complete sequence of plasma prothrombin, the 3′ untranslated sequence, and a poly(A) tail (FIG. 1). The initiator methionine was identified by translating prothrombin mRNA in a rabbit reticulocyte lysate in the presence of radiolabeled amino acids. The resulting translation product was isolated by immunoprecipitation and analyzed by automatic Edman degradations in a Sequenator. The resulting partial sequence agreed well with that predicted from the cDNA sequence.[15]

Degen *et al.* used the bovine prothrombin cDNA as a hybridization probe to isolate human prothrombin cDNAs.[16] The hybridizations were performed under conditions of reduced stringency to allow for mismatches between the bovine and human sequences. Three of the positives were characterized (FIG. 1). The longest clone, pHII3, contained DNA coding for part of a leader peptide of 36 amino acids as well as the entire coding region of the plasma protein, a 3′ untranslated sequence of 97 bp and a poly(A) tail (FIG. 1).

To isolate a human prothrombin cDNA clone coding for the remainder of the leader peptide, we screened a different cDNA library[17] using pBII111 as a hybridization probe. One hundred and twenty thousand colonies were screened by colony hybridization[18] using the same conditions as Degen *et al.*[16] Eight of the positives were characterized further. By restriction endonuclease mapping, pIIH13 appeared to be a full-length cDNA for human prothrombin. The DNA sequence of the 5′ region of pIIH13 was determined as shown in FIG. 2. The DNA sequence was determined on both strands by using the chain termination method.[19] Translation of the cDNA sequence using the standard genetic code showed that pIIH13 did indeed contain DNA coding for human prothrombin. Nucleotides 157-327 (FIG. 2) encoded amino acid residues 1-57 of plasma prothrombin. Nucleotides 49-156 (FIG. 2) encode the part of the leader sequence in pHII3 as reported by Degen *et al.*[16] Upstream of nucleotide 49 is an ATG codon (nucleotides 28-30, FIG. 2) that is in the same position as the initiator methionine found in bovine prothrombin.[15] Six nucleotides upstream of this ATG codon is a TGA stop codon (nucleotides 19-21, FIG. 2) strongly suggesting that the ATG at nucleotides 28-30 encodes the initiator methionine for human prothrombin mRNA. In that case, human prothrombin is synthesized as a precursor containing a leader peptide of 43 amino acid residues. This is the same length as the bovine prothrombin leader peptide. There are seven differences between the amino acid sequences of the bovine and human prothrombin leader peptides (FIG. 3).

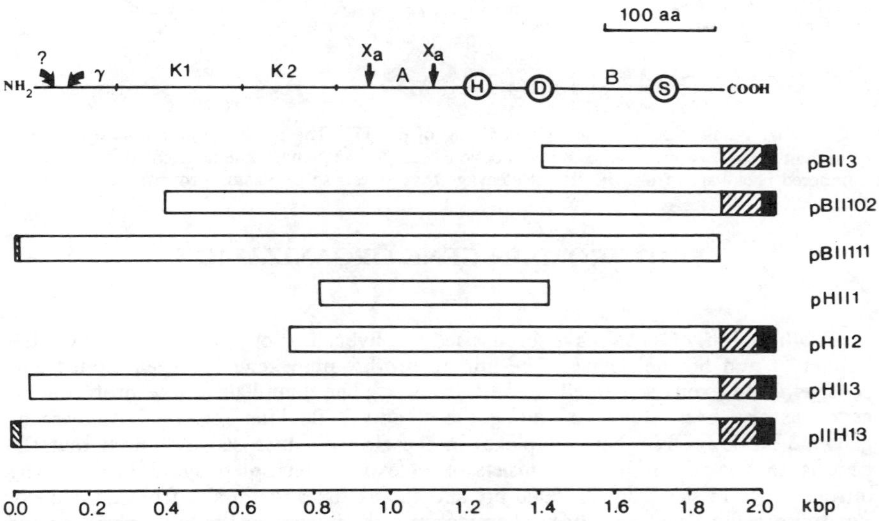

FIGURE 1. Bovine and human prothrombin cDNA clones. The prepro-prothrombin polypeptide chain is represented at the top and includes the proposed signal peptidase cleavage site (➘), the putative proprotease cleavage site (➚), the γ-carboxyglutamic acid region (γ), the two kringle regions (K1 and K2), the factor Xa cleavage sites (↓), the B and A chains of thrombin, and the histidine, aspartic acid, and serine residues at the active site of thrombin (H, D, and S). The bars underneath the protein represent the cDNAs including the 5′ untranslated region (slashed bar), preproprothrombin coding region (open bar), 3′ untranslated region (slashed bar) and poly (A) tail (solid bar). The scale at the top represents 100 amino acids, and the scale at the bottom is in kilobase pairs (kbp). Data are from references 14-16 and this paper. See text for details.

As has been found for the other vitamin K dependent clotting factors (see ref. 20), human prothrombin is synthesized as a preproprotein. Presumably, signal peptidase cleaves the leader peptide during the transfer of the nascent chain across the rough endoplasmic reticulum membrane giving rise to a proprothrombin molecule. Swanson and Suttie[21] have reported the isolation of such a species from rat liver microsomes and showed that it contained a basic M_r 1500 peptide that was missing from the plasma form of prothrombin. The function of the propiece is not clear, but because the amino acid sequences of the propieces of the vitamin K-dependent clotting factors and osteocalcin are homologous,[22] it is possible that this region may be involved in the vitamin K-dependent carboxylation of these proteins.

```
                                    -43         -40                                         -30
                                    Met Ala Arg Ile Arg Gly Leu Gln Leu Pro Gly Cys Leu Ala Leu Ala
CCC TAG TGA CCC AGG AGC TGA CAC ACT ATG GCC CGC ATC CGA GGC TTG CAG CTG CCT GGC TGC CTG GCC CTG GCT
                 15                  30                  45                  60                  75

                        -20                                     -10
Ala Leu Cys Ser Leu Val His Ser Gln His Val Phe Leu Ala Pro Gln Gln Ala Arg Ser Leu Leu Gln Arg Val
GCC CTG TGT AGC CTT GTG CAC AGC CAG CAT GTG TTC CTG GCT CCT CAG CAA GCA CGG TCG CTG CTC CAG CGG GTC
                 90                 105                 120                 135                 150

    -1  +1                              10                                      20
Arg Arg Ala Asn Thr Phe Leu Glu Glu Val Arg Lys Gly Asn Leu Glu Arg Glu Cys Val Glu Glu Thr Cys Ser
CGG CGA GCC AAC ACC TTC TTG GAG GAG GTG CGC AAG GGC AAC CTG GAG CGA GAG TGC GTG GAG GAG ACG TGC AGC
                165                 180                 195                 210                 225

                            30                                      40
Tyr Glu Glu Ala Phe Glu Ala Leu Glu Ser Ser Thr Ala Thr Asp Val Phe Trp Ala Lys Tyr Thr Ala Cys Glu
TAC GAG GAG GCC TTC GAG GCT CTG GAG TCC TCC ACG GCT ACG GAT GTG TTC TGG GCC AAG TAC ACA GCT TGT GAG
                240                 255                 270                 285                 300

    50
Thr Ala Arg Thr Pro Arg Asp Lys Leu
ACA GCG AGG ACG CCT CGA GAT AAG CTT
                315                 327
```

FIGURE 2. Nucleotide sequence of the 5′ end of pIIH13. The predicted amino acid sequence of human preproprothrombin is shown above the cDNA sequence. The leader peptide has been numbered backwards from the site of cleavage that gives rise to plasma prothrombin.

PROTHROMBIN GENE ORGANIZATION

Prothrombin cDNAs have been used as hybridization probes to isolate the human[16,23] and bovine[24] genes. The human prothrombin gene has been cloned and consists of 14 exons separated by 13 introns.[16,23] The complete bovine prothrombin gene has also been cloned including the 5′ and 3′ flanking regions.[24] Analysis of genomic DNA/cDNA heteroduplexes in the electron microscope showed that the gene is 15 kbp in length and consists of 14 exons interrupted by 13 introns. The introns range in size from 75-6900 bp, and the exons range in size from 25-315 bp. For those regions that have been characterized, the introns in the human and bovine genes are located in identical positions.[16,23–25]

EXPRESSION OF THE PROTHROMBIN GENE

The successful expression of a cloned gene in a heterologous system depends upon the ability of the cell line to process the primary translation product correctly, and upon the ability of the polypeptide chain to fold into the correct conformation. In the case of prothrombin gene expression, the cell line must be able to remove the pre- and propieces and carboxylate certain glutamic acid residues before functional pro-

```
         -43         -40                                     -30
BOVINE:  Met Ala Arg Val Arg Gly Pro Arg Leu Pro Gly Cys Leu Ala Leu Ala Ala Leu Phe Ser Leu Val
HUMAN :  Met Ala Arg Ile Arg Gly Leu Gln Leu Pro Gly Cys Leu Ala Leu Ala Ala Leu Cys Ser Leu Val

             -20                                     -10                                 -1  +1
BOVINE:  His Ser Gln His Val Phe Leu Ala His Gln Gln Ala Ser Ser Leu Leu Gln Arg Ala Arg Arg Ala
HUMAN :  His Ser Gln His Val Phe Leu Ala Pro Gln Gln Ala Arg Ser Leu Leu Gln Arg Val Arg Arg Ala
```

FIGURE 3. Comparison of the amino acid sequences of the leader peptides of bovine[15] and human prothrombin. Residues that are different between the two sequences are boxed.

thrombin can be formed. In addition, plasma prothrombin is glycosylated,[26] but the carbohydrate moiety has no effect on the enzymic[27,28] and nonenzymic[8] properties of thrombin.

Three groups have successfully expressed a cloned human factor IX gene. Anson *et al.*[29] used a human factor IX cDNA under the control of the promoter of the long terminal repeat of Moloney murine leukemia virus. The transcription unit was completed by placing the Simian virus 40 (SV40) small t antigen intron and polyadenylation signal downstream of the cDNA. This expression plasmid produced factor IX antigen in fibroblasts and in the rat hepatoma cell line H4-11-E-C3, although only the hepatoma cell line produced functional factor IX (*i.e.* carboxylated factor IX). A different approach was used by de la Salle *et al.*[30] who inserted a factor IX cDNA into a vaccinia virus-derived vector. Again, active factor IX was produced after infection of the human hepatoma cell line HepG2, but little factor IX activity was produced after infection of fibroblasts. Finally, Bubsy *et al.*[31] placed a human factor IX cDNA under the control of the adenovirus 2 major late promoter and obtained active factor IX after introduction of the clone into baby hamster kidney cells. Thus, it appears that

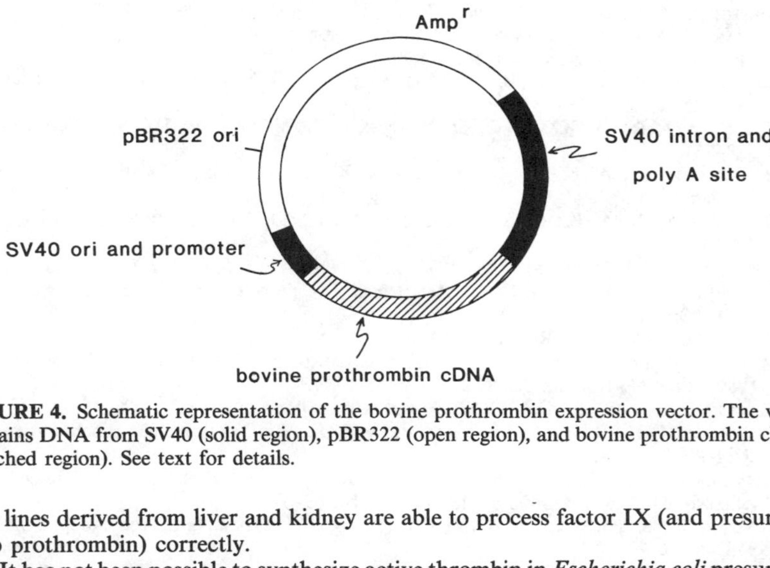

FIGURE 4. Schematic representation of the bovine prothrombin expression vector. The vector contains DNA from SV40 (solid region), pBR322 (open region), and bovine prothrombin cDNA (hatched region). See text for details.

cell lines derived from liver and kidney are able to process factor IX (and presumably also prothrombin) correctly.

It has not been possible to synthesize active thrombin in *Escherichia coli* presumably because the protein does not fold properly.[32] For this reason, we have chosen to express the prothrombin cDNA in eukaryotic cells. If we can express functionally active prothrombin, we will be able to use *in vitro* mutagenesis techniques to study the steps involved in the biosynthesis of prothrombin. We will also be able to generate thrombin by proteolysis of the prothrombin, thereby allowing a study of structural/functional relationships in thrombin.

We have constructed a prothrombin expression plasmid as shown in FIGURE 4. The hybrid vector is based on pSV2gpt,[33] which contains a pBR322 origin of replication and β-lactamase gene (allowing selection and growth in *E. coli*) joined to a segment of SV40 DNA containing the SV40 early promoter upstream of *Ecogpt* (the *E. coli* gene coding for xanthine-guanine phosphoribosyltransferase). The *Ecogpt* segment is followed by another SV40 DNA segment containing the small t antigen intervening sequence, the early region polyadenylation site, and the 3′ terminal segment of SV40's late region. The *Ecogpt* gene was excised and replaced with a full-length bovine prothrombin cDNA. This was derived from the cDNA inserts of pBII102 and pBII111 after removal of the polydeoxyguanosine/cytosine tails (from the cloning procedure) and the polydeoxyadenosine/thymidine tail. We are currently using this expression vector to transform HepG2 cells. If we can obtain high levels of functional bovine prothrombin, we will initiate similar experiments using human prothrombin cDNA.

REFERENCES

1. JACKSON, C. M., C. T. ESMON & W. G. OWEN. 1975. *In* Proteases and biological control. E. Reich, D. B. Rifkin & E. Shaw, Eds.: 95-109, Cold Spring Harbor Laboratory. Cold Spring Harbor, New York.
2. JACKSON, C. M. & Y. NEMERSON. 1980. Annu. Rev. Biochem. **49:** 765-811.
3. ESMON, C. T. 1978. J. Biol. Chem. **254:** 964-973.
4. NESHEIM, M. E. & K. G. MANN. 1978. J. Biol. Chem. **254:** 1326-1334.
5. VEHAR, G. A. & E. W. DAVIE. 1980. Biochemistry **19:** 401-410.
6. ESMON, C. T. 1983. Blood **62:** 1155-1158.
7. BAR-SHAVIT, R., A. KAHN, J. W. FENTON II & G. D. WILNER. 1983. J. Cell Biol. **96:** 282-285.
8. BAR-SHAVIT, R., A. KAHN, G. D. WILNER & J. W. FENTON II. 1983. Science **220:** 728-731.
9. BAR-SHAVIT, R., A. KAHN, G. D. WILNER, K. G. MANN & J. W. FENTON II. 1984. Biochemistry **23:** 397-400.
10. BAR-SHAVIT, R., A. KAHN, J. W. FENTON II & G. D. WILNER. 1983. Lab. Invest. **49:** 702-707.
11. CHEN, L. B. & J. M. BUCHANAN. 1975. Proc. Natl. Acad. Sci. USA **72:** 131-135.
12. BAR-SHAVIT, R., A. KAHN, K. G. MANN & G. D. WILNER. 1986. Proc. Natl. Acad. Sci. USA. **83:** 976-980.
13. SMITH, M. 1985. Annu. Rev. Genet. **19:** 423-462.
14. MACGILLIVRAY, R. T. A., S. J. F. DEGEN, T. CHANDRA, S. L. C. WOO & E. W. DAVIE. 1980. Proc. Natl. Acad. Sci. USA **77:** 5153-5157.
15. MACGILLIVRAY, R. T. A. & E. W. DAVIE. 1984. Biochemistry **23:** 1626-1634.
16. DEGEN, S. J. F., R. T. A. MACGILLIVRAY & E. W. DAVIE. 1983. Biochemistry **22:** 2087-2097.
17. PROCHOWNIK, E. V., A. F. MARKHAM & S. H. ORKIN. 1983. J. Biol. Chem. **258:** 8389-8394.
18. HANAHAN, D. & M. MESELSON. 1980. Gene **10:** 63-67.
19. SANGER, F., S. NICKLEN & A. R. COULSON. 1977. Proc. Natl. Acad. Sci. USA **74:** 5463-5467.
20. FUNG, M. R., C. W. HAY & R. T. A. MACGILLIVRAY. 1985. Proc. Natl. Acad. Sci. USA **82:** 3591-3595.
21. SWANSON, J. C. & J. W. SUTTIE. 1985. Biochemistry **24:** 3890-3897.
22. PAN, L. C. & P. A. PRICE. 1985. Proc. Natl. Acad. Sci. USA **82:** 6109-6113.
23. DEGEN, S. J. F., B. RAJPUT, E. REICH & E. W. DAVIE. 1985. Protides Biol. Fluids Proc. Colloq. **33:** 47-50.
24. IRWIN, D. M., K. G. AHERN, G. D. PEARSON & R. T. A. MACGILLIVRAY. 1985. Biochemistry **24:** 6854-6861.
25. IRWIN, D. M. & R. T. A. MACGILLIVRAY. 1986. Manuscript submitted.
26. MAGNUSSON, S., T. E. PETERSEN, L. SOTTRUP-JENSEN & H. CLAEYS. 1975. *In* Proteases and biological control. E. Reich, D. B. Rifkin & E. Shaw, Eds.: 123-149. Cold Spring Harbor Laboratory. Cold Spring Harbor, New York.
27. HORNE III, MCD. K. & H. R. GRALNICK. 1984. Blood **63:** 188-194.
28. ROSENFELD, L. & I. DANISHEFSKY. 1984. Arch. Biochem. Biophys. **229:** 359-367.

29. ANSON, D. S., D. E. G. AUSTEN & G. G. BROWNLEE. 1985. Nature (London) **315:** 683-685.
30. DE LA SALLE, H., W. ALTERBURGER, R. ELKAIM, K. DOTT, A. DIETERLE, R. DRILLIEN, J-P. CAZENAVE, P. TOLSTOSHEV & J-P. LECOCQ. 1985. Nature (London) **316:** 268-270.
31. BUSBY, S., A. KUMAR, M. JOSEPH, L. HALFPAP, M. INSLEY, K. BERKNER, K. KURACHI & R. WOODBURY. 1985. Nature (London) **316:** 271-273.
32. THORNEGATE, F., P. GREEN, R. T. A. MACGILLIVRAY & D. FOWLKES. 1985. Thromb. Haemostasis **54:** 46.
33. SOUTHERN, P. J. & P. BERG. 1982. J. Mol. Appl. Genet. **1:** 327-341.

PART II. SUBSTRATE SPECIFICITY AND ACTIVE-SITE MODELING OF THROMBIN

Thrombin: Active-Site Topography[a]

LAWRENCE J. BERLINER, JENS J. BIRKTOFT, THEODORE L. MILLER, GIOVANNI MUSCI, JULIE E. SCHEFFLER, YUAN YUAN SHEN, AND YOSHIAKI SUGAWARA[a]

Department of Chemistry
The Ohio State University
Columbus, Ohio 43210

INTRODUCTION

In this paper, we will focus principally on the applications of spectroscopic and enzymological techniques for learning about binding sites and functionalities in the human thrombins. In particular, we will present evidence for the bioregulation of thrombin functions. Our approach has been to mimic thrombin-macromolecule binding *in vivo* as its component interactions; that is, when thrombin interacts with another coagulation factor, for example, protein C, there are specific interactions with thrombin binding loci that are critical to this interaction. These loci may be localized to interactions involving a few amino acid residues at most. Thus, these sites are related to small ligands or metabolites that bind specifically to thrombin and elicit distinct effects on its functionality. Surprisingly, much of our insight about the structural features of α-thrombin came first from the spin-labeling technique.[1] This has resulted in a concerted effort in designing specific active site (and exosite) probes of varying geometry, which enable the various regions of the α-thrombin structure and their interrelationships to be identified.

In particular, knowledge of the details of the thrombin-fibrinogen interaction is critical to our understanding both of the structural aspects of events directly preceding clot formation, as well as its relevance to other thrombin-macromolecule interactions. Some useful tools for studying the fibrinogen binding and cleavage reactions include modified thrombins that lack essentially only clotting activity. Under microbially sterile conditions for three days at pH 8, 25°C, a pure α-thrombin preparation converts to a mixture of α, β, and γ forms. The latter two forms completely retain esterase activity, whereas no clotting activity remains.[2] The same conversion may also be effected by passing pure human α-thrombin over trypsin-Sepharose, wherein complete α to γ conversion is accomplished.[2,3] The two specific cleavages that yield the noncovalently associated β and γ forms have been characterized in both the human and bovine species.[4] Whereas γ-thrombin does not bind fibrinogen, it binds hirudin more

[a]Supported in part by a Grant from the U.S. Public Health Service (HL 24549).

weakly and behaves otherwise identically to α-thrombin in other hemostatic events such as antithrombin III-heparin complex formation, factor XIII activation, and several plasma related reactions (*e.g.* complement C3 and C5, mitogenic stimulation[5]). Thus the γ form truly approaches the model for α-thrombin that does not clot while retaining most other catalytic features.

SPIN LABELING AS A SPECTROSCOPIC PROBE OF THROMBIN CONFORMATION

The spin labeling method uses electron spin resonance (ESR) spectroscopy to monitor the spectral lineshape of selectively targeted affinity labels based on the organic nitroxide ring structure. The information derived from the ESR experiment is dynamic, that is, of the rotational freedom (or restricted mobility) of the nitroxide moiety.[1] FIGURE 1 depicts a spin label-derived thrombin binding site topography map.[6] The results surmised in this map came from the incorporation of specific fluorosulfonyl-phenyl substituted nitroxide derivatives as depicted in FIGURE 2. Each of these derivatives reacts specifically and uniquely with the active serine 195 of thrombin, and in precisely the same fashion as other phenylsulfonyl fluoride inhibitors react with thrombin, α-chymotrypsin, trypsin, elastase, protein C (PC), and other serine proteases.[7] Thus, by studying the broad series of spin-labeled sulfonyl fluorides depicted in FIGURE 2, we were able to elucidate two general binding loci in human α- and γ-thrombins:

(a) One series of these fluorosulfonyl spin labels (indole site), which were all linear in shape, experienced distinct environmental changes (as manifested in a decrease in the mobility of the nitroxide) upon the binding of apolar ligands such as indole and tryptamine. Whereas it cannot be stated explicitly that this binding site was coincidental with the binding locus of the nitroxide spin label, one can at least state that the environment of the spin label was changed (or affected) by binding of the apolar ligand. The mechanism behind this change, in the case where the apolar (or indole) site is distant from the active site, is an indole-induced conformational change that is expressed at the binding locus of the nitroxide. This apolar binding affects several other functions of thrombin, which include inactivation of esterase kinetics and clotting rates, to be discussed later.

(b) The second binding region was found from a series of spin labels (α-γ site) with bent structures, that is, where the nitroxide was substituted at the meta position of the phenylsulfonyl fluoride. This site detected subtle structural differences between the coagulant α- and noncoagulant γ-human thrombin forms as shown in FIGURE 3.

We have thus far shown that the conformation of the γ-thrombin active site is identical to that of the α form except for one region about 8-14 Å away from the active serine where a small structural obstruction has occurred.[6] Furthermore, we also demonstrated that the three- (noncovalently associated) fragment γ form could be denatured, dissociated, and then shown to recombine with full activity even though each one of the three critical groups of the catalytic triad (Asp-His-Ser) exists on a separate chain.[8]

Because no x-ray crystal structure is yet available that might explain which features of the γ-thrombin structure contribute to its obliterated coagulation ability, this result was of much importance. Specifically, all nitroxides that detected the γ-thrombin structural differences were more immobilized, that is, hindered in their motion, than

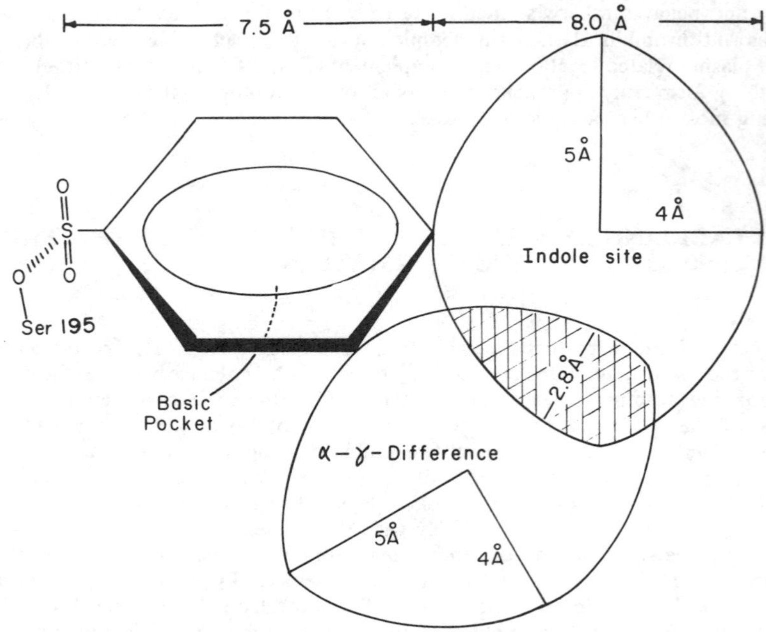

FIGURE 1. Two-dimensional representation of human thrombin active site topography as a map constructed from the accessible volume of rotation of each nitroxide moiety with respect to the phenylsulfonyl group. The distances, which include van der Waals radii, were measured from Corey-Pauling-Koltun models. The distance marker at the phenyl ring bisects the covalent bond between the ring and the nitroxide moiety. The two oblate ellipsoids of revolution approximate those of the smallest spin label that senses the designated thrombin structural feature. The volume of intersection excludes either the indole or α-γ difference sites.[6]

in the corresponding α-thrombin derivative. It is again important to emphasize that these spin labels are in a sense isomorphous; that is, they are covalently linked to precisely the same serine in a catalytic site that appears to be identical by several criteria in both species.[9,10] Perhaps the obstruction in nitroxide rotation is related to the obstruction of binding of the fibrinogen molecule to γ-thrombin, explaining the totally obliterated fibrinogen clotting activity of this thrombin derivative.[6] The development in this article will focus on these various binding loci, including other binding loci that have been discovered from enzymological and physical measurements.

THE α- TO γ-THROMBIN STRUCTURAL CHANGE

The spin-label studies located a site close to the active serine where α- and γ-thrombin differed significantly.[6] On the other hand, adjacent regions of the α- and γ-thrombin active site were identical by several criteria: The apolar site-sensitive spin labels showed essentially identical mobility and changes upon indole binding for the several labels tested. The intrinsic fluorescence of both forms as well as the properties of two small active site-directed (irreversible) fluorescent inhibitors were identical in λ_{em}^{max}, quantum yield, and energy transfer efficiency.[10] The fluorophore, bis-ANS, binds to γ-thrombin threefold stronger with a quantum yield threefold greater than that observed for the α-species, although the λ_{em}^{max} was identical for both.[11]

The spin-label results with the thrombins were also compared closely to trypsin: The immediate active site conformation, as reflected by sulfonyl fluoride spin label mobility between α-thrombin and trypsin, was quite similar for *m*-substituted spin labels. The basic specificity binding pocket must be deeper in trypsin, however, because benzamidine and other basic trypsin inhibitors did not displace nor alter any spin label probe from its orientation over the pocket, whereas for both α- and γ-thrombin, every spin label underwent a conformational shift upon benzamidine binding. Trypsin was not affected by indole binding.[6]

With the absence of a thrombin x-ray crystal structure, we employed molecular computer graphics modeling of the thrombin B chain, based on the atomic coordinates of porcine trypsin.[12] The structure was generated by aligning homologous regions of

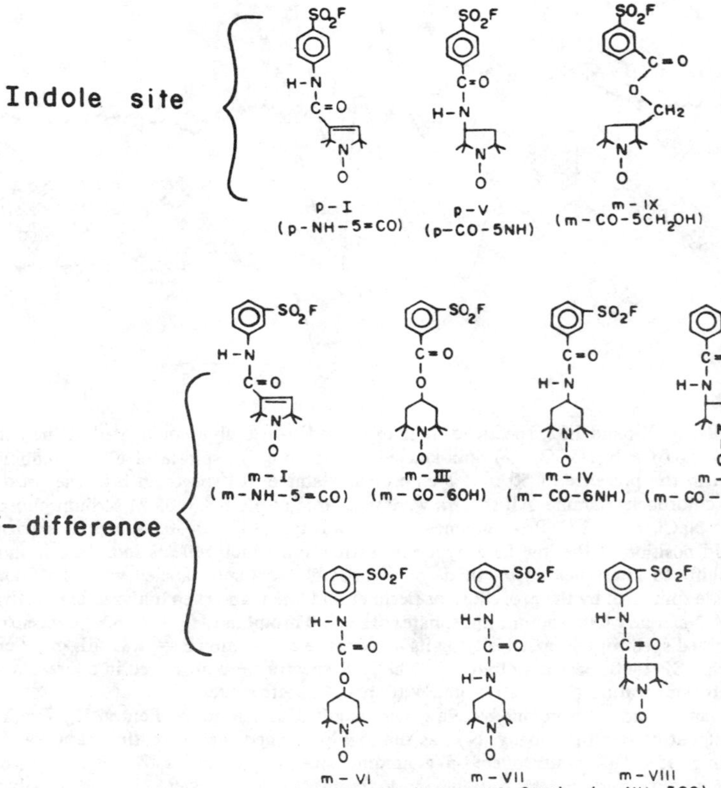

FIGURE 2. Structure of spin-labeled sulfonyl fluorides. Compounds that are isomers of the same structure are designated by the same Roman numeral. The two classes of label, indole site and α-γ difference, respectively, are related to the tumbling domains in space of each nitroxide group relative to the sulfonyl substituent on the ring.[6]

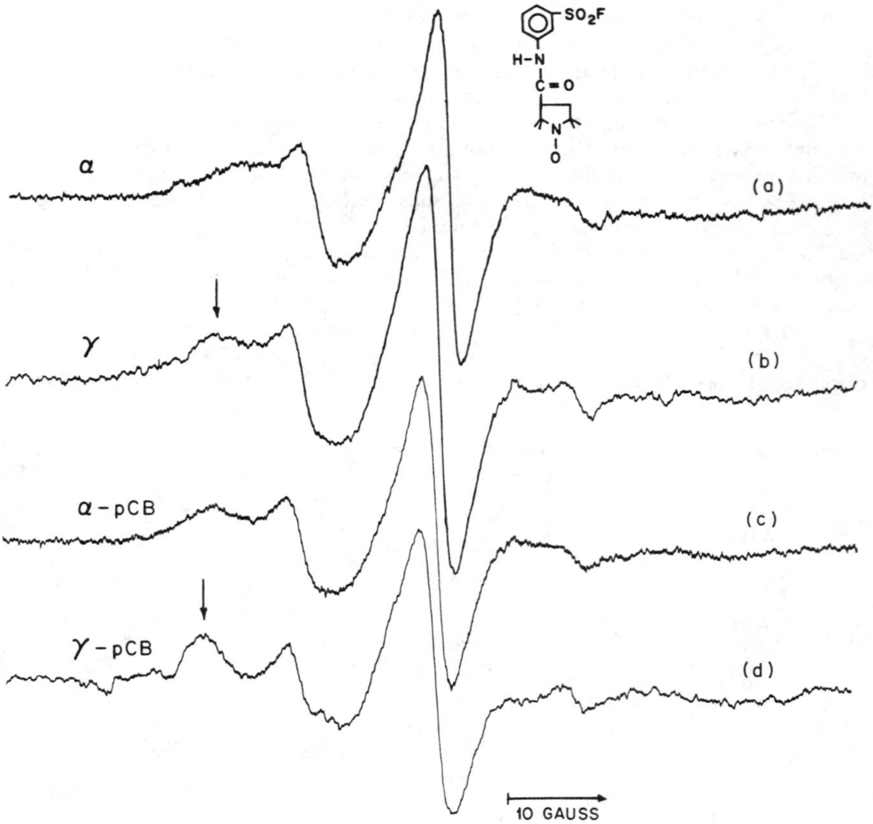

FIGURE 3. X-band ESR spectra of human α- and γ-thrombin conjugated at the active serine with *m*-VIII (*m*-NH-5CO). (**a**) Spin-labeled α-thrombin; (**b**) spin-labeled γ-thrombin; (**c**) spectrum a in the presence of 50 mM *p*-chlorobenzylamine; (**d**) spectrum b in the presence of 50 mM *p*-chlorobenzylamine. All spectra were measured at pH 6.5, 0.05 M sodium phosphate, and 0.75 M NaCl, 26 ± 2°C. Protein concentration was typically 0.07-0.08 mM. The arrows denote the field position of the low field hyperfine extremum, which reflects increased immobilization as it shifts to lower field. Human α- or γ-thrombin was spin labeled with the fluorosulfonyl nitroxide spin label by the procedure of Berliner and Shen[7] and then dialyzed exhaustively versus 0.75 M NaCl and 0.05 sodium phosphate, pH 6.5. Thrombin (M_r = 36,600) concentration was determined spectrophotometrically by its absorbance at 280 nm (E = 1.83 mL mg^{-1} cm^{-1}) with a Unicam SP 1800 spectrophotometer.[3] The ESR spectra were measured in quartz flat cells near ambient temperature (26 ± 1°C) on a Varian E-4 spectrometer.

Human α- and γ-thrombins were a generous gift of Dr. John W. Fenton II, New York State Department of Health, Albany, NY, as the highly purified species (α-thrombin was 3000 NIH units/mg, 95−98% *p*-nitrophenyl-*p*′-guanidinobenzoate [NPGB] active sites). Enzyme purity, specific activity, and analysis of polypeptide fragment structure were checked in Albany and in our laboratories by sodium dodecyl sulfate gel electrophoresis (nonreducing, reducing); clotting and esterase (Tos-Arg-OMe) activities and active-site concentration (NPGB) were checked by described procedures.[2] The enzyme was stored in 0.75 M NaCl at −72°C and thawed only immediately before use. Standard thrombin (lot B-3), 21.7 NIH units/mg, was supplied by Dr. D. Aronson, Bureau of Biologics, FDA, Bethesda, MD.

bovine or human thrombin with the serine protease family. Particular emphasis was placed on evaluating probable orientations of the *m*- or *p*-substituted phenylsulfonyl fluoride spin labels discussed above.[13] One of the most useful views of a general serine protease structure was accomplished by rotating the standard view 90° up (about the horizontal axis) to form a "bowl" or "crown" view with the catalytic center at the bottom of the bowl, the major structural differences between the serine proteases, and especially the β- and γ-insertion loops in the thrombins (FIGURE 4).

Analysis of the potential interactions of the spin labels with α- or γ-thrombin did not necessarily suggest that the proteolytic cleavages to yield γ-thrombin should have a direct effect on the positioning of the spin labels; rather, the cleavage might afford the spin label much greater freedom to adopt even more preferential binding inter-

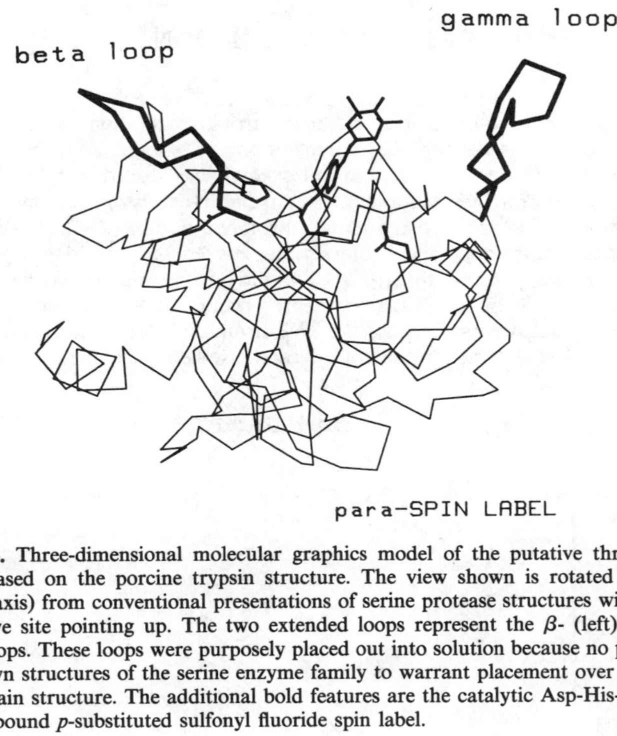

FIGURE 4. Three-dimensional molecular graphics model of the putative thrombin B-chain structure based on the porcine trypsin structure. The view shown is rotated 90° (about the horizontal axis) from conventional presentations of serine protease structures with the entrance to the active site pointing up. The two extended loops represent the β- (left) and γ- (right) insertion loops. These loops were purposely placed out into solution because no precedent exists in the known structures of the serine enzyme family to warrant placement over specific regions of the B-chain structure. The additional bold features are the catalytic Asp-His-Ser triad and a covalently bound *p*-substituted sulfonyl fluoride spin label.

actions. Because the *m*-substituted labels were more immobilized in γ- than α-thrombin (FIG. 3), we concluded that the cleaved γ- and/or β-loops somehow participated in the formation of additional hydrophobic binding loci accessible to the nitroxide. Binding of benzamidine in the basic pocket sterically disrupts the sulfonyl oxygen:oxyanion hole interaction, forcing all spin labels into an alternate orientation consistent with the ESR results that showed a large change in mobility.[6]

A major question that resulted from these modeling studies was to what extent the β- and/or γ-loops penetrate into the "bowl" or active site because they are involved to some extent in spin label interactions. We were intrigued by reports published fifteen years ago that claimed that trypsin-inhibitor proteins did not affect thrombin.[14,15] After examining a putative thrombin-bovine pancreatic trypsin inhibitor

(BPTI) complex by molecular graphics, based on an isomorphous trypsin-BPTI structure, it was clear that the γ- and/or β-loop must fold down into the "crown" (active site region) in order to block BPTI binding.[13] We have carefully reexamined α- as well as noncoagulant γ-thrombin for binding to soybean trypsin inhibitor (STI), ovomucoid (egg white) trypsin inhibitor, and BPTI[16] (FIGURE 5). To our surprise we observed very weak BPTI and STI inhibition of both α- and γ-thrombin amidase activity (using the chromogenic tripeptide anilide, S-2238) with K_i values up to six to nine orders of magnitude weaker than that for trypsin (see TABLE 1).[17] The ovomucoid protein was ineffective, which may be a reflection of the large molecular weight of this inhibitor.

THROMBOMODULATION

The phenomenon of homotropic and heterotropic regulation in biochemistry is well documented and fascinating. Thrombin, of course, should be without exception as a bioregulated enzyme. A most unusual system was discovered by Esmon and colleagues for the heterotropic stimulation of thrombin-catalyzed activation of PC by a specific protein, which adopted the name, thrombomodulin (TM).[18,19] Whereas the molecular details of this noncovalent interaction between TM and α-thrombin are not completely known at present, the (*ca* 20,000-fold) activation of bovine thrombin/bovine PC (*ca* 800-fold in the human system)[20] occurs by not occluding the active site from access by substrates. Because the TM:thrombin interaction is probably quite extensive and involves several component interactions, we have coined the term throm-

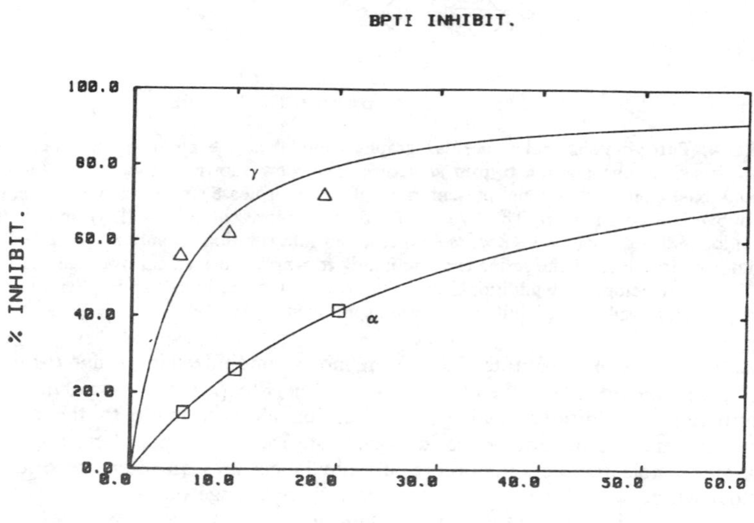

FIGURE 5. Inhibition of human α-thrombin (□) or γ-thrombin (△) catalyzed hydrolysis of S-2238 by increasing concentrations of BPTI. Conditions were 2.5 nM α-thrombin, 0.1 M NaCl, 0.05 M Tris-HCl, pH 8.3, 25°C.

TABLE 1. Inhibition of Human Thrombins by Various Trypsin Inhibitors

	K_i(app), amidase[a]			
Inhibitor	α-Thrombin	γ-Thrombin	Clotting	Trypsin[17]
STI	85 μM	85 μM	8.7 μM	2×10^{-10} M
BPTI	2.0 mM	0.3 mM	0.16 mM	$10^{-11}-10^{-12}$ M
Ovomucoid	NI[b]	NI	NI	5×10^{-9} M

[a] Assayed by S-2238 hydrolysis, pH 8.3, 0.1 M NaCl, 0.05 M Tris-HCl.
[b] NI, no inhibition observed up to 2.1 mM ovomucoid.

bomodulation to describe conformational changes caused by binding interactions at one or more loci that are not at the catalytic center. This is manifested in catalytic rate enhancements (*e.g.*, amidase, esterase, clotting, PC activation); a part of the fibrinogen A chain may serve as a thrombomodulator. We present some examples below of thrombomodulators, which are small compounds that elicit heterotropic activation (or inhibition) of various thrombin functions.

APOLAR THROMBOMODULATORS (INDOLE ANALOGS)

The importance of apolar or hydrophobic binding regions in thrombin structure and function has been shown from spectroscopic as well as kinetic investigations. These studies were, in part, stimulated from speculations about the nature and importance of, for example, an invariant Phe residue in the ninth penultimate amino residue position to the Arg-Gly bond cleaved in the fibrinogen Aα chain.[21] The evidence for an apolar binding locus (from the spectroscopic work outlined earlier[7]) led to the discovery of several small apolar thrombomodulators.[22] For example, both indole and tryptamine were found to activate both human α- and γ-thrombin catalyzed Tos-Arg-OMe esterase activity by a factor of two to three.[7,22] Of even more interest were their effects on fibrinogen hydrolysis and clotting. FIGURE 6 shows the effects of tryptamine (○), serotonin (●), and 5-fluoroindole (□) on fibrinogen clotting time. The data reflect activation at the lower concentrations of ligand followed by inhibition by binding to additional site(s). The clotting data for the most potent thrombomodulator, 5-fluorotryptamine, is shown in FIGURE 7, plotted as percent inhibition. Here, a negative value corresponds to rate activation, which was *ca* 25% or more. In all of the cases shown above, it was impossible to fit the results to a simple additive model of activation/inhibition, as the data obviously fit some cooperative ligand binding model, that is, involving conformational change(s).

The true test, then, for a thrombomodulator should be its ability to mimic the properties of the macromolecular analog. In a fascinating study, Musci and Berliner examined the rate of human α-thrombin activation of human PC to activated PC in the presence and absence of the ligands: tryptamine, 5-fluorotryptamine, and 6-fluorotryptamine.[24] The observed rate enhancements in the presence of 0.16 μM α-thrombin and 1.4 μM PC were tryptamine, 2.8; 5-fluorotryptamine, 4.0; and 6-fluorotryptamine, 7.0. Whereas the conditions were well below the K_m(app) for α-thrombin:PC, the observed relative rate enhancements versus the control (in the absence of effector) are probably close to the actual rate constant ratios. Considering

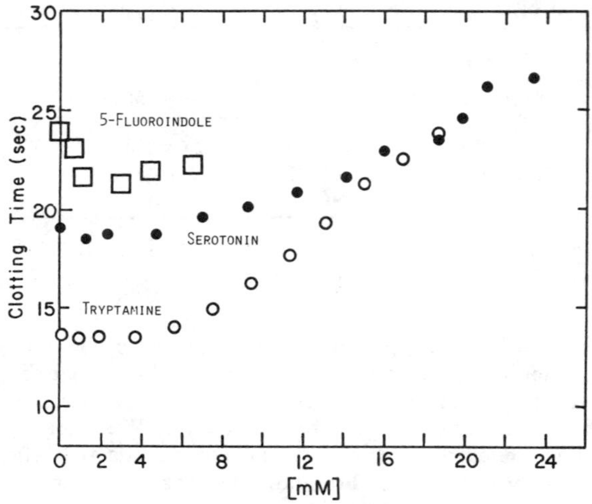

FIGURE 6. Activation/inhibition of human α-thrombin catalyzed fibrinogen clotting in the presence of the effectors: tryptamine (0), serotonin (●), or 5-fluoroindole (□). Conditions were 0.024 M sodium phosphate, pH 7.0, 0.1 M NaCl, 0.66% (w/v) PEG 6000. Note the decrease in clotting time at lower effector. The reaction for thrombin-catalyzed clotting of fibrinogen is a two-step process: hydrolysis followed by fibrin polymerization. It is not totally valid to construe changes in clotting time to alterations in enzyme activity unless it is ascertained that the hydrolysis step is always rate limiting. Cases where the polymerization step becomes rate limiting have been reported, albeit under fairly high concentrations of group 1A salts or with calcium.[23] On the other hand, the inclusion of PEG 6000 in clotting assays was always chosen because of its pronounced accelerating affect on the fibrin polymerization rate whereby thrombin-catalyzed hydrolysis is usually rate limiting. Additional evidence for the relevance of the clotting results comes from the close correlation of the kinetic data with Tos-Arg-OMe or tosyl-chromozymTH and direct physical evidence, such as proflavin or spin label spectra.

the fact that these ligands probably bind to just one locus on the thrombin surface and that the α-thrombin:TM interaction is most likely "multidentate," the *ca* sevenfold rate enhancements observed here were quite significant. If this effect were expressed in concert with other thrombin ligand binding interactions, the net activation might easily approach the *ca* 800-fold enhancement found with TM.[20]

This apolar ligand-rate enhancement phenomenon appears to be quite general with several thrombin ligands including those that also possess anionic moieties (*e.g.*, ATP); these are discussed in the next section.

ANIONIC THROMBOMODULATORS (ATP)

Another class of sites exists on human α-thrombin that recognizes, in part, anionic group(s) on a ligand. As discussed below, the complex cooperative binding found with several of these anionic thrombomodulators was primarily an inhibitory phenomenon, but where the ligand also contained an apolar moiety, activation/inhibition of catalytic function was observed. ATP binds cooperatively to at least two sites in human thrombin. Clotting inhibition occurs with K_i(app) values of *ca* 1.6 and *ca* 2-5 mM.[22] On the other hand, as shown in FIGURE 8, ATP activates the tosyl-chromozymTH hydrolysis in the 0-2 mM range followed by inhibition in the 8-20 mM range.[25] Note that, by proflavin displacement measurements, ATP binds with a K_d(app) of 2.3 mM. Incorporation of a di- or trivalent cation to the pyrophosphate linkage (*e.g.*, Ca(II)-, Zn(II)-, or Co(III)-ATP) emphasizes the inhibitory binding, as depicted in FIGURE 9. For example, Co(III)-ATP inhibits both clotting and amidase activity very strongly (K_i[app] = 0.7 mM) and displaces proflavin with a similar K_d value. This "proflavin site" may correspond to the strong clotting inhibition and amidase activation site(s) above. It appears that the site that displaces the proflavin strongly prefers metal coordinated ATP. The inhibitory effect is propagated by the pyrophosphate linkage, because Co(III)-tripolyphosphate has a K_i(app) of *ca* 0.8 mM, whereas adenosine is a very weak inhibitor of clotting or amidase activity even though it binds to the proflavin site ($K_d \leq$ 4.0 mM).[24] It is also interesting to note that ATP binds to chymotrypsin and other proteases as well.[26]

Several direct pieces of physical evidence were found for this cooperative binding with the fluorescent probe bis-ANS (4,4′-bis-[1-phenylamino-8-naphthalene sulfonate]), which binds in a 1:1 complex with K_d = 14.8 ± 2.2 μM for α-thrombin at pH 7.0 (25 mM Tris, 0.15 M NaCl).[11] Fluorescence changes upon complexation included a considerable (~30 nm) blue shift in the fluorescence emission maximum as well as a 70-fold enhancement in the fluorescence emission intensity. A number of

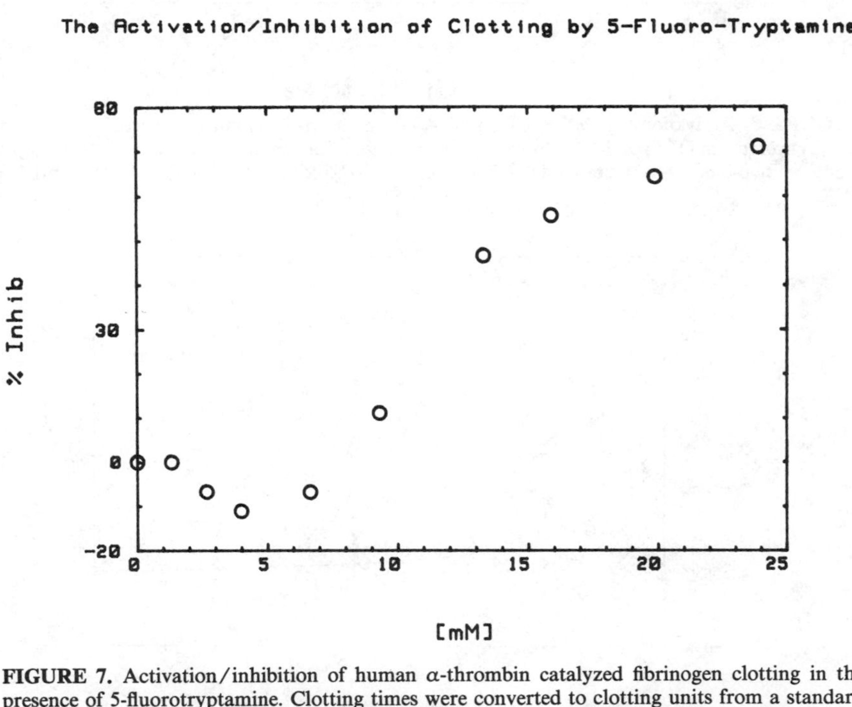

FIGURE 7. Activation/inhibition of human α-thrombin catalyzed fibrinogen clotting in the presence of 5-fluorotryptamine. Clotting times were converted to clotting units from a standard curve. The activity is plotted as a percent of the clotting activity in the absence of effector, such that negative values correspond to rate activation. All other conditions were identical to those in FIGURE 6.

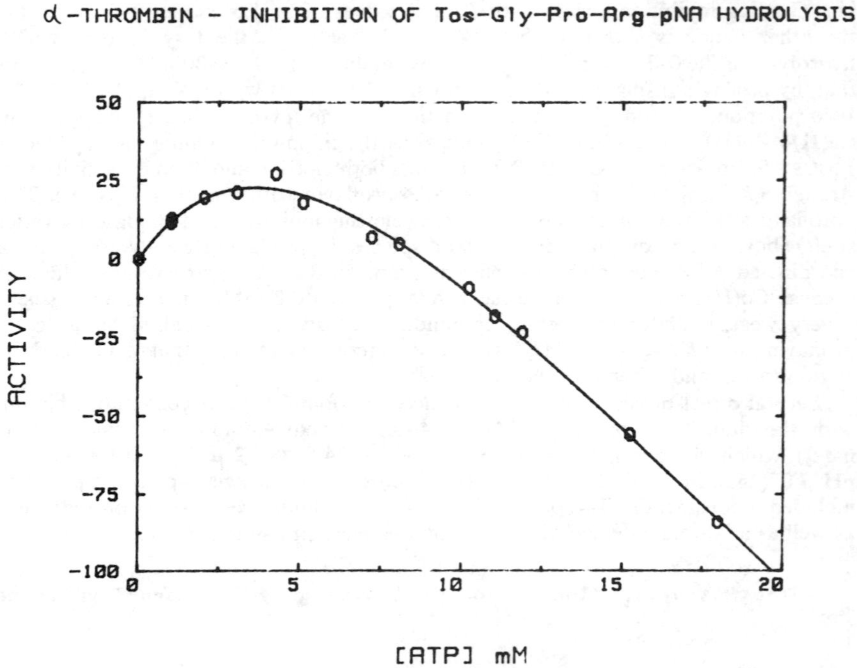

FIGURE 8. Activation/inhibition effects of ATP on the α-thrombin catalyzed hydrolysis of tosyl-chromozymTH (Tosyl-Gly-Pro-Arg-*p*-nitroanilide). The curves could not be fit to a simple, additive, two-independent site model. Conditions were 0.05 mM Tris-HCl, 0.1 M NaCl, pH 8.3, 25°C.

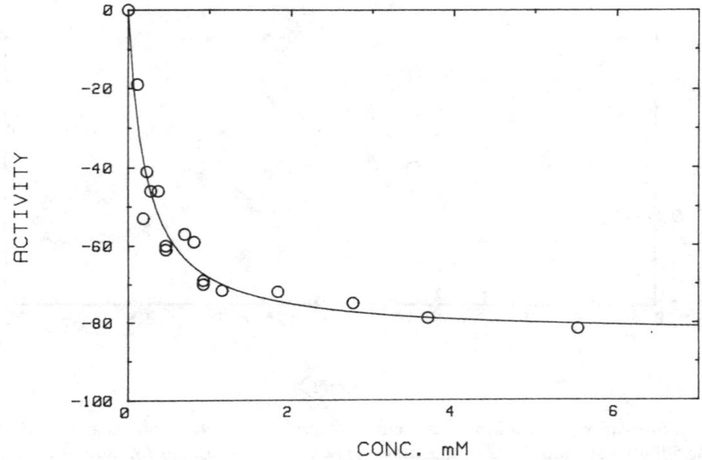

FIGURE 9. Inhibition of α-thrombin catalyzed hydrolysis of tosyl-chromozymTH (Tosyl-Gly-Pro-Arg-*p*-nitroanilide) by Co[III]$(NH_3)_4$-ATP. A K_I(app) of 0.33 mM was fit to these data. Conditions were as in FIGURE 8.

known anionic thrombin effectors (ATP, Ca(II)-ATP, Co(III)-ATP, phosphate, and pyrophosphate) caused further enhancement of the bis-ANS:α-thrombin fluorescence. FIGURE 10A shows an ATP titration of a bis-ANS-α-thrombin complex. The sigmoidal nature of this plot indicates cooperative binding to at least two ATP sites. The additional enhancement of fluorescence emission (~80 fold) in the bis-ANS-α-thrombin-ATP complex extrapolated to a 5600-fold enhancement versus free bis-ANS. In another experiment, shown in FIGURE 10B, active serine-labeled dansyl α-thrombin[10] was titrated with Co(II)-ATP, where first a tenfold enhancement in dansyl fluorescence was observed (0-2 mM range), quite similar to the enhancements of bis-ANS-thrombin in the previous FIGURE 10A. A second, cooperative phase of the titration (2-20 mM)

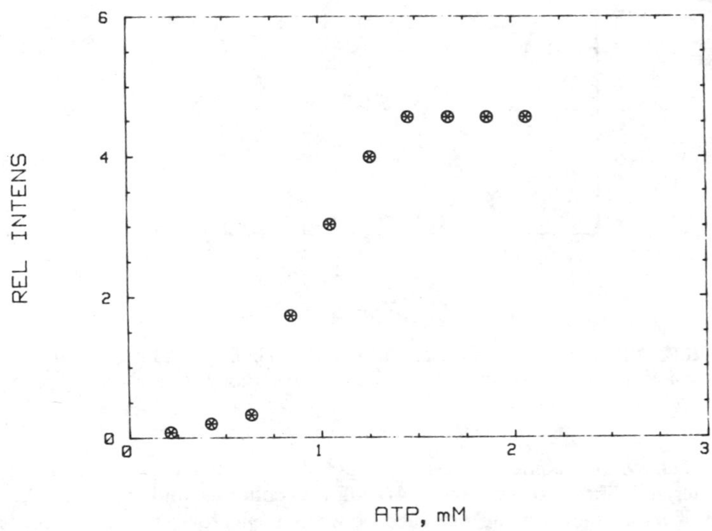

FIGURE 10A. ATP induced fluorescence changes upon binding to human α-thrombin. ATP titration of α-thrombin (0.54 μM)-bis-ANS (1.83 μM) complex at pH 7.0 (25 mM Tris HCl, 0.75 M NaCl, 25°C, λ_{ex} = 375 nm, λ_{em} = 485 nm.[24]

resulted in quenching of the fluorescence, which leveled out at about 40-50% of the maximum intensity where the fluorescence intensity was still four- to fivefold higher than for dansyl-thrombin alone. These results again confirmed the cooperative binding of ATP and its derivatives. Approximate distances between the dansyl moiety and the closest ATP binding locus were in the 6 to 8 Å range.[25] Similar results were also obtained with DAPA (dansylarginine piperidine amide)-α-thrombin, another dansyl fluorophore that binds very tightly to the active center.[25]

The use of clotting measurements for determining whether thrombin or a modified thrombin has altered binding or catalytic behavior with fibrinogen may always raise some ambiguities: if the fibrinogen binding (recognition) site were intact while the catalytic center was inactive, the clotting measurement could not distinguish the above possibility from totally denatured enzyme. Furthermore, one must always verify whether the rate-limiting step in the clotting measurement was indeed the thrombin catalyzed cleavage of fibrinogen and not secondary fibrin association. Several of these

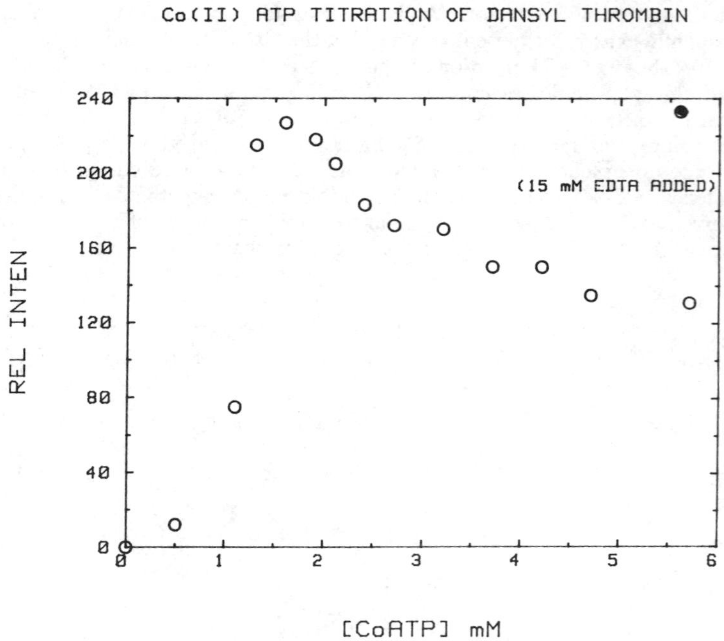

FIGURE 10B. ATP induced fluorescence changes upon binding to human α-thrombin Co(II)-ATP titration of dansyl-α-thrombin, pH 7.0 (50 mM Tris-HCl, 0.75 M NaCl, 25°C, λ_{ex} = 360 nm, λ_{em} = 520 nm).

problems can be overcome because it is possible to covalently bind fibrinogen or nonpolymerized fibrin to Sepharose 4B affinity columns and examine the elution behavior of α-thrombin in the presence of various effectors such as those discussed earlier. Where the complex elutes with the void volume, fibrin-thrombin binding has been obliterated. Reduced binding affinity may be quantitated relative to controls from their respective elution volumes. In a detailed study, several ionic ligand-thrombin complexes were evaluated for their eluting behavior on fibrin-sepharose. The results, found in TABLE 2, list the NaCl concentration required for eluting α-thrombin at

TABLE 2. Elution Concentration of NaCl from Fibrin-Sepharose[16]

	NaCl[a]	$K_{release}$(app), mM	K_i of ligand[b], mM
α-thrombin alone	170		
10 mM serotonin in eluate	165	—	4
10 mM tryptamine in eluate	150	—	7-16
50 mM phosphate in eluate	125	20	<50
10 mM pyrophosphate in eluate	95	3.5	1.8-2.3
4 mM ATP or ADP in eluate	80	1.8	1.6-1.8

[a] pH 7.6, 50 mM Tris-HCl. The conductivity of each fraction was measured and then converted to the corresponding NaCl concentration of the same conductivity.
[b] From clotting, amidase, and esterase results.

saturating ligand.[27] When the elution NaCl concentration was measured versus varying ATP, pyrophosphate (PP_i), or phosphate (P_i) concentrations, an apparent dissociation constant, K_d(app), was estimated from each curve: 1.8 mM for ATP, 3.5 mM for PP_i, and 20 mM for P_i. Further examination of TABLE 2 indicates that the nucleotide ADP was clearly similar to ATP. Such effects were not due to the chelation of Ca^{2+}

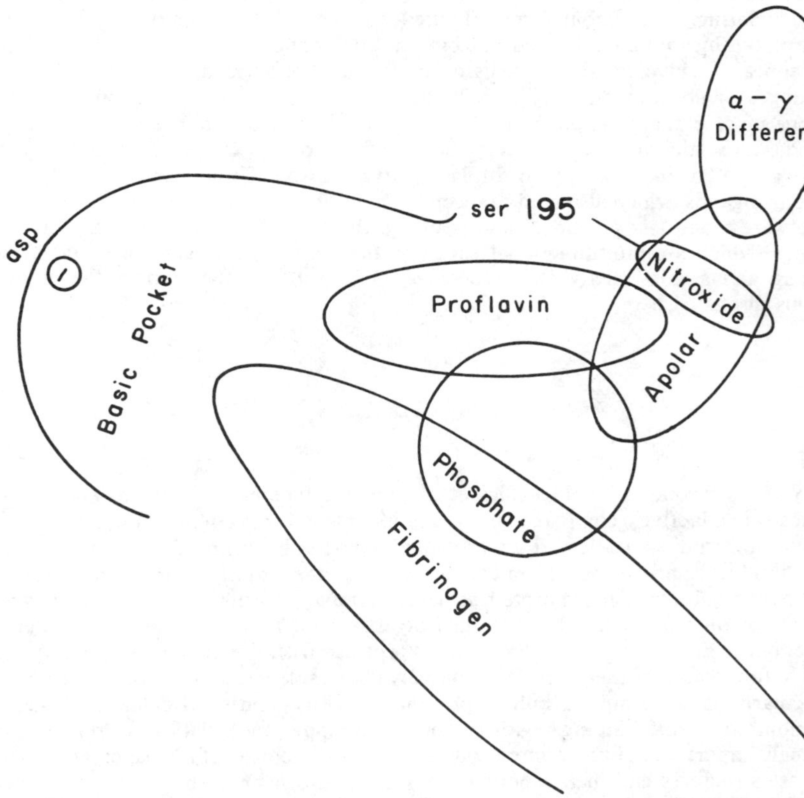

FIGURE 11. Binding site map of human thrombin. The relative sizes of binding loci are not to scale, but are drawn to show overlaps. The apolar (indole) binding region overlaps a Tos-Arg-OMe activation site, which effects proflavin binding, certain apolar site spin labels, and the adenosyl moiety of adenine nucleotides (the latter group also overlaps proflavin binding). The nitroxide locus signifies either a spin label of bent conformation, which overlaps the α-γ difference site or a nitroxide spin label of linear conformation, which senses apolar binding. The phosphate site, shown here with an adenine nucleotide is one of at least two (ATP) phosphate sites that effect clotting and fibrinogen binding. The relative location of the second (ATP) phosphate site is not known exactly at present. The basic specificity pocket is overlapped by proflavin and the susceptible Arg-Gly bonds in fibrinogen.[5]

ion from the fibrin, because inclusion of 1 mM EGTA (which is adequate to remove all Ca^{2+} from the fibrin) did not effect the desorption of α-thrombin from the fibrin column. The K_d(app) values derived from these fibrin column experiments were in remarkable agreement with the apparent equilibrium constants derived from inhibition or activation of estero/amidolytic or clotting activity and proflavin displacement measurements. That is, the similarity between the fibrin resin binding data and activity measurements above strongly suggests that the ligand/inhibitor binding effects were at identical sites in each case.

Catalytically inactivated forms of α-thrombin (with *e.g.*, diisopropyl phosphorofluoridate, phenylmethanesulfonyl fluoride, or methanesulfonyl fluoride) bind to nonpolymerized fibrin resin but elute similarly to that of the native enzyme. Furthermore, the nonclotting γ-thrombin form exhibited markedly reduced binding, whereas the α-thrombin-hirudin complex did not bind at all.[28] Thus, the fibrin binding site does not appear to involve the immediate active site, but instead, a region related to fibrinogen or fibrin binding. The results indicated that thrombin-fibrin binding interactions involve charge interactions that may be blocked by the presence of charged ligands, especially anions. Note that the specific thrombin inhibitor, pyrophosphate, was very potent in its ability to displace thrombin from fibrin monomer Sepharose. Cationic ligands, which also bind to specific regions in thrombin (principally the apolar site), were much less potent inhibitors of the thrombin-fibrin complex, except ATP analogs, which are multifunctional effectors, that is, inhibitors and/or activators of clotting and amidase activities, respectively.[27] FIGURE 11 summarizes the binding regions discussed here.

CONCLUSIONS

Whereas thrombin is a less efficient enzyme and whereas it shows a relative lack of substrate adaptivity compared to trypsin, its unique interactions, for example, with fibrinogen, hirudin, platelets, α_2-macroglobulin, α-1-antitrypsin, and its ability to induce fibroblast and splenocyte mitogenicity, and other interactions,[5] suggest that it must have a quite specialized protein structure compared with the pancreatic esterases. Whereas many researchers have studied digestive enzymes in the past, thrombin is probably the most important bioregulatory protease with the most diverse number of specific functions. Furthermore, it is an easily obtainable and most abundant enzyme, particularly as it pertains to human physiology. Thus, continued detailed studies of thrombin active-site binding regions, their topography, and relation to function are of much importance. Furthermore, our background knowledge of pancreatic serine protease structures and their function serves as an excellent starting point for understanding thrombin and its noncoagulant derivatives.

REFERENCES

1. BERLINER, L. J., Ed. 1976, 1979. Spin Labeling: Theory and Applications. Vols. 1, 2. Academic Press. New York.
2. FENTON II, J. W., B. H. LANDIS, D. A. WALZ & J. S. FINLAYSON. 1977. *In* Chemistry and Biology of Thrombin. R. L. Lundblad, J. W. Fenton II & K. G. Mann, Eds.: 43-70. Ann Arbor Science. Ann Arbor, MI.
3. FENTON II, J. W., M. J. FASCO, A. B. STACKROW, D. L. ARONSON, A. M. YOUNG & J. S. FINLAYSON. 1977. J. Biol. Chem. **252:** 3587-3598.
4. BOISSEL, J. P., B. LEBONNIE, M. J. RABIET, D. LABIE & J. ELION. 1984. J. Biol. Chem. **259:** 5691-5697.
5. BERLINER, L. J. 1984. Mol. Cell. Biochem. **61:** 159-172.

6. BERLINER, L. J., R. S. BAUER, T.-L. CHANG, J. W. FENTON II & Y. Y. L. SHEN. 1981. Biochemistry **20:** 1831-1837.
7. BERLINER, L. J. & Y. Y. L. SHEN. 1977. Biochemistry **16:** 4622-4626.
8. CHANG, T.-L., R. S. BAUER & L. J. BERLINER. 1980. J. Biol. Chem. **255:** 5904-5906.
9. LOTTENBERG, R., J. A. HALL, J. W. FENTON II & C. M. JACKSON. 1982. Thromb. Res. **28:** 313-332.
10. BERLINER, L. J. & Y. Y. L. SHEN. 1977. Thromb. Res. **12:** 15-25.
11. MUSCI, G., G. D. METZ, H. TSUNEMATSU & L. J. BERLINER. 1985. Biochemistry **24:** 2034-2039.
12. BODE, W. & P. SCHWAGER. 1975. J. Mol. Biol. **98:** 693-717.
13. BIRKTOFT, J. J. & L. J. BERLINER. 1986. Submitted to Biochemistry.
14. FEENEY, R. E., G. E. MEANS & J. D. BIGLER. 1969. J. Biol. Chem. **244:** 1957-1960.
15. LANCHANTIN, G. F., J. A. FRIEDMANN & D. W. HART. 1969. J. Biol. Chem. **244:** 865-875.
16. SUGAWARA, Y., J. J. BIRKTOFT & L. J. BERLINER. 1986. Semin. Thromb. Hemostasis **12:** 209-212.
17. LASKOWSKI JR., J. & R. W. SEALOCK. 1971. *In* The Enzymes **3:** 403-405.
18. ESMON, C. T. & N. L. ESMON. 1984. Semin. Thromb. Hemostasis **10:** 122-130.
19. ESMON, N. L., W. G. OWEN & C. T. ESMON. 1982. J. Biol. Chem. **257:** 859-864.
20. SALEM, H. H., I. MARUYAMA, H. ISHII & P. W. MAJERUS. 1984. J. Biol. Chem. **259:** 12246-12251.
21. BLOMBACK, B. 1967. *In* Blood Clotting Enzymology. W. H. Seegers, Ed.: 143-215. Academic Press. New York.
22. CONERY, B. G. & L. J. BERLINER. 1983. Biochemistry **21:** 369-375.
23. LANDIS, B. H., K. A. KOEHLER & J. W. FENTON II. 1981. J. Biol. Chem. **250:** 4604-4610.
24. MUSCI, G. & L. J. BERLINER. 1986. Submitted to Biochemistry.
25. SCHEFFLER, J. E., T. E. MILLER & L. J. BERLINER. 1986. Unpublished results.
26. CHANG, C. T-L., J. E. SCHEFFLER & L. J. BERLINER. 1986. Unpublished results.
27. BERLINER, L. J., Y. SUGAWARA & J. W. FENTON II. 1985. Biochemistry **24:** 7005-7009.
28. FENTON II, J. W. 1981. Ann. N.Y. Acad. Sci. **370:** 468-495.

Heparin Binding in Proximity to the Catalytic Site of Human α-Thrombin[a]

TIMOTHY A. OLSON, STEVEN A. SONDER,
GEORGE D. WILNER, AND JOHN W. FENTON II[b]

Wadsworth Center for Laboratories and Research
New York State Department of Health
Albany, New York 12201
and
Department of Pathology
Washington University
School of Medicine
St. Louis, Missouri 63110

INTRODUCTION

Although heparin interacts with both thrombin and antithrombin III, its acceleration of thrombin inactivation is believed to result from interactions with antithrombin III.[1,2] Furthermore, both human α-thrombin with high fibrinogen clotting activity and γ-thrombin with essentially no clotting activity are inactivated at similar rates by antithrombin III in the presence of heparin, suggesting that heparin functions are independent of requirements for clotting activity.[3] The amino acid residues immediately preceding the arginine at the functional cleavage site in antithrombin III constitute a hydrophobic cluster[4] and should correspondingly bind through the apolar binding site[5] in the fibrinopeptide groove adjacent to the catalytic site.[6] This active-site region is largely conserved in nonclotting thrombin forms, and does not account for additional requirements for clotting activity.[7,8]

Various catalytically inactivated forms of α-thrombin, like the fully active native enzyme, incorporate into fibrin clots and bind to nonpolymerized fibrin agarose, whereas γ-thrombin does not incorporate[9] and binds only weakly.[10] Because binding to fibrin agarose involves an anionic binding site in α-thrombin,[11] we examined binding to heparin agaroses[12] with various thrombin forms in order to assess if a similar site was accountable for binding to this negatively charged resin. In these experiments, hirudin complexing blocked a major anionic binding site, which is independent of the carbohydrate attachment, the catalytic site, and the apolar binding site. This anionic

[a]This work was supported in part by NIH Grant HL 13160 and SCOR Grant HL 14147 from the National Heart, Lung, and Blood Institutes.

[b]To whom correspondence should be addressed at the Wadsworth Center for Laboratories and Research.

binding site appears to be involved in fibrinogen clotting and other biological functions of α-thrombin.

MATERIAL AND METHODS

Material Sources

Human fraction III paste was obtained through Dr. James Cavanaugh as a gift from Armour Pharmaceutical Co. (Kankakee, IL); porcine heparin (162 U/mg) was a gift through Dr. William H. Holleman from Abbott Laboratories (North Chicago, IL). The following were purchased: concanavalin A agarose and α-methyl-D-mannoside from Sigma Chemical Co. (St. Louis, MO); D-phenylalanyl-L-prolyl-L-arginine chloromethyl ketone (D-Phe-Pro-Arg-Ch_2-Cl) from Calbiochem-Behring (San Diego, CA); hirudin from American Diagnostica, Inc. (Greenwich, CT); 2-(*N*-morpholino) ethane sulfonic acid (MES) from Research Organics, Inc. (Cleveland, OH); diisopropyl phosphorofluoridate (*i*-Pr_2P-F) from Aldrich Chemical Co. (Milwaukee, WI); *p*-nitrophenyl-*p*′-guanidinobenzoate (NPGB) from ICN Pharmaceuticals, Inc. (Cleveland, OH); polyethylene glycol (PEG) 6,000 from MCB Reagents (Gibbstown, NJ); and Sepharose 4B from Pharmacia Fine Chemicals (Piscataway, NJ).

TABLE 1. Specifications of Thrombin Preparations

Property		Preparation			
		α-Thrombin	γ-Thrombin	*i*-Pr_2P-α-thrombin	D-Phe-Pro-Arg-CH_2-α-thrombin
Thrombin form	percent α	96.6	0.0	(98.2)[a]	(100.0)[a]
	percent β	2.7	0.7	(1.1)	(0.0)
	percent γ	0.7	99.3	(0.7)	(0.0)
NPGB active-site titration, percent active enzyme		100	100	< 1.0	1.3
Fibrinogen-clotting activity, U/mg		3,400	6.3	0.38	<0.2

[a] Values in parenthesis are those of the initial α-thrombin preparation.

Thrombin Preparations

Human α-thrombin was prepared from fraction III paste employing thromboplastin activation and was stored frozen at −70°C in 0.75 M NaCl at protein concentrations of 2 to 4 mg/mL, pH 6.[8] The preparation used in the present experiments met criteria for the highly pure and active enzyme (TABLE 1). Essentially nonclotting γ-thrombin with <0.5% original clotting activity was made by controlled passage through a column of trypsin agarose equilibrated in 0.75 M NaCl and 10 mM MES at pH 6.2 and 23°C.[7] Inactivated *i*-Pr_2P-α-thrombin was made by adding 0.2 M *i*-Pr_2P-F (in acetone) at an ~1:1 molar ratio to α-thrombin in 1.0 M Tris at pH 8.0 until clotting activity declined to <2 percent. Affinity labeled D-Phe-Pro-Arg-Ch_2-α-thrombin was prepared by reaction with a 6-fold molar excess of reagent in 0.75 M NaCl buffered with 100 mM Tris at pH 8.0 for 30 minutes. Both inactivated α-thrombin preparations were dialyzed overnight against 0.75 M NaCl at 4°C prior to frozen storage at −70°C.[6] Hirudin complexes were formed by adding the inhibitor to the various forms at an ~1:1 molar ratio (unit per unit for α-thrombin). Protein concentrations were calculated from the absorbance at 280 nm, assuming an extinction coefficient of 1.83 mL mg^{-1} cm^{-1} for human α-thrombin in 0.1 M NaOH and an M_r of 36,500 for all forms.[8]

Resin Preparations and Chromatography

Concanavalin A agarose was equilibrated in 0.15 M NaCl containing 1.0 mM Tris, 1.0 mM $MgCl_2$, 1.0 mM $CaCl_2$, 6 mg/mL of PEG 6,000, and 2 mg/mL of sodium azide at pH 8.0. Thrombin preparations were dialyzed overnight against the equilibration buffer at 4°C, and 1 mL samples were applied to a 1.5 cm (i.d.) by 3.2 cm column of the resin at ~23°C. The resin was washed with 3 column volumes of the equilibration buffer, prior to eluting thrombin preparations, with 200 mM α-methyl-D-mannoside in the buffer. Eluates were withdrawn with an LKB 12000 peristaltic pump and passed through an ISCO UA-5 UV monitor, equipped with a 10 nm path flow-through cell, and absorbencies were measured at 280 nm. Individual 1 to 2 mL fractions were collected at 0.6 mL/minute.

Heparin agarose was prepared by modification of the conventional methods.[12,13] Briefly, 75 g of Sepharose 4B in 150 mL of water were activated with 12 g of CNBr while maintaining the pH at 10.5 by the addition of 4 M NaOH. The activated resin was washed with 2 L of water, then resuspended in 150 mL of 0.1 M $NaHCO_3$ at pH 9.0, and 160 mg of heparin dissolved in 80 mL of the $NaHCO_3$ buffer were added. This conjugation mixture was slowly stirred overnight at 4°C, and the reaction was terminated by the addition of 7.5 mL of ethanolamine, allowing the mixture to stir for an additional 3 hours. The conjugated resin was washed with 2 L of water and subsequently equilibrated in 0.05 M NaCl buffered with 10 mM HEPES at pH 7.4. Thrombin preparations were dialyzed overnight against the equilibration buffer at 4°C, and 1 mL samples were applied to 1.5 cm i.d. by 4.5 cm columns of the resin. The resin was developed at 23°C with a linear salt gradient generated by addition of 100 mL of 0.25 M NaCl buffered with 10 mM HEPES at pH 7.4 (reservoir chamber) to 100 mL of the equilibration buffer (mixing chamber). Fractions were collected and monitored as described above. In addition, conductivity was measured with a Yellow Springs Instrument Model #32 Conductance Meter. Conductivity measurements were converted into salt concentrations from calibration plots.

RESULTS AND DISCUSSION

Human α-thrombin bound to concanavalin A agarose in 0.15 M NaCl and was eluted by addition of 200 mM α-methyl-D-mannoside (FIGURE 1a). The recovered enzyme retained >95% of its original clotting activity and was quantitatively eluted on the basis of recovered clotting units and the observation that 1 M NaCl did not elute additional 280 nm absorbing materials. When nonclotting γ-thrombin was similarily applied to the resin, this enzymic form bound (FIGURE 1b). When eluted with α-methyl-D-mannoside and with 94% of recovered protein, only 12 to 15% of the original esterolytic activity was found by NPGB titration. This suggests that concanavalin A binding of the single carbohydrate side chain in the human enzyme[14] causes the γ-thrombin form to undergo denaturation. In this regard, the B chain of the

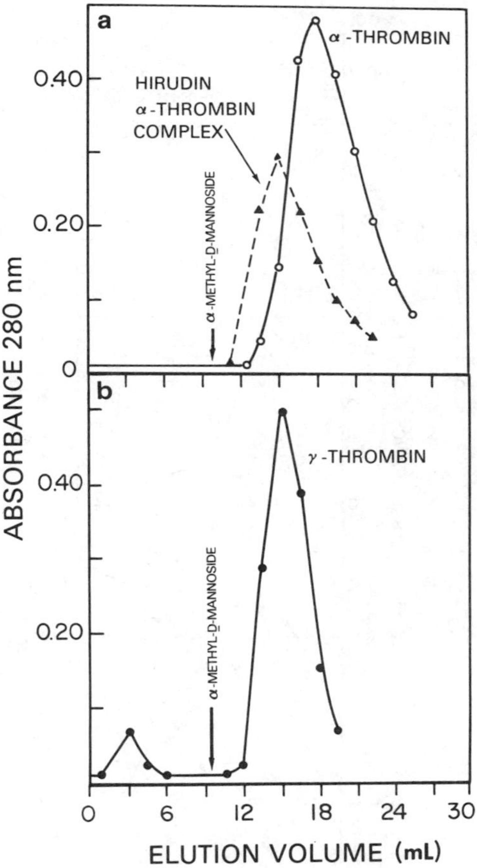

FIGURE 1. Elution of human thrombins from concanavalin A agarose. Experiments were performed at pH 8.0 and 23°C. See text for experimental details. The panels are a) α-thrombin and its hirudin complex (dashed line), and b) γ-thrombin.

human enzyme is cleaved into roughly thirds, where the functional histidine (His_{57} in chymotrypsin) and the carbohydrate attachment reside in the first noncovalently associated B-chain fragment.[7] This histidine is furthermore situated 9 residues preceding the carbohydrate attachment,[15] which precedes the β-cleavage sites by an additional 9 and 19 residues.[16] Thus, cleavage at these sites may destabilize the protein structure, such that binding of concanavalin A to the carbohydrate side chain may induce irreversible changes.

When α-thrombin was premixed with an equivalent amount of hirudin (unit per unit), clotting activity was abolished. Despite the proximity of the functional histidine to the carbohydrate attachment (see above), however, the hirudine α-thrombin complex bound to concanavalin A and was eluted with α-methyl-D-mannoside in the same manner as the native enzyme (FIGURE 1a). The eluted complex was intact based on the absence of clotting activity. Therefore, hirudin complexing does not mask the

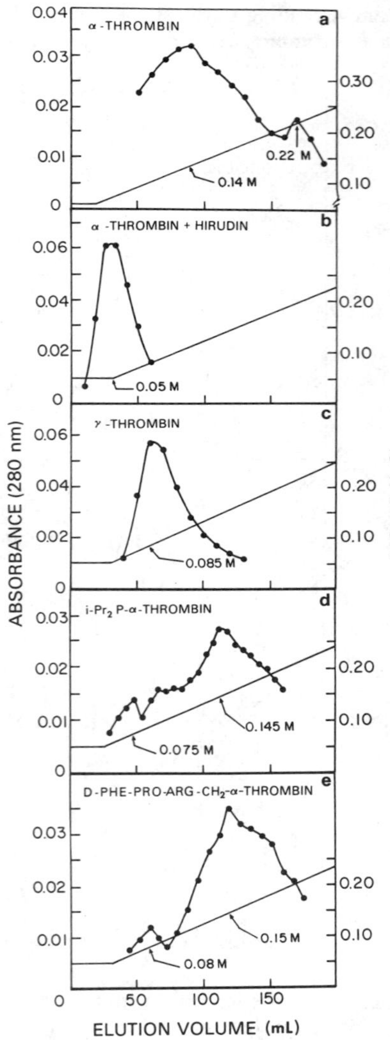

FIGURE 2. Elution of human thrombins from heparin agarose. Experiments were performed at pH 7.4 and 23°C. See text for experimental details. The panels are a) α-thrombin, b) hirudin α-thrombin complex, c) γ-thrombin, d) i-Pr_2P-α-thrombin, and e) D-Phe-Pro-Arg-CH_2-α-thrombin.

carbohydrate side chain nor presumptively the surface domain adjacent to the carbohydrate attachment.

In marked contrast, whereas α-thrombin bound to heparin agarose, its hirudin complex did not, demonstrating that hirudin complexing masks the heparin binding site (FIGURES 2a and b). Unlike the native enzyme, γ-thrombin bound weakly to the resin (FIGURE 2c), suggesting that its reduced affinity for heparin was related to its loss of clotting activity, due to obstruction or destruction of the fibrin(ogen) recognition exosite (Fenton, 1981). On the other hand, both *i*-Pr_2P- and D-Phe-Pro-Arg-Ch_2-α-thrombins bound to the resin in a manner similar to the parent enzyme (FIGURES 2d and e). Although the former has an obstructing group conjugated to the functional serine (Ser_{195}), the latter has a tripeptide ligand occupying the fibrinopeptide groove adjacent to the catalytic site (His_{57} and Ser_{195}). The D-Phe-Pro- portion of this ligand is notably hydrophobic and occupies a prominent apolar binding site.[6] Inasmuch as heparin is a highly negatively charged sulfonated polysaccharide, it should not associate with this site, but rather with an anionic binding site elsewhere in the enzyme.

Hirudin is a small protein derived from the salivary glands of the European medicinal leech and is a highly specific thrombin inhibitor.[17] The first two-thirds from the amino terminus of hirudin consists predominantly of hydrophobic amino acid residues and has three disulfide bridges forming an apolar knot. The final third constitutes a tail and contains the Pro-Lys-Pro sequence, which presumably binds at active-site regions neighboring the catalytic site. This sequence is followed by a highly negatively charged cluster, which contains a sulfonated tyrosine.[18] Proteolytic cleavage of varying segments of the tail destroys activity,[19] as does reduction of disulfide bridges.[20] Thus, both the knot structure and the tail are essential for thrombin complexing, as if the knot bound to the apolar binding site and the tail to an anionic binding site. In this regard, hirudin displaces proflavin from the apolar binding site of α- and γ-thrombins,[6] whereas heparin does not.[3,21] On the other hand, heparin inhibits NPGB binding and is a hyperbolic competitive inhibitor of N_α-tosyl-L-arginine methyl ester hydrolysis, suggesting that heparin binds in the proximity of the catalytic site.[21]

Hirudin noncovalently complexes with human α-thrombin in a noncompetitive manner with an exceedingly high affinity (K_i of $\sim$60 pM), but it complexes with γ-thrombin with a 200-fold reduced affinity in a competitive manner.[22] The loss of clotting activity of γ-thrombin appears, therefore, to be related to reductions in hirudin affinity[22] binding to nonpolymerized fibrin agarose,[23] polymethylacrylic acid resin,[24] and heparin agarose (FIGURES 2a and c). Such binding furthermore appears attributable to a common exosite region within the fibrin side of the thrombin active site.[10]

Despite their differences in heparin affinities, human α- and γ-thrombins react similarly with antithrombin III in the presence of heparin.[3] This suggests that heparin thrombin interactions are less important than heparin antithrombin III interactions in heparin acceleration of thrombin inactivation, as was previously indicated by other experimental approaches.[1,2] The anionic binding site of α-thrombin appears to be required for clotting activity[11] and most likely is involved in interactions with high-affinity receptors on certain cells, where α-thrombin may function nonenzymically in a hormone-like manner.[25] Thrombin chemotactic activity is also nonenzymic,[26] where this activity resides in a unique protein domain.[27] The anionic binding site, which requires a cluster of arginyl and/or lysyl residues, may also be part of the thrombin chemotactic domain.[28]

REFERENCES

1. ROSENBERG, R. D. & P. S. DAMUS. 1973. The purification and mechanism of action of human antithrombin-heparin cofactor. J. Biol. Chem. **248:** 6490-6505.
2. LI, E. H. H., J. W. FENTON II & R. D. FEINMAN. 1976. The role of heparin in the thrombin antithrombin III reaction. Arch. Biochem. Biophys. **175:** 153-159.

3. CHANG, T-I., R. D. FEINMAN, B. H. LANDIS & J. W. FENTON II. 1979. Antithrombin reactions with α- and γ-thrombins. Biochemistry **18:** 113-119.
4. BJORK, I., A. DANIELSSON, J. W. FENTON II & H. JORNVALL. 1981. The site in human antithrombin for functional proteolytic cleavage by human thrombin. FEBS Lett. **126:** 257-260.
5. BERLINER, L. J. & Y. Y. L. SHEN. 1977. Physical evidence for an apolar binding site near the catalytic center of human α-thrombin. Biochemistry **16:** 4622-4626.
6. SONDER, S. A. & J. W. FENTON II. 1984. Proflavin binding within the fibrinopeptide groove adjacent to the catalytic site of human α-thrombin. Biochemistry **23:** 1818-1823.
7. BING, D. H., M. CORY & J. W. FENTON II. 1977. Exo-site affinity labeling of human thrombins. Similar labeling on it and B chain/fragments of clotting α- and nonclotting γ/β-thrombins. J. Biol. Chem. **252:** 8027-8034.
8. FENTON II, J. W., M. J. FASCO, A. B. STACKROW, D. L. ARONSON, A. M. YOUNG & J. S. FINLAYSON. 1977. Human thrombins. Production, evaluation, and properties of α-thrombin. J. Biol. Chem. **252:** 3587-3598.
9. WILNER, G. D., M. P. DANITZ, M. S. MUDD, K-H. HSIEH & J. W. FENTON II. 1981. Selective immobilization of α-thrombin by surface-bound fibrin. J. Clin. Med. **97:** 403-411.
10. FENTON II, J. W., M. P. ZABINSKI, K. HSIEH & G. D. WILNER. 1981. Thrombin non-covalent-protein binding and fibrin(ogen) recognition. Thromb. Haemostasis **46:** 177.
11. BERLINER, L. J., Y. SUGAWARA & J. W. FENTON II. 1985. Human α-thrombin binding to non-polymerized fibrin-sepharose: evidence for an anionic binding region. Biochemistry **24:** 7005-7009.
12. MILLER-ANDERSSON, M., H. BORG & L-O. ANDERSSON. 1974. Purification of antithrombin III by affinity chromatography. Thromb. Res. **5:** 439-452.
13. IVERIUS, P. H. 1971. Coupling of glycosaminoglycans to agarose beads (Sepharose 4B). Biochem. J. **124:** 677-683.
14. NILSON, B., MCD. K. HORNE III & H. R. GRALNICK. 1983. The carbohydrate of human thrombin: structural analysis of glycoprotein oligosaccharides by mass spectrometry. Arch. Biochem. Biophys. **224:** 127-133.
15. DEGEN, S. J. F., R. T. A. MACGILLIVRAY & E. W. DAVIE. 1983. Characterization of the complementary deoxyribonucleic acid and gene coding for human prothrombin. Biochemistry **22:** 2087-2097.
16. BOISSEL, J. P., B. LEBONNIEC, M-J. RABIET, D. LABIE & J. ELION. 1984. Covalent structures of and autolytic derivatives of human α-thrombin. J. Biol. Chem. **259:** 5691-5697.
17. MARKWARDT, F. 1970. Hirudin as an inhibitor of thrombin. Methods Enzymol. **19:** 924-932.
18. DODT, J., H-P. MULLER, V. SEEMULLER & J-Y. CHANG. 1984. The complete amino acid sequence of hirudin, a thrombin specific inhibitor. FEBS Lett. **165:** 180-183.
19. CHANG, J-Y. 1983. The functional domain of hirudin, a thrombin-specific inhibitor. FEBS Lett. **1044:** 307-313.
20. BAGDY, D., E. BARBAS, L. GRAFF, T. E. PETERSEN & S. MAGNUSSON. 1976. Hirudin. Methods Enzymol. **45:** 669-678.
21. LI, E. H. H., C. ORTON & R. D. FEINMAN. 1974. The interaction of thrombin and heparin. Proflavine dye binding studies. Biochemistry **13:** 5012-5017.
22. LANDIS, B. H., M. P. ZABINSKI, G. J. M. LAFLEUR, D. H. BING & J. W. FENTON II. 1978. Human α- and γ-thrombin differential inhibition with hirudin. Fed. Proc. Fed. Am. Soc. Exp. Biol. **37:** 1445.
23. FENTON II, J. W. 1981. Thrombin specificity. Ann. N. Y. Acad. Sci. **370:** 468-495.
24. FENTON II, J. W., B. H. LANDIS, D. A. WALZ, D. H. BING, R. D. FEINMANN, M. P. ZABINSKI, S. A. SONDER, L. J. BERLINER & J. S. FINLAYSON. 1979. Human thrombin: preparative evaluation, structural properties and enzymic specificity. *In* The Chemistry and Physiology of the Human Plasma Proteins. D. H. Bing, Ed.: 151-183. Pergamon Press. New York.
25. CARNEY, D. H., J. STIERNBERG & J. W. FENTON II. 1984. Initiation of proliferative events by human α-thrombin requires both receptor binding and enzymic activity. J. Cell. Biochem. **26:** 181-195.

26. BAR-SHAVIT, R., A. KAHN, G. D. WILNER & J. W. FENTON II. 1983. Unique exosite region in thrombin stimulates monocyte chemotaxis. Science **220:** 728-731.
27. BAR-SHAVIT, R., A. KAHN, M. S. MUDD, G. D. WILNER, K. G. MANN & J. W. FENTON II. 1984. Localization of a chemotactic domain in human thrombin. Biochemistry **23:** 397-400.
28. BAR-SHAVIT, R., D. H. BING, A. J. KAHN & G. D. WILNER. 1985. Thrombin-medicated chemotaxis: relationship of ligand structure to biological activity. *In* UCLA Symposium on Molecular and Cellular Biology. M. P. Czech and C. R. Kahn, Eds.: **23:** 329-338. Alan R. Liss. New York.

Structure-Function Relationships of Thrombin Based on the Computer-Generated Three-Dimensional Model of the B Chain of Bovine Thrombin[a]

DAVID H. BING,[b,c] RICHARD J. FELDMANN,[d] AND JOHN W. FENTON II[e]

[c]*Beth Israel Hospital*
Cambridge Research Laboratory
Cambridge, Massachusetts 02139

[d]*Division of Computer Research and Technology*
National Institutes of Health
Bethesda, Maryland 20205

[e]*Wadsworth Center for Laboratories and Research*
New York State Department of Health
Albany, New York 12201

INTRODUCTION

The study of enzyme function has been greatly facilitated by having available a three-dimensional model of the protein that is based on X-ray crystallographic diffraction data. Such representations of protein structure can be used to design experiments and evaluate data obtained from studies of the enzyme in solution. Insights derived from the study of such models have been used to elucidate structural and functional relationships of many proteins. The family of mammalian serine proteinases, which include the pancreatic enzymes trypsin, chymotrypsin, and elastase, have been studied and analyzed extensively with the aid of such models. The comparison of these three enzymes reveals that they have an identical enzyme mechanism that involves the same three amino acids: serine 195, histidine 57, and aspartate 102.[f] They also exhibit secondary and tertiary structural homology, in spite of significant differences in primary structure and a dramatic difference in terms of substrate specificity.[1–5]

The realization that the folding pattern (*e.g.* the secondary, tertiary, and quaternary structural features) remains conserved within a family of proteins that exhibited similar

[a]This work was supported by Grants from the National Institutes of Health, HL 13160 and AM 34028.

[b]To whom correspondence should be addressed. Mailing address: CBR Laboratories Inc., 800 Huntington Ave., Boston, MA 02115.

[f]The numbering for chymotrypsin is used for amino acid sequence in the serine proteinases.[43]

function and enzyme mechanism(s) led to the development of a method, which we called protein extension, that allowed for the construction of three-dimensional models of proteins for which there was no suitable crystallographic solution.[6] The method is based on the empirical observation that the folding pattern of the protein is maintained in a family of proteins that exhibits similar functions. This apparently occurs because in families of proteins there is a high degree of amino acid homology within the inner core of the protein, and this leads to characteristic architectural features for the protein. By contrast, most of the changes in proteins within a family, occur on surfaces that are exposed to the solvent as well as at locations where the changes lead directly to differences in ligand binding specificity of the protein.

The initial description of a computer-generated three-dimensional model for thrombin was based on the similarities between the bovine thrombin B chain and bovine trypsin and chymotrypsin.[7,8] In the 32 kDa B chain of bovine thrombin, which contains the active-site catalytic triad of Ser 195, His 57, and Asp 102, the homology at the primary sequence level between thrombin and these two pancreatic serine proteinases is high at the region of the active center—69% for thrombin versus trypsin and 66% for thrombin versus chymotrypsin. There is, furthermore, a high degree of homology of thrombin with these enzymes with respect to the amino acids that line the binding pocket where the P_1 residue in the substrate binds;[g] thrombin specificity for arginine at this site makes it resemble trypsin, but it is more restricted with respect to possible protein substrates.[9,10] Unlike either trypsin or chymotrypsin, thrombin retains a 4.6 kDa A chain that remains covalently bonded by a disulfide bond with Cys 122 after limited proteolysis of the activation peptide(s) in prothrombin. This small peptide has no structural homolog in the pancreatic serine proteinases and thus cannot be modeled by way of the protein extension method.[9]

The precedence for the protein extension method with respect to the mammalian serine proteinases was set by Kiel *et al.* in 1968 when they constructed a model of trypsin based on the then newly described structure of *N*-tosyl-α-chymotrypsin. As reported in that study, a comparison of trypsin with chymotrypsin demonstrated a 44-50% primary structural homology with the substitution of an aspartate for serine at position 189 at the bottom of the pocket binding the P_1 residue in the substrate; this accounts for the preferred substate specificity of trypsin for cationically charged arginine or lysine residues.[11-13] Subsequent crystallographic studies on both enzymes demonstrated the striking similarities between the two enzymes.[1,2,14-17] Both are globular molecules in which the secondary structure is characterized by the presence of extensive beta structure and little alpha helix. The internal beta structure is organized into two, six-stranded beta barrels composed of mostly hydrophobic amino acids. There is also homology with respect to the position of the interchain disulfide bridges; whereas trypsin contains six and chymotrypsin contains five, four of these are at identical positions, and the additional two cysteines in trypsin join the beta barrels of trypsin in a manner that is consistent with the secondary structure of chymotrypsin. Trypsin also differs from chymotrypsin in that it is a single polypeptide chain and has 13 fewer amino acids in its primary structure.

Magnusson *et al.* based their model of the B chain of thrombin on the primary sequence similarity between chymotrypsin and thrombin.[18] They identified the similarities at the catalytic center and a possible site for the binding of fibrinopeptides. Although there were no pictures published of the model, the description was similar to the model for thrombin that we subsequently constructed based on more generalized

[g] The usual terminology for referring to substrate residue is to call the residue in the specificity binding pocket P_1, the residue extending towards the N terminus from the arginine P_2, P_3, et cetera, and the residue for the C terminus side of the arginine P_1, P_2, P_3, et cetera.[8a]

rules developed in the protein extension method.[6-8] In their model a position for the A chain was described that was consistent with its participating in restricting access to the active site of thrombin by protein substrates.

DESCRIPTION OF THE COMPUTER GENERATED MODEL OF THE THROMBIN B CHAIN

Primary, Secondary, and Tertiary Structural Features

The primary, secondary, and tertiary structural features of the thrombin model have been described previously,[6-8] and the model generated by the protein extension method is similar to models of the mammalian serine proteinases described by Greer.[19,20] We noted early that there was an advantage to using the chymotrypsin peptide backbone for generating a model of the B chain of thrombin, as it minimized the size and number of deletions and insertions that were required to obtain a structural model. Chymotrypsin, however, contains three polypeptide chains linked by disulfide bonds and lacks residues 147 and 148 as opposed to trypsin, which not only has residues at these positions but is also a single polypeptide chain. Because the bovine thrombin B chain resembles trypsin in terms of primary binding specificity as well as also being a single polypeptide chain, we decided to incorporate favorable structural features from trypsin into a hybrid structure that would contain aspects of both chymotrypsin and trypsin.[8] This included inserting the 147-148 segment of trypsin and deleting residue 218 of chymotrypsin in order to make Cys 220 trypsin-like in its spatial orientation (see FIGURE 1). The B chain of bovine thrombin has 259 amino acids as compared to 238 residues in the hybrid molecule on which it was modeled. To accommodate the extra polypeptide structure, amino acids had to be inserted into the overall sequence. With one exception, these were made outside of the regions that constitute a strand in the beta sheet. Likewise, at certain steps in the construction of the model, it was apparent that deletions had to be made to avoid disrupting both the beta structure and alpha helix. The inserts and deletions are as follows:

Two deletions were made at positions 76 and 218. Insertion of one amino acid at positions 35, 84, 95, and 223, and an insertion of nine amino acids at position 60 were made. Five amino acids were inserted at positions 146 and 185, three amino acids at positions 126, and two amino acids at 204, and at the C terminus at position 245. The insertion at 84 is in the middle of the fifth strand of the first beta barrel. The deletion at 76, however, offset this change and permitted maximizing amino acid homology in this region of the protein. These changes are present schematically in FIGURE 1.

The resulting thrombin model has areas where there is both low and high degrees of homology with the primary structure of chymotrypsin. Overall, the beta chain of bovine thrombin exhibits 36% and 38% homology with bovine alpha chymotrypsin and bovine trypsin, respectively. In the area that corresponds to the activation domain of trypsin as described by Huber and Bode,[2] (residues 16-19, 142-145, 193-194, and 216-223), there is only 27% and 28% with chymotrypsin and trypsin. By contrast, a similar comparison in the region of the charge relay triad and the amino acids that line the binding pocket (189-201, 211-220, 55-60, and 99-104) shows a 66% and 69% homology respectively with the two enzymes. Between residues 211 and 220, an

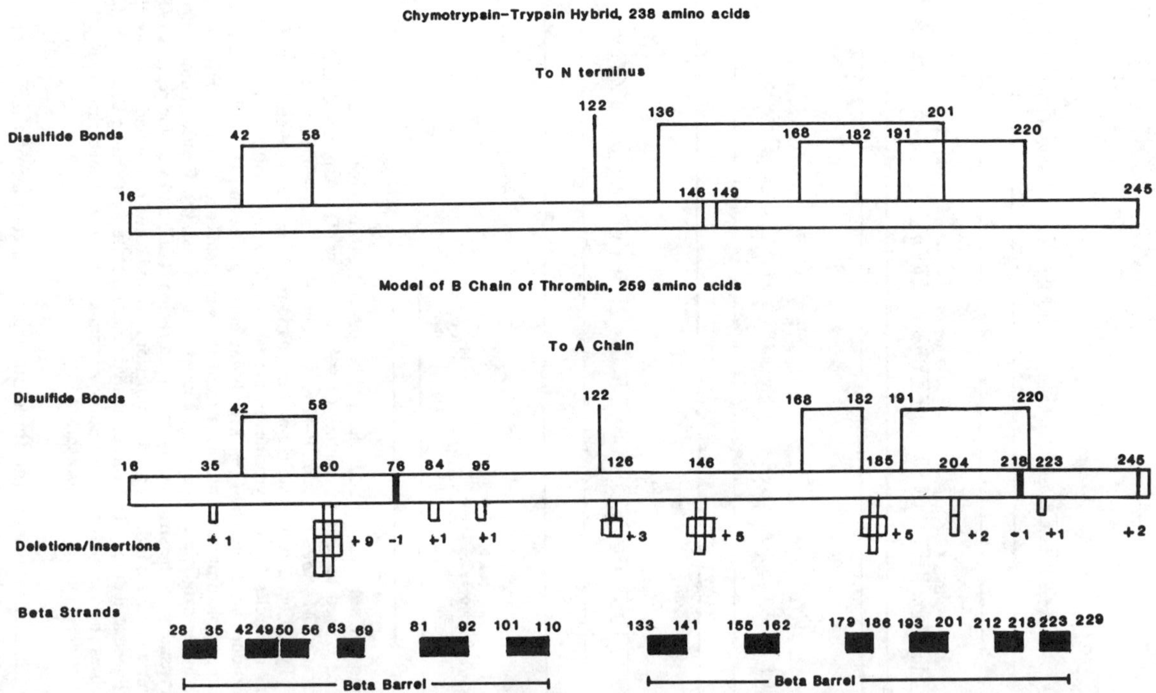

FIGURE 1. Schematic representation of the linear structure of the proposed model of the B chain of bovine thrombin. Top, chymotrypsin-trypsin hybrid structure used to model the thrombin molecule. Middle, proposed model of the B chain with deletions and insertions. The numbers designate the positions in the primary structure of the disulfide bonds and the deletions and insertions. Bottom, beta structure; the solid blocks represent the location of the strands that constitute the beta structure in chymotrypsin. See text for details.

area that is part of the secondary binding site for protein substrates, there is 86% and 88% homology with chymotrypsin and trypsin. The amino acid sequence of the B chain of bovine thrombin with the inserts, presented as loops of amino acids, is presented in FIGURE 2.

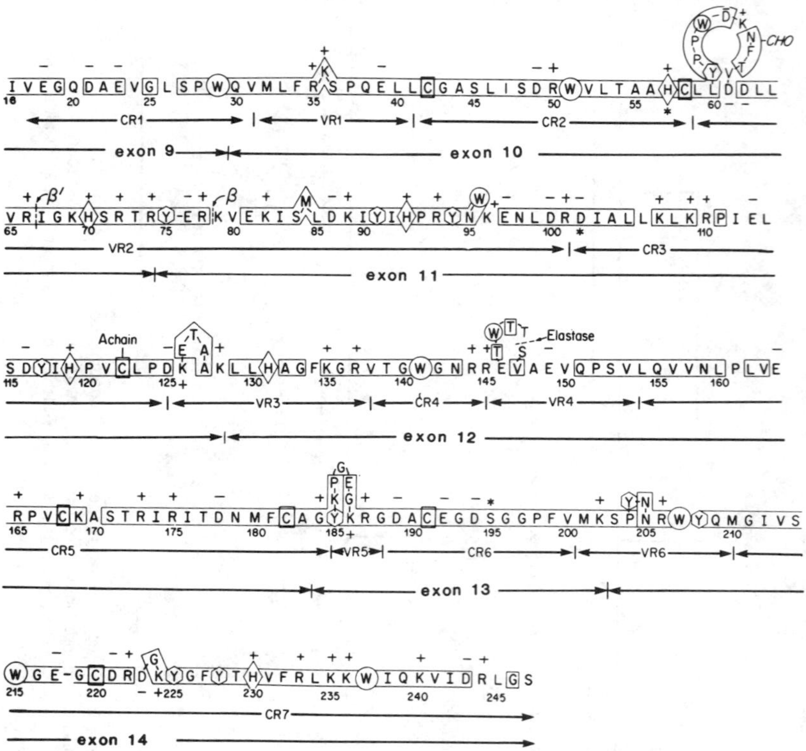

FIGURE 2. Amino acid sequence of the B chain of bovine alpha thrombosin. The single amino acid and letter code is used to refer to residues (A=Ala, C=Cys, D=Asp, E=Glu, H=His, I=Ile, K=Lys, L=Leu, M=Met, N=Asn, P=Pro, Q=Glu, R=Arg, S=Ser, T=Thr, V=Val, W=Trp, and Y=Tyr). Location of cysteines and aromatic residues: the cysteines are in boxes (C), tryptophans in circles (W), tyrosines in hexagons (Y), and histidines in diamonds (H). Charged residues are shown by (+) for lysine and arginine and (−) for glutamate and aspartate. The carbohydrate attachment is from the gene sequence. Residues His 57, Ser 195, and Asp 102 in the catalytic triad are marked with an asterisk (*). Residue numbering is based on chymotrypsinogen. The structurally conserved regions (CR) and variable regions (VR) as described by Furie *et al.* are indicated. Exon junctions are indicated below and based on the recently described gene structure.[28] The autoproteolytic cleavage site for forming beta thrombin is indicated as well as the secondary site for autolyzed snake venom-activated thrombin.[34] The site for pancreatic elastase cleavage is also shown.[40]

The resulting model represents the three-dimensional structure of the B chain of bovine thrombin as a globular protein that retains the segments that constitute the beta barrels and alpha-helix structures found in bovine alpha chymotrypsin. The position of the cysteine disulfide bonds is retained exactly as in chymotrypsin, and the architecture of the core of chymotrypsin is likewise conserved almost exactly in the thrombin model. With the exception of two residues in the primary binding pocket, almost all of the changes in amino acids seen in the thrombin model have occurred on what are surface-exposed amino acid residues. These are both hydrophobic and hydrophilic in nature.

In the final stages of modeling by the protein extension method, the side chains of the amino acids are rotated in order to minimize contacts between side chains that would be inside the van der Waals radii of atoms that constitute the side chains. This leads to maximizing the exposure, on the surface of the protein, of those amino acid side chains that are located at positions where there has been an insertion or deletion of amino acids in the polypeptide backbone of the hybrid structure that was used to model the final structure. The net effect is a highly irregular surface as compared to the rather compact models of the mammalian serine proteinases that are based entirely on X-ray crystallographic data, (compare FIGURES 3A-3F to FIGURES 4A-4F) but overall, the thrombin B-chain model retains many of the characteristic structural features seen in this family of enzymes.

Relationship of the Gene Structure of Bovine Thrombin to the Computer-Generated Three-Dimensional Model

In the study that described the construction of computer-generated models of the blood coagulation proteinases, we described an alignment of the amino acid sequences of factor IXa, Factor Xa, and thrombin with trypsin and chymotrypsin that was based on placing insertions and deletions in areas that were outside the stretches of amino acids and that constituted the beta barrels and the alpha helix.[8] Once the amino acids were aligned, we noted that there were regions that were well conserved as well as regions that were highly variable in terms of amino acid sequence homology. These were called the conserved regions (CR) and variable regions (VR).

Greer had previously identified structurally CR and VR in elastase, trypsin, and chymotrypsin based on a comparison of amino acid sequence homology between these three enzymes.[20] He noted that these regions could be placed at approximately the same locations in the entire family of mammalian serine proteinases. He also identified 23 constant regions that were sections that corresponded to sequences of amino acids that constitute the beta structure (as identified in the models based on X-ray crystallographic data) and 11 variable regions that contained the majority of the differences in amino acid sequences that were seen between the entire family of proteins. These variable regions uniformly fell between the beta-strand segments. By contrast, Furie *et al.* identified seven conserved regions and six variable regions based solely on consideration of the final three-dimensional models of the five proteins studied.[8] These regions were termed CR1-CR7 and VR1-VR6 (see FIGURE 2).

Since publication of the reports of the computer graphic models of the family of mammalian serine proteinases, data has been obtained on the gene structure of these proteins. Serine proteinases for which there are gene structures include rat trypsin, rat chymotrypsin, rat elastase, human factor IX, human and bovine prothrombin, pig urokinase, human plasminogen activator, mouse kallikrein, human complement factor B, C1r and C1s, and human haptoglobin.[21,22] Based on these data, Craik *et al.*[23–25] have suggested that exon-intron junctions map to surface loops of the serine proteinases. In a separate study on chicken pyruvate kinase, Lonberg and Gilbert have also suggested that introns are located at junctions between secondary structural features—the alpha helices and beta sheets.[26]

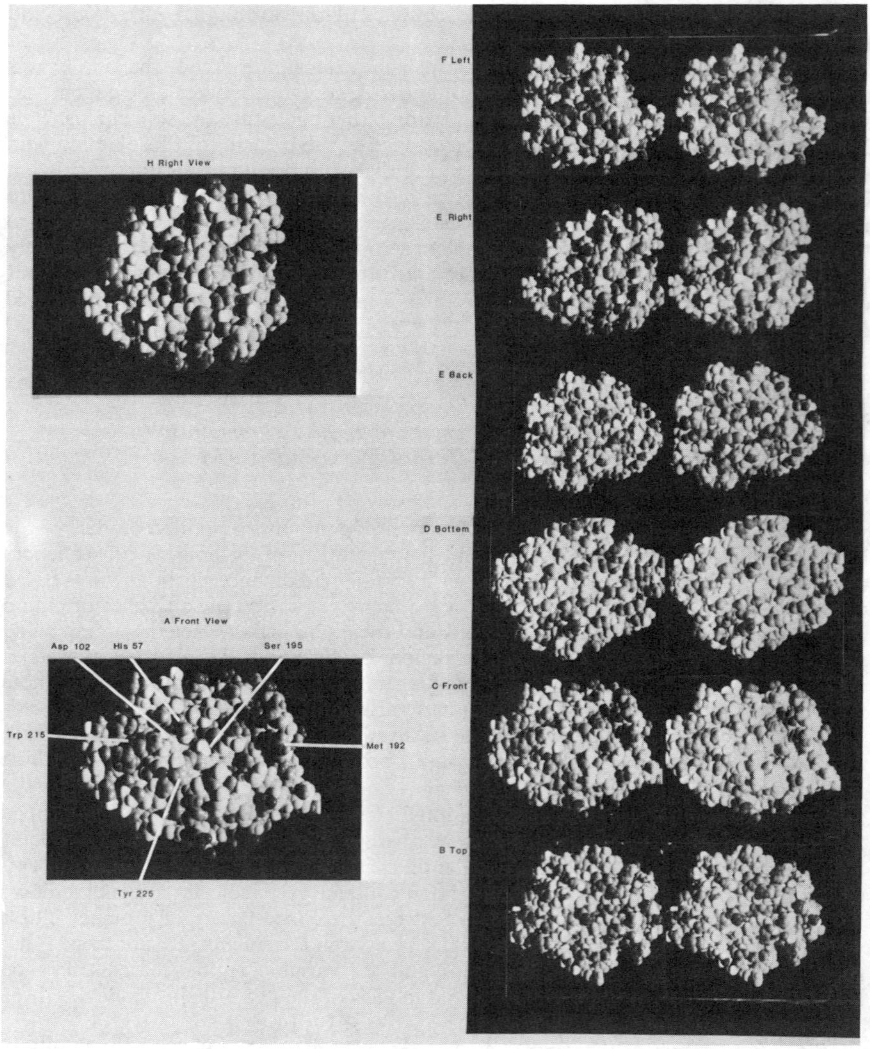

FIGURE 3. Computer-generated graphic representation of the model of alpha-chymotrypsin based on the crystallographic data set of Tulinsky *et al.*[41] Preparation of these models has been previously described.[6] The catalytic triad of Ser 195, His 57, and Asp 102 is taken as the center and is called the front (see A). With this orientation the stereo pairs are as follows: B is the top, C is the front (same view as A), D is the bottom, E is the back, F is the left, and G is the right. H is a nonstereo presentation of the right view (G) and shows an apparent open cavity in the front of the molecule. The amino acids are labeled. See text for details.

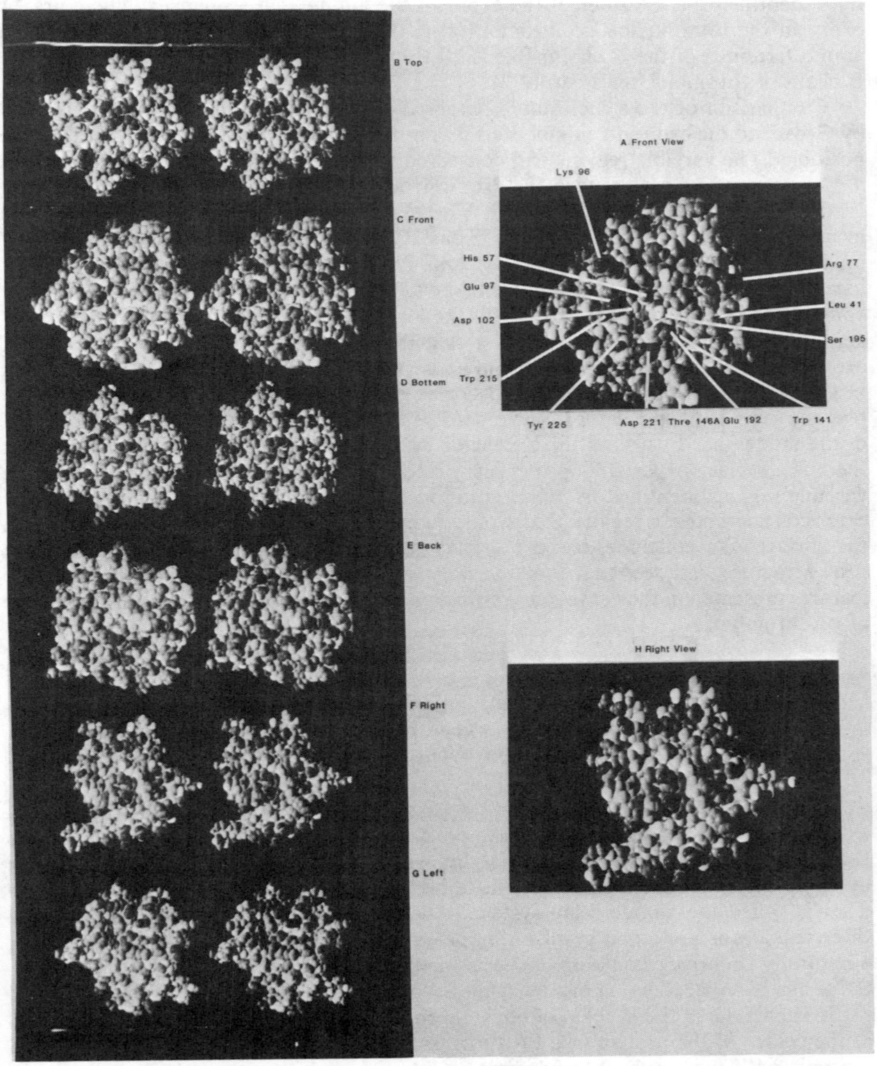

FIGURE 4. Computer-generated graphic representations of the proposed model of the B chain of bovine alpha thrombin. The model has been previously described.[6,8] The catalytic triad of Ser 195, His 57, and Asp 102 is taken as the center and called the front (see A). With this orientation, the stereo pairs are as follows: B is the top, C is the front (same view as A), D is the bottom, E is the back, F is the right view, and G is the left view. H is a nonstereo presentation of the right view (F) and shows an apparent open cavity in the front of the molecule. Compare this to the same view of chymotrypsin (3G and 3H). Chymotrypsinogen numbering is used for labeling the amino acids.

MacGillivray and coworkers[27] recently described the bovine prothrombin gene and have identified the locations of the exons in the amino acid sequence.[28] There are 14 exons in the total bovine prothrombin gene. Exon 9 codes for the A chain and the amino terminus of the B chain. Exons 10 through 14 are located entirely within the B chain of thrombin (see FIGURE 2).

Comparison of the structurally conserved regions and variable regions described by Greer[20] to the exon-intron junctions do not reveal an obvious correlation with these positions. The variable regions and conserved regions, however, identified by Furie *et al.*[8] correspond very closely to the exon-intron map for bovine prothrombin. Examination of the model shows that VR1, VR3, VR5, and VR6 begin at almost the same locations in the primary sequence as exons 10, 12, 13, and 14 (see FIGURE 2). Based on the predictions of Craik *et al.*[23–25] and Lonberg and Gilbert,[26] these should be located at surface-exposed regions on loops. This is what is seen in the model.[8] A comparison of amino acid sequences at the location of the exon junctions and the VR and CR regions would at first suggest that this analysis breaks down in the case of exon 11. Exon 11 begins at Tyr 75 and ends at Lys 128 (53 amino acids). VR2 begins at Leu 59 and ends at Arg 100; CR3 begins at Asp 102 and ends at about the same place as exon 11 (Asp 125 for CR3 versus Lys 128 for exon 11). Examination, however, of the model (see FIGURE 3 in reference 8 and FIGURE 4 in reference 39) shows that there is a surface-exposed loop that just precedes the beginning of exon 11. Thus, the variable regions identified by Furie *et al.*[8] in the model constructed with the protein extension method are regions that would likewise be inferred to be external loops on the surface. We conclude, based on what is known about the relationship between gene structure and secondary and tertiary structural features of proteins, that the features presented in the computer graphic model are consistent with the gene structure of prothrombin.

The Active Site of Thrombin as Defined in the Computer-Generated Model of the Thrombin B Chain

The active site of serine proteinases consists of two parts, the catalytic center and the extended binding site(s). The catalytic center in this family of enzymes is defined by three amino acids, serine 195, histidine 57, and aspartate 102. They constitute what is called the charge relay system.[1] The geometric spatial relationship of these three residues is preserved in all serine proteinases.[1–3] This is apparently even true in a naturally occurring homolog of the serine proteinases, haptoglobin. In this protein, the serine is replaced by an alanine, thus accounting for the lack of enzyme activity.[29]

In the model of the B chain of bovine thrombin, these three amino acids are placed at the center of the protein (see FIGURES 4A and 4B), and Asp 189, which forms an ion pair with positively charged amino acid side chains in the substrate, is at the bottom of a pocket that extends into the interior of the protein, 13.5 nm away from the hydroxyl oxygen of serine 195. It is buried and not visible in this view of the model. The region of the protein that contains these four amino acids is called the primary binding site. As previously noted by Bing *et al.*,[7] there are two changes in thrombin in this region, a serine to alanine change at 190 and a glycine to threonine change at 219. Both of these changes are consistent with the lower binding energy that thrombin (as opposed to trypsin) exhibits towards the small benzamidine inhibitors, as the alanine substitution would eliminate a possible hydrogen bond that trypsin forms with benzamidine at this position.

The extended or secondary binding site includes those portions of the enzyme on either side of the primary site (catalytic center) that interact at secondary positions in polypeptide inhibitors or substrates, as well as in other kinds of inhibitors or binding ligands. This covers an extended surface of the protein and can involve amino acids that are often widely spaced in the primary sequence. It can also involve only a small fraction of the total surface area of the proteinase. The enzyme trypsin has been studied quite extensively with regard to this aspect of its structure.[30] In trypsin, this secondary binding site can be roughly described according to those amino acids outside the primary binding site that are in actual contact with specific amino acid side chains in the protein inhibitors that form a complex with trypsin. Two such inhibitors that have been analyzed in terms of interaction with bovine trypsin are soybean trypsin inhibitor and pancreatic trypsin inhibitor. As analyzed by Janin and Chothia, only 29 out of the 224 residues in trypsin are in contact with the soybean trypsin inhibitor in the complex between the two proteins ($\geq$ 10 nm^2 of the available surface of the amino acid is buried), and of these (Phe 41, His 57, Leu 99, Gln 192, Ser 195, Trp 215, and Gly 216) 7 account for 70% of the interactions between the two proteins in a region that spans P_3 to $P_{3'}$.[31] Huber and Bode have additionally identified binding roles for Asn 143, Ser 217, Gly 217, and Ala 221 in complexes formed between trypsin and pancreatic trypsin inhibitor.[2]

We have used the information on the secondary binding site of trypsin to define a region in the thrombin B-chain model that can be hypothesized to correspond to the secondary binding site for protein substrates and inhibitors as well as other kinds of binding ligands. The hypothesis is that the restricted substrate activity of thrombin might be ascribed to amino acids located in this region of the model. In chymotrypsin, this region can be seen as an open cavity that extends on both sides of the catalytic center (compare the front view of chymotrypsin, FIGURE 3B, to the left and right views, FIGURE 3E, 3F, and 3H).

In the thrombin model, a similar groove is retained in about the same orientation (see FIGURE 4B front and 4E, 4F, and 4H, left and right side). The interior of this apparent groove contains the identical or functionally same amino acids as found in chymotrypsin as well as the hybrid structure used to model the thrombin B. Starting from right to left (FIGURES 4A and 4B), there is Tyr 225 (proline in chymotrypsin) and Trp 215, the catalytic center consisting of Ser 195, His 57, and Asp 102 at the center, and then down to the right, Trp 141. The primary binding pocket extends up and back, and Asp 189 replaces Ser 189 at the bottom of this pocket and is not immediately apparent in this view. At the far left hand side of the apparent groove are Leu 41 (phenylalanine in chymotrypsin) and Leu 99 (isoleucine in chymotrypsin). Thus, this groove retains structurally similar amino acids that presumably participate in the binding of polypeptide substrates.

By contrast, there are many changes on the surface outside of this apparent groove. These changes appeared to be localized in clusters of functionally similar amino acids. To the left and below the hypothesized active site groove is a series of charged amino acids (FIGURES 4B, 4G, and 5A). These include Glu 217, Asp 221, and Glu 192. To the right and above the groove is Glu 39 and at the lower right end is Glu 76. Above the catalytic center are two amino acids of opposite charge, Lys 96 and Glu 97. The cluster of anionically charged amino acids near the apparent groove have been ascribed to participating in the specific recognition of fibrin(ogen) and hirudin[32] (see FIGURES 4A and 5A).

In an area above the active site is found a cluster of hydrophobic amino acids. This includes Trp 95A, Tyr 60A, and Trp 60D. These are amino acids not found in trypsin or chymotrypsin, and the letters refer to the fact that they represent new loops of amino acids that are part of the variable regions described previously (see FIGURE

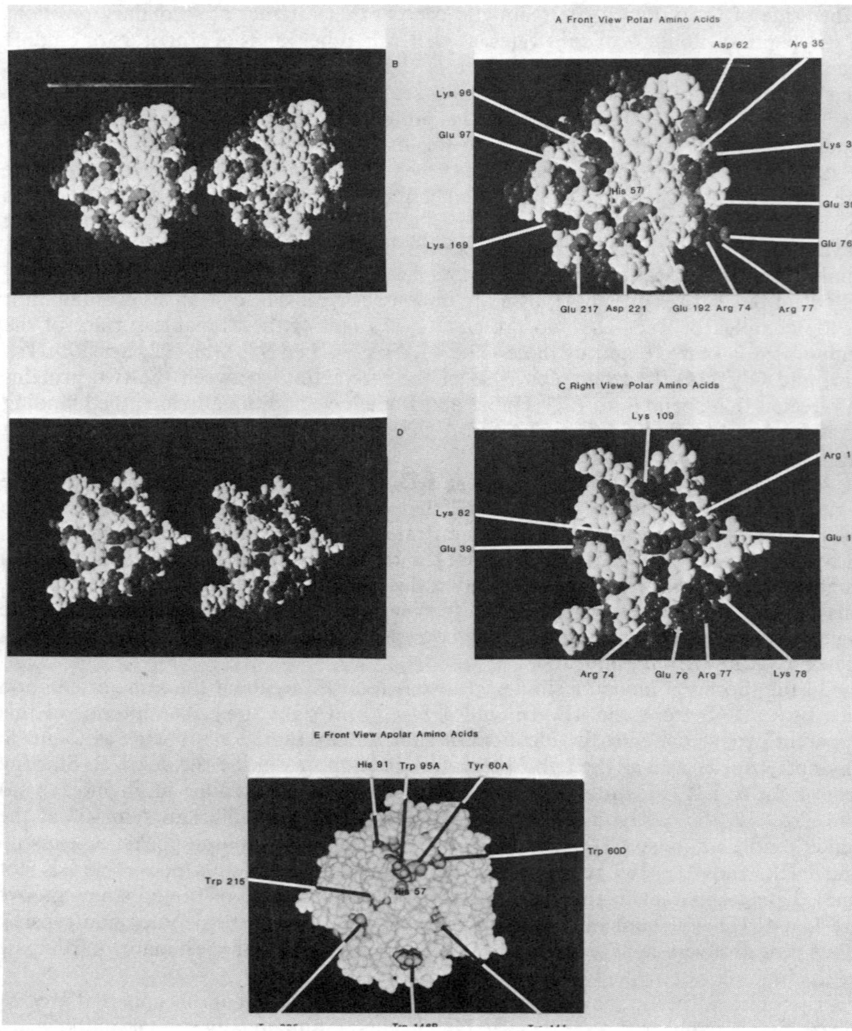

FIGURE 5. Computer-generated graphic representations of the B chain of bovine thrombin. A is the front view of thrombin, showing charged amino acids near active center. Dark residues are arginines or lysines, and lighter residues are glutamates and aspartates. The remainder is white. His 57 is marked to identify the active center. B is the stereo pair of the view presented in A. C is the right view of thrombin (see FIGURES 4F and 4H) depicting charged amino acids near the beta cleavage site; the color is the same as A. D is the stereo pair of the view presented in C. E is the front view of thrombin (see FIGURES 4A and 4C) depicting polar amino acids near the catalytic center in dark shading. His 57 identifies the active center. Chymotrypsinogen numbering is used. The letters represent additional amino acids found in thrombin, but not in chymotrypsin, and represent insertions (see FIGURES 1 and 2). See text for details.

2). In the same area is found Tyr 94, which is a tryptophan in trypsin but is also a tyrosine in chymotrypsin. The existence of a hydrophobic cluster near the active site is consistent with the observed inhibition of thrombin by proflavin and other apolar ligands.[9,32] An additional, apparently exposed hydrophobic residue that is seen in the front view of the model, (FIGURE 4A), is Trp 146B, below the hypothesized active site groove; FIGURES 4A and 5E show an area near the elastase cleavage site (see below), which may not participate in the binding of apolar inhibitors (see FIGURE 5E).

The Mapping of Bioregulatory Functions to Sites in the Model of the B Chain of Thrombin

In addition to its function in the coagulation pathway, thrombin possesses bioregulatory and growth-promoting functions.[32–38] Studies on the structural and functional relationships have allowed assignment of some of these functions of thrombin to specific segments of the primary amino acid sequence. Two bioregulatory functions for which there is such specific information are (1) the site of limited proteolysis in the B chain that leads to loss of clotting activity[33–35] and (2) the portion of the polypeptide chain that imparts chemotactic and growth factor activity to thrombin.[36–38]

The coagulant active form of thrombin, termed alpha thrombin, consists of the two-chain form of the enzyme; the A chain is about a 4 kDa protein and the B chain is about a 32 kDa protein for both the bovine and human species of this enzyme. The loss of clotting activity of bovine alpha thrombin is associated with limited proteolysis C terminal to Arg 77, but this new form retains full esterolytic activity as well as the ability to bind to antithrombin III, alpha 2-macroglobulin, and factor XIII.[9,2] In human thrombin, in addition to this proteolytic site, there is a second proteolytic site, Lys 149, which apparently is accessible only after the beta cleavage. This form of human thrombin is called gamma thrombin. The bovine enzyme has a glutamate at this position and does not undergo the beta-to-gamma transition.[33] A secondary beta cleavage site at Arg 66 by snake venom enzyme has recently been described[34] (see FIGURE 2).

In the thrombin B-chain model, the site of the beta cleavage is prominently displayed on the surface (see FIGURE 5C, right view). This represents another area where there is a cluster of charged amino acids that may relate to the activity of the enzyme. The Arg 77-Lys 78 residues, which are the sites of the beta cleavage, are readily apparent in the model (see FIGURE 5C). To the left somewhat buried are Glu 113 and Arg 110. Directly below Arg 110 is Lys 82. To the front is Lys 35A, which in this view obscures Arg 35. This latter amino acid, however, is apparent in the front view of the enzyme (see FIGURE 5A). Up to the left in the front view is Asp 62. Thus, there is a cluster of cationic residues, Arg 74, Arg 77, and Lys 78, in an area that corresponds to the site that is associated with the loss of clotting activity.

Presumably the beta cleavage site in the human enzyme will be the same, as there is a high degree of conservation of amino acids at all the positions mentioned above. The only difference, with respect to charged amino acids, is a replacement of Lys 78 by Asn 78 in human thrombin. By contrast, the gamma cleavage site is less clearly seen in the thrombin B-chain model, because the amino acid sequence homology between the two proteins is quite different. Not only is there little homology in sequence (Gly 148-Lys 149-Gly 150 in human versus Ala 148-Glu 149-Val 150 in bovine), there are significant charge differences at 144 and 145 (Leu-Lys in human versus Arg-Arg in bovine). Recently, another site in bovine thrombin has been described where proteolytic cleavage by elastase leads to loss of coagulant activity.[9,32] This site is located at the 146D and is on a prominently displayed surface loop that is readily apparent in the model (see lower left loop in FIGURES 4H and 5C). In the front view of the model site, this is located at the area of the protein where the Thr 146A (FIGURE 4A) and Trp 146B (FIGURE 5E) are identified.

Based on the assumption that the bovine and human thrombins will have approximately the same configuration, an analysis was made of the possible location of the chemotactic/growth factor domain in the model of the B chain of thrombin. Wilner *et al.* have shown that this activity can be ascribed entirely to the sequence encompassed in a cyanogen bromide peptide that covers the region from Leu 34 to Met 84A.[36-39] This part of the sequence spans almost all of VR1, all of CR2, and most of VR2 and is almost entirely within exon 10 (FIGURE 2). Thus, it can be ascribed to a distinct area in the gene as well as to distinct structural regions defined in the model of the thrombin B chain. A carbon alpha representation of this part of thrombin is presented in FIGURE 6. In the model, the segment from Leu 41 to Ala 56, as well as the disulfide bond Cys 42 to Cys 58 is internalized. There is a bend at Ala 56 that positions His 57 to be part of the catalytic center. The remainder of the sequence (the amino terminal part of VR2 or the C terminal part of exon 10) is a portion that in the model is surface exposed. This includes the site in the sequence to which the carbohydrate is attached. Because blockage of the active-site histidine, as well as loss of the carbohydrate moiety, does not effect the chemotactic/growth factor activity, it would appear that the amino terminal boundary of this activity coincides with about the beginning of VR2, for example, at or about Asp 61. It was predicted that Arg 74 and perhaps Arg 72 would not be required, whereas Arg 66 would be required, because the latter amino acid was part of the beta barrel secondary structure.[38] The fact that exon 10 ends at Arg 74 is consistent with this hypothesis. Currently, experiments are underway that use synthetic peptides as analogs of the naturally occurring peptide in order to define more exactly the structural requirements for this particular biological activity of thrombin.

SUMMARY

The advent of sophisticated computer graphics systems that permit the representation of macromolecular structure has made it possible to examine protein structure in detail. We have used one aspect of this technology to develop a model of thrombin. The model is based on structural and functional similarities this enzyme exhibits with respect to proteins found in the family of serine proteinases.

This review has covered interpretations of the structure of the model based on analyses of data that had been collected before and after the model was developed. On one hand, the conceptualization of primary and secondary features in the model of the active site of thrombin has for the most part been preceded by data from experiments on the interaction of thrombin with naturally occurring substrates and inhibitors. The features of the model explain these data adequately. On the other hand, the model has been more recently used in an interactive way to derive information about the bioregulatory aspects of thrombin. The realization that the amino-terminus portion of the cyanogen-bromide fragment was probably not part of the chemotactic activity, because it was probably internalized in the native protein, has suggested that

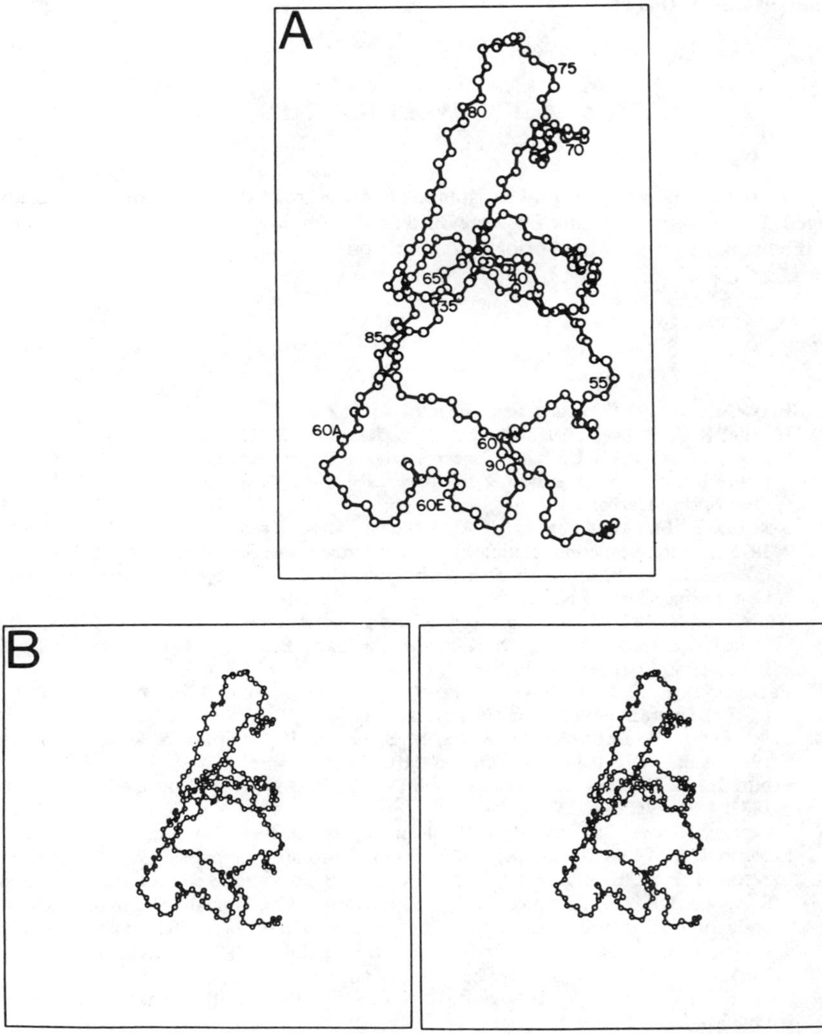

FIGURE 6. Computer-generated graphic representation of the cyanogen bromide fragment of thrombin, which has chemotactic and hormonal activity. **A** is the carbon alpha backbone with numbering. **B** is the stereo view of what is presented in **A.** Chymotrypsinogen numbering is used. The letters represent additional amino acids found in thrombin, but not in chymotrypsin, and represent insertions (see FIGURES 1 and 2).

synthetic analogs should focus more on the carboxyterminus of the peptide. It is hoped that in the future the model will continue to serve more in this function and that it can be used to explore further other aspects about the structural and functional relationships of this enzyme.

ACKNOWLEDGMENTS

The secretarial and editorial assistance of Ms. Noreen Ryan is gratefully acknowledged. We also wish to thank Dr. MacGillivray for sending us the amino acid sequence of the exon-intron junctions prior to publication.

REFERENCES

1. Blow, D. M. 1976. Accts. Chem. Res. **9:** 145-152.
2. Huber, R. & P. Bode. 1978. Accts. Chem. Res. **11:** 114-122.
3. Walsh, K. A. 1975. Unifying concepts among Proteases. *In* Proteases and Biological Control. E. Reich, D. Rifkin & E. Shaw, Eds.: 1-12. Cold Spring Harbor Laboratory. Cold Spring Harbor, N.Y.
4. Stroud, R. M., M. Kreiger, R. E. Koeppe, A. A. Kossiakoff & J. L. Chambers. 1975. Structure-function relationships in the serine proteases. *In* Proteases and Biological Control. E. Reich, D. Rifkin & E. Shaw, Eds.: 13-32. Cold Spring Harbor Laboratory. Cold Spring Harbor, N.Y.
5. Neurath, H. 1975. Limited proteolysis and zymogen activation. *In* Proteases and Biological Control. E. Reich, D. Rifkin & E. Shaw, Eds.: 51-64. Cold Spring Harbor Laboratory, Cold Spring Harbor, N.Y.
6. Feldmann, R. J., D. H. Bing, M. Potter, C. Mainhardt, B. Furie, B. C. Furie & L. H. Caporale. 1985. Ann. N.Y. Acad. Sci. **439:** 12-43.
7. Bing, D. H., R. Laura, D. J. Robison, B. Furie, B. C. Furie & R. J. Feldmann. 1981. Ann. N.Y. Acad. Sci. **370:** 496-510.
8. Furie, B., D. H. Bing, R. J. Feldmann, D. J. Robinson, J. P. Burner & B. C. Furie. 1982. J. Biol. Chem. **257:** 3875-3882.
8a. Shecter, S. & A. Berger. 1967. Biochem. Biophysics Res. Commun. **27:** 157-162.
9. Fenton II, J. W. & D. H. Bing. 1986. Semin. Thromb. Hemostasis **12:** 200-208.
10. Fenton II, J. W., B. H. Landis, D. A. Walz, D. H. Bing, R. D. Feinman, P. Zabinski, S. A. Sonder, L. J. Berliner & J. S. Finlayson. 1979. Human thrombin: Preparative evaluation, structural properties, and enzymic specificity. *In* The Chemistry and Physiology of the Human Plasma Proteins. D. H. Bing, Ed.: 151-184. Pergamon Press. New York.
11. Keil, B. P., V. Couhá, V. Holeyšuvský & F. Sorm. 1968. Coll. Czech. Chem. Commun. **33:** 2307-2315.
12. Keil, B. 1970. Structural aspects of interaction of trypsin with macromolecular inhibitors. *In* Structure-Function Relationships of Proteolytic Enzymes. P. Desnuella, H. Neurath & M. Ottesen, Eds.: 102-112. Academic Press. New York.
13. Neurath H. & K. A. Walsh. 1976. The role of proteases in biological regulation. *In* Proteolysis and Physiological Regulation. D. W. Ribbons & K. Brew, Eds. Miami Winter Symposia. Vol. **11:** 29-42. Academic Press. New York.
14. Neurath H., K. A. Walsh & W. P. Winter. 1967. Science **158:** 1638-1644.
15. Kreiger, M., L. M. Kay & R. M. Stroud. 1974. J. Mol. Biol. **83:** 209-230.
16. Stroud, R. M., L. M. Kay & R. E. Dickerson. 1974. J. Mol. Biol. **83:** 185-208.

17. HUBER, R. D., D. KUKLA, W. BODE, P. SCHWAGER, K. BARTELS, J. DEISENHOFER & W. STERGMANN. 1974. J. Mol. Biol. **89:** 73-101.
18. MAGNUSSON, S., T. E. PETERSEN, L. SOTTRUP-JENSEN & H. CLAEYS. 1975. Complete primary structure of prothrombin: Isolation, structure and reactivity of ten carboxylated glutamic acid residues and regulation of prothrombin activation by thrombin. *In* Proteases and Biological Control. E. Reich, D. Rifkin & E. Shaw, Eds.: 123-150. Cold Spring Harbor Laboratory. Cold Spring Harbor, N.Y.
19. GREER, J. 1981. J. Mol. Biol. **153:** 1027-1042.
20. GREER, J. 1981. J. Mol. Biol. **153:** 1043-1053.
21. ROGERS, J. 1985. Nature (London) **315:** 458-489.
22. TOSI, M., A. JOURNET, M. COLUMB & T. MEO. 1985. Complement **2:** 229. (Abstract).
23. CRAIK, C. S., S. SPRANG, R. FLETTERICK & W. J. RUTTER. 1982. Nature (London) **299:** 180-182.
24. CRAIK, C. S., W. J. RUTTER & R. FLETTERICK. 1983. Science **220:** 1125-1129.
25. CRAIK, D., Q. L. CHOO, G. H. SWIFT, C. QUINTO, R. J. MACDONALD & W. J. RUTTER. 1984. J. Biol. Chem. **259:** 14255-14264.
26. LONBERG, N. & W. GILBERT. 1985. Cell **40:** 81-90.
27. IRWIN, D. M., K. G. AHERN, G. D. PEARSON & R. T. A. MACGILLIVRAY. 1985. Biochemistry **24:** 6854-6861.
28. MACGILLIVRAY, R. T. A., D. M. IRWIN, E. R. GUINTO & J. C. STONE. 1987. Ann. N.Y. Acad. Sci. This volume.
29. KUROSKY, A., D. R. BARNET, T. H. LEE, B. TOUCHSTONE, R. HAY, M. S. ARNOTT, B. H. BOWMAN & W. M. FITCH. 1980. Proc. Natl. Acad. Sci. USA **77:** 3388-3392.
30. FENTON II, J. W. & S. H. SONER. 1984. Ann. N.Y. Acad. Sci. **435:** 412-414.
31. JANIN, J. & C. CHOTHIA. 1976. J. Mol. Biol. **100:** 197-211.
32. FENTON II, J. W. 1985. Structural regions and bioregulatory functions of thrombin. *In* Cell Proliferation: Recent Advances. A. L. Boynton & H. L. Leffert, Eds.: Vol. 2. Academic Press. New York.
33. FENTON II, J. W., M. J. FASCO, A. B. STOCKROW, D. L. ARONSON, A. M. YOUNG & J. S. FINLAYSON. 1977. J. Biol. Chem. **252:** 3587-3598.
34. BOISSEL, J-P., N. LE BONNIEE, M-J. RABIET, D. LABIE & J. ELION. 1984. J. Biol. Chem. **259:** 5691-5697.
35. FENTON II, J. W. & B. H. LANDIS. 1981. Prothrombin and thrombin transformations: bioregulatory and functions. *In* Perspectives in Hemostasis. J. Fareed, H. L. Messmore, J. W. Fenton & K. M. Brinkhouse, Eds.: 31-52. Pergammon Press. New York.
36. BAR-SHAVIT, R., K. HIRUSKA, A. J. KAHN & G. D. WILNER. 1983. Science **220:** 728-731.
37. BAR-SHAVIT, R., A. KAHN, M. S. MULD, G. D. WILNER, G. MANNIK & J. W. FENTON II. 1984. Biochemistry **23:** 397-400.
38. BAR-SHAVIT, R., D. H. BING, A. J. KAHN & G. D. WILNER. 1985. Thrombin-medicated chemotoxis: relationship to biological activity. *In* Membrane Receptors and Cellular Recognition. 329-338. Alan R. Liss. New York.
39. KAWATATA, S., T. U. MORITA, S. IWANUGA & H. IGARASKI. 1985. J. Biochem. **97:** 325-331.
40. OLSON, T. A., D. A. WALZ & J. W. FENTON II. Unpublished data.
41. TULINSKY, A., N. Y. MANI, C. N. MORINOTO & R. L. VANDLEN. 1973. Acta Crystallogr. Sect. B. Struct. Crystallogr. Cryst. Chem. **B29:** 1309-1322.

Specificity of Thrombin and Its Action on Fibrinogen

BIRGER BLOMBÄCK

Karolinska Institutet
Stockholm, Sweden
and
The New York Blood Center
New York, New York 10036

In 1876 Olof Hammarsten suggested that the action of thrombin on fibrinogen was by limited proteolysis.[1] Firm evidence of this was obtained about 70 years later.[2] We know now that although thrombin has a narrow specificity of action, it can digest a large number of protein substrates in addition to fibrinogen. This is exemplified by the recent review on protein substrates for thrombin compiled by Muszbek and Laki.[3] This list of substrates can be lengthened to include factor VIII,[4] and immunoglobulins.[5] The study of the cleavage points in these substrates shows that arginyl bonds are the preferred ones in all substrates. Furthermore, the presence of hydrophobic residues in P sites near the arginyl residue and usually small apolar residues in P′ positions, is evident. Otherwise, there are no similarities in the sequences preceding or succeeding the arginyl bond. It should, however, be stressed that a comparison of this kind is hampered by the lack of kinetic analyses of bond cleavage in most of the substrates.

In fibrinogen, a peptide bond is split at a considerable rate in the Aα- and Bβ-chain, respectively, releasing fibrinopeptides A and B (FPA and FPB) from the NH_2-terminal end of the peptide chains. The release of FPA is by far the fastest.[6] There is also a slow but complete release of a Gly-Pro-Arg peptide from the NH_2-terminal of the α chain of fibrin.[7] Kinetic analyses by several groups have shown that with regard to the Aα chain, the structural elements responsible for binding of thrombin reside within the first 50 amino acids of the chain. The most important elements are confined to three regions of this structure, that is, Aα 1-23, 33-44, and 40-51, the last being of least significance.[8–10] It has also been suggested that acidic residues in positions P′6-8 are of importance.[11] In the Aα 1-23 segment, the interest became focused early in the study on a nonapeptide sequence preceding the COOH-terminal in FPA, because this sequence was shown to be selected during mammalian evolution.[12] In the Bβ chain, it is impossible at the present time to recognize a similarly preserved recognition sequence for thrombin. It should be pointed out that in purified fibrinogen-thrombin systems, the FPB is released at a very slow initial rate. Subsequent to cleavage of FPA and once polymerization has started, however, there is usually a dramatic increase in its rate of release.[13,14] Conformational changes in the substrate as a result of polymerization have been offered as an explanation for this phenomenon.

A search for structures in FPA having affinity for thrombin was investigated in our laboratory some 20 years ago.[12] Based on the phylogenetic studies, we considered the hydrophobic residues in the COOH-terminal part to be of considerable importance, and in particular, the phenylalanine residue at P_9. It occurred to us that this residue was very likely part of an ordered structure that brought it near and in a fixed space relationship to the thrombin-susceptible arginyl bond in the Aα chain.[12] We tested this hypothesis by synthesis of peptides with phenylalanine at different positions from Val-Arg-OH.[15] The Bz-nonapeptide methyl ester (with Phe in position 9 from the COOH-terminal arginine) inhibited thrombin action. A tripeptide ester, Bz-Phe-Val-Arg-OMe inhibited thrombin almost as much as the nonapeptide ester. We assumed that this was due to the proximity of the phenylalanine to the arginine residue. The recent studies by Marsh *et al.*[16] give evidence for a β-bond structure in the COOH-terminal part of the Aα chain, which would bring the phenylalanine at P_9 close to the hydrolyzable Arg-Gly bond. On the basis of the above-mentioned assumption,[12] paranitroanilide tripeptide substrates for thrombin were synthesized.[17] It turned out that when position P_2 was replaced by a proline analogue, pipecolic acid, and P_3 by D-Phe, an even better substrate was obtained.[18] As mentioned above, there is an additional bond in the Aα chain, which is cleaved at an extremely slow rate in fibrinogen or fibrin. A synthetic Cbo analogue of this sequence, however, turned out to be a good substrate for thrombin.[19] This again points to the importance of a hydrophobic milieu around the bond being cleaved. The slow cleavage of the Aα 19-20 bond in the natural human substrate is not understood. Could the bulky residue at position 21 in the Aα chain possibly be responsible?

Several studies on isolated fibrinogen-thrombin systems have shown that the crucial event in fibrinogen gelation is activation of fibrinogen by release of FPA.[2,6,20,21] It is also evident that release of FPA leads to unfolding of a polymerization domain in the NH_2 terminal part of fibrinogen. This domain interacts with domains in the COOH-terminal part of other activated fibrinogen molecules.[22–26] Part of the complementary site is possibly located in the COOH-terminal part of the γ chain.[27–29] As a result of the interactions between the domains, linear polymers are formed (fibrin I polymers). In the polymers, the protomers are aligned in a half-staggered fashion. This model is supported by both hydrodynamic and electromicroscopic studies (see references cited in 30). These polymers subsequently interact and form the network structures that include water in its pores and thus form a gel. The incorporation of activated fibrinogen into polymers and gel matrix is stoichiometrically related to the release of FPA.[31] In purified thrombin-fibrinogen systems the initial rate of release of FPB is much slower than the release of FPA. The role of release of FPB in the initial polymer formation is therefore uncertain. Some facts, however, point to the importance of release of FPB for polymerization and gelation. Thus, in fibrinogen Detroit, having a point mutation (Aα 19 Arg $\rightarrow$ Ser), release of FPA does not produce clotting, which only occurs after FPB has been released.[13] In another fibrinogen, fibrinogen Aarhus, a similar phenomenon is found.[32] Light-scattering experiments have also indicated that polymers formed after the release of FPA and FPB have a larger average width than those formed after release of FPA alone.[22] Liquid permeation of gels produced after release of FPA and FPA plus FPB, respectively, also show differences in structure.[33] These findings suggest that release of FPB unfolds a second unique polymerization site in the fibrinogen molecule. This site is most likely unfolded by release of FPB from polymers formed subsequent to release of FPA and would result in interaction between polymeric species leading to increase in strand width of polymers and fibers.[31] It is also possible that for the complete unfolding of one polymerization site, both events, that is, release of FPA as well as of PFB, are necessary. In any case, it is appropriate at the present time to describe fibrin formation as a two-step process.

The initial release of FPB in recalcified platelet poor plasma is, like in isolated fibrinogen-thrombin systems, much slower than the release of FPA.[34] In platelet-rich plasma and in whole blood, the release of FPB appears to be dramatically accelerated.[34] Thus, in addition to changes in the substrate induced by polymer formation, factors in blood may change the susceptibility of certain bonds for thrombin. An apparent change in substrate specificity of thrombin occurs also when it is bound to thrombomodulin.[35] In this case, the enzyme has almost completely lost its capacity to clot fibrinogen, but has retained its capacity to split the specific arginyl bond in protein C that leads to its activation. In fact, the activation by the complex is several orders faster than by the free enzyme.

Finally, we should address the question of the effect of thrombin on the quality of the gels being formed. It has recently been found by liquid permeation experiments that thrombin regulates the size of the pores in the gels in such a way that high concentrations of thrombin give small pores, and low concentrations give large pores.[36] The pores in these gels have a remarkable uniformity, which can be shown by particle permeation studies and by scanning electronmicroscopy of gel matrices.[31,36] It is unlikely that one can obtain these ordered structures in random mixtures of polymers of varying lengths. We have therefore suggested that polymerization starts at initiation periods in the solution, and that the number of these foci are determined by the thrombin concentration.[31] Conformational changes in connection with the activation of fibrinogen may create density heterogeneity in the solution phase, resulting in the flow of nonactivated fibrinogen to the initiation points as a first step in the creation of order out of an initially chaotic situation. When polymers growing from these initiation points come in contact with each other, a three-dimensional network structure is established.

REFERENCES

1. Hammarsten, O. 1876. Nova Acta Regiae Soc. Sci. Ups. Ser. III. **10:** 1-130.
2. Bailey, K., F. R. Bettelheim, L. Lorand & W. R. Middlebrook. 1951. Nature (London) **167:** 233-234.
3. Muszbek, L. & K. Laki. 1984. Interaction of thrombin with proteins other than fibrinogen (thrombin-susceptible bonds). Activation of factor VIII. *In* The thrombin. R. Machovich, Ed. Vol. **1:** 83-102.
4. Vehar, G. A., B. Keyt, D. Eaton, H. Rodriguez, D. P. O'Brien, F. Rotblat, H. Oppermann, R. Keck, W. I. Wood, R. N. Harkins, E. G. D. Tuddenham, R. M. Lawn & D. J. Capon. 1984. Nature. (London) **312:** 337-342.
5. Chang, J. Y., S. S. Alkan, N. Hilschmann & D. G. Braun. 1985. Eur. J. Biochem. **151:** 225-230.
6. Blombäck, B. & A. Vestermark. 1958. Ark. Kemi. **12:** 173-182.
7. Blombäck, B., M. Blombäck, B. Hessel & S. Iwanaga. 1967. Nature (London) **215:** 1445-1448.
8. Hogg, D. H. & B. Blombäck. 1974. Thromb. Res. **5:** 685-693.
9. Blombäck, B., B. Hessel, D. Hogg & G. Claesson. 1977. Substrate specificity of thrombin on proteins and synthetic substrates. *In* Chemistry and Biology of Thrombin. R. L. Lundblad, J. W. Fenton II & K. G. Mann, Eds.: 275-290. Ann Arbor Science Publishers Inc., Ann Arbor, MI.
10. Marsh Jr., H. C., Y. C. Meinwald, S. Lee & H. A. Scheraga. 1982. Biochemistry **21:** 6167-6171.
11. Walz, D. A., W. H. Seegers, J. Reuterby & L. E. McCoy. 1974. Thromb. Res. **4:** 713-717.
12. Blombäck, B., M. Blombäck, N. J. Gröndahl & E. Holmberg. 1966. Ark. Kemi. **25:** 411-428.
13. Blombäck, B., B. Hessel, D. Hogg & L. Therkildsen. 1978. Nature (London) **257:** 501-505.
14. Martinelli, R. A. & H. A. Scheraga. 1980. Biochemistry **19:** 2343-2350.

15. Blombäck, B., M. Blombäck, P. Olsson, L. Svendsen & G. Åberg. 1969. Scand. J. Clin. Lab. Invest. (Suppl. 107) **24:** 59-64.
16. Marsh Jr., H. C., Y. C. Meinwald, S. Lee, R. A. Martinelli & H. A. Scheraga. 1985. Biochemistry **24:** 2806-2812.
17. Svendsen, L., B. Blombäck, M. Blombäck & P. I. Olsson. 1972. Thromb. Res. **1:** 267-278.
18. Claeson, G., L. Aurell, G. Karlsson & P. Friberger. 1977. *In* New Methods Anal. Coagulation Using Chromogenic Substrates. Proc. Symp. Dtsch. Ges. Klin. Chem. 1976. I. Witt, Ed.: 37-54. W. deGruyter. Berlin and New York.
19. Svendsen, L. 1978. Haemostasis **7:** 97.
20. Blombäck, B. 1958. Ark. Kemi. **12:** 321-335.
21. Blombäck, B. & T. C. Laurent. 1958. Ark. Kemi. **12:** 137-146.
22. Laurent, T. C. & B. Blombäck. 1958. Acta Chem. Scand. **12:** 1875-1877.
23. Blombäck, B. & M. Blombäck. 1972. Ann. N. Y. Acad. Sci. **202:** 77-97.
24. Kudryk, B. J., D. Collen, K. R. Woods & B. Blombäck. 1974. J. Biol. Chem. **249:** 3322-3325.
25. York, L. & B. Blombäck. 1976. Thromb. Res. **8:** 607-618.
26. Olexa, S. A. & A. Z. Budzynski. 1980. Proc. Natl. Acad. Sci. USA **77:** 1374-1378.
27. Olexa, S. A. & A. Z. Budzynski. 1981. J. Biol. Chem. **256:** 3544-3549.
28. Varadi, A. & H. A. Scheraga. 1986. Biochemistry **25:** 519-528.
29. Southan, C., E. Thompson, M. Panico, T. Etienne, H. R. Morris & D. A. Lane. 1985. J. Biol. Chem. **260:** 13095-13101.
30. Blombäck, B. 1985. Fibrinogen to fibrin—an overview. *In* Fibrinogen-Structural Variants and Interactions. A. Henschen, B. Hessel, J. McDonagh & T. Saldeen, Eds.: 33-42. Walter de Gruyter & Co. Berlin and New York.
31. Blombäck, B., M. Okada, B. Forslind & U. Larsson. 1984. Biorheology **21:** 93-104.
32. Hessel, B., S. Stenbjerg, J. Dyr, B. Kudryk, L. Therkildsen & B. Blombäck. 1986. Thromb. Res. **42:** 21-37.
33. Blombäck, B. & M. Okada. 1982. Thromb. Res. **25:** 51-70.
34. Blombäck, B., B. Hessel, M. Okada & N. Egberg. 1981. Ann. N.Y. Acad. Sci. **370:** 536-544.
35. Esmon, C. T., N. L. Esmon & K. W. Harris. 1982. J. Biol. Chem. **257:** 7944-7947.
36. Okada, M. & B. Blombäck. 1983. Ann. N. Y. Acad. Sci. **408:** 233-253.

Chemical Basis of Thrombin Interactions with Fibrinogen[a]

HAROLD A. SCHERAGA

Baker Laboratory of Chemistry
Cornell University
Ithaca, New York 14853-1301

INTRODUCTION

Thrombin plays many physiological roles, one of which is its proteolytic action to release 2 mol each of fibrinopeptides A and B (FPA and FPB, respectively) from 1 mol of fibrinogen. The proteolysis is very specific, occurring at particular Arg-Gly bonds of the Aα and Bβ chains of fibrinogen (FIGURE 1).[1,2] The purpose of this proteolysis is to expose one of the regions that is involved in the subsequent polymerization of the fibrin monomer produced by the action of thrombin; the complementary polymerization site, which is available even in the intact fibrinogen molecule, involves the C-terminus of the γ chain[3] (FIGURE 2). Immunoelectron microscopy[4] reveals that the site of thrombin action (and hence one of the polymerization sites) is in the central nodule of the linear trinodular structure of fibrinogen, and that residues 240-424 of the Aα chains[5] [and, presumably, the C-terminal portions of the γ chains containing the other polymerization sites (FIGURE 2)] are in the two outer nodules. It appears that the release of only FPA is sufficient to initiate polymerization, and that the release of FPB may uncover additional polymerization sites.[6-9] Our studies of the chemistry of the thrombin-fibrinogen interaction have been limited primarily to the proteolytic action on the Aα chain, although some of our experiments also concern the action on the Bβ chain. Some of these studies are summarized here, and further details are given in reference 2.

SOME PROPERTIES OF PROTHROMBIN

Before discussing the chemistry of thrombin, it is of interest to cite some properties of its precursor, prothrombin.

There is a disulfide-bonded loop near the N-terminus of prothrombin, at residues 18-23 (Cys-Leu-Gla-Gla-Pro-Cys in the bovine species), which binds Ca^{2+} ions.[10,11] (Gla is γ-carboxyglutamic acid.) The binding of Ca^{2+} to bovine prothrombin induces conformational changes detectable by intrinsic fluorescence,[12-15] circular dichroism,[16,17]

[a] This work was supported by a research Grant from the National Heart, Lung, and Blood Institute of the National Institutes of Health, U.S. Public Health Service (HL-30616).

and immunochemical methods.[18,19] Nelsestuen[14] and Marsh *et al.*[15] suggested that the Ca^{2+}-binding region of prothrombin might exist in two conformational states involving *cis-trans* isomerism about the Gla-21-Pro-22 peptide bond, with Ca^{2+} being bound only to the *cis* form. In this proposal, the binding of Ca^{2+} would induce a transition from the *trans* to the *cis* form. Eastman *et al.*[20] have begun to address the question of such a Ca^{2+}-induced conformational change by computing the low-energy conformational states of the 18-23 loop of bovine prothrombin in both the presence and absence of Ca^{2+}. In the absence of Ca^{2+}, the lowest-energy form has a *trans* Gla-21-Pro-22 peptide bond (FIGURE 3). However, when Ca^{2+} is bound to this Gla residue, the *cis* form has a slightly lower energy (FIGURE 3). These computations support the hypothesis that the binding of Ca^{2+} ions to the *cis* form shifts the *trans*-to-*cis* equilibrium to favor the *cis* conformation.

The bovine prothrombin molecule actually consists primarily of three domains: the 156 N-terminal amino acids (prothrombin fragment 1) which can be cleaved from the rest of the molecule (prethrombin 1) by thrombin; amino acid residues 157-274 (prothrombin fragment 2) which can be cleaved from the rest of prethrombin 1 by factor Xa to produce prethrombin 2 (the third domain). Cleavage of the Arg-323-Ile-324 peptide bond of prethrombin 2 by factor Xa (without the loss of any amino acids) produces α-thrombin, where residues 275-323 constitute the A chain and residues 324-582 the B chain of thrombin; the A and B chains of α-thrombin are linked by

A D S G E G D F L A E G G G V R ↓ G P R V V E R

Z G V N D N E E G F F S A R ↓ G H R P L D K

FIGURE 1. Amino acid sequences of the N-terminal portions of the Aα (top) and Bβ (bottom) chains of human fibrinogen.[1] The arrows indicate the thrombin cleavage sites.

a disulfide bond. The three domains of prothrombin are thought to be independent of each other.[21–31] Keeping in mind this proposed independence of the domains of prothrombin, we have begun an investigation of the folding of the reduced proteins (prothrombin, prethrombin 1, and prethrombin 2) to determine whether the domains can fold independently.[32]

Prothrombin and prethrombins 1 and 2 were first reduced and sulfonated by a method previously used for ribonuclease.[33] Next, the S-sulfocysteine residues of the reduced proteins were completely exchanged with glutathione in the presence of a denaturant (2 M guanidine thiocyanate), and refolding was initiated by a 20-fold dilution and incubation at 4°C for 1 hr. The use of a totally glutathione-blocked protein to initiate oxidative refolding was reported previously.[34] The resultant proteins were then activated with factor Xa in the presence of appropriate cofactors, and analyzed for thrombin activity by a standard clotting assay. The percentage recovery (relative to activated prothrombin that had not been modified) represents that amount of prothrombin, prethrombin 1, and prethrombin 2 that was correctly folded and recognized by factor Xa.

The amount of activity measured by these procedures varied inversely with the prothrombin concentration used in the refolding step, suggesting that interchain disulfide bonds are formed at high protein concentration. The recovery was only 40% (±5%) when the concentration of prothrombin was 4.8 μM, and as high as 93% (±5%) when this concentration was reduced by a factor of 10. Refolding of pre-

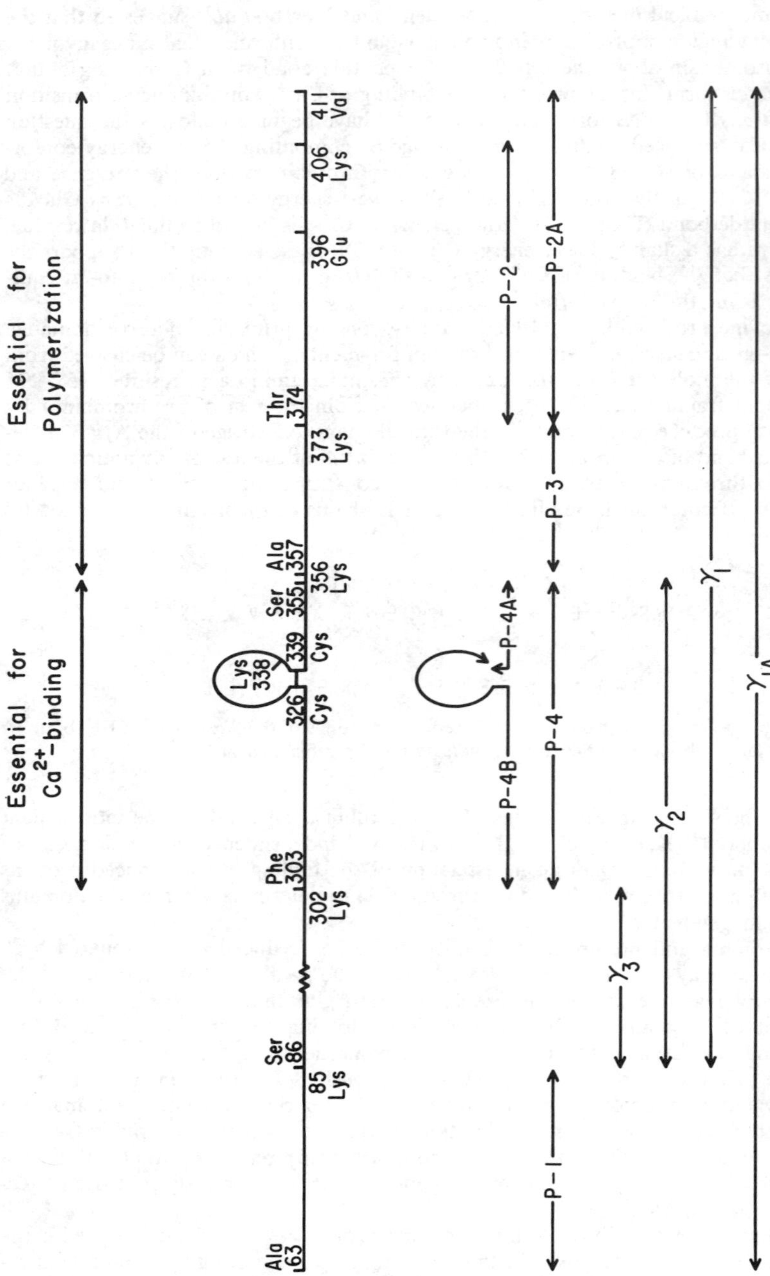

FIGURE 2. Schematic representation of the amino acid sequence of various fragments at the C-terminus of the γ chain of human fibrinogen.[3] The region essential for polymerization of the fibrin monomer is indicated.

thrombin 1 and prethrombin 2 at similar low protein concentrations led to similar recoveries (90 and 85%, respectively, with a standard deviation of ±5%). These results indicate that residues 1-274 are not required for the folding of the thrombin-containing domain (prethrombin 2). This is consistent with the view that prethrombin 2 is an independent domain in the prothrombin molecule. It must be emphasized that these results do not imply that prothrombin fragments 1 or 2 have necessarily been refolded in these experiments because the assay for thrombin activity provides information only about the folding of prethrombin 2 (and the factor Xa-binding site of prethrombin 1). However, other experiments are in progress to assess the refolding of these two N-terminal domains of prothrombin.

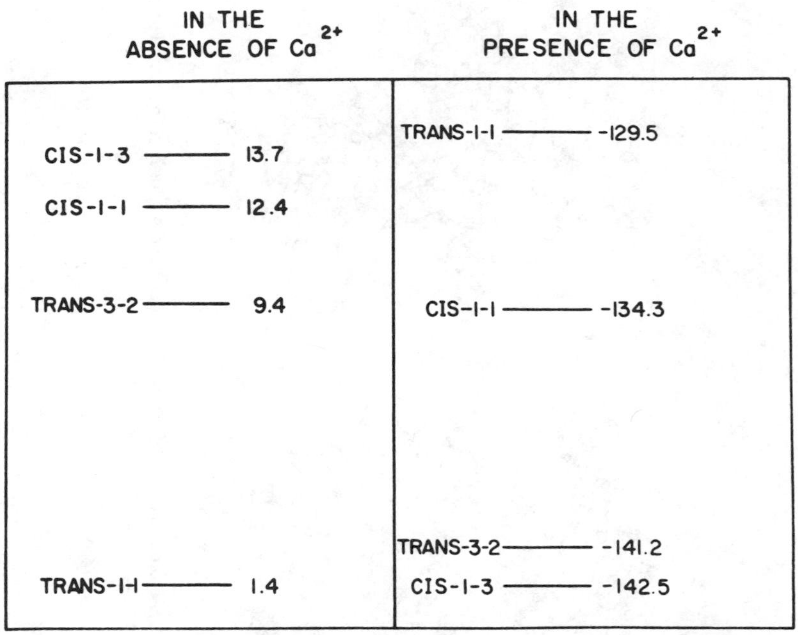

FIGURE 3. Relative energies (in kcal/mol) of the low-energy conformations of the 18-23 residue loop of bovine prothrombin in the absence and presence of Ca^{2+}. The two numbers following the words *cis* and *trans* designate specific conformations of the backbone and side chains, respectively.[20]

KINETICS OF THE THROMBIN-FIBRINOGEN REACTION

Generation of a fibrin clot from purified thrombin and fibrinogen is initiated by the proteolytic action of the enzyme and proceeds by means of three *reversible*[35-39] steps: the thrombin-induced conversion of fibrinogen to fibrin monomer, the formation of intermediate polymers from fibrin monomer, and the incorporation of the intermediate polymers into the fibrin gel network.[35-41] We shall confine our discussion here to the first step, the proteolytic action of thrombin on fibrinogen.

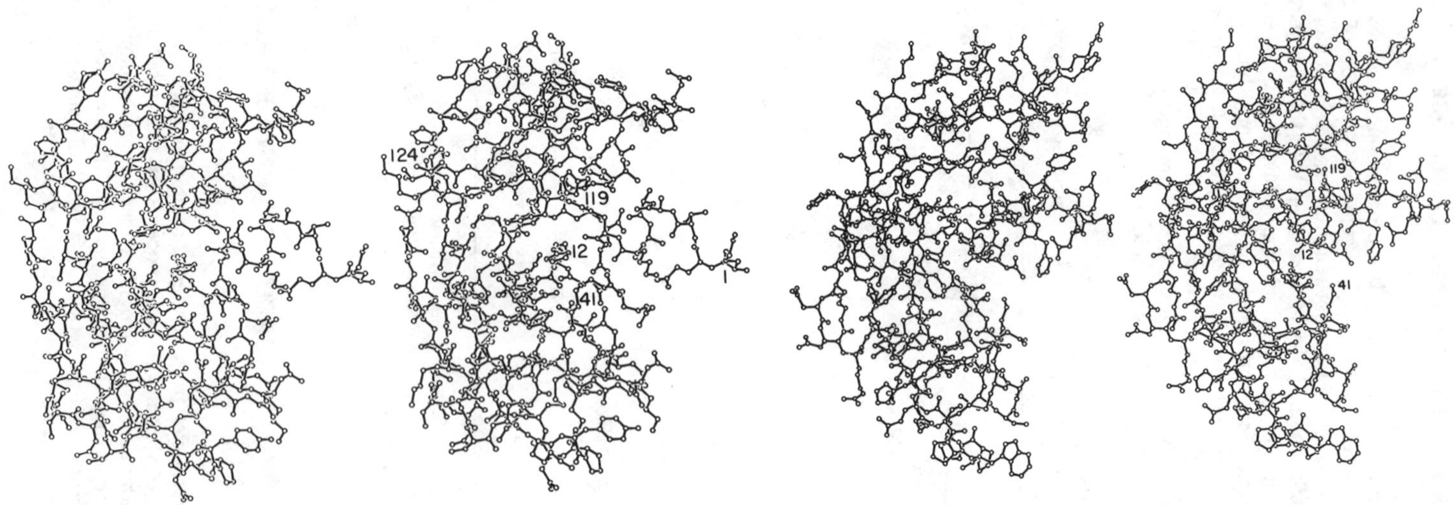

FIGURE 4. Stereo ORTEP diagrams of the full (heavy)-atom structures of ribonuclease (left) and angiogenin (right).[49] The active-site residues His-12, Lys-41, and His-119 (bovine ribonuclease numbering) are labeled in each structure.

An ultimate understanding of the thrombin-fibrinogen reaction will require knowledge of the three-dimensional structures of thrombin and fibrinogen. Since neither of these is yet available, we have to resort to various chemical and physical chemical approaches to try to elucidate the mechanism of this reaction. From its amino acid sequence homology to trypsin, chymotrypsin, and elastase,[42–44] it has been possible to suggest a preliminary three-dimensional structure of thrombin.[45,46] The computational methodology used for this purpose has also been applied to determine the three-dimensional structures of several other proteins, viz., the structure of α-lactalbumin from that of lysozyme,[47] the structures of several snake venom toxins from that of pancreatic trypsin inhibitor,[48] and a preliminary structure of angiogenin[49] based on its homology to pancreatic ribonuclease (FIGURE 4). Pending the acquisition of an X-ray crystal structure of thrombin, such models will have to serve to interpret experimental data on the thrombin-fibrinogen interaction.

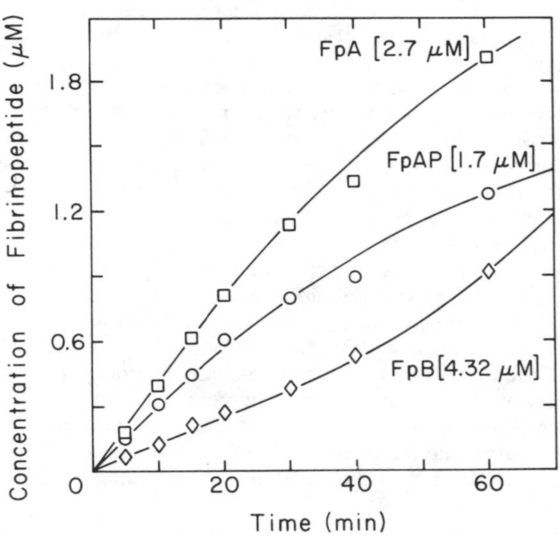

FIGURE 5. Typical experimental data showing rate of release of (□) FPA, (○) FPAP, and (◇) FPB from human fibrinogen at pH 8.0 and 25°C.[50] Values in brackets are the concentrations at infinite time. The initial concentrations were: fibrinogen, 2.15 μM; thrombin, 0.01 unit/ml; sodium phosphate, 0.05 M; KCl, 0.15 M; and ϵ-aminocaproic acid, 0.1 M. Clotting time was ~ 2 hr.

The kinetics of the thrombin-induced release of fibrinopeptides A and B from human fibrinogen have been studied under conditions where the subsequent polymerization of fibrin monomer is minimal, i.e. *before* t_c, the clotting time.[50] Some of the FPA was present as FPAP (phosphorylated at Ser-3 of the Aα chain; see FIGURE 1), and FIGURE 5 illustrates typical experimental data for the rates of release of FPA, FPAP, and FPB. The intrinsic rates of release (as measured by k_{cat}/K_M) are in the order FPAP > FPA > FPB (TABLE 1). It appears in FIGURE 5 that FPA is released faster than FPAP. However, under the conditions of the experiment, the concentration of FPAP was lower than that of FPA, and the kinetic constants of TABLE 1 demonstrate that FPAP (with a lower value of K_M and a higher value of k_{cat}/K_M) is a slightly better substrate than FPA.

TABLE 1. Kinetic Constants[a] for the Hydrolysis of Arg-Gly Bonds of Human Fibrinogen by Thrombin at pH 8.0 and 25°C

Peptide Released	$K_M \times 10^6$ (M)	$k_{cat} \times 10^{11}$ [M[(NIH units/liter)sec]$^{-1}$]	$k_{cat}/K_M \times 10^7$ [[(NIH units/liter)sec]$^{-1}$]
FPA	9.5 ± 0.5	50.0 ± 5.0	525 ± 50
FPAP	4.8 ± 0.3	32.0 ± 3.0	670 ± 30
FPB	15.5 ± 0.5	16.0 ± 0.5	105 ± 10

[a]See Reference 50.

A kinetic analysis of the data showed that the reaction is a competitive rather than a sequential one; i.e., the Arg-Gly bonds of both the Aα and Bβ chains are exposed to thrombin and compete with each other for the enzyme. Thus, FPA (FPAP) and FPB are released, without any observable lag time, from the start of the reaction, with FPB being released more slowly. The availability of the Arg-Gly bonds of both the Aα and Bβ chains is supported by immunochemical studies in which antibodies to the Arg-Gly regions of both chains were found to bind to the intact fibrinogen molecule.[51,52] Further evidence for this mechanism was provided by Ebert *et al.*,[53] working with fibrinogen Seattle II in which a His residue is substituted for Arg at position 16 of the Aα chain; only 40% of the FPA is released from this fibrinogen, whereas essentially all of the FPB is released by thrombin.

At longer times (e.g., later than 30 min in FIGURE 5), the rate of release of FPB seems to increase. It appears[54] that polymerization of fibrin monomer (which takes place after a sufficient concentration of fibrin monomer has been produced) may induce a conformational change which increases the rate of release of FPB and makes the reaction *appear* to be sequential (this latter process is of no concern in the above interpretation of the *initial* rates of release of these peptides, i.e., during the first 20 min). Further, Hurlet-Jensen *et al.*[54] showed that, in the *early* stages (where presumably very little polymerization of fibrin monomer occurs), the addition of a polymerization inhibitor does not affect the *initial* rates of release of FPA and FPB. Therefore, the initial rates in the first 20 min of the reaction were not influenced by any subsequent polymerization.

ACTIVE-SITE MAPPING

An active-site mapping technique has been used to assess the suitability of small synthetic polypeptides as substrates for thrombin. Polypeptides of various sizes, having sequences of portions of the Aα chain (FIGURE 1), were treated with thrombin, and the values of k_{cat} and K_M for the hydrolysis of the Arg-Gly bond were determined. The data are summarized in reference 55. As one adds residues, moving from the Arg-Gly bond toward the N-terminus of the Aα chain, the peptides are poor substrates until Phe-8 is incorporated. Then the value of k_{cat}/K_M begins to approach, but does not yet attain, the value for the Aα chain of fibrinogen (shown in TABLE 1). Addition of Asp-7 further increases the value of k_{cat}/K_M. The kinetic data were interpreted in terms of the hairpin-like model shown in FIGURE 6. This model places Phe-8 near the Arg-Gly bond, with the Phe presumably being required for hydrophobic interactions with thrombin in the enzyme-substrate complex. This structure is thought to be stabilized by a salt link between Asp-7 and Arg-19 and, because FPAP is a slightly better substrate than FPA (see TABLE 1), also by a salt link between the phosphate on Ser-3 and Arg-23. The absence of such salt links, as in fibrinogen Lille[56] (in which Asn replaces Asp at position 7) or in fibrinogen Munich[57] (in which Asn replaces Arg at position 19), would impair the effectiveness of the corresponding fibrinogen molecule as a substrate for thrombin.

Attempts were made,[58] using nuclear magnetic resonance (NMR) measurements, to obtain direct evidence for the hairpin-like structure shown in FIGURE 6. While linear polypeptides, such as those used in the kinetic and NMR experiments, undoubtedly exist as ensembles of many conformational states of similar free energy (i.e., they do not adopt a single native, low-energy form as do their larger protein counterparts), the NMR data[58] suggest the presence of a detectable amount of a hairpin-like structure resembling that of FIGURE 6. However, instead of the bend being at Gly-13-Gly-14 (as in FIGURE 6), the NMR data suggest that it is at Gly-12-Gly-13. Such a shift would bring the required Phe-8 even closer to the Arg-Gly peptide bond, and improve the alignment of the residues in the alleged salt links at Asp-7...Arg-19 and phosphorylated Ser-3...Arg-23. The proposed structure (i.e., the revision of FIGURE 6) would place the Gly-17-Val-20 portion of the chain close to the Asp-2-Asp-7 portion; in fact, such an interaction, but a *bimolecular* one (between the Asp-2-Asp-7 portion of fibrinopeptide A and the tetrapeptide Gly-Pro-Arg-Pro, a Gly-17-Val-20 analog), has been demonstrated by NMR measurements.[59] In summary, it appears that the specificity of thrombin may reside in a unique hairpin-like structure in the Aα chain of fibrinogen to bring Phe-8 into a hydrophobic pocket close to the groups on the enzyme that play the direct role in catalyzing the hydrolysis of the Arg-Gly bond.

It is of interest to note that the sequence -Gly-Gly-Gly- appears in the Aα chain of the fibrinogens of almost all animal species in positions corresponding to 12-13-14 of human fibrinogen.[60] This suggests that the -Gly-Gly-Gly- tripeptide may serve a structure/function role in accomodating a β-bend in this position of the Aα chain.

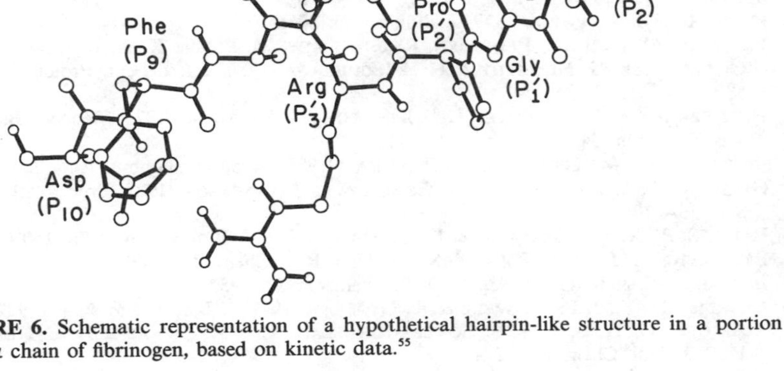

FIGURE 6. Schematic representation of a hypothetical hairpin-like structure in a portion of the Aα chain of fibrinogen, based on kinetic data.[55]

SOME PERSPECTIVES

Until we have X-ray structures of thrombin and fibrinogen, we shall continue our physical chemical studies of the interactions between these two molecules. Kinetic measurements on the hydrolysis of the Arg-Gly bonds of various polypeptide analogues of the sequences in FIGURE 1, two-dimensional NMR measurements on the polypeptides, and enzyme-substrate complexes thereof, offer hope of gaining information about the interactions between thrombin and fibrinogen.

REFERENCES

1. HENSCHEN, A., F. LOTTSPEICH, M. KEHL & C. SOUTHAN. 1983. Ann. N.Y. Acad. Sci. **408:** 28.
2. SCHERAGA, H. A. 1983. Ann. N.Y. Acad. Sci. **408:** 330.
3. VÁRADI, A. & H. A. SCHERAGA. 1986. Biochemistry **25:** 519.
4. TELFORD, J. N., J. A. NAGY, P. A. HATCHER & H. A. SCHERAGA. 1980. Proc. Natl. Acad. Sci. USA **77:** 2372.
5. HARFENIST, E. J. & R. E. CANFIELD. 1975. Biochemistry **14:** 4110.
6. BLOMBÄCK, B., B. HESSEL, D. HOGG & L. THERKILDSEN. 1978. Nature **275:** 501.
7. HANTGAN, R. R. & J. HERMANS. 1979. J. Biol. Chem. **254:** 11272.
8. OLEXA, S. A. & A. Z. BUDZYNSKI. 1980. Proc. Natl. Acad. Sci. USA **77:** 1374.
9. WILTZIUS, P., G. DIETLER, W. KÄNZIG, V. HOFMANN, A. HÄBERLI & P. W. STRAUB. 1982. Biophys. J. **38:** 123.
10. HENRIKSEN, R. A. & C. M. JACKSON. 1975. Arch. Biochem. Biophys. **170:** 149.
11. FURIE, B. C., M. BLUMENSTEIN & B. FURIE. 1979. J. Biol. Chem. **254:** 12521.
12. PRENDERGAST, F. G. & K. G. MANN. 1977. J. Biol. Chem. **252:** 840.
13. NELSESTUEN, G. L. 1976. J. Biol. Chem. **251:** 5648.
14. NELSESTUEN, G. L. 1977. *In* Calcium-Binding Proteins and Calcium Function. R. H. Wasserman, R. A. Corradino, E. Carafoli, R. H. Kretsinger, D. H. Maclenan & F. L. Siegel, Eds.: 23. Elsevier/North-Holland. New York, N.Y.
15. MARSH, H. C., M. E. SCOTT, R. G. HISKEY & K. A. KOEHLER. 1979. Biochem. J. **183:** 513.
16. BLOOM, J. W. & K. G. MANN. 1978. Biochemistry **17:** 4430.
17. MARSH, H. C., P. ROBERTSON, JR., M. E. SCOTT, K. A. KOEHLER & R. G. HISKEY. 1979. J. Biol. Chem. **254:** 10268.
18. STENFLO, J. & P. O. GANROT. 1972. J. Biol. Chem. **247:** 8160.
19. FURIE, B. & B. C. FURIE. 1979. J. Biol. Chem. **254:** 9766.
20. EASTMAN, M. A., L. G. PEDERSEN, R. G. HISKEY, M. PIQUE, K. A. KOEHLER, K. E. GOTTSCHALK, G. NÉMETHY & H. A. SCHERAGA. 1986. Int. J. Pept. Protein Res. **27:** 530.
21. HELDEBRANT, C. M., C. NOYES, H. S. KINGDON & K. G. MANN. 1973. Biochem. Biophys. Res. Commun. **54:** 155.
22. BENSON, B. J., W. KISIEL & D. J. HANAHAN. 1973. Biochim. Biophys. Acta **329:** 81.
23. GITEL, S. N., W. G. OWEN, C. T. ESMON & C. M. JACKSON. 1973. Proc. Natl. Acad. Sci. USA **70:** 1344.
24. BAJAJ, S. P., R. J. BUTKOWSKI & K. G. MANN. 1975. J. Biol. Chem. **250:** 2150.
25. PRENDERGAST, F. G. & K. G. MANN. 1977. J. Biol. Chem. **252:** 840.
26. BLOOM, J. W. & K. G. MANN. 1979. Biochemistry **18:** 1957.
27. NESHEIM, M. E., J. B. TASWELL & K. G. MANN. 1979. J. Biol. Chem. **254:** 10952.
28. ROSING, J., G. TANS, J. W. P. GOVERS-RIEMSLAG, R. F. A. ZWAAL & H. C. HEMKER. 1980. J. Biol. Chem. **255:** 274.

29. MANN, K. G., J. ELION, R. J. BUTKOWSKI, M. DOWNING & M. E. NESHEIM. 1981. Methods Enzymol. **80:** 286.
30. PLOPLIS, V. A., D. K. STRICKLAND & F. J. CASTELLINO. 1981. Biochemistry **20:** 15.
31. VAN RIJN, J. L. M. L., J. W. P. GOVERS-RIEMSLAG, R. F. A. ZWAAL & J. ROSING. 1984. Biochemistry **23:** 4557.
32. HANNA, L. S., T. W. THANNHAUSER & H. A. SCHERAGA. To be submitted for publication.
33. THANNHAUSER, T. W. & H. A. SCHERAGA. 1985. Biochemistry **24:** 7681.
34. DUDA, C. T. & A. LIGHT. 1982. J. Biol. Chem. **257:** 9866.
35. LASKOWSKI, M., JR., D. H. RAKOWITZ & H. A. SCHERAGA. 1952. J. Am. Chem. Soc. **74:** 280.
36. DONNELLY, T. H., M. LASKOWSKI, JR., N. NOTLEY & H. A. SCHERAGA. 1955. Arch. Biochem. Biophys. **56:** 369.
37. SCHERAGA, H. A. & M. LASKOWSKI, JR. 1957. Adv. Protein Chem. **12:** 1.
38. SCHERAGA, H. A. 1958. Ann. N.Y. Acad. Sci. **75:** 189.
39. LASKOWSKI, M., JR., S. EHRENPREIS, T. H. DONNELLY & H. A. SCHERAGA. 1960. J. Am. Chem. Soc. **82:** 1340.
40. BLOMBÄCK, B. 1979. *In* Plasma Proteins. B. Blombäck & L. A. Hanson, Eds.: 221. John Wiley & Sons. New York, N.Y.
41. DOOLITTLE, R. F., H. BOUMA III, B. A. COTTRELL, D. STRONG & K. W. K. WATT. 1979. *In* The Chemistry and Physiology of the Human Plasma Proteins. D. H. Bing, Ed.: 77. Pergamon Press. Elmsford, N.Y.
42. HARTLEY, B. S. 1970. Philos. Trans. R Soc. London Ser. B **257:** 77.
43. MAGNUSSON, S. 1971. *In* The Enzymes. 3rd edit. P. D. Boyer, Ed. **3:** 277. Academic Press. New York, N.Y.
44. MAGNUSSON, S., T. E. PETERSEN, L. SOTTRUP-JENSEN & H. CLAEYS. 1975. *In* Proteases and Biological Control. E. Reich, D. B. Riffin & E. Shaw, Eds.: 123. Cold Spring Harbor Laboratory. Cold Spring Harbor, N.Y.
45. ENDRES, G. F., M. K. SWENSON & H. A. SCHERAGA. 1975. Arch. Biochem. Biophys. **168:** 180.
46. BING, D. H., R. LAURA, D. J. ROBISON, B. FURIE, B. C. FURIE & R. J. FELDMANN. 1981. Ann. N.Y. Acad. Sci. **370:** 496.
47. WARME, P. K., F. A. MOMANY, S. V. RUMBALL, R. W. TUTTLE & H. A. SCHERAGA. 1974. Biochemistry **13:** 768.
48. SWENSON, M. K., A. W. BURGESS & H. A. SCHERAGA. 1978. *In* Frontiers in Physicochemical Biology. B. Pullman, Ed.: 115. Academic Press. New York, N.Y.
49. PALMER, K. A., H. A. SCHERAGA, J. F. RIORDAN & B. L. VALLEE. 1986. Proc. Natl. Acad. Sci. USA. **83:** 1965.
50. HANNA, L. S., H. A. SCHERAGA, C. W. FRANCIS & V. J. MARDER. 1984. Biochemistry **23:** 4681.
51. NAGY, J. A., Y. C. MEINWALD & H. A. SCHERAGA. 1982. Biochemistry **21:** 1794.
52. NAGY, J. A., Y. C. MEINWALD & H. A. SCHERAGA. 1985. Biochemistry **24:** 882.
53. EBERT, R. F., W. E. SCHREIBER & W. R. BELL. 1986. Thromb. Res. **43:** 7.
54. HURLET-JENSEN, A., H. Z. CUMMINS, H. L. NOSSEL & C. Y. LIU. 1982. Thromb. Res. **27:** 419.
55. MARSH, H. C., JR., Y. C. MEINWALD, T. W. THANNHAUSER & H. A. SCHERAGA. 1983. Biochemistry **22:** 4170.
56. MORRIS, S., M. H. DENNINGER, J. S. FINLAYSON & D. MENACHE. 1981. Thromb. Haemostasis **46:** 104, Abstr. 315.
57. HENSCHEN, A., C. SOUTHAN, M. KEHL & F. LOTTSPEICH. 1981. Thromb. Haemostasis **46:** 181, Abstr. 559.
58. MARSH, H. C., JR., Y. C. MEINWALD, S. LEE, R. A. MARTINELLI & H. A. SCHERAGA. 1985. Biochemistry **24:** 2806.
59. ROOT-BERNSTEIN, R. S. & F. C. WESTALL. 1984. Proc. Natl. Acad. Sci. USA **81:** 4339.
60. DAYHOFF, M. O. 1972. Atlas of Protein Sequence and Structure. Vol. 5, p. D-90. National Biomedical Research Foundation. Silver Spring, Md.

Effect of Fibrinogen and Ca^{2+} on the Thrombin-Catalyzed Proteolytic Event That Triggers Activation of Factor XIII

JULES A. SHAFER,[a] SIDNEY D. LEWIS,[a]
TODD J. JANUS,[b] AND LASZLO LORAND[b]

[a]*Department of Biological Chemistry*
The University of Michigan
Ann Arbor, Michigan 48109

[b]*Department of Biochemistry and Molecular and Cell Biology*
Northwestern University
Evanston, Illinois 60201

Formation of stable blood clots requires formation of glutamyl-ϵ-lysyl peptide cross-links between certain glutamyl and lysyl residues in fibrin. Formation of these cross-links is catalyzed by the transamidase factor XIII_a. Production of this enzyme is initiated by thrombin-catalyzed limited proteolysis of the inactive zymogen factor XIII during the final stage of the blood clotting cascade.[1] This initial proteolytic event in the reaction pathway for conversion of factor XIII to factor XIII_a involves cleavage at Arg-a36 and release of a 36 amino acid residue activation peptide from the a chains of the a_2b_2 molecules comprising plasma factor XIII.[2]

Using an HPLC procedure developed to monitor the release of peptides upon treatment of human factor XIII with human α-thrombin, two peptides, AP and AP′, with amino acid compositions consistent with that reported[2] for activation peptide (TABLE 1), were produced upon treatment of factor XIII with thrombin.[3] The appearance in lower amounts ($< 20\%$) of the second activation peptide (AP′) may reflect the presence of a factor XIII variant in the pooled plasma from which the protein was purified, or it could reflect partial hydrolysis at a Gln or Asn residue during purification. Treatment of factor XIII, or isolated AP and AP′, with alkaline phosphatase had no effect on the relative amounts or elution positions of AP and AP′, suggesting that activation peptide does not exist in different states of phosphorylation as does fibrinopeptide A (FPA). Incubation of acidified mixtures of AP and AP′ for several hours prior to HPLC resulted in the appearance of a shoulder on both the AP and AP′ peaks, but no interconversion of the AP and AP′. The appearance of the shoulder may well reflect an N-O acyl shift in the *N*-acetylseryl residue at the amino terminus of the activation peptide. Additional studies are required, however, to determine the structural basis for the different elution positions of AP and AP′ and for the acid catalyzed alterations of these peptides. All kinetic parameters reported in this work are for the release of the major activation peptide, AP.

Studies of the dependence of the time dependence of the release of AP on the concentration of factor XIII indicated a value of 0.14 × $10^6 M^{-1}s^{-1}$ for the specificity constant k_{cat}/K_m for thrombin-catalyzed release of AP. The value of K_m, which was too high to determine accurately, was estimated to be 84 (± 30) μM. Comparison of the K_m value for this process with estimates[4] of 20 nM for the factor XIII concentration in blood plasma, suggested thrombin-catalyzed activation of factor XIII might be too inefficient to be physiologically significant unless the process was enhanced by other plasma constituents. FIGURE 1 shows that the presence of 0.45 μM fibrinogen produces a dramatic enhancement in the thrombin-catalyzed release of activation peptide. The promoting effect of fibrinogen increased with its concentration, and under the experimental conditions a near maximal effect was obtained at 0.9 μM fibrinogen, well below the plasma fibrinogen concentration (~ 8 μM). When the concentration of fibrinogen was not in large excess of the factor XIII, there was a clearly discernible lag in the release of activation peptide. Under these conditions FPA appeared prior to activation peptide, which in turn appeared prior to fibrinopeptide B, FPB (FIGURE 2). This observation suggested that fibrin I or FPA, rather than fibrinogen, might be the immediate promoter of thrombin-catalyzed activation of factor XIII. Whereas FPA had no effect, fibrin I and II promoted thrombin-catalyzed release of AP from factor XIII. More importantly, as illustrated in FIGURE 3, the lag in the release of AP seen with fibrinogen was eliminated when fibrin I or II was the promoter. A kinetic analysis of the time dependence of the release of AP with fibrinogen as the promoter indicated that both fibrin I and II were equally effective in promoting thrombin-catalyzed activation of factor XIII.

TABLE 1. Amino Acid Composition of Activation Peptides Derived from the Reaction of Human Factor XIII with Human Thrombin

Amino acid	AP	AP′	Literature[a]
Aspartic acid	4.4	4.7	5
Glutamic acid	3.9	4.2	4
Arginine	3.6	3.5	4
Serine	3.0	2.6	3
Glycine	3.3	2.8	3
Threonine	2.8	2.7	3
Proline	4.0	4.0	4
Alanine	4.0	3.7	4
Valine	3.0	3.1	3
Leucine	1.8	2.7	2
Phenylalanine	1.0	1.0	1

[a] From the amino acid sequence for the activation peptide reported in reference 2.

FIGURE 4 illustrates that the inhibitor of fibrin polymerization, glycyl-L-prolyl-L-arginyl-L-proline (GPRP),[5,6] antagonized the promoting effect of fibrinogen. Because GPRP does not inhibit thrombin-catalyzed release of FPA from fibrinogen,[7] the simplest explanation of the antagonism by GPRP, is that fibrin monomer is not a promoter of thrombin-catalyzed release of AP from factor XIII, and that the ability

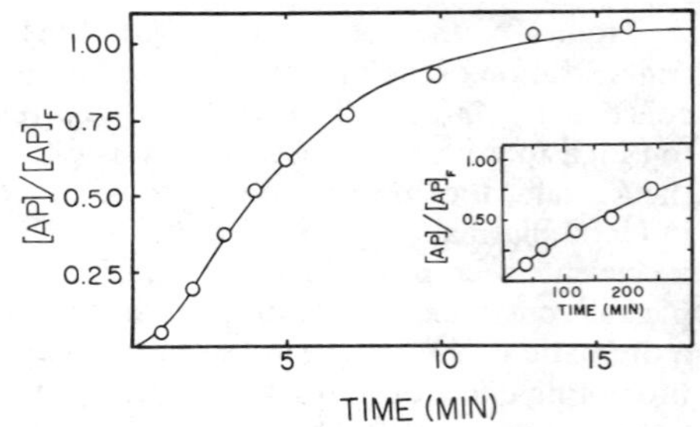

FIGURE 1. Thrombin-mediated release of activation peptide from 0.194 μM factor XIII protomer in the presence and absence (inset) of 0.45 μM fibrinogen at pH 7.4 (37°C, μ = 0.15), 0.1% PEG, and 0.565 nM thrombin. (Janus *et al.*[3] With permission from *Biochemistry*.).

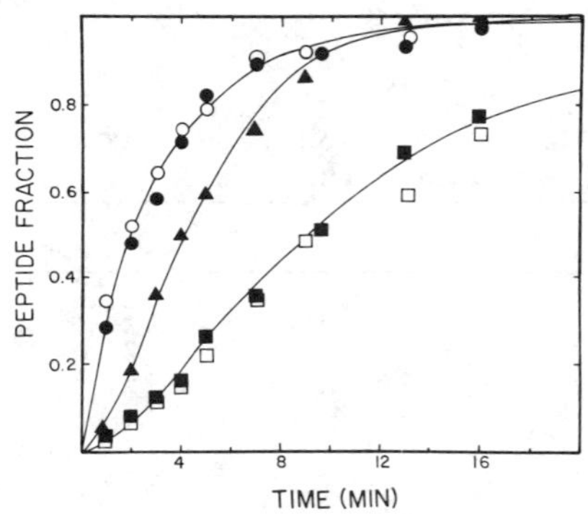

FIGURE 2. Sequence of release of fibrinopeptides and activation peptide from factor XIII at pH 7.4 (37°C, μ = 0.15) in 0.1% PEG by using 0.565 nM thrombin, 0.445 μM fibrinogen, and 0.258 μM factor XIII protomer. FPA, circles; FPB, squares; AP, triangles. The open circles and squares are data points obtained for the release of FPA and FPB in the absence of factor XIII. The ordinate (peptide fraction) is the quotient between the amount of peptide released at the indicated time and that released at completion of the reaction. (Janus *et al.*[3] With permission from *Biochemistry*.)

FIGURE 3. Time dependence of the release of AP, containing factor XIII and either fibrinogen (△) or polymeric fibrin I (▲) or fibrin II (○). Reaction mixtures contained 0.29 nM thrombin, 0.1 μM factor XIII, and 0.1 μM fibrinogen or 0.1 μM (with respect to fibrin monomer) polymeric fibrin. Reactions were carried out in 9.5 mM phosphate buffer, pH 7.4, 0.14 M NaCl, and 0.1% PEG, 37°C. (Lewis *et al.*[8] With permission from *Biochemistry*.)

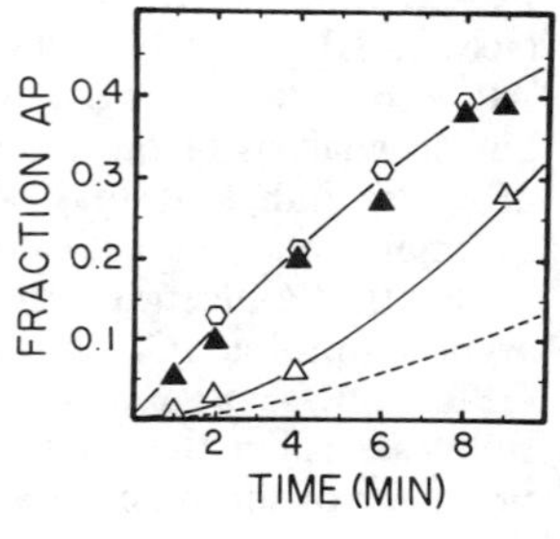

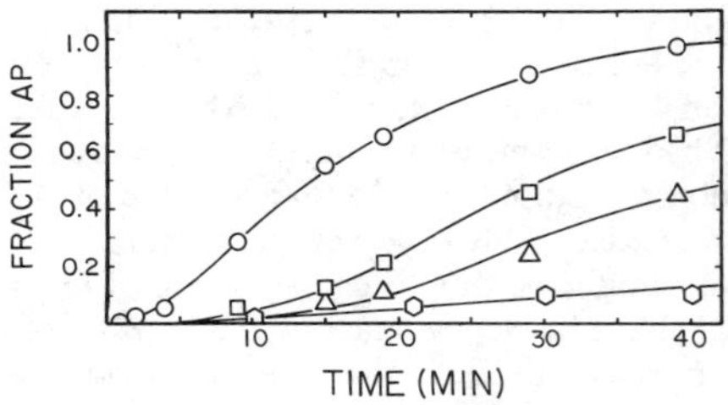

FIGURE 4. Thrombin-catalyzed release of AP from 0.10 μM factor XIII, with 0.10 μM fibrinogen added, in the absence (○) and presence of 0.10 (□), 0.21 (△), and 0.490 mM (⬡) GPRP. Reactions were carried out as described in FIGURE 3. (Lewis *et al.*[8] With permission from *Biochemistry.*)

of GPRP to act as an antagonist is due to its suppression of the polymerization of fibrin.

These studies of the fibrin-promoted thrombin-catalyzed release of AP from factor XIII were done in the absence of calcium. In the absence of added calcium, enzymically active factor XIII_a is not generated, because Ca^{2+} is required for steps subsequent to initial proteolysis in the reaction pathway for the conversion of factor XIII to factor XIII_a. Thus, in the absence of added Ca^{2+}, the fibrin in the reaction mixture remains non-cross-linked during measurements of the time dependence of AP release. Ca^{2+}-promoted cross-linking of fibrin, however, could well alter its competence as a promoter. Therefore, we were prompted to determine the effect of Ca^{+} on thrombin-catalyzed release of AP. The plots in FIGURE 5 show that the presence of 1.4 mM Ca^{2+} dramatically reduced the effectiveness of fibrinogen. FIGURE 6 shows that the effect of Ca^{2+} can be partially reversed by the presence of plasma levels of fibrinogen. Interestingly, 1.4 mM Ca^{2+} had no effect on the unpromoted rate of release of AP

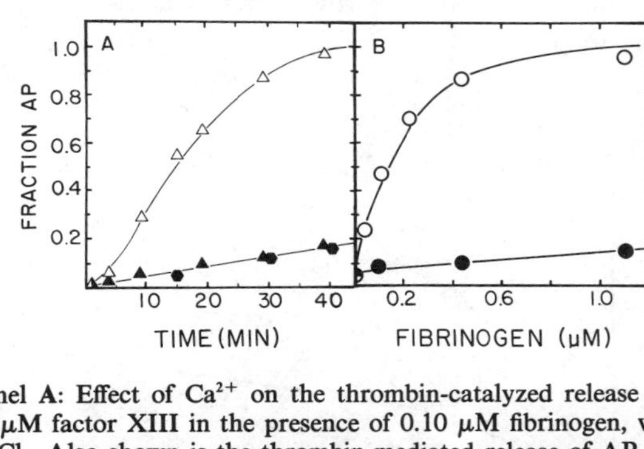

FIGURE 5. Panel **A**: Effect of Ca^{2+} on the thrombin-catalyzed release of activation peptide (AP) from 0.10 μM factor XIII in the presence of 0.10 μM fibrinogen, with (▲) and without (△) 1.4 mM $CaCl_2$. Also shown is the thrombin-mediated release of AP from 0.10 μM factor XIII without fibrinogen and in the presence of 1.4 mM $CaCl_2$ (⬢). Reactions were carried out as described in FIGURE 3. Panel **B**: Dependence of thrombin-catalyzed release of AP from 0.10 μM factor XIII on the fibrinogen concentration in the absence (○) and presence (●) of added 1 mM $CaCl_2$. The ordinate is the fraction of AP released in 15 minutes. The reaction conditions are as described in FIGURE 3, except the buffer contains 0.01 M Tris instead of 9.5 mM phosphate. Control experiments showed that the fibrinogen-promoted release of AP from factor XIII was the same in both buffers when Ca^{2+} was absent and that Ca^{2+} at 1 mM antagonized the effect of 0.1 μM fibrinogen to the same extent in 0.01 M Tris and 9.5 mM phosphate buffer. (Lewis *et al.*[8] With permission from *Biochemistry.*)

from factor XIII observed in the absence of fibrinogen. The data in FIGURE 6 indicate that only a fraction of the AP is released at an enhanced rate in the presence of Ca^{2+}. Thus, in the presence of 6 μM fibrinogen and 1 mM Ca^{2+}, the rate of AP release fell to the unpromoted rate after 20% of the AP had been released, whereas in the absence of added Ca^{2+}, the presence of 6 μM fibrinogen resulted in an enhanced rate of AP release until well over 90% of the AP was released. This observation indicated that the time-dependent loss in promoting activity might be due to cross-linking of fibrin by the activated factor XIII. Comparison of the time dependence of AP release and cross-linking of fibrin revealed that in the presence of Ca^{2+} the rate of AP release decreased to that seen in the absence of fibrin when 40% of the γ chains of fibrin had become cross-linked. This result suggests that if non-cross-linked fibrin is a promoter and cross-linked fibrin is not, the promoting activity of fibrin must involve the interaction of more than one repeating unit of fibrin with each molecule of factor XIII.

Consistent with the notion that formation of cross-links inactivated fibrin as a promoter of thrombin-catalyzed release of AP from factor XIII, the thiol reagent methyl methanethiosulfonate (MMTS) inactivated the activated factor XIII and substantially blocked the effect of Ca^{2+} (FIGURE 7). The failure of MMTS to block completely the inhibitory effect of Ca^{2+} suggests that Ca^{2+} may have secondary inhibitory effects on the fibrin-promoted reaction.

Preliminary studies of the dependence of thrombin-catalyzed AP release on the concentration of factor XIII and fibrin indicate that fibrin reduces the K_m for the thrombin-catalyzed reaction, consistent with the possibility that fibrin forms a complex with factor XIII, which exhibits a high affinity for thrombin. Interestingly, γ-thrombin, a form of thrombin that interacts poorly with fibrinogen, did not exhibit fibrin-promoted release of AP, although in the absence of fibrin, the rate of γ-thrombin-catalyzed release of AP from factor XIII was only fivefold lower than that of normal α-thrombin. This observation suggests the possibility that in fibrin-promoted α-thrombin-catalyzed release of AP from factor XIII, the fibrin interacts with both the factor XIII and thrombin and thereby presents the factor XIII scissile bond to the active site of thrombin.

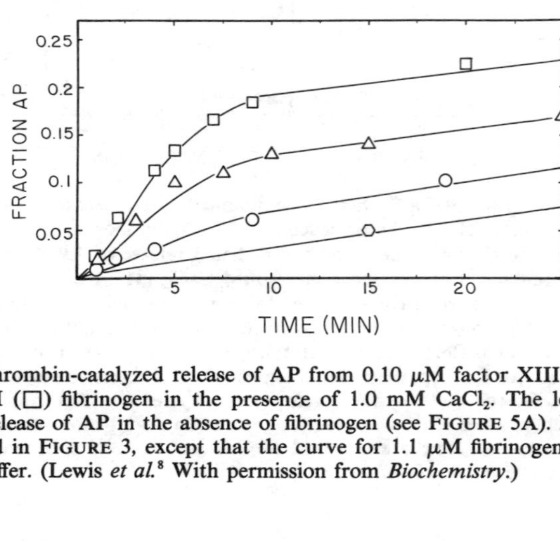

FIGURE 6. Thrombin-catalyzed release of AP from 0.10 μM factor XIII with 0.10 (○), 1.1 (△), and 6 μM (□) fibrinogen in the presence of 1.0 mM $CaCl_2$. The lowest line and (○) represent the release of AP in the absence of fibrinogen (see FIGURE 5A). Reaction conditions are as described in FIGURE 3, except that the curve for 1.1 μM fibrinogen was determined in 0.01 M Tris buffer. (Lewis *et al.*[8] With permission from *Biochemistry.*)

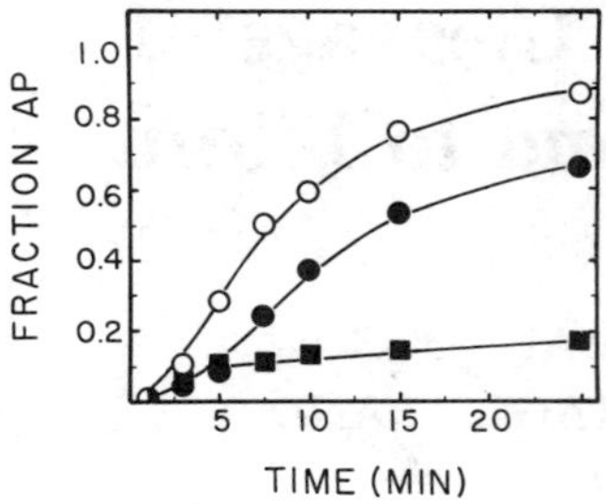

FIGURE 7. Ability of MMTS to block the inhibitory effects of Ca^{2+} on thrombin-catalyzed release of AP from factor XIII. Reaction mixtures contained 0.29 nM thrombin, 1.1 μM fibrinogen, 0.1 μM factor XIII, and (■) no MMTS and 1 mM Ca^{2+}, (●) 1.2 mM MMTS and 1 mM Ca^{2+}, or (○) 1.2 mM MMTS and no added Ca^{2+}. Reaction conditions are as described in FIGURE 3 except the buffer species was 0.01 M Tris. (Lewis *et al.*[8] With permission from *Biochemistry*.)

The unique ability of polymeric non-cross-linked fibrin to promote thrombin-catalyzed release of AP could ensure that production of factor XIII_a is initiated when its substrate is present and that production of additional factor XIII_a is terminated upon cross-linking of fibrin γ chains. This mode of regulation may serve to ensure against wasteful and possibly deleterious activation of factor XIII. It is our hypothesis that the final degree of cross-linking of a fibrin clot should increase with the amount of fibrin-associated factor XIII_a, because the ability of a molecule of factor XIII_a to catalyze formation of cross-links should be lost as the factor XIII_a becomes enmeshed in the network of cross-links it produces. If this contention is correct, a high density of factor XIII_a might be expected to result in a more heavily cross-linked clot, which would be more difficult for plasmin to dissolve, and more likely to lead to thrombosis. Thus, the regulation of factor XIII_a described in this paper may be an important determinant for the formation of stable fibrin blood clots, which can later be efficiently dissolved by plasmin. Investigations are in progress to test this hypothesis.

REFERENCES

1. LORAND, L. & K. KONISHI. 1984. Arch. Biochem. Biophys. **105:** 58-67.
2. TAKAGI, T. & R. F. DOOLITTLE. 1974. Biochemistry **13:** 750-756.
3. JANUS, T. J., S. D. LEWIS, L. LORAND & J. A. SHAFER. 1983. Biochemistry **22:** 6269-6272.
4. SKRZYNIA, C., H. M. REISNER & J. MCDONAGH. 1982. Blood **60:** 1089-1095.
5. LAUDANO, A. P. & R. F. DOOLITTLE. 1978. Proc. Natl. Acad. Sci. USA **75:** 3085-3089.
6. LAUDANO, A. P. & R. F. DOOLITTLE. 1980. Biochemistry **19:** 1013-1019.
7. HIGGINS, D. L., S. D. LEWIS & J. A. SHAFER. 1983. J. Biol. Chem. **258:** 9276-9282.
8. LEWIS, S. D., T. J. JANUS, L. LORAND & J. A. SHAFER. 1985. Biochemistry **24:** 6772-6777.

Regulation of Thrombin Cleavage of Plasma Factor XIII Bound to Fibrin

CHARLES S. GREENBERG, KOMANDOOR E. ACHYUTHAN, CHARLES C. MIRAGLIA, AND JOSEPH V. DOBSON

Departments of Medicine and Pathology
Duke University Medical Center
Durham, North Carolina 27710

The regulation of thrombin cleavage of plasma factor XIII is an important step in hemostasis. Thrombin cleavage of factor XIII is required to generate factor XIII_a, the fibrin stabilizing enzyme, during blood coagulation. Thrombin cleaves a 4,000 dalton activation peptide from both A chains of plasma factor XIII,[1] which in the presence of calcium and fibrinogen causes both B chains to dissociate producing factor XIII_a.[2,3] During clotting, factor XIII_a makes fibrin resistant to mechanical disruption and plasminolysis by covalently cross-linking fibrin molecules to each other and cross-linking α_2-plasmin inhibitor to fibrin.

During the clotting of platelet-rich plasma, thrombin cleaves fibrinogen 43-fold faster than plasma factor XIII, causing factor XIII_a to form during fibrin polymerization.[4] Gly-Pro-Arg-Pro, an inhibitor of fibrin polymerization, inhibits thrombin cleavage of plasma factor XIII without modifying thrombin cleavage of fibrinogen.[4–6] Fibrin polymers derived from des A or des A,B fibrinogen enhance the rate of α-thrombin cleavage of plasma factor XIII in afibrinogenemic plasma.[5] Furthermore, sodium chloride and glycerol, compounds, which inhibit fibrin polymerization, also delay thrombin cleavage of factor XIII in the presence of fibrin polymers.[7] Fibrinogen degradation products (fragments D and E) produced by plasmin neither polymerize nor enhance thrombin cleavage of factor XIII.[7] Therefore, plasmin regulates factor XIII_a formation by degrading fibrinogen, an important cofactor for factor XIII_a formation. Recently, Lewis *et al.* found that factor XIII_a-cross-linked fibrin polymers no longer promote thrombin cleavage of factor XIII.[6] This may also provide a mechanism for regulating factor XIII_a formation. Kinetic studies using purified plasma factor XIII and des A,B fibrinogen demonstrate that fibrin polymers reduce the K_m for thrombin-catalyzed cleavage of plasma factor XIII by at least 130-fold.[6] Furthermore, there is limited dependence of the initial rate of thrombin cleavage of plasma factor XIII on the factor XIII concentration.[6] These results provide further support for the formation of a complex between fibrin polymers and factor XIII, which has a higher affinity for thrombin than free plasma factor XIII.[6] These studies document the importance of fibrin polymers as cofactors for thrombin cleavage of plasma factor XIII. They do not explain, however, the mechanism by which fibrin polymers promote thrombin cleavage of factor XIII.

Plasma factor XIII binds specifically to fibrin polymers during blood clotting in the presence or absence of divalent cations.[8] Therefore, the association of plasma factor XIII (a_2b_2) with the fibrin polymer surface may be important in regulating thrombin cleavage of factor XIII. Furthermore, platelet factor XIII, which is composed only of A chains, also binds to fibrin polymers.[8] To investigate whether the B chains regulate thrombin cleavage of factor XIII A chains bound to fibrin, we studied the effect of fibrin polymers on α-thrombin cleavage of platelet and plasma factor XIII. Another mechanism by which thrombin cleavage of plasma factor XIII may be enhanced is through thrombin binding to fibrin. α-Thrombin binds to both fibrin and fibrinogen.[9,10] By contrast, γ-thrombin, a trypsin-modified form of α-thrombin, which cleaves factor XIII to factor XIII_a,[11] does not bind to fibrin(ogen).[9,10] To test the hypothesis that α-thrombin binding to fibrin regulates thrombin cleavage of factor XIII, we studied the effect of fibrin polymers on α- and γ-thrombin cleavage of plasma factor XIII.

Human α-thrombin, γ-thrombin, and DIP-thrombin were supplied by Dr. John Fenton II, Albany, NY. Fibrinogen, des A,B fibrinogen, plasma, and platelet factor XIII were prepared using previously described methods.[5,12] Thrombin concentrations were based upon protein concentrations.

Measurement of α- and γ-thrombin cleavage of platelet and plasma factor XIII was performed in the presence and absence of des A,B fibrinogen. α- or γ-Thrombin concentrations from 0.01 to 1000 nM were incubated with platelet factor XIII (6 nM) or plasma factor XIII (9 nM) for 5 minutes at 37°C in the presence or absence of des A,B fibrinogen (0.62 nM) in either 0.02 M Tris-HCl, 0.13 M NaCl, 5 mM $CaCl_2$ pH 7.4 or bentonite-adsorbed factor XIII-deficient plasma.[13] Thrombin was inhibited by adding 100-fold molar excess of D-phenylalanyl-L-prolyl-arginine-chloromethylketone (PPACK). The amount of factor XIII that was cleaved by thrombin was determined by a [^{3}H]putrescine incorporation assay.[14] Results from the [^{3}H]putrescine assay correlated with the amount of factor XIII cleaved by thrombin[14] when analyzed by sodium dodecyl sulfate polyacrylamide gel electrophoresis (SDS-PAGE). Less than 5% of the factor XIII preparations used in this study exhibited activity in the absence of thrombin. SDS-PAGE of thrombin-cleaved factor XIII demonstrated that over 90% of the A chains were cleaved by thrombin.

Des A,B fibrinogen reduced by 20-fold the α-thrombin concentration required to convert plasma factor XIII to factor XIII_a in bentonite-adsorbed afibrinogenemic plasma and in Tris-buffered saline. When a 10-fold molar excess of DIP- or PPACK-modified thrombins were added to reaction mixtures containing purified plasma factor XIII, des A,B fibrinogen, and thrombin, α-thrombin cleavage of factor XIII was inhibited by greater than 90 percent.

In the absence of fibrin polymers, the thrombin concentration necessary to activate plasma factor XIII was 10-fold higher than that required to activate platelet factor XIII. γ-Thrombin cleavage of plasma factor XIII was not modified by the presence of fibrin polymers. In addition, the α- or γ-thrombin concentration required to activate platelet factor XIII was not modified by fibrin polymers. When platelet factor XIII was added, however, to plasma containing only factor XIII B chains, the α-thrombin concentration required to cleave the newly formed a_2b_2 complex was lowered 20-fold by fibrin polymers.

Based upon the findings that both plasma and platelet factor XIII bind to fibrin polymers and soluble fibrinogen,[8,12] and that fibrin polymers accelerated thrombin cleavage of plasma factor XIII,[4–6] we proposed that plasma factor XIII binding to fibrin(ogen) regulates thrombin cleavage of factor XIII.[5,13] A trimeric complex between plasma factor XIII, α-thrombin, and fibrin polymers may facilitate factor XIII_a formation during hemostasis.[13] Trimeric complexes have been demonstrated for other hemostatic reactions, including tissue plasminogen activator cleavage of plasminogen bound to either fibrin[15] or thrombospondin.[16] Results obtained with γ-thrombin and active site modified thrombin show that thrombin binding to fibrin is necessary for fibrin polymers to promote thrombin cleavage of factor XIII.[13] Furthermore, because the α- and γ-thrombin concentrations required to cleave platelet factor XIII were not reduced by fibrin polymers, α-thrombin binding to fibrin was not sufficient to promote thrombin cleavage of the A chains bound to fibrin unless the B chains were also present.

It is well recognized that plasma factor XIII A chains and B chains interact with fibrin polymers.[2] Credo *et al.* demonstrated that fibrin(ogen) binding to thrombin-cleaved plasma factor XIII promotes the dissociation of the B chains.[2] Because intact plasma factor XIII (a_2b_2 complex) binds to fibrin polymers,[8] the B chains may function to regulate α-thrombin cleavage of the A chains bound to fibrin. Results demonstrating that factor XIII B chains, in the presence of soluble fibrin polymers, lower the thrombin concentration required to cleave platelet factor XIII A chains support this hypothesis.[13]

In conclusion, the fibrin polymer surface functions as an important cofactor for α-thrombin cleavage of plasma factor XIII by providing binding sites for both α-thrombin and plasma factor XIII. Furthermore, the binding of the plasma factor XIII a_2b_2 complex to fibrin polymers promotes thrombin cleavage of plasma factor XIII A chains. Studies characterizing the fibrin binding domain on factor XIII A chains are in progress and may improve our understanding of this important physiologic event that regulates fibrin stabilization.

REFERENCES

1. TAKAGI, T. & R. F. DOOLITTLE. 1974. Amino acid sequence studies on factor XIII and the peptide released during its activation by thrombin. Biochemistry **13:** 750-756.
2. CREDO, R. B., C. G. CURTIS & L. LORAND. 1978. Ca^{2+}-related regulatory function of fibrinogen. Proc. Natl. Acad. Sci. USA **75:** 4234-4237.
3. JANUS, T. J., S. D. LEWIS, L. LORAND & J. A. SHAFER. 1983. Promotion of thrombin-catalyzed activation of Factor XIII by fibrinogen. Biochemistry **26:** 6269-6272.
4. GREENBERG, C. S., C. C. MIRAGLIA, F. R. RICKLES & M. A. SHUMAN. 1985. Cleavage of blood coagulation Factor XIII and fibrinogen by thrombin during *in vitro* clotting. J. Clin. Invest. **75:** 1463-1470.
5. GREENBERG, C. S. & C. C. MIRAGLIA. 1985. The effect of fibrin polymers on thrombin-catalyzed plasma Factor XIIIa formation. Blood **66:** 466-469.
6. LEWIS, S. D., T. J. JANUS, L. LORAND & J. A. SHAFER. 1985. Regulation of formation of Factor XIII_a by its fibrin substrates. Biochemistry **24:** 6772-6777.
7. GREENBERG, C. S., C. C. MIRAGLIA & K. E. ACHYUTHAN. 1985. The effect of fibrinogen degradation products on thrombin catalyzed plasma Factor XIIIa formation. Thromb. Haemostasis **54:** 42 (Abstr.)
8. GREENBERG, C. S., J. V. DOBSON & C. C. MIRAGLIA. 1985. Regulation of plasma Factor XIII binding to fibrin *in vitro.* Blood **66:** 1028-1034.
9. WILNER, G. D., M. P. DANITZ, S. MUDD, K. S. HSIEH & J. W. FENTON II. 1981. Selective immobilization of α-thrombin by surface-bound fibrin. J. Lab. Clin. Med. **97:** 403-411.
10. FENTON II, J. W., M. P. ZABINSKI, K. HSIEH & G. D. WILNER. 1981. Thrombin non-covalent-protein binding and fibrin(ogen) recognition. Thromb. Haemostasis **46:** 177 (Abstr).
11. LORAND, L. & R. B. CREDO. 1977. Thrombin and fibrin stabilization. *In* Chemistry and Biology of Thrombin. R. L. Lundblad, J. W. Fenton II & K. G. Mann, Eds.: 311-323. Ann Arbor Science Publishers, Inc. Ann Arbor, MI.
12. GREENBERG, C. S. & M. A. SHUMAN. 1982. The zymogen forms of blood coagulation Factor XIII bind specifically to fibrinogen. J. Biol. Chem. **257:** 6096-6101.

13. Greenberg, C. S., K. E. Achyuthan & J. W. Fenton II. 1987. Factor XIII_a formation promoted by complexing of α-thrombin, fibrin, and plasma factor XIII. Blood. In press.
14. Miraglia, C. C. & C. S. Greenberg. 1985. Measurement of blood coagulation Factor XIIIa formation in plasma containing glycyl-L-prolyl-L-arginyl-L-proline. Anal. Biochem. **144:** 165-171.
15. Holyaerts, M., D. C. Rijken, H. R. Lignen & D. Collen. 1982. Kinetics of the activation of plasminogen by human tissue plasminogen activator. Role of fibrin. J. Biol. Chem. **257:** 2912-2919.
16. Silverstein, R. L., L. L. K. Leung, P. C. Harper & R. L. Nachman. 1984. Complex formation of platelet thrombospondin with plasminogen. J. Clin. Invest. **74:** 1625-1633.

Activation of Blood Coagulation Factor XIII[a]

LASZLO LORAND

Department of Biochemistry
Molecular Biology and Cell Biology
Northwestern University
Evanston, Illinois 60201

Limited proteolysis is the common motif for activating enzyme precursors of the blood coagulation cascade, and activation of the fibrin stabilizing factor, that is, factor XIII, is no exception. Yet the conversion of this zymogen, giving rise to a transamidating enzyme with cysteine as the catalytic residue, is markedly different from that of the other clotting factors, all of which generate serine proteases. In fact, the factor XIII to XIII_a transition provides a rather unique and fascinating study in biological regulation. If one were to ask what was the critical step for activating factor XIII, the answer must be that it was the dissociation of the heterologous protomer unit. Proteolysis of one of the two subunits by thrombin merely serves the purpose of somewhat loosening the attraction between the two different subunits so that dissociation can take place in the physiological milieu (for background references, see the review by Lorand *et al.)*[1]

Throughout this discussion, factor XIII will be presented as an [ab] structure with an approximate protomer weight of 2 × 80,000 or 160,000. There is some support for such a value from sucrose density centrifugation,[2] but other thorough investigations yielded a molecular weight of about 320,000, corresponding to the $[a_2b_2]$ tetramer.[3] Whereas it would be nice to decide whether the 160,000 or 320,000 value would best represent the functional molecule at the low concentration of the protein existing in plasma, physical estimates obtained in the absence of fibrinogen have limited significance. Because factor XIII seems to form an extremely tight complex with fibrinogen[4] and because the latter is present at a molar concentration 20- to 100-fold in excess of the former, it may be assumed that there is essentially no free factor XIII circulating in plasma.[b] Considering the fact that fibrinogen (Φ) itself is a disulfide-linked duplex of three chains $[A\alpha_2B\beta_2\gamma_2]$, the truly relevant question is whether the combination of factor XIII with fibrinogen would be Φ··[ab], Φ··2[ab], or some other stoichiometry of the two proteins. Would an $[a_2b_2]$ oligomeric formulation be at all meaningful for factor XIII in the presence of fibrinogen? Depending on individual variations in factor XIII, one in one hundred to one in twenty of fibrinogen molecules in plasma would be bound to factor XIII; would this complexed fibrinogen be Φ··[ab], Φ··2[ab] as shown in FIGURE 1A, or Φ··$[a_2b_2]$? I doubt that we have the means to distinguish

[a]This work was aided by a USPHS Research Career Award (HL-03512) and by Grants from the National Institutes of Health (HL-02212 and HL-16346).

[b]Nevertheless, it is interesting to observe that the half-life of factor XIII in the circulation appears to be about 12 days,[1] as measured by clearance of the zymogen injected into factor XIII-deficient individuals. This is considerably longer than that of fibrinogen.

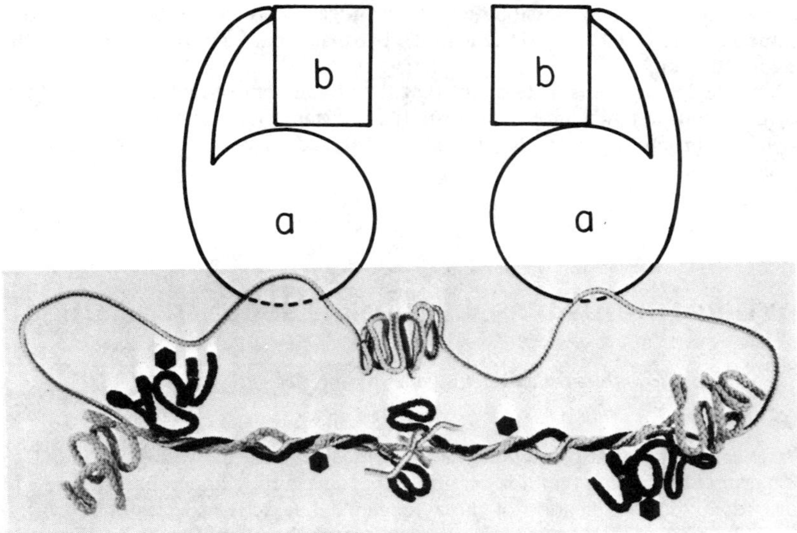

FIGURES 1A and 1B. Illustration of possibilities for the attachment of two [ab] protomers (panel A) and two $[a_2b_2]$ oligomers (panel B) of factor XIII to the model of fibrinogen presented by Weisel *et al.*[5] Binding of the zymogen to the Aα-chain domain of the fibrinogen molecule was chosen on account of the observed regulatory role of this region, present in fibrinogen as well as in fibrin, on factor XIII activation.[6]

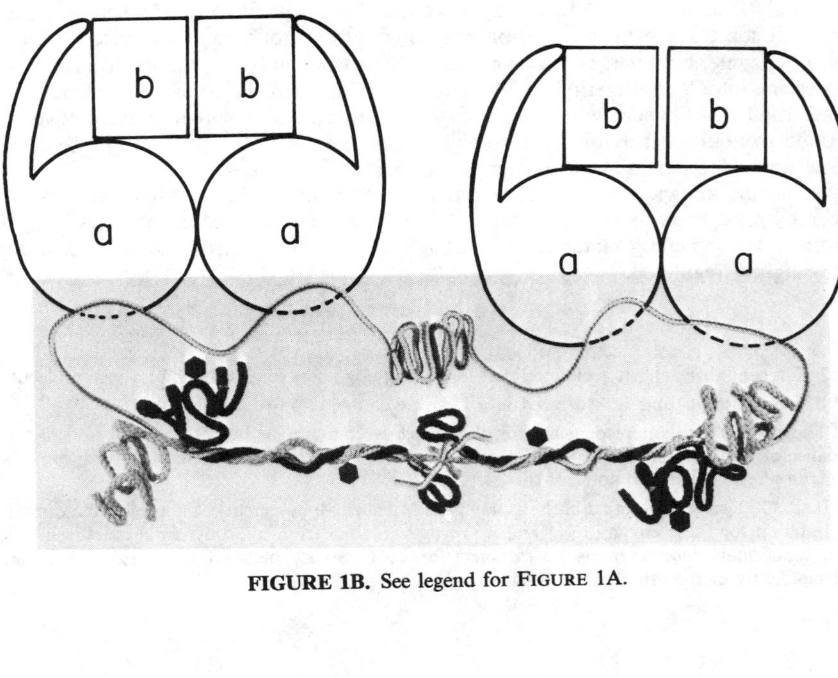

FIGURE 1B. See legend for FIGURE 1A.

between the latter two possibilities. If fibrinogen were to be decorated with two tetrameric units of factor XIII (FIGURE 1B), that would surely be a case of the tail wagging the dog.[c]

Nevertheless, there is little doubt that the attachment of factor XIII to fibrinogen and, even more significantly, to fibrin is important because the latter serves as a midwife in promoting both the thrombin-catalyzed hydrolysis of the zymogen[d] and the dissociation of subunits.[e]

HETEROLOGOUS DISSOCIATION OF SUBUNITS IS THE KEY

A Thrombin-Independent Pathway for Activating Factor XIII

The conclusion that dissociation is the critical step for activating factor XIII rests on experiments showing that it is possible to produce a fully functional enzyme without prior proteolytic modification of the zymogen.[8,9] The active species obtained by this route is denoted as a° in order to distinguish it from the a^* enzyme, which is generated following thrombin treatment. Thrombin-independent activation can be accomplished with great ease by exposure of factor XIII to a relatively high concentration of Ca^{2+} at rather high ionic strength, suggesting that salt linkages contribute to the stability of [ab]. Chaotropic agents, thought to disorganize water structure around proteins, aid in breaking up the heterologous combination of [ab] to a° + b (FIGURE 2). Active center titration of a° with [^{14}C]iodoacetamide was shown to label the same cysteine-containing peptide that becomes unmasked in the thrombin-dependent activation pathway.

Catalytic constants for the a° enzyme are indistinguishable from a^* when measured on small substrates[10,11] such as β-phenylpropionylthiocholine and dansylcadaverine.[f] The a° enzyme, however, is somewhat less efficient in catalyzing the incorporation of putrescine into *N,N'*-dimethylcasein,[12] showing a higher K_m(app) for the protein substrate than a^*. Thus, it would seem that the removal of the *N*-terminal activation peptide from the *a* subunit by thrombin, as in the course of producing a^*, would allow for a better binding of the enzyme to protein substrates.

It is not known whether there might be circumstances, perhaps pathological, whereby an a° enzyme could be generated in plasma. In any case, the physiological pathway for activating factor XIII is thought to be entirely thrombin dependent and more tightly regulated.

[c] In a recent abstract,[6a] it is claimed that four [a_2b_2] oligomers bind to one fibrinogen molecule.

[d] This important topic is addressed in a separate contribution to this Volume.[7]

[e] The protein domain responsible for this effect is common to both fibrinogen and fibrin.[6] Because of the temporal sequence of reactions, however, fibrin rather than fibrinogen must be the true physiological promoter of this step.

[f] It should also be noted that both display pure Michaelis-type kinetics. Thus, even if a dimeric formulation for these enzymes (a_2° and a_2^*) was suggested from hydrodynamic measurements, in a functional sense, there is no evidence for cooperativity between subunits, each acting independently of the other in catalysis.

THE THROMBIN-DEPENDENT, PHYSIOLOGICAL ACTIVATION OF FACTOR XIII

Two methods should be mentioned for evaluating the attack of thrombin on the zymogen. One is sodium dodecylsulfate-polyacrylamide gel electrophoresis, introduced into this field by Schwartz *et al.*[3] and useful in monitoring the difference between the hydrolytically altered *a'* and the original *a* subunit (FIGURE 3); the other procedure, employing high pressure liquid chromatography, measures the release of the activation peptide during the conversion of [ab] to [a'b]. The latter approach was used extensively in recent kinetic studies.[14,15]

Earlier work on thrombin led to a suggestion[16] that there might be a positively charged area on thrombin constituting a secondary binding domain outside the catalytic pocket, to complement some negative patches on its best protein substrates. Albeit the original illustration was given for the anchoring of the fibrinopeptide A moiety in fibrinogen (FIGURE 4), it should not go unnoticed that the activation peptide that is to be removed from the *N*-terminus of the *a* subunit of factor XIII is also rich

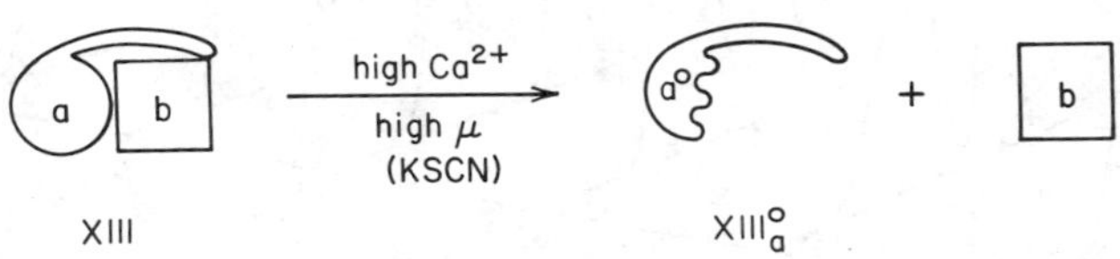

FIGURE 2. Pac-Man-like model, showing generation of a transmidating enzyme (a°) without hydrolytic cleavage of the *a* subunit of factor XIII. This experiment proves that dissociation of the [ab] protomer to *a* plus *b*, and the consecutive conformational change of *a* to a° are the key ingredients for activating the zymogen.

in unneutralized negatively charged side chains (FIGURE 5) and could conceivably bind at the same site. The existence of such positively charged domains for the binding of anions outside the active center region of thrombin is strongly reinforced by the recent studies of Berliner *et al.*,[17] even though the location of positive charges relevant for the binding of fibrinopeptide is as yet unknown.

The thrombin-modified factor XIII, called XIII', still retains the heterologous subunit structure; it is still a zymogen[g] with the catalytic-cysteine residue remaining inaccessible. Nevertheless, the [a'b] ensemble is much better poised for dissociation and expression of enzymatic activity than the original [ab] structure. In the presence of fibrinogen or fibrin, simple exposure to physiological concentrations of Ca^{2+} (1.5 mM) at the ionic strength of 0.15 produces dissociation of the subunits and unmasking of the active center thiol group, generating the functional transamidase: a^*.

Heterologous dissociation of the subunits could be demonstrated by nondenaturing electrophoresis,[20,21] developed in conjunction with the dansylcadaverine-staining procedure to reveal the active or potentially active subunit (FIGURE 6).

According to our present estimates, dissociation of the [a'b] heterodimer to $a'+b$ appears to be the rate-limiting step in the conversion of the zymogen; the confor-

[g] The hydrolytically modified factor could properly be designated an "allozymogen."

mational change leading to the unmasking of active center cysteine during the $a' \rightarrow a^*$ transition is much faster. The lag phase noted in kinetic studies, with thrombin-modified factor XIII′ as the starting material, is a reflection on the relatively slow pace of dissociation; it can be shortened, however, by increasing the Ca^{2+} concentration and/or the ionic strength of the medium (FIGURE 7).[h]

The dissociated, hydrolytically modified a' subunit is presumed to have only a fleeting existence in the presence of Ca^{2+} before being transformed to the active a^*

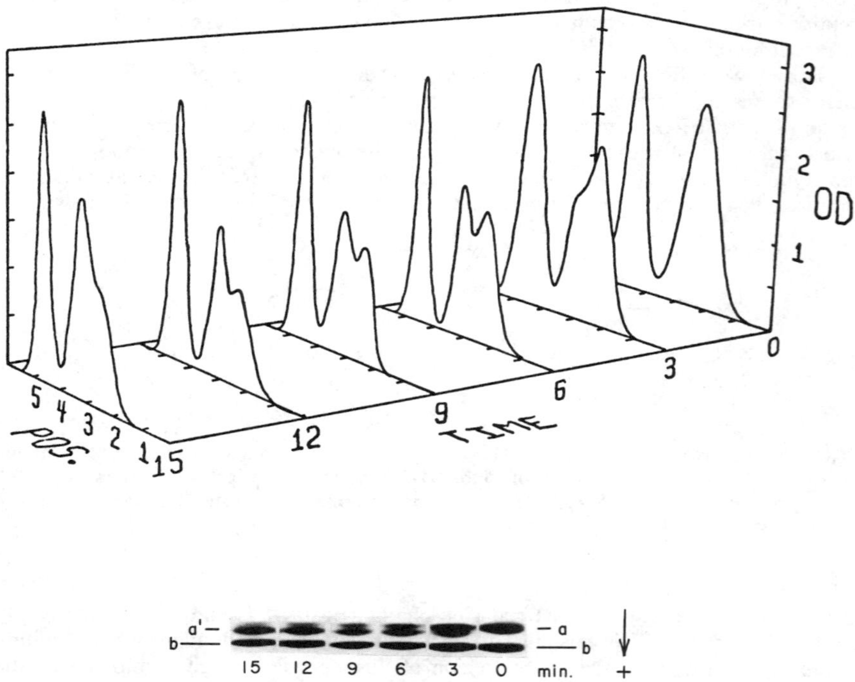

FIGURE 3. Sodium dodecylsulfate-polyacrylamide gel electrophoresis reveals the change of *a* to *a′* in one of the subunits of factor XIII, due to cleavage by thrombin (Schwartz *et al.*[3]). Proteolysis by thrombin was terminated at the times indicated by the addition of excess of hirudin over thrombin. Densitometric tracings of the Coomassie blue-stained gels are presented in the three-dimensional computer drawing, with optical density (OD) on the ordinate and position of bands (POS) in cm on one of the abscissae.[13]

species. With fibrin in the medium, both a' and a^* would, of course, remain attached to the clotting protein. In the test tube, it is possible to mix a^* with ethylenediaminetetraacetate (EDTA) to reverse the conformational change in the sense that the transamidase activity disappears and that the active center cysteine becomes buried

[h] It could be suggested that, on account of its sialic acid content, the role of the *b* subunit was to protect the *a* subunit in the circulation. Its true physiological *raison d'être*, however, may be the regulation of the rate of a^* formation.

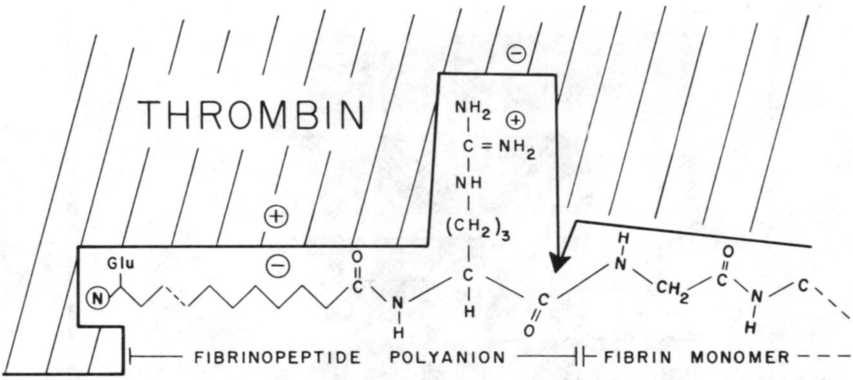

FIGURE 4. An early drawing[16] postulating the existence of an anionic binding domain on thrombin outside the catalytic pocket. The latter accommodates the arginyl residue, reacting with the active center serine of the enzyme, represented by the arrow. The anionic domain of thrombin might be the recognition site for the negatively charged fibrinopeptide moiety at the *N*-terminus of the Aα chain of fibrinogen, as illustrated by the drawing, and also for the *N*-terminal activation peptide in the *a* subunit of factor XIII. As shown in FIGURE 5, the distribution of negative charges is quite similar in these two peptides.

again; there is no guarantee, however, that such an a'_{EDTA} species would be truly the equivalent of the natural a' molecule.

Zn^{2+} is very potent in blocking the expression of a^* activity[22] by apparently competing against Ca^{2+} both in terms of enzyme activity and titratability with [^{14}C]iodoacetamide (FIGURES 8 and 9). Remarkably, however, Zn^{2+} does not seem to prevent Ca^{2+} from causing the dissociation of [a'b] to $a' + b$, suggesting that the Ca^{2+}-binding sites that must be filled for the heterologous dissociation of subunits are different from the ones that are to be occupied for producing the conformational change in a' to become converted to a^*.

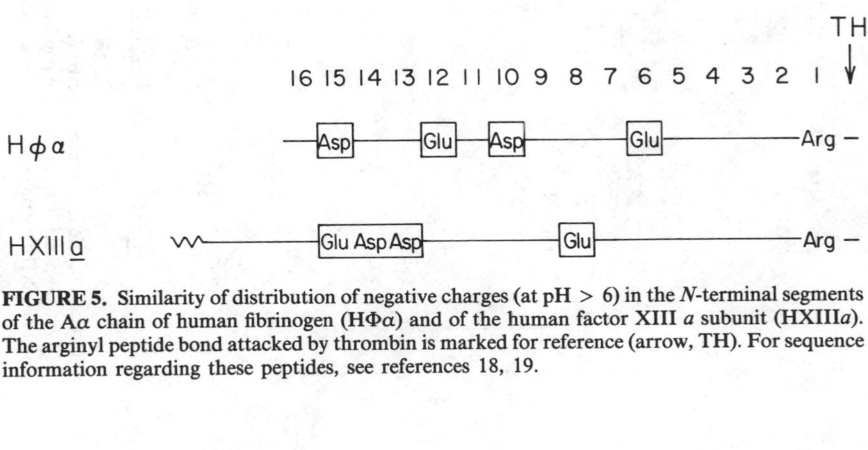

FIGURE 5. Similarity of distribution of negative charges (at pH > 6) in the *N*-terminal segments of the Aα chain of human fibrinogen (H$\Phi\alpha$) and of the human factor XIII *a* subunit (HXIII*a*). The arginyl peptide bond attacked by thrombin is marked for reference (arrow, TH). For sequence information regarding these peptides, see references 18, 19.

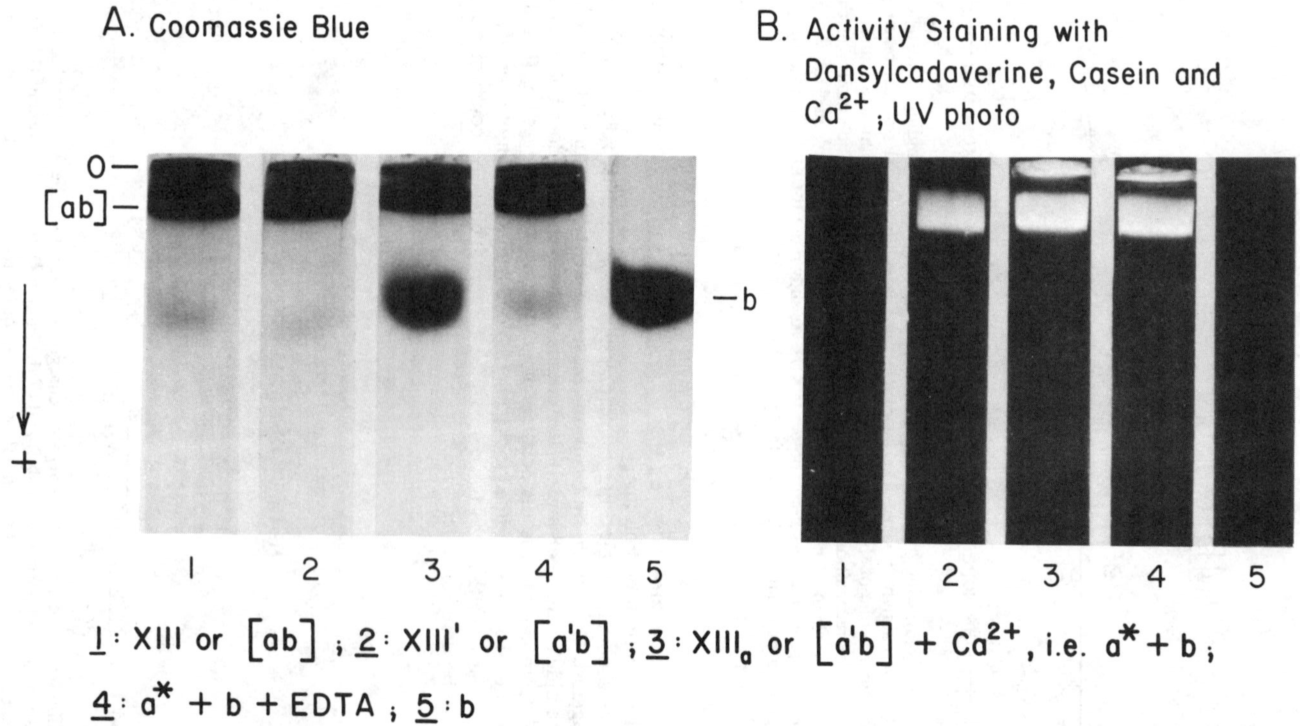

FIGURE 6. Nondenaturing electrophoresis of various molecular species derived from the activation of human factor XIII. Panel **A** shows distribution of protein; panel **B** is the staining pattern obtained with the enzyme-catalyzed incorporation of fluorescent dansylcadaverine into casein.[20] The thrombin-modified XIII′ zymogen is denoted as [a′b] and the active XIII_a enzyme as *a**.

IS THERE A PUSH-OFF MECHANISM FOR THE RELEASE OF THE *B* SUBUNIT?

A more precise formulation of this question would be to ask whether, concomitant with generating transamidase activity, the dissociating *b* subunit would itself serve as a substrate for the *a** enzyme. The latter could modify specific endo-γ-glutaminyl residues in the *b* subunit either by hydrolysis or by aminolysis. The outlines for such possibilities are presented in FIGURE 10, bearing in mind that factor XIII_a-catalyzed reactions proceed by acylation-deacylation pathways, with the active center thiol group on *a** forming thiolester acyl-enzyme intermediates with γ-carbonyl groups of the

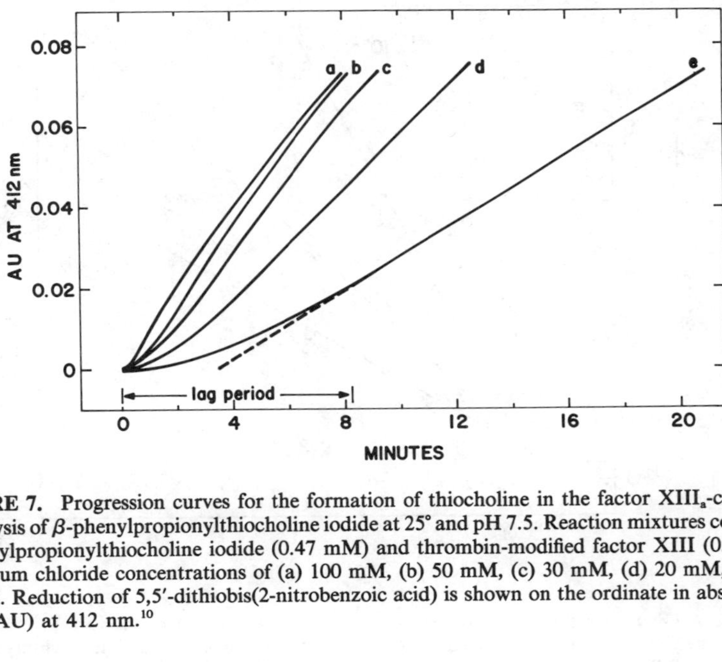

FIGURE 7. Progression curves for the formation of thiocholine in the factor XIII_a-catalyzed hydrolysis of β-phenylpropionylthiocholine iodide at 25° and pH 7.5. Reaction mixtures contained β-phenylpropionylthiocholine iodide (0.47 mM) and thrombin-modified factor XIII (0.16 μM) at calcium chloride concentrations of (a) 100 mM, (b) 50 mM, (c) 30 mM, (d) 20 mM, and (e) 10 mM. Reduction of 5,5′-dithiobis(2-nitrobenzoic acid) is shown on the ordinate in absorbancy units (AU) at 412 nm.[10]

relevant side chain residues in substrates. Indeed, when the Ca^{2+}-mediated conversion of [a′b] to *a** and *b* was allowed to occur in the presence of dansylcadaverine, a time-dependent labeling of the *b* subunit with the fluorescent amine could be demonstrated[24] (FIGURE 11). This shows that the *b* subunit can, in fact, become modified in the medium in which the transamidase is generated, though it would be difficult to assess the concertedness of the two events; nor could one claim that alteration of the specific glutamine residues in *b* was essential for the release of this subunit. Nevertheless, the creation of a novel *b* species would shift the equilibrium for the heterologous dissociation of subunits, and it should be anticipated that altered forms of free *b* subunit (denoted as $\bar{b}$) may appear as by-products of the factor XIII activation process in blood.[i]

[i] With the modification of *b* subunits, ammonia would also be a by-product (see FIGURE 10).

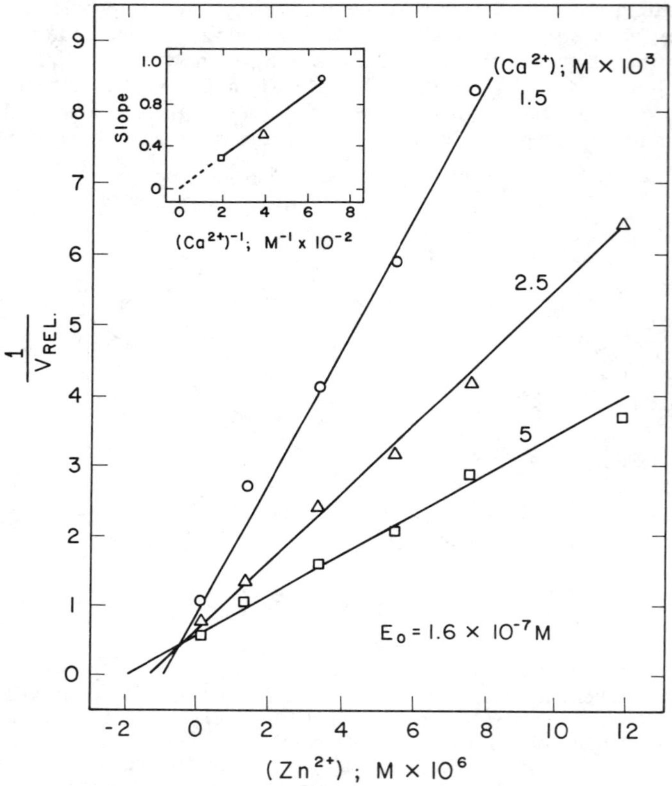

FIGURE 8. Dixon-plot for the inhibition of factor XIII_a by Zn^{2+}-ions (abscissa) at 25°C, μ = 0.25, and pH 7.5. The enzyme (E) was generated from the thrombin-modified zymogen [a′b], at 1.6×10^{-7}M, by addition of different concentrations of Ca^{2+} (1.5, 2.5 and 5 mM). The insert is a plot of slopes, measured with Zn^{2+}, as a function of the reciprocal Ca^{2+} concentration. It should be noticed that the line extrapolates back to zero, suggesting a true competition between Zn^{2+} and Ca^{2+}.[22] Reciprocal velocities for the reaction of β-phenylpropionylthiocholine and dansylcadaverine, measured by the production of the fluorescent coupling product,[23] were computed from relative fluorescence values.

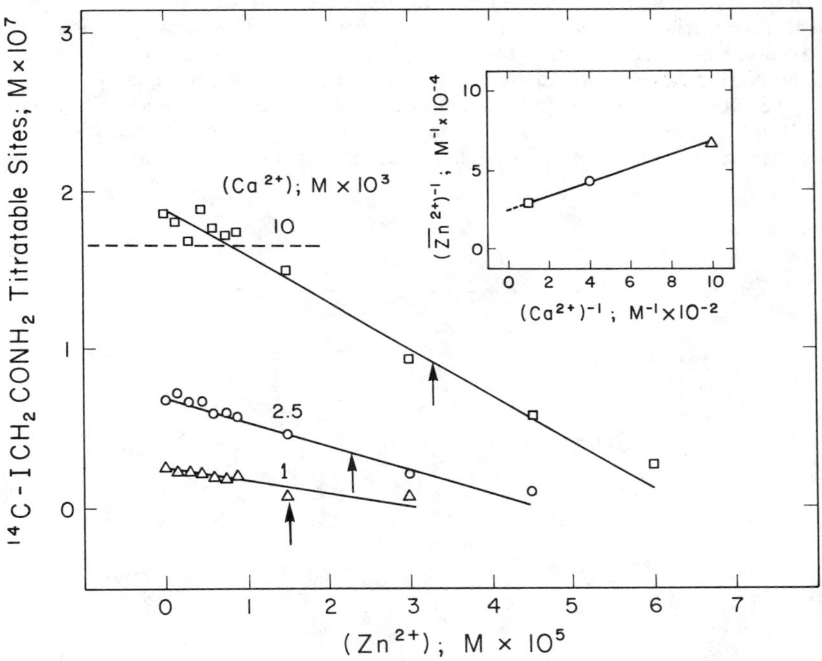

FIGURE 9. Alkylation of active-center cysteine residues with [^{14}C]iodoacetamide upon treatment of thrombin-modified factor XIII, that is, [a'b] in the presence of various concentrations of both Ca^{2+} (1, 2.5, and 10 mM) and Zn^{2+}-ions (0 to 6 $\times$ 10^{-5}M). Arrows denote Zn^{2+}-concentrations that, for each of the Ca^{2+}-concentrations examined, lowered iodoacetamide-titratable sites by 50 percent. The double reciprocal relationship between this concentration of Zn^{2+} ($\overline{Zn}^{2+}$) and the pertinent Ca^{2+}-concentration is given in the insert. Experiments were carried out with [a'b] = 1.6 $\times$ 10^{-7}M, at pH 7.5, μ = 0.34 and 25°C.[22]

CONCLUDING REMARKS

As illustrated in FIGURE 12, it is now possible to assemble essentially all the important elements of molecular transformations necessary for the conversion of the factor XIII zymogen. A reconstruction of the regulation by fibrin within the context of the clotting in blood is shown in FIGURE 13. After what has already been presented, no further clarification of individual reaction steps should be required. What needs to be emphasized, however, is that throughout the process of the conversion of the factor XIII zymogen [ab] to the thrombin-modified allozymogen [a′b] and the *a** enzyme, all species are thought to remain tightly bound to the fibrinogen-fibrin matrix. The only components released into the clot liquor would be the activation peptide and the *b* subunit, perhaps in its virgin as well as in its modified form. The *a** enzyme

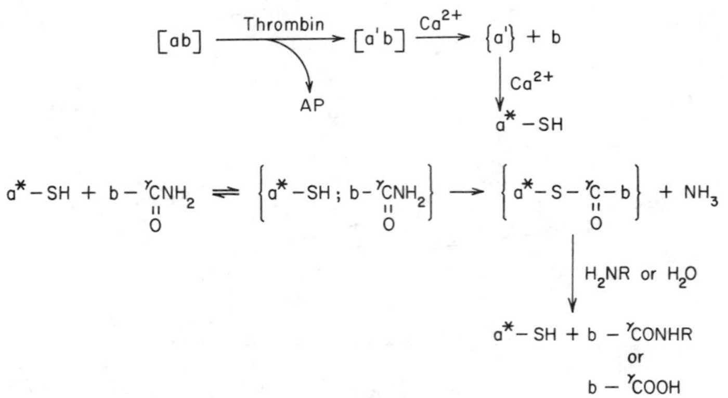

FIGURE 10. Kinetic scheme showing the site-specific modification of the dissociated *b* subunit of factor XIII during conversion of the zymogen to the transamidating enzyme: *a**. The active center cysteine thiol group is marked as a*-SH. The reactive γ-glutamine residue of the *b* subunit is denoted as: *b*-$^{\gamma}CONH_2$. The illustration shows possibilities for hydrolytic as well as aminolytic alterations at this endo-glutaminyl site.

would roll over anywhere between twenty to one hundred fibrin molecules in the clot network, attacking susceptible endo-glutaminyl residues first in the γ- then in the α-chains, for a total of four to six hits per fibrin.[25] There is no reason to assume that the mechanistic steps of enzyme action, that is, Michaelis complex formation with fibrin, and consecutive acylation and deacylation by aminolysis, would be different from those established for the transamidase activity of *a** in solution.[10,23] Accordingly, the favorable affinity of the enzyme for the γ chain over the α-chain site should account for the ordered reactivities of the cross-linking of fibrin chains by ε(γ-glutamyl)lysine bonds. Considering the fact that fibronectin[26] and α_2-plasmin inhibitor[27] may also become cross-linked to fibrin, it is not surprising that the actual enzymatic organization of the clot by factor XIII_a requires a much longer period than reflected in the clinically measured "clotting time".

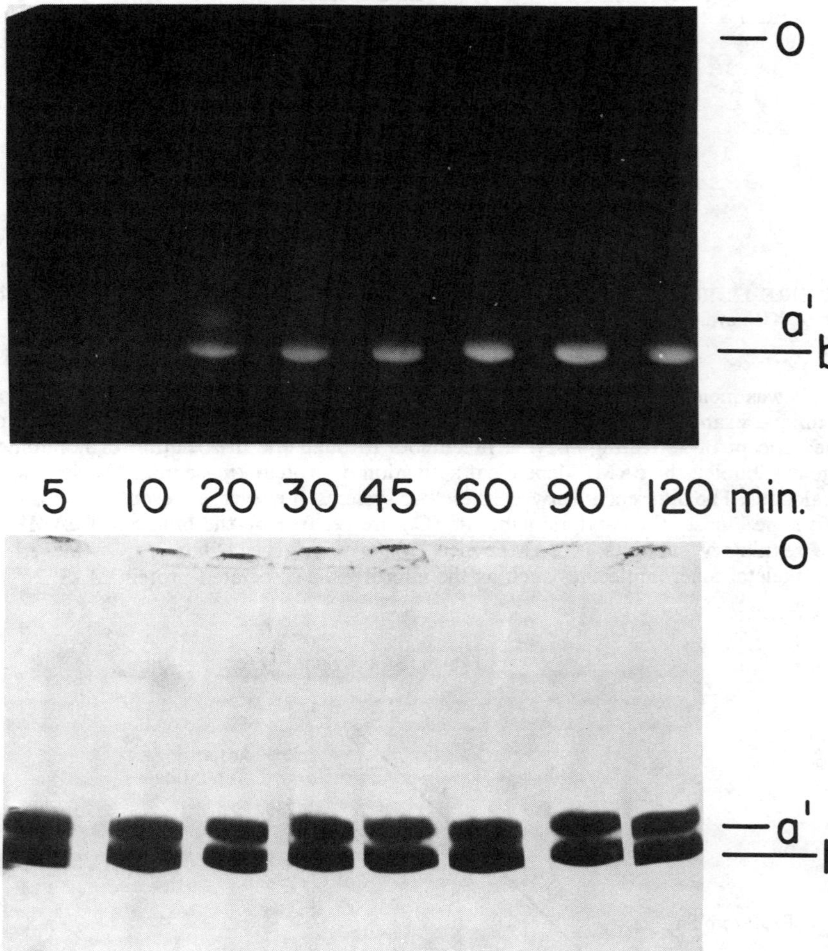

FIGURE 11. Time-dependent incorporation of dansylcadaverine into the dissociated *b* subunit of factor XIII, concomitant with generation of transamidating activity in *a**.[24] Top panel: electrophoretic gels after sodium dodecylsulfate electrophoresis in polyacrylamide, under UV illumination. Bottom panel: protein staining with Coomassie blue.

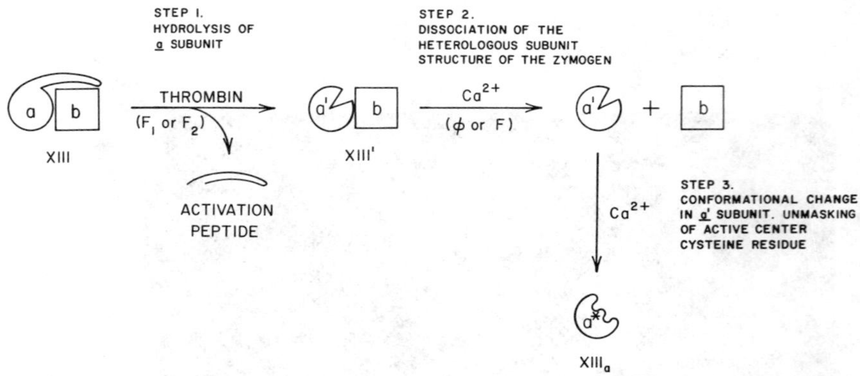

FIGURE 12. Illustration of molecular transformations in the physiological conversion of the factor XIII zymogen by the thrombin-dependent activation pathway.

It was mentioned in the introduction that the activation of factor XIII represents a unique example of biological regulation at the molecular level. Focusing only on the concept of activating enzyme precursors through the dissociation of nonhomologous subunits, the cAMP-dependent activation of protein kinase might be somewhat analogous. The differences between these two systems, however, are even more obvious. With the kinase, the catalytic subunits (C_2) are set free by the binding of cAMP to the regulatory subunits (4 cAMPs per R_2), even when the latter are attached to cytoskeletal macromolecules such as the microtubule-associated protein MAP 2.[28] In

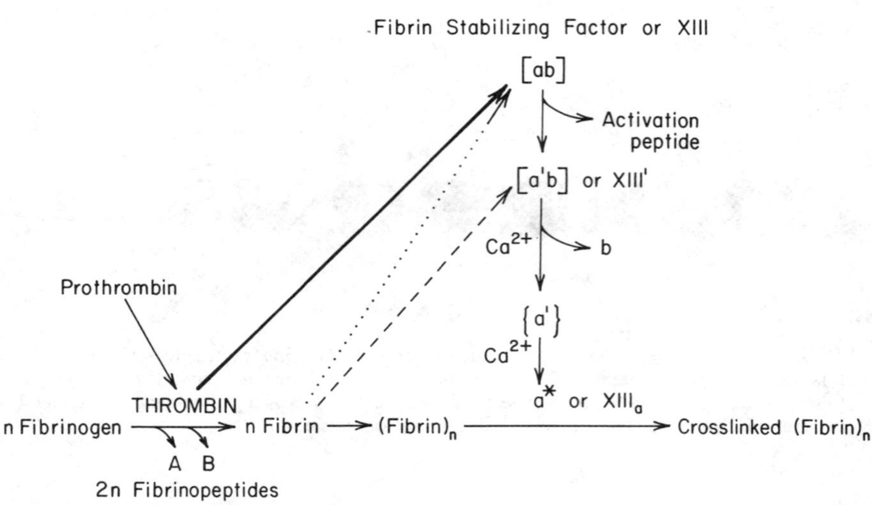

FIGURE 13. Reconstruction of the physiological pathway of factor XIII conversion and fibrin stabilization, emphasizing the "feed-forward" regulatory aspects by fibrin in promoting the reaction of factor XIII with thrombin[14,15] and in reducing the Ca^{2+} requirement for the dissociation of the hydrolytically modified [a'b] allozymogen.[6,8]

the case of factor XIII, the catalytic *a* subunit undergoes a limited proteolytic cleavage, which by itself is a rather more permanent alteration than regulation through the reversible binding of cAMP. More significantly, following the activation of factor XIII, the catalytic *a** subunit remains attached to the fibrin matrix, whereas the inert *b* subunit is released into the medium.

REFERENCES

1. LORAND, L., M. S. LOSOWSKY & K. J. M. MILOSZEWSKI. 1980. Human factor XIII: Fibrin-stabilizing factor. *In* Progress in Hemostasis and Thrombosis, T. H. Spaet, Ed., **5:** 245-290. Grune and Stratton, Inc. New York.
2. LORAND, L., J. DOWNEY, T. GOTOH, A. JACOBSEN & S. TOKURA. 1968. The transpeptidase system which cross-links fibrin by γ-glutamyl-ε-lysine bonds. Biochem. Biophysics Res. Commun. **31:** 222-230.
3. SCHWARTZ, M. L., S. V. PIZZO, R. L. HILL & P. A. MCKEE. 1971. The subunit structures of human plasma and platelet factor XIII (fibrin stabilizing factor). J. Biol. Chem. **246:** 5851-5854.
4. GREENBERG, C. S. & M. A. SHUMAN. 1982. The zymogen forms of blood coagulation factor XIII bind specifically to fibrinogen. J. Biol. Chem. **257:** 6096-6101.
5. WEISEL, J. W., C. V. STAUFFACHER, E. BULLITT & C. COHEN. 1985. A model for fibrinogen: Domains and sequence. Science **230:** 1388-1391.
6. CREDO, R. B., C. G. CURTIS & L. LORAND. 1981. α-Chain domain of fibrinogen controls generation of fibrinoligase (coagulation factor XIII_a). Calcium ion regulatory aspects. Biochemistry **20:** 3770-3778.
6a. CHUNG, S. I. & M. C. LEWIS. 1986. Fed. Proc. Fed. Am. Soc. Exp. Biol. **45:** 1639. (Abst. 924).
7. SHAFER, J. A., S. D. LEWIS, T. J. JANUS & L. LORAND. 1986. Effect of fibrinogen and Ca^{2+} on the thrombin-catalyzed proteolytic event that triggers activation of factor XIII. Ann. N. Y. Acad. Sci. This volume.
8. CREDO, R. B., C. G. CURTIS & L. LORAND. 1978. Ca^{2+}-related regulatory function of fibrinogen. Proc. Natl. Acad. Sci. USA **75:** 4234-4237.
9. LORAND, L., R. B. CREDO & T. J. JANUS. 1981. Factor XIII (fibrin stabilizing factor). *In* Methods in Enzymology **80:** 333-341.
10. CURTIS, C. G., P. STENBERG, K. L. BROWN, A. BARON, K. CHEN, A. GRAY, I. SIMPSON & L. LORAND. 1974. Kinetics of transamidating enzymes. Production of thiol in the reactions of thiol esters with fibrinoligase. Biochemistry **13:** 3257-3262.
11. JANUS, T. J., R. B. CREDO, C. G. CURTIS, L. HAGGROTH & L. LORAND. 1981. Novel model of activating human factor XIII zymogen without the hydrolytic cleavage of the *a* subunits. Fed. Proc. Fed. Am. Soc. Exp. Biol. **40:** 1585 (Abst. #258).
12. JANUS, T. J. 1985. Doctoral Dissertation. Northwestern University.
13. DOMANIK, R. A. 1974. Doctoral Dissertation. Northwestern University.
14. JANUS, T. J., S. D. LEWIS, L. LORAND & J. A. SHAFER. 1983. Promotion of thrombin-catalyzed activation of factor XIII by fibrinogen. Biochemistry **22:** 6269-6272.
15. LEWIS, S. D., T. J. JANUS, L. LORAND & J. A. SHAFER. 1985. Regulation of the formation of factor XIIIa by its fibrin substrates. Biochemistry **24:** 6772-6777.
16. LORAND, L. 1965. Physiological roles of fibrinogen and fibrin. Fed. Proc. Fed. Am. Soc. Exp. Biol. **24:** 784-793.
17. BERLINER, L. J., Y. SUGAWARA & J. W. FENTON II. 1985. Human α-thrombin binding to nonpolymerized fibrin-sepharose: Evidence for an anionic binding region. Biochemistry **24:** 7005-7009.
18. DOOLITTLE, R. L., K. W. K. WATT, B. A. COTTRELL, D. D. STRONG & M. RILEY. 1979. The amino acid sequence of the α-chain of human fibrinogen. Nature (London) **280:** 464-468.

19. TAKAGI, T. & R. F. DOOLITTLE. 1974. Amino acid sequence studies on factor XIII and the peptide released during its activation by thrombin. Biochemistry **13:** 750-756.
20. LORAND, L., A. J. GRAY, K. BROWN, R. B. CREDO, C. G. CURTIS, R. A. DOMANIK & P. STENBERG. 1974. Dissociation of the subunit structure of fibrin stabilizing factor during activation of the zymogen. Biochem. Biophysics Res. Commun. **56:** 914-922.
21. CURTIS, C. G., K. L. BROWN, R. B. CREDO, R. A. DOMANIK, A. GRAY, P. STENBERG & L. LORAND. 1974. Calcium-dependent unmasking of active center cysteine during activation of fibrin stabilizing factor. Biochemistry **13:** 3774-3780.
22. CREDO, R. B., P. STENBERG, Y. S. TONG & L. LORAND. 1976. Inhibition of fibrinoligase and transglutaminase by zinc ions. Fed. Proc. Fed. Am. Soc. Exp. Biol. **35:** 1630 (Abst. #1390).
23. STENBERG, P., C. G. CURTIS, D. WING, Y. S. TONG, R. B. CREDO, A. GRAY & L. LORAND. 1975. Transamidase kinetics. Amide formation in the enzymic reactions of thiol esters with amines. Biochem. J. **147:** 155-163.
24. GRAY, A. & L. LORAND. 1974. Selective modification of the *b* subunit of fibrin stabilizing factor during activation of the zymogen. Fed. Proc. Fed. Am. Soc. Exp. Biol. **33:** 1474 (Abst. #1419).
25. LORAND, L., D. CHENOWETH & A. GRAY. 1972. Titration of the acceptor cross-linking sites in fibrin. Ann. N. Y. Acad. Sci. **202:** 155-171.
26. MOSHER, D. F. 1975. Cross-linking of cold-insoluble globulin by fibrin stabilizing factor. J. Biol. Chem. **250:** 6614-6621.
27. ICHINOSE, A. & N. AOKI. 1982. Reversible cross-linking of α_2-plasmin inhibitor to fibrinogen by fibrin-stabilizing factor. Biochim. Biophys. Acta **706:** 158-164.
28. NAIRN, A. C., H. C. HEMMINGS JR. & P. GREENGARD. 1985. Protein kinases in the brain. Annu. Rev. Biochem. **54:** 931-976.

Thrombin/Prothrombin Interactions with Very Low Density Lipoproteins[a]

WILLIAM A. BRADLEY, JIAN-NAN SONG,[b] AND SANDRA H. GIANTURCO[c]

Department of Medicine
Baylor College of Medicine
and
The Methodist Hospital
Houston, Texas 77030

INTRODUCTION

We have been involved in studying the most common form of hyperlipidemia, hypertriglyceridemia, and trying to find and understand mechanisms by which the triglyceride-rich lipoproteins that accumulate in these disorders may be involved in the atherogenic processes.

TABLE 1 illustrates some of the *in vivo* observations that have been made concerning hypertriglyceridemia and that we believe make this an important area of study. Very low density lipoproteins (VLDL) are the major lipoproteins that carry triglyceride. In hypertriglyceridemia, it is catabolized abnormally[1] when compared to the same VLDL subfractions from normal subjects. In certain forms of hypertriglyceridemia, both premature atherosclerosis and foam cell formation can occur. Hypertriglyceridemia has been associated with hypercoagulability in several recent studies,[2-4] and hypertriglycerdemia is a risk factor for myocardial infarction.[5]

Our recent *in vitro* work has focused on what we believe may be some of the mechanisms by which the *in vivo* observations may be explained. For example, Gianturco *et al.*,[6] were the first to show that there is an abnormal interaction of large VLDL ($S_f > 60$) from hypertriglycerdemic patients with two lipoprotein receptors, the low density lipoproteins (LDL) and β-VLDL receptors,[7] when compared to normal subjects. It was also shown that the VLDL from hypertriglyceridemic (HTG) patients converted macrophages into foam cells and were cytotoxic to endothelial cells when compared to the VLDL of normal subjects. Finally, we have recently been able to demonstrate that HTG-VLDL can contain coagulation factors. It is our hypothesis that these *in vitro* observations yield important clues concerning the above-mentioned *in vivo* observations.

[a] This work is supported in part by a SCOR Grant in Arteriosclerosis, HL27341, and by the American Heart Association.

[b] Dr. Jian-nan Song is a Fellow of the World Health Organization.

[c] Dr. Sandra H. Gianturco is an Established Investigator of the American Heart Association.

TABLE 1. *In Vivo* Observations in Hypertriglyceridemia

Abnormal catabolism of very low density lipoproteins
Premature atherosclerosis
Foam-cell accumulation
Hypercoagulability
Myocardial infarction

LIPOPROTEINS

Lipoproteins are complexes of protein and lipid that are found in blood and are the major transporters of water-insoluble cholesteryl esters (CE) and triglyceride (TG). Because of their characteristic sizes, densities, and compositions, the three major classes of lipoproteins are called the very low density lipoproteins (or VLDL), the low density lipoproteins (LDL), and the high density lipoproteins (HDL). Each of these major classifications has subsets, and the lipoproteins are highly heterogeneous. This report emphasizes VLDL, because these are the triglyceride-rich lipoproteins that accumulate in hypertriglyceridemia.

Large VLDL (S_f > 100-400) are lipoproteins with an average diameter of 50 nm and are composed of a protein, phospholipid monolayer surrounding a water-insoluble core of triglyceride TG and CE. The cholesterol is thought to be located just below the protein-phospholipid monolayer. The apoproteins in the surface serve as part of the polar monolayer to make these particles water soluble, but in addition, two of the apoproteins, apoE and apoB, can serve as ligands for specific cell-surface receptors for the removal of VLDL from plasma in hypertriglyceridemia.

LIPOPROTEIN RECEPTORS FOR LARGE VLDL (S_f > 60)

The two lipoprotein receptors that concern our attention are the LDL and the β-VLDL receptor of macrophages. The LDL receptor is ubiquitous in cellular distribution and has been elegantly described by Goldstein and Brown and reviewed many times.[8–10] The β-VLDL receptor was also described by these workers in 1980 (reviewed in Brown and Goldstein,[11]) and is present on monocytes/macrophages, endothelial cells, and cells of reticuloendothelial origin. The β-VLDL receptor does not appear to be highly regulated like the LDL receptor and can engorge macrophages with lipid causing them to take on the appearance of foam cells often associated with the atherosclerotic process. The receptors and the known lipoproteins that bind to these receptors are listed in TABLE 2.

LDL RECEPTOR

When apoB or apoE of lipoproteins bind to the LDL receptor on the plasma membrane of cultured human fibroblasts, the receptor localizes in a coated pit. The lipoprotein-receptor complex is then internalized through a coated endocytic vesicle; the lipoprotein is dissociated from the receptor, which returns to the plasma membrane to interact with another lipoprotein. The endocytic vesicle then can fuse with a lysosome, where the protein is degraded and the amino acids secreted into the medium (which is a measure of degradation), while the CE are hydrolyzed. The cholesterol, thus generated, stimulates the activity of ACAT (acyl Co-A:cholesterol transferase), which reesterifies the cholesterol to cholesteryl oleate for storage in the cytoplasm. In addition, the sterol signals the suppression of 3-hydroxy-3-methylglutaryl (HMG)-CoA reductase so that the cell stops producing cholesterol and thus maintains a balance between endogenous and exogenous cholesterol. In addition, the sterol entry into the cell by way of this pathway provides a signal for a down-regulation of the LDL receptor, again providing an exquisite control system for cholesterol homeostasis in the cell.

FIGURE 1 illustrates schematically several important points concerning the binding of LDL and HTG-VLDL to the LDL receptor. The lipoproteins, receptor, and membrane are drawn to scale based on known values for diameters of the lipoproteins and molecular weights for the proteins. LDL, a relatively small particle, binds to the receptor by way of apoB, the exclusive apoprotein of this lipoprotein particle. Even though apoB is a major constituent of large VLDL, we have shown that apoB is incapable of binding to the LDL receptor in these large particles.[12] This has been confirmed.[13] Large VLDL from HTG patients bind to the receptor by way of apoE of a specific conformation.[14] We have also shown that thrombin cleaves one peptide bond of a particular conformation of apoE of HTG-VLDL and that this specific cleavage of apoE destroys binding of HTG-VLDL to the LDL receptor. Although thrombin also cleaves apoB, it does not affect its ability to interact with the LDL receptor in small particles where it is the ligand for receptor-mediated uptake, as in VLDL (S_f 20-60), IDL, and LDL.[15]

As just mentioned, unlike LDL, the binding of HTG-VLDL is mediated by a particular conformation of apolipoprotein E. Using human α-thrombin as a probe, we were able to cleave this apoE on the surface of HTG-VLDL and render the particle incapable of binding to the LDL receptor. Thrombin cleavage of apoE is highly specific, even when the apoprotein is bound to the phospholipid surface of VLDL. A comparison of the cleavage site of apoE (TABLE 3) with the cleavage site of fibrinopeptide A shows that the region of apoE actually cleaved by thrombin is highly homologous to a native thrombin cleavage site in fibrinogen and partially explains the high specificity of thrombin for this specific domain of apoE. The E-22 fragment of the apoE (the *N*-terminal two/thirds of the apoprotein produced by thrombin cleavage) contains the receptor binding domain, whereas the carboxyterminal E-12 fragment contains a major lipid binding domain. We have shown that the E-12 region not only anchors the apoprotein to the lipoprotein, but that it probably is involved in the proper orientation of apoE for interaction with the LDL receptor.[14]

Thrombin changes the binding of HTG-VLDL to the LDL receptor, from saturable, high affinity (FIGURE 2), to linear, low affinity (FIGURE 3), with little evidence

TABLE 2. Lipoprotein Receptors for apoB/apoE-Containing Lipoproteins

Receptor	Lipoproteins
LDL Receptor	LDL, HTG-VLDL, β-VLDL
β-VLDL	β-VLDL, HTG-VLDG, Chylomicrons

of internalization. The binding and uptake of thrombin-inactivated HTG-VLDL by fibroblasts has the characteristics of VLDL of the same subclass of normal subjects, which also are not taken up by high-affinity mechanisms. Because the LDL receptor high-affinity binding domain in HTG-VLDL is abolished by thrombin, thrombin-inactivated HTG-VLDL (designated TI-HTG-VLDL) no longer are capable of suppressing HMG-CoA reductase activity.[14] To further verify that apoE was responsible for this interaction with the receptor, we added intact apoE back to the TI-HTG-VLDL, reconstituting its ability to bind to the receptor and to suppress HMG-CoA reductase.[14]

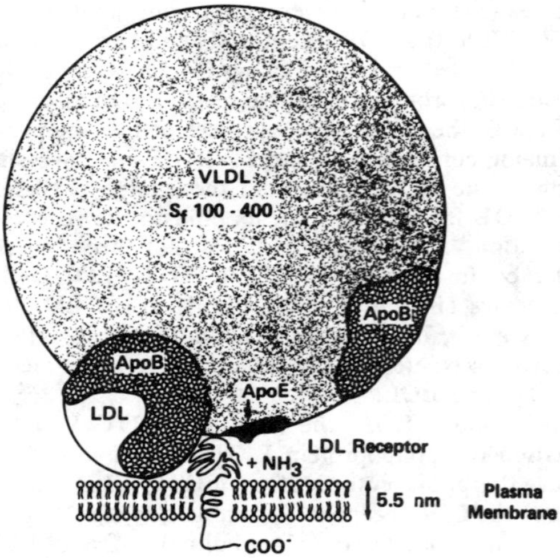

FIGURE 1. Schematic of the interaction of either LDL or HTG-VLDL S_f 100-400 with the low density lipoprotein receptor. This is drawn to scale to demonstrate the differences in which each of these lipoproteins approach the LDL receptor residing in the plasma membrane. Values for the size of HTG-VLDL and LDL are taken from both compositional data,[12,15] physical measurements, and the molecular weights of the apoproteins and receptor (apoE, 34,350; apoB, 389,000; LDL receptor, 95,000). The consequences of these differences are discussed in the text.

THE β-VLDL RECEPTOR PATHWAY OF MACROPHAGES

As stated earlier, a second receptor for some large TG-rich lipoproteins is the β-VLDL receptor. Triglyceride can accumulate in macrophages when certain HTG-VLDL ($S_f > 60$) are incubated with the murine macrophage line P388D_1 for as little as 4 hours. The triglyceride accumulation is dramatic. HTG-VLDL at 25 μg/ml of protein can produce a 10-20-fold increase in cellular triglyceride, from 10-20 μg/mg cell protein up to 200 μg TG/mg cell protein. Triglyceride accumulates in a curvilinear

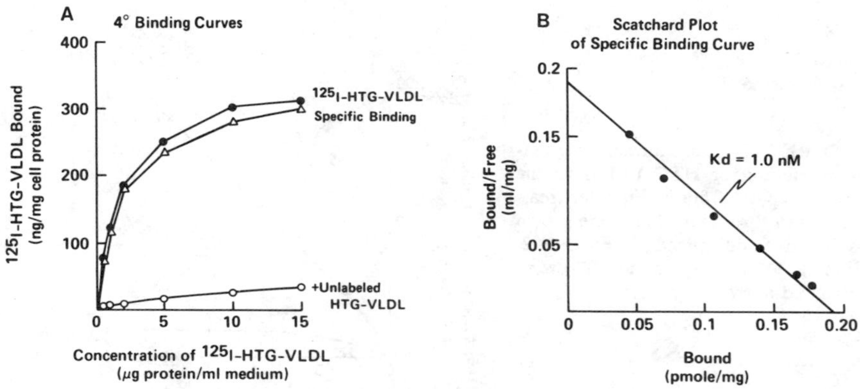

FIGURE 2. Saturable, high-affinity binding of HTG-VLDL S_f 100-400 to the LDL receptor of human fibroblasts at 4° C. **A**: Binding curve: cells were grown to approximately 75% confluency. Medium containing the indicated quantities of radioiodinated [^{125}I]HTG-VLDL, in the absence (●) and in the presence (○) of unlabeled homologous HTG-VLDL, 50 μg/ml, were added to duplicate dishes with and without cells and incubated for 2 hr at 4°C. Cells were washed extensively and dissolved in 2.0 ml of 0.1 ml NaOH. Radioactivity associated with each dish represents [^{125}I]HTG-VLDL bound, corrected for nonspecific binding to empty dishes. Each point represents the average of values from two dishes, which varied by less than 5%, expressed as ng [^{125}I]HTG-VLDL per mg cell protein. The calculated difference between the curves, representing binding of [^{125}I]HTG-VLDL in the absence and in the presence of unlabeled HTG-VLDL, represents specific binding (△). **B**: Scatchard analysis of the specific binding data from **A**.

manner, indicating receptor mediation, with half-maximal binding and maximal binding at 8 μg protein/ml and 30 μg/ml, respectively.[16] Direct binding and competition binding analyses confirm that this is a receptor-mediated interaction. Normal VLDL and LDL do not cause triglyceride loading in these macrophages.[7,16]

A more dramatic, but less quantitative, picture of this lipid loading by the macrophage is obtained by staining with Oil red O for neutral lipid in the P388D$_1$ murine macrophage after incubation with HTG-VLDL. Incubating with either normal VLDL or LDL under the same conditions does not show such lipid accumulation within these cells, as shown previously in the unstimulated murine macrophage.[7]

When HTG-VLDL are treated with thrombin to abolish binding to the LDL receptor, this treatment does not diminish the binding, uptake, or the ability to load macrophage with lipid.[16] In fact, not only does thrombin not abolish binding, but rather, it can enhance uptake.[17] This demonstrates that the ligands for β-VLDL receptor recognition are different from those for the LDL receptor. FIGURE 4 sche-

TABLE 3. Homology of the Primary Thrombin Cleavage Sites of apoE and Fibrinopeptide A (FPA)

	191 192
apoE:	PRO-*LEU*-VAL-*GLU*-GLN-*GLY*-ARG-*VAL-ARG*--ALA-ALA
	16, 17
FPA:	PHE-**LEU**-ALA-**GLU**-GLY-**GLY**-GLY-**VAL-ARG**--GLY-PRO

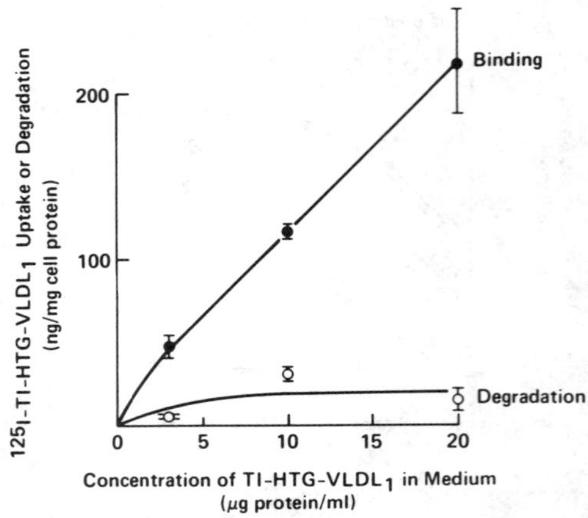

FIGURE 3. Loss of saturable, high affinity binding of HTG-VLDL to the LDL receptor of fibroblasts after treatment with thrombin. Cells were grown as described in legend of FIGURE 2. Binding (●) and degradation (○) were measured at 37° C.

matically summarizes these findings. Furthermore, thrombin can activate a native lipoprotein that does not normally interact with the macrophage receptor: normal VLDL S_f 60-400 can bind to the β-VLDL receptor and load macrophages with lipid after, but not prior, to thrombin processing.[17]

To summarize, hypertriglyceridemic VLDL bind to both the LDL receptor and the β-VLDL receptor. Normal VLDL bind to neither lipoprotein receptor. After thrombin treatment, HTG-VLDL lose their ability to bind to the LDL receptor, but not their ability to bind to the macrophage receptor. VLDL from normal subjects bind to neither receptor prior to treatment with thrombin; after thrombin treatment, the lipoprotein still no longer binds to the LDL receptor (the apoE of appropriate conformation is not present), but it now can bind to the macrophage receptor. The overall result, then, is that thrombin processing of the VLDL can cause interaction of VLDL with the macrophage receptor. When overloaded, uptake of triglyceride-rich lipoproteins by this route causes lipid engorgement and foam-cell formation. Thrombin proteolysis of these lipoproteins is either destroying apoprotein receptor binding domains, as in the case of apoE on HTG-VLDL necessary for LDL receptor binding, or it is creating (or unmasking) a receptor binding domain for the β-VLDL receptor as in the case of its effect on normal VLDL. The questions then arise: Can thrombin process VLDL apoproteins *in vivo*? and What are the consequences?

OBSERVATIONS CONCERNING *IN VIVO* BREAKDOWN OF apoB AND apoE

We have observed that HTG-VLDL, when isolated by identical procedures used for normal VLDL, often contain large, specific apoB fragments and apoE fragments[18] that are not found in normal VLDL or LDL. ApoB-100 is the only apoB species found in VLDL and LDL from normal subjects. Also, the apoB-100 in LDL from the same HTG-subject is also intact and not degraded.

Furthermore, we can mimic the fragmentation of apoB in HTG-VLDL by thrombin cleavage of apoB-100-containing lipoproteins.[15] Recently, we have shown that both prothrombin and thrombin can associate with the VLDL phospholipid surface.

Therefore, it is our current working model that prothrombin can associate with VLDL in hypertriglyceridemia, and when it is activated to thrombin, it can degrade apoE, which destroys VLDL interaction with the LDL receptor, and may process apoB for recognition by the macrophage β-VLDL receptor.

ENDOGENOUS PROTEASE ACTIVITY OF HTG-VLDL

The VLDL-associated protease activity and endogenous degradation of the apoprotein B of HTG-VLDL have been previously described.[15,18] HTG-VLDL, which show partial degradation after isolation, show increased degradation by the endogenous, thrombin-like protease activity, when incubated for 2 hours at 37° C with 5 mM Ca^{2+}. Controls show that this is a proteolytic degradation and not oxidative cleavage of apoB. ApoB of HTG-VLDL is a good substrate for thrombin and can be processed even at low physiological levels with exogenous thrombin (1 unit/ml, for 2 hr).

BOTH THROMBIN AND PROTHROMBIN CAN BIND TO VLDL

Thrombin, in this case an inactivated thrombin, can bind to the surface of VLDL (FIGURE 5). The experiment is carried out in the following way. Using a salt density gradient, the lipoproteins are placed in the bottom 2 ml of the ultracentrifuge tube, and because they are less dense than water, they will float to the top of the tube in 120 minutes. FIGURE 5 shows the distribution of radiolabeled diisopropylphosphofluoridate (DFP)-inactivated thrombin (a gift from John Fenton) in the presence and absence of the VLDL subfractions, $VLDL_1$ (S_f 100-400), $VLDL_2$ (S_f 60-100), and $VLDL_3$ (S_f 20-60). In the absence of VLDL, thrombin is found only in the bottom 2 mls of the tube, as indicated by the open circles, whereas in the presence of physiological concentrations of VLDL, thrombin binds to the VLDL subclasses, at ratios that reflect the amount of each subfraction of the VLDL.

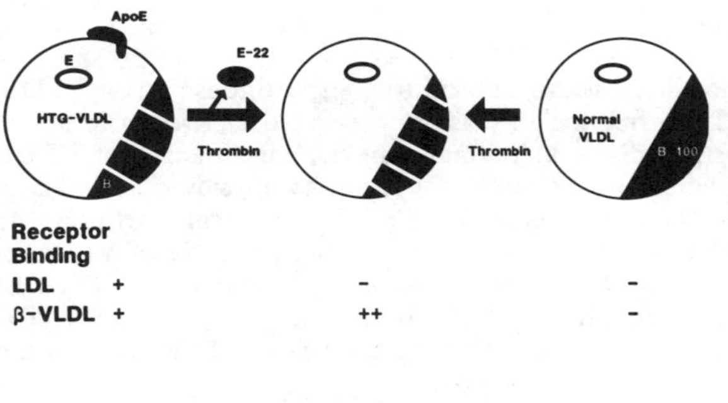

FIGURE 4. Schematic summary of the functional effects of thrombin degradation of apoE and apoB in VLDL S_f 100-400.

We have also been able to show that prothrombin binds to large VLDL at physiological concentrations of prothrombin, VLDL, and Ca^{2+}. TABLE 4 illustrates the incorporation of radiolabeled prothrombin at different concentrations of VLDL. The prothrombin-VLDL complexes were isolated using density gradient flotation of the lipoproteins, the method we normally use to isolate VLDL subfractions from plasma or unfractionated VLDL. In this experiment, highly purified VLDL (S_f 100-400), the largest VLDL subclass, was used. Recovery of the VLDL was greater than 90% of starting material. Several points can be made: (1) Under these particular conditions we did not reach the saturation of prothrombin for the VLDL phospholipid surface.

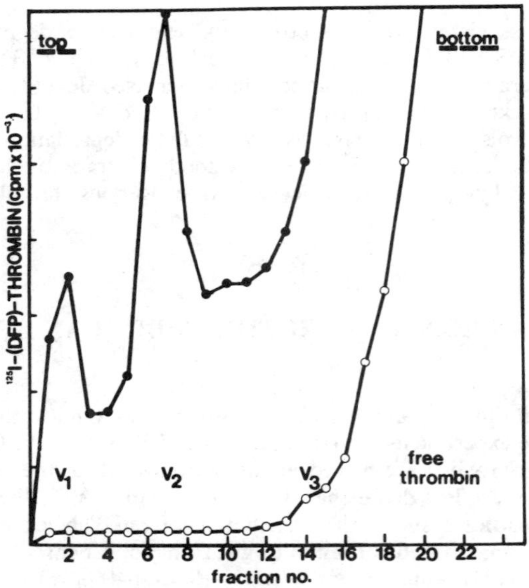

FIGURE 5. Thrombin binding to the HTG-VLDL. [^{125}I](DFP)-thrombin was placed in the bottom of a salt density gradient in the absence (○) or presence (○) of HTG-VLDL S_f 20-400. After centrifugation, the gradient was fractionated and the radioactivity measured. [^{125}I](DFP)-thrombin is found associated with each of the VLDL subclasses, S_f 100-400 (V_1), S_f 60-100 (V_2), and S_f 20-60 (V_3).

(2) As the VLDL concentration increases, more prothrombin partitions into the VLDL. This suggests that as the VLDL fraction in plasma is elevated *in vivo,* as in severe hypertriglyceridemia, or postprandially in normal subjects, this fraction of VLDL could compete for the circulating prothrombin. (3) At these physiological levels of VLDL and prothrombin, stoichiometric amounts of prothrombin can partition into the VLDL phospholipid surface (up to 2 moles prothrombin per mole of VLDL in this study). This indicates that this native circulating phospholipid surface (VLDL) has high capacity for binding prothrombin. VLDL from normal subjects have equivalent capacity to bind prothrombin. In normal subjects, however, the amount of the

TABLE 4. Isolated Prothrombin-VLDL (S_f 100-400) Complexes

VLDL[a] (picomoles) i[b]	PT (nmoles) i[b]	PT/VLDL[c]
23	0.3	0.2
23	1.0	0.5
23	2.7	1.6
46	2.7	0.8
92	2.7	0.5
0	2.7	0.0

[a] Based on VLDL-triglyceride content of 0.65, protein 0.059, and molecular weight of 30,000,000.

[b] i = initial incubation quantities of each component.

[c] Complexes isolated by Lingren density ultracentrifugation; this ratio is picomole of prothrombin (PT)/picomole of isolated VLDL S_f (100-400).

large VLDL subclasses present in plasma, and thus the phospholipid surface provided by these lipoproteins, are from 2.5 to 10 times less than in hypertriglyceridemic subjects.

When one isolates VLDL in the absence of the Ca^{2+} chelator, EDTA, which may yield a more native-state lipoprotein, both immunological electrophoretic blot methods and radioimmunoassay reveal that prothrombin is indeed associated with highly purified VLDL; that is, prothrombin coisolates and copurifies with VLDL. The amount of prothrombin associated with the VLDL fraction appears to be a function of the levels of VLDL in the individual. The amount of prothrombin actually observed in VLDL is a function of the isolation conditions, as indicated by the decreased levels of prothrombin when VLDL are isolated in the presence of Ca^{2+} chelators.

SUMMARY

FIGURE 6 summarizes our current thoughts on the interaction of prothrombin with the VLDL surface. We have shown that VLDL have the capacity to bind both

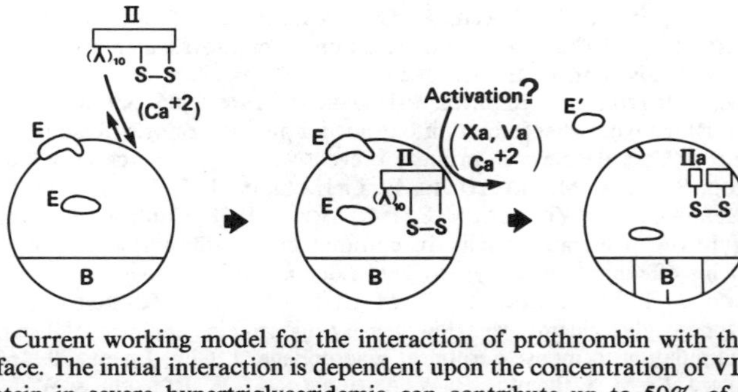

FIGURE 6. Current working model for the interaction of prothrombin with the VLDL phospholipid surface. The initial interaction is dependent upon the concentration of VLDL in plasma. This lipoprotein in severe hypertriglyceridemia can contribute up to 50% of the circulating phospholipid surface in blood. Once prothrombin is bound, it can cocirculate with the HTG-VLDL and can be activated by unknown mechanisms and at unknown sites. When this occurs, minimally, the apoproteins of the VLDL are processed with consequences discussed in the text.

prothrombin and thrombin. As indicated here, when the VLDL levels in plasma are increased in hypertriglyceridemia or postprandially, the fraction of circulating prothrombin partitioned into the VLDL phospholipid surface can increase. The lipoprotein can then circulate with prothrombin bound. VLDL-associated prothrombin could be activated to thrombin *in vivo,* by as yet unknown mechanisms and at unknown sites. Castellino and coworkers[19] have demonstrated that factor Xa can convert prothrombin to thrombin on the surface of VLDL; VLDL was the only lipoprotein capable of this. We are currently working to demonstrate that VLDL will support the prothrombinase complex. Nonetheless, whatever the mechanism, if thrombin is generated on the surface of VLDL, it can minimally degrade specifically the apoproteins of VLDL. This apoprotein processing causes a loss of receptor binding determinants for the LDL receptor, diverting these lipoproteins for interaction with the β-VLDL receptor of macrophages that, in turn, can cause foam-cell formation—an initiating event of the atherosclerotic process.

ACKNOWLEDGMENTS

The authors would like to thank Alice Lin, Shiah-Lian Huang, Jill Young, and Flora Brown for excellent technical help and Rosetta Ray for manuscript preparation. We thank Dr. John W. Fenton II for his continued encouragement and for human α-thrombin. Dr. J. Probstfield, Dr. J. Guyton, and Dr. P. Jones are gratefully acknowledged for supplying hypertriglyceridemic plasma.

REFERENCES

1. Reardon, J. F., N. H. Fidge & P. J. Nestel. 1978. Catabolism of very low density lipoprotein B apoprotein in man. J. Clin. Invest. **61:** 850-860.
2. Simpson, H. C. R., T. W. Meade, Y. Stirling, J. I. Mann, R. Chakrabarti & L. Woolf. 1983. Hypertriglyceridemia and hypercoagulability. Lancet **1(8328):** 787-790.
3. Elkeles, R. S., R. Chakrabarti, M. Vickers, Y. Stirling & T. W. Meade. 1980. Effect of treatment of hyperlipidaemia on haemostatic variables. Br. Med. J. **281(6246):** 973.
4. Meade, T. W., W. R. S. North, R. Chakrabarti, Y. Stirling, A. P. Haines & S. G. Thompson. 1980. Haemostatic function on cardiovascular death: Early results of prospective study. Lancet **1:** 1050-1054.
5. Aberg, H., H. Lithell, I. Selinus & H. Hedstrand. 1985. Serum triglycerides are a risk factor for myocardial infarction but not for angina pectoris: Results from a 10-year follow-up of Uppsala, Sweden primary preventive study. Atherosclerosis **54:** 89-97.
6. Gianturco, S. H., A. M. Gotto Jr., R. L. Jackson, J. R. Patsch, O. D. Taunton, H. D. Sybers, D. L. Yeshurun & L. C. Smith. 1978. Control of 3-hydroxy-3-methylglutaryl-CoA reductase activity in cultured human fibroblasts by very low density lipoproteins of subjects with hypertriglyceridemia. J. Clin. Invest. **61:** 320-328.
7. Gianturco, S. H., W. A. Bradley, A. M. Gotto Jr., J. D. Morrisett & D. L. Peavy. 1982. Hypertriglyceridemic very low density lipoproteins enhance triglyceride synthesis and accumulation in mouse peritoneal macrophage. J. Clin. Invest. **70:** 168-178.
8. Goldstein, J. L., M. S. Brown, R. W. Anderson, D. W. Russell & W. J. Schneider. 1985. Receptor-mediated endocytosis: Concepts emerging from the LDL receptor system. Annu. Rev. Cell Biol. **1:** 1-39.

9. Mahley, R. W. & T. L. Innerarity. 1983. Lipoprotein receptors and cholesterol-homeostasis. Biochim. Biophys. Acta **737:** 197-222.
10. Brown, M. S. & J. L. Goldstein. 1985. The LDL receptor and HMG-CoA reductase—Two membrane molecules that regulate cholesterol homeostasis. *In* Current Topics in Cellular Regulation. **26:** 3-15. Academic Press.
11. Brown, M. S. & J. L. Goldstein. 1983. Lipoprotein metabolism in the macrophage: Implication for cholesterol deposition in atherosclerosis. Annu. Rev. Biochem. **52:** 223-261.
12. Gianturco, S. H., F. B. Brown, A. M. Gotto Jr. & W. A. Bradley. 1982. Receptor-mediated uptake of hypertriglyceridemic very low density lipoproteins by normal human fibroblasts. J. Lipid Res. **23:** 984-993.
13. Krul, E. S., M. J. Tikkanen, T. G. Cole, J. M. Davie & G. Schonfeld. 1985. Roles of apolipoprotein B and E in the cellular binding of very low density lipoproteins. J. Biol. Chem. **75:** 361-369.
14. Gianturco, S. H., A. M. Gotto Jr., S.-L. C. Hwang, J. B. Karlin, A. H. Y. Lin, S. C. Prasad & W. A. Bradley. 1983. Apolipoprotein E mediates uptake of S_f 100-400 hypertriglyceridemic very low density lipoproteins by the low density lipoprotein receptor pathway in normal human fibroblasts. J. Biol. Chem. **258:** 4526-4533.
15. Bradley, W. A., S.-L. C. Hwang, J. B. Karlin, S. C. Prasad, A. M. Gotto Jr. & S. H. Gianturco. 1984. Low-density lipoprotein receptor binding determinants switch from apolipoprotein E to apolipoprotein B during conversion of hypertriglyceridemic very-low-density lipoproteins to low-density lipoproteins. J. Biol. Chem. **259:** 14728-14735.
16. Gianturco, S. H., S. A. Brown, D. P. Via & W. A. Bradley. 1986. The β-VLDL receptor pathway in murine P388D cells. J. Lipid Res. **27:** 412-420.
17. Gianturco, S. H., A. M. Gotto Jr. & W. A. Bradley. 1985. Hypertriglyceridemia: lipoprotein receptors and atherosclerosis. Adv. Exp. Med. Biol. **183:** 47-71.
18. Bradley, W. A., E. B. Gilliam, A. M. Gotto Jr. & S. H. Gianturco. 1982. Apolipoprotein-E degradation in human very low density lipoproteins by plasma protease(s): chemical and biological consequences. Biochem. Biophysics Res. Commun. **109:** 1360-1367.
19. Bajaj, S. P., J. A. K. Harmony, M. Martinez-Carrion & F. J. Castellino. 1976. Human plasma lipoproteins as accelerators of prothrombin. J. Biol. Chem. **251:** 5233-5236.

Choices among the Possible Reaction Routes Catalyzed by Thrombin[a]

RAYMUND MACHOVICH[b]

Semmelweis University Medical School
Second Institute of Biochemistry
Puskin 9, H-1444 Budapest, POB. 262, Hungary

INTRODUCTION

Thrombin, as a multifunctional enzyme,[1] may play several roles in hemostasis,[2,3] and it is the most powerful trigger for thrombus formation. Activities of thrombin, however, are strictly controlled by different means. Its biological functions may be determined by apparent kDa values and the concentrations of the "substrates" present in blood and on the blood vessel wall. Moreover, thrombin produced from prothrombin may have various conformations, influencing thereby its affinity toward various substrates. To control thrombin activities, a relevant candidate may be the endothelial cell that is present at all places where thrombin can be formed.

Thrombin, not bound to an endothelial cell (T_f), has the capacity to clot fibrinogen,[4] to activate platelets,[5] factor XIII,[6] and/or accelerate its own formation by activation of factor V and factor VIII_c through a positive feedback control mechanism.[1] Under these conditions, thrombus formation develops in a few seconds. T_f can also react with plasma proteinase inhibitors,[7] primarily with antithrombin III, α_2-macroglobulin, heparin cofactor II, and α_1-proteinase inhibitor, although these reactions are relatively slow compared with its action on fibrinogen and/or platelets.

Thrombin, bound to endothelial cells (T_b), on the other hand, is modified in conformation and/or in orientation, and as a consequence, its reactivity with the various substrates is altered. Thrombin may bind to endothelial cells through several structures. If thrombin binds to the cells by way of heparin-like structures, that is, heparan sulfate, its inactivation by antithrombin III is accelerated on the cell surface,[8–10] resulting in thrombin-antithrombin III complex formation, in which the enzyme loses all of its proteolytic activities.[11]

If thrombin binds to an endothelial cell by way of thrombomodulin, its capacity to activate protein C increases, resulting in a rate enhancement of several orders of magnitude.[12] Activated protein C formed, in turn, inhibits thrombin formation from prothrombin by a negative feedback control mechanism[13] and, in addition, if thrombus has already formed, activated protein C initiates fibrinolysis.[14] Thrombin, in this bound form, loses its activity toward fibrinogen, factor V, and platelets.[12] Finally, thrombin

[a]This work was supported partly by the Hungarian Ministry of Health and the Hungarian Academy of Sciences, Grant no. 20, 057/85.

[b]Present address: Mayo Clinic, Hematology Research, Rochester, Minnesota 55905.

may bind to endothelial cells by way of an active site-dependent receptor, and this form of enzyme is internalized by the cell. (For details see below.) The reactions discussed above are briefly summarized in FIGURE 1.

THROMBIN STRUCTURE REQUIRED FOR BINDING TO ENDOTHELIAL CELLS

One of the questions arising is, What is the domain(s) of the thrombin molecule responsible for the interaction with endothelial cells? Several earlier studies used

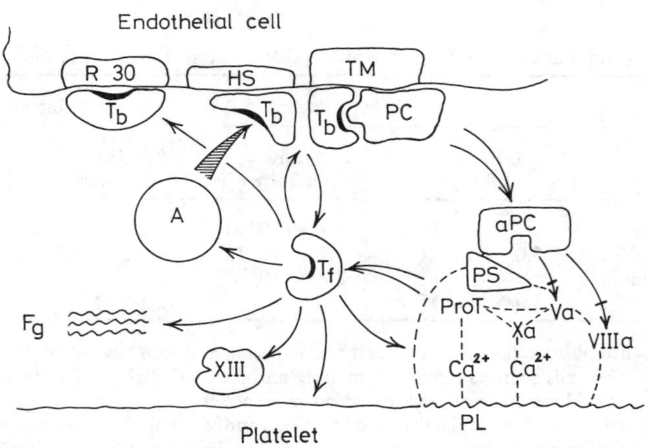

FIGURE 1. Functions of free and endothelial cell-bound thrombin. Thrombin (T_f), formed from prothrombin (ProT) can react easily with fibrinogen (Fg), factor XIII (XIII), or with platelets, can activate factor V (V) and factor VIII (VIII) in the prothrombinase complex, and may select among three receptors of endothelial cell surface. Interaction of thrombin (T_b) with thrombomodulin (TM) or heparan sulfate (HS) is reversible, whereas its binding to a membrane protein with M_r 30 000 (R-30) is irreversible. Thrombin bound to HS is facilitated to react with antithrombin III (A), whereas thrombin bound to TM is more reactive towards protein C (PC), resulting in the activation of the latter. Activated protein C (aPC) formed, in turn, inactivates activated factor V (Va) as well as activated factor VIII (VIIIa), and these reactions are accelerated by protein S (PS) on the phospholipid (PL) surface of the activated platelet. Not all the possible substrates for thrombin are shown.

chemically modified thrombin to probe the structure of the enzyme necessary to bind to fibrinogen, platelets, antithrombin III, heparin, or endothelial cell. Thus, thrombin modified at the active center binds to heparin,[15] platelets,[16] or endothelial cells,[17] but not to antithrombin III,[18] indicating that the active site of the enzyme is not required for a rapid, reversible and high-affinity binding to endothelial cells. On the other hand, when a lysine residue of thrombin involved in the heparin binding site[19] is modified by pyridoxal 5′-phosphate, thrombin loses not only its affinity to heparin but also the high-affinity binding site for endothelial cells[9] (TABLE 1). It is also known that heparin binds tightly to thrombin,[21,22] and the presence of heparin inhibits the binding of the enzyme to endothelial cells.[9,23] Heparin, however, binds to endothelial cells as well[9] (TABLE 1). Thus the question arises, whether heparin exerts its effect by interfering with the heparin-binding domain of thrombin or with the heparin-binding site of the endothelial cell. Because the interaction between heparin and cells develops slowly (see FIGURE 5), that is, it takes hours,[9] and the formation of the heparin-thrombin complex takes only seconds,[24] we conclude that it is the thrombin-heparin rather than the endothelial cell-heparin interaction that interferes with the binding of thrombin to the cells. These, and additional data in the literature,[16] suggest a model for the binding regions of thrombin.[1] Namely, the active center serine residue of the enzyme participates in the reaction with antithrombin III,[25] whereas the fibrinogen binding site extends over a large part of the enzyme molecule, involving the low-affinity platelet-binding site as well. The high-affinity platelet-binding site overlaps with both the fibrinogen and heparin binding sites, and the heparin binding site is at least partially involved in the domains responsible for endothelial cell binding.

TABLE 1. Binding Parameters for Phosphopyridoxylated Thrombins and Heparin[a]

	kDa		Sites/cell	
	High affinity	Low affinity	High affinity	Low affinity
Native-thrombin	2.7×10^{-8}M	2.1×10^{-6}M	2.7×10^{4}	3.3×10^{6}
PLP-thrombin[b]	3.0×10^{-8}M	1.7×10^{-6}M	3.3×10^{4}	1.5×10^{6}
PLP_2-thrombin[c]	—	2.2×10^{-6}M	—	7.5×10^{5}
Heparin	3.0×10^{-7}M	—	1.4×10^{6}	—

[a] Human α-thrombin or heparin used for these experiments were labeled by ^{125}I or tritiated, respectively.[9,20] The cells represent cultured minipig aortic endothelial cells. Data are calculated by use of the Klotz-Hunston equations, based on reference 9.

[b] PLP-thrombin, thrombin modified in a one-lysine residue involved in fibrinogen binding.

[c] PLP_2-thrombin, enzyme phosphopyridoxylated in two lysine residues responsible for fibrinogen as well as heparin binding.

RECEPTOR(S) OF ENDOTHELIAL CELLS FOR THROMBIN

Thrombin binds to endothelial cells very rapidly and with high affinity.[17] After the rapid and reversible binding, however, a slower interaction of thrombin with endothelial cells takes place. The second step is irreversible, active site specific with the formation of a covalent bond between thrombin and a protein of endothelial cell membranes having an M_r of 30 000.[26] The latter may serve as a receptor for uptake, internalization, and degradation of thrombin.[27,30] Hence, the endothelium may contribute directly to thrombin inactivation (FIGURE 2).

Another possible mechanism for thrombin inactivation by endothelial cells may occur by way of an interaction of the enzyme with the heparin-like membrane receptor(s). Several data in the literature suggest that heparin-like substances, that is, heparan sulfate and dermatan sulfate with anticoagulant nature,[19,28] are available on endothelium,[10,29–32] and thrombin inactivation by antithrombin III is accelerated on the endothelial cell surface[8–10,32,33] (FIGURE 3).

A third candidate for the thrombin receptor of the endothelial cell surface is the thrombomodulin, an unusually stable protein with an M_r of 74 000,[34,35] having high

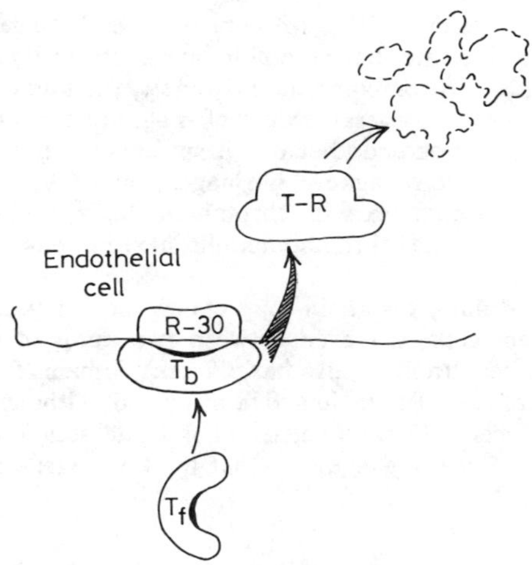

FIGURE 2. Endothelial cell receptors for thrombin: the binding site responsible for the irreversible interaction of the enzyme with the cell. Thrombin (T_f), bound to an endothelial cell surface with low affinity (T_b), forms an irreversible bond by way of its active site serine with a 30 000-dalton cell membrane protein (R-30). The reaction is slow, compared with the high affinity, reversible binding, and is followed by the uptake and degradation of the thrombin-receptor complex (T-R) by the cell.

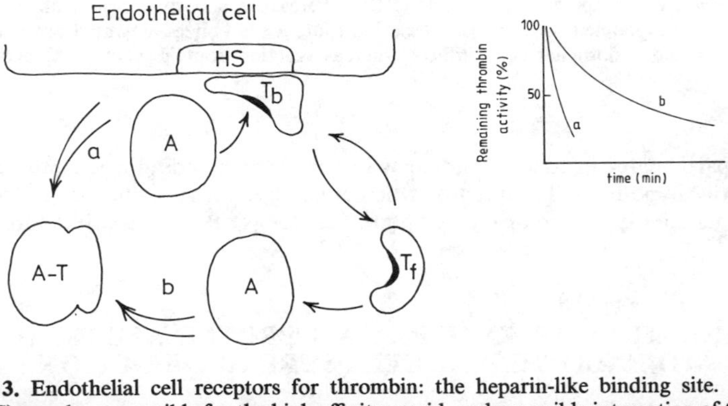

FIGURE 3. Endothelial cell receptors for thrombin: the heparin-like binding site. Heparan sulfate (HS) may be responsible for the high affinity, rapid, and reversible interaction of thrombin (T_f) with endothelial cells. The inactivation of the bound form of enzyme (T_b) by antithrombin III (A) is facilitated on the cell surface, resulting in thrombin-antithrombin III complex (A-T) formation. Reaction **a** symbolizes thrombin inactivation by antithrombin III on the endothelial cell surface or in the presence of heparin, whereas reaction **b** represents thrombin inactivation by antithrombin III in solution or in blood plasma.

affinity for thrombin[36] (K_m: 5×10^{-10} M, approximately). Experimental results published in the literature indicate that thrombin specificity to its substrates is changed when the enzyme binds to thrombomodulin. Namely, the rate of protein C activation by thrombin is enhanced by several orders of magnitude in the presence of either isolated thrombomodulin[36] or endothelial cell surfaces.[37] Thrombin activity, on the other hand, is highly restricted against fibrinogen, factor V, and platelet activation when the enzyme is in a complex with thrombomodulin[38,39] (FIGURE 4). Moreover, our recent results indicate that thrombomodulin also inhibits factor XIII activation by thrombin.[46]

According to these data, thrombin may choose not only among several soluble substrates and different cells, but even between two kinds of receptors on a single endothelial cell. Whether thrombin also has different domains for the interaction with the various receptors of the cells remains to be answered. Although the heparin binding domain of thrombin seems to be involved in the interaction with the heparin-like receptor of endothelial cells, a suggestion that the fibrinogen-binding domain of the

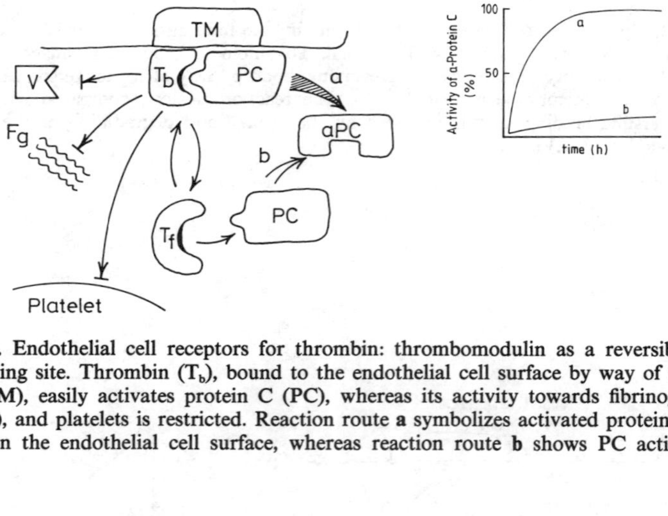

FIGURE 4. Endothelial cell receptors for thrombin: thrombomodulin as a reversible, high-affinity binding site. Thrombin (T_b), bound to the endothelial cell surface by way of thrombomodulin (TM), easily activates protein C (PC), whereas its activity towards fibrinogen (Fg), factor V (V), and platelets is restricted. Reaction route **a** symbolizes activated protein C (aPC) formation on the endothelial cell surface, whereas reaction route **b** shows PC activation in solution.

enzyme participates in the interaction with the thrombomodulin receptor would be an attractive hypothesis. The question whether endogeneous modifiers bound to thrombin alter its affinity to one of the receptors has not yet been properly addressed.

CONTRIBUTION OF SOME PLASMA PROTEINASE INHIBITORS TO ENDOTHELIAL CELL-SURFACE FUNCTION

Interaction of thrombin with endothelial cells occurs almost always in the presence of a high, micromolar concentration of plasma proteinase inhibitors.[7] Some of the inhibitors may also bind to these cells with different rates and affinities. Therefore, it is reasonable to ask how the interactions of thrombin with endothelial cells are altered in the presence of the inhibitors.

Rates of binding and dissociation of thrombin, antithrombin III, thrombin-antithrombin III complex, or heparin on endothelial cells are schematically shown in FIGURE 5a and b. Although the affinity of antithrombin III for endothelial cells is similar to that of thrombin, the rate of binding, and the amount of ligand bound at equilibrium is smaller for antithrombin III than for thrombin. Intermediate values characterize the thrombin-antithrombin III complex. As to the reverse reaction, thrombin dissociates fastest ($t_{1/2}$ is approximately 1 minute), and the complex dissociates slowest, and in addition, complete dissociation of the latter needs trypsin treatment.[42] Heparin, as indicated earlier, displays a very slow binding rate, with one order of magnitude lower affinity (see TABLE 1) than that of thrombin or antithrombin III. Moreover, heparin is taken up by endothelial cells;[43] therefore, the precise measurement of the dissociation is rather difficult.

Binding of Thrombin to Endothelial Cells in the Presence of Antithrombin III and/or α_2-Macroglobulin

There are conflicting reports in the literature regarding the receptor(s) of endothelial cells for thrombin and antithrombin III, namely it is not clear if a heparin-like substance, for example, heparan sulfate, is involved in thrombin and antithrombin III binding.[10,30–33] The question is crucial; if both thrombin and antithrombin III bind to heparan sulfate of the endothelial cell surface, but at a distinct part of the molecule, then a putative catalytic action of the receptor, similar to the mechanism proposed for heparin as a template,[44,45] seems to be possible. Our recent experimental results indicate that there is no competition between thrombin and antithrombin III in their binding to endothelial cells (TABLE 2). Antithrombin III inhibits the binding of the native thrombin, whereas it does not affect the interaction of active center-blocked thrombin with endothelial cells. These data suggest that if both thrombin and antithrombin III bind to endothelial cells by way of heparan sulfate, the binding sites are different for enzyme and inhibitor, and a catalytic role of heparin-like receptors in the thrombin-antithrombin III reaction is likely.

The participation of α_2-macroglobulin in the interaction of thrombin with endothelial cells is another interesting question. There are two reasons to study that point. One is that α_2-macroglobulin is present in blood plasma at a relatively high concentration and may contribute to the function of antithrombin III. The second reason is that α_2-macroglobulin may be considered a modifier of thrombin function (see above), because thrombin, in the complex with the inhibitor, retains some of its activity and may still have a biological function. *In vitro* experiments show that although the binding of thrombin decreased when complexed with α_2-macroglobulin (TABLE 3) and although the thrombin-α_2-macroglobulin complex formation proceeds in the medium of endothelial cells, the amount of thrombin bound to endothelial cells does not change during a 20-minute incubation period (FIGURE 6). α_2-Macroglobulin also binds to endothelial cells, and the rate of binding is similar to that of thrombin, that is, to attain equilibrium between free and bound inhibitor molecules takes only a few seconds (FIGURE 6, inset). These data suggest that although the affinity of the thrombin-α_2-macroglobulin complex for endothelial cells is lower than that of thrombin alone, thrombin, if formed from prothrombin, can bind to endothelial cells easily because its reaction is faster with the cells than with the inhibitor.

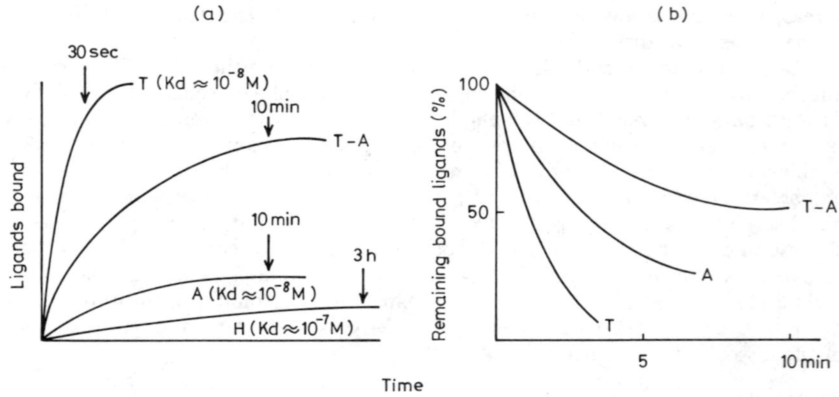

FIGURE 5. Schematic representation of the rate of association (**a**) and dissociation (**b**) of thrombin, antithrombin III, thrombin-antithrombin III complex, and heparin with the endothelial cell surface. Binding kinetics are shown on an arbitrary scale. At equilibrium, the amount of ligands bound to endothelial cells is in order of magnitude of fentomoles per 10^5 cells. Total ligand concentrations are in the nanomolar range, except for heparin, which is at micromolar level. Proteins are of human, whereas endothelial cells are of minipig or of bovine aortic origin. Methods for isolation of proteins and their isotopic labeling, as well as those of heparin, and details of the binding studies have been described in references 9, 20, 40, and 42. Because heparin is internalized by endothelial cells, its dissociation is not shown. Abbreviations: T, thrombin; A: antithrombin III; T-A, thrombin-antithrombin III complex; H, heparin.

Effect of Heparan Sulfate and Thrombomodulin on the Reaction of Thrombin with Antithrombin III and α_2-Macroglobulin

Heparin, as well as heparan sulfate, accelerate thrombin inactivation by antithrombin III as detailed earlier. Thrombomodulin, on the other hand, does not influence the inactivation rate of thrombin by antithrombin III. That is, a maximum twofold increase in the *in vitro* reaction was measurable,[47] and this moderate effect may be

TABLE 2. Competition between Thrombin and Antithrombin III for Binding to Endothelial Cells[a]

	Thrombin bound (fmole/10^5 cells)			
		Antithrombin III added (μM)		
[^{125}I]Thrombin	none	0.5	1	2
Native-thrombin	200	50	50	50
PMSF-thrombin	195	175	170	160

[a] Bovine aortic endothelial cells (2 × 10^5) were preincubated with various concentrations of antithrombin III at 22°C for 1 minute. Thereafter [^{125}I]thrombin (40 nM) was added (either native or active center modified by phenylmethyl sulfonyl-fluoride (PMSF)), and cell bound radioactivity was determined after 30 sec incubation.[42]

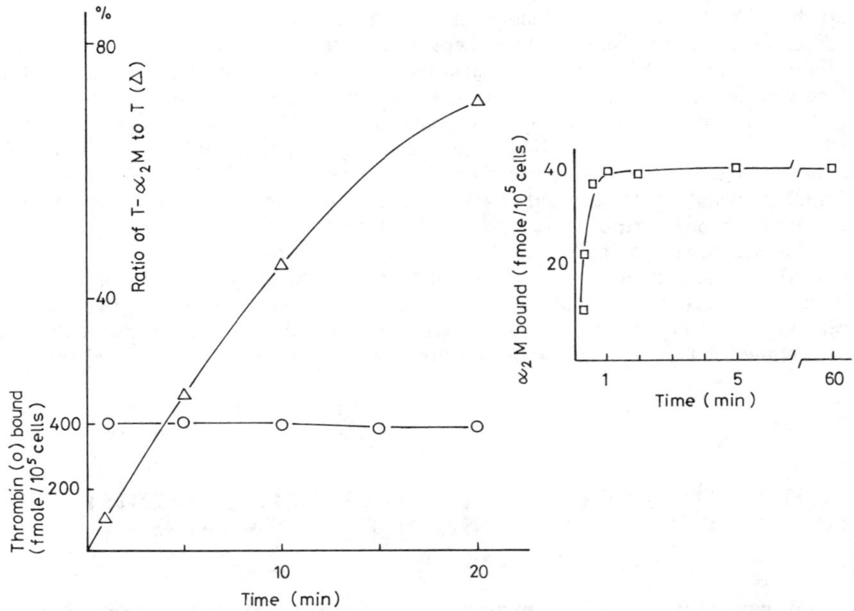

FIGURE 6. Binding of thrombin to endothelial cells in the presence of α_2-macroglobulin. Endothelial cells (bovine aortic) were preincubated with human α_2-macroglobulin (240 nM) at 22°C for 2 minutes; thereafter human [^{125}]α-thrombin (100 nM) was added and incubated further as indicated in the figure. Cell-bound radioactivity was determined and the amount of enzyme bound calculated.[49] The ratio of thrombin-α_2-macroglobulin complex (T-α_2M) to free thrombin (T) in the cell medium was also determined by electrophoresis according to the Laemmli system.[41] Inset: time dependence of the binding of isolated, ^{125}I-labeled α_2-macroglobulin (α_2-M) to endothelial cells, at a concentration of 40 nM.

TABLE 3. Binding of Thrombin and Thrombin-α_2-Macroglobulin Complex to Endothelial Cells[a]

	Preincubation (min) of [^{125}I]thrombin with α_2-macroglobulin for					
	zero	1	5	10	20	30
Thrombin bound to cell (percent)	100	90	73	50	30	15

[a] Human α-thrombin and α_2-macroglobulin, in a molar ratio of 1 to 2.4, were preincubated at 22°C for 30 minutes. At the indicated times, aliquots were taken and added to endothelial cells (2×10^5) and incubated for a further 5 minutes. Final concentration of thrombin in medium was 100 nM. Thereafter cells were washed three times, and the cell-bound radioactivity was determined.[49] For experimental details see references 9 and 40. The results are duplicates and expressed as a percentage of thrombin bound to endothelial cells without preincubation with α_2-macroglobulin.

attributed to heparin contamination of thrombomodulin isolated from rabbit lung.

Regarding the possible effect of heparan sulfate and thrombomodulin on the inhibition of thrombin activity by α_2-macroglobulin, data are lacking in the literature. One can, however, extrapolate from observations made on the thrombin-α_2-macroglobulin-heparin system. Namely, thrombin is protected by heparin against inactivation by α_2-macroglobulin.[48] According to our recent experimental results, thrombomodulin appears to exert a similar protective effect. When the thrombin-α_2-macroglobulin complex formation is measured *in vitro* in the presence of isolated thrombomodulin, an inhibition of the reaction can be found (FIGURE 7).

These data suggest that if thrombin binds to endothelial cells by way of thrombomodulin, the enzyme in protected against inactivation by α_2-macroglobulin, whereas its reaction with antithrombin III is neither facilitated nor inhibited. If bound to these cells by way of heparan sulfate, the reaction of thrombin with α_2-macroglobulin may be inhibited, but its reaction with antithrombin III can be extremely accelerated.

THE INTERACTION OF THROMBIN WITH ENDOTHELIAL CELLS IN THE PRESENCE OF FIBRINOGEN

Fibrinogen, the specific thrombin substrate circulates inside the blood vessel at a high level,[4] at a concentration of about 10 μM. Hence, if thrombin is formed, the enzyme is saturated by that substrate. Fibrinogen, on the other hand, binds to endothelial cells, too, with a kDa of approximately 2×10^{-7} M. The interaction is reversible, and it takes about 10 minutes[50] to attain equilibrium between free and cell-bound molecules. Thus, it is possible that thrombin *in vivo* binds to endothelial cells not only by way of the endothelial cell receptors but also through fibrinogen bound to endothelial cells. If so, fibrinogen, thrombomodulin, and heparan sulfate can mutually influence thrombin functions.

In vitro experiments show that fibrinogen inhibits, in a concentration-dependent manner, the binding of thrombin to endothelial cells (TABLE 4). When the endothelial cells are preincubated with fibrinogen, the amount of thrombin bound to endothelial cells does not increase, indicating that the enzyme has no affinity to the cell-bound fibrinogen. Thus, the action by which fibrinogen competes with the binding of thrombin to the cells seems to be a consequence of a direct interaction between the enzyme and its substrate.

Fibrinogen, however, may also interfere with endothelial cell-bound thrombin, thereby influencing thrombin functions localized on the cell surface. Because thrombin bound to thrombomodulin is restricted to act on fibrinogen, as mentioned earlier, the question emerges whether fibrinogen also affects the activation of protein C by thrombin bound to endothelial cells. Experiments with fibrinogen degradation products and with chemically modified fibrinogen that cannot be clotted by thrombin show that the activation of protein C by thrombin or by thrombomodulin-bound thrombin is inhibited by these products (TABLE 5). In addition, preliminary experiments indicate that when α-thrombin is modified by pyridoxal 5′-phosphate, resulting in a decrease in the affinity of heparin binding domain for heparin as well as for endothelial cell binding, the enzyme does not lose its ability to activate protein C either in the absence or presence of thrombomodulin (I. Léránt, B. Papp, T. Kovács, and R. Machovich, unpublished). These data allow us to suppose that the heparin-binding domain (which is the same as the endothelial cell binding domain) of thrombin is distinguished from the thrombomodulin and protein C binding domains. The latter, on the other hand, are partially involved in the fibrinogen-binding domain of the enzyme.

CONCLUSION

On the basis of the data discussed above, it is suggested that the endothelial cells play a decisive role in the regulation of thrombin functions. Furthermore, with the

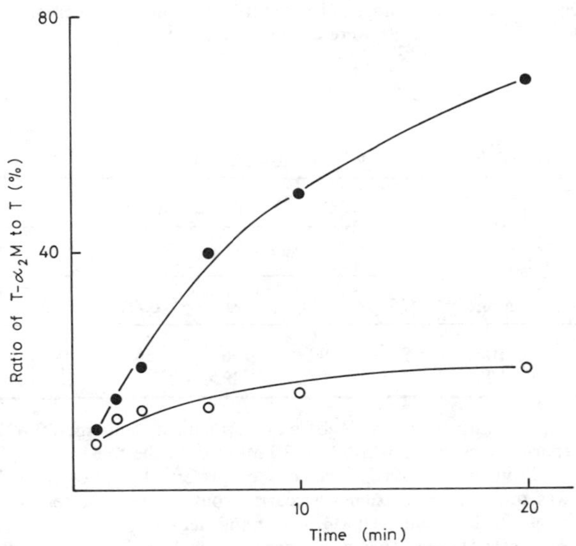

FIGURE 7. Effect of thrombomodulin on thrombin-α_2-macroglobulin complex formation. Human [^{125}I]α-thrombin (14 μg/ml) was preincubated at 37°C for 1 minute with thrombomodulin (150 μg/ml) isolated from rabbit lung;[36] thereafter human α_2-macroglobulin (670 μg/ml) was added and incubated further. At various indicated times, aliquots of reaction mixture were taken and applied to SDS-polyacrylamide gel electrophoresis. The gels were sliced and determined for radioactivity to calculate the ratio of thrombin-α_2-macroglobulin complex (T-α_2M) to free thrombin (T).[49] Thrombomodulin: none (●), added (○).

more detailed information now available, our model of the different binding domains of the thrombin molecule described earlier,[1] can be improved further.

Because thrombin binds to thrombomodulin with high affinity,[36] and the bound form of enzyme is restricted to acting on fibrinogen[38] and/or platelets,[39] the thrombomodulin-binding domain of thrombin may be located somewhere at the fibrinogen and platelet-binding region of the enzyme, or at least, this region is influenced by a conformational change induced by the thrombin-thrombomodulin interaction. The possibility that the lysine residues responsible for fibrinogen and heparin binding are

TABLE 4. Effect of Fibrinogen on the Binding of Thrombin to Endothelial Cells[a]

	Fibrinogen (μg/ml)					
			present			preincubated[b]
	None	10	50	100	1000	1000
Thrombin bound (fmoles/10^5 cells)	600	535	470	389	308	366

[a] Bovine aortic endothelial cells (2×10^5) were preincubated with fibrinogen, at concentrations indicated, for 1 minute at 22°C; thereafter, 100 nM of [^{125}I] human α-thrombin blocked in its active center by diisopropyl fluorophosphate (DFP-thrombin) was added and incubated for 10 minutes further. Cells were washed three times, and the cell-bound radioactivity was determined.[49]

[b] Cells were preincubated with fibrinogen (1 mg/ml) for 20 minutes; thereafter, free molecules were removed. Otherwise, experiments were carried out as above.

TABLE 5. Activation of Protein C by Thrombin in the Presence of Fibrinogen[a]

	Fibrinogen (μg/ml)							
		FDP				Fg-Lys		
Thrombomodulin	None	75	150	300	600	150	300	600
Added	100	98	90	66	55	90	60	50
None	100			38				

[a] Human α-thrombin (10 μg/ml) was incubated with rabbit thrombomodulin (26 μg/ml) and human protein C (partially purified) at 37°C for 10 minutes in the presence of plasmin-digested fibrinogen (FDP) or fibrinogen modified chemically by pyridoxal 5′-phosphate (Fg-Lys). When thrombomodulin was omitted, incubation was carried out for 60 minutes. The reaction was stopped by addition of antithrombin III (40 μg/ml) and heparin (8 μg/ml). Activated protein C was assayed by substrate H-D-phenylalanyl-L-arginine-p-nitroanilide as described.[34,49] Results are shown in percentage of protein C activity of sample without fibrinogen.

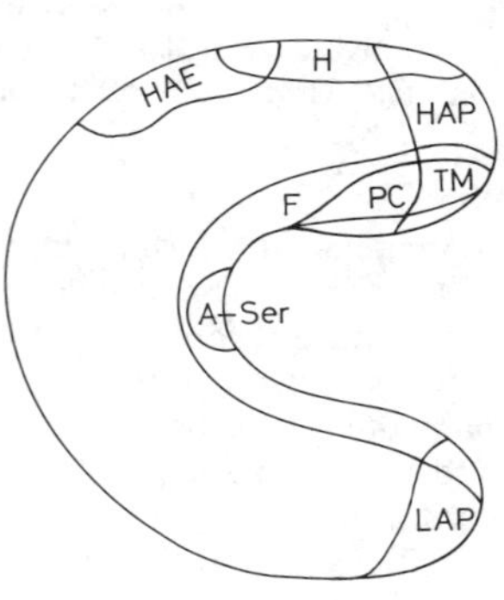

FIGURE 8. Schematic model for the possible binding domains of thrombin. Abbreviations for binding domains: A, active center and antithrombin III; F, fibrinogen; PC, protein C; TM, thrombomodulin; HAP, high-affinity platelet; H, heparin; HAE, high-affinity endothelial cell; LAP, low-affinity platelet.

not involved in the protein C-binding domain is supported by the finding that the chemical modification of these amino acid residues does not inhibit enzyme activity towards protein C and also does not diminish the protein C activation accelerated by thrombomodulin. Our present conception, thus, is that the domains of thrombin for interaction with endothelial cells are distinct for thrombomodulin and heparan sulfate. Finally, as fibrinogen or fibrinogen degradation products inhibit protein C activation, both protein C and thrombomodulin binding domains seem to overlap with the fibrinogen-binding domain. The schematic model for the various binding domains of thrombin is shown in FIGURE 8.

There is, however, one important unanswered question: Does thrombin select among receptors of endothelial cells randomly, or is its action determined by factors emerging step by step during the blood coagulation process?

ACKNOWLEDGMENTS

I am indebted to Dr. P. Arányi and Dr. J. Mandl for critical reading of the manuscript. I also wish to thank Mrs. Ágnes Himer and Mrs. Ida Horváth for tissue culture and for excellent assistance in experiments.

REFERENCES

1. MACHOVICH, R. 1984. Thrombin and hemostasis. *In* The Thrombin. R. Machovich, Ed. Vol. I: 1-22. CRC Press Inc. Boca Raton, Florida.
2. FENTON II, J. W. 1981. Thrombin specificity. Ann. N. Y. Acad. Sci. **370:** 468-495.
3. MACHOVICH, R. & I. HORVÁTH. 1981. Thrombin and hemostasis: regulation of the biological functions of thrombin. Haematologia **14:** 339-359.
4. SMITH, G. F. 1984. Fibrinogen—The specific thrombin substrate. *In* The Thrombin. R. Machovich, Ed. Vol. I: 55-82. CRC Press Inc. Boca Raton, Florida.
5. WHITE, G. C., C. L. KNUPP & R. L. LUNDBLAD. 1984. The interaction of thrombin with platelets. *In* The Thrombin. R. Machovich, Ed. Vol. II: 25-42. CRC Press Inc. Boca Raton, Florida.
6. MUSZBEK, L. & K. LAKI. 1984. Interaction of thrombin with proteins other than fibrinogen. Activation of Factor XIII. *In* The Thrombin. R. Machovich, Ed. Vol. I: 83-102. CRC Press Inc. Boca Raton, Florida.
7. MACHOVICH, R. 1984. Inactivation of thrombin by plasma proteinase inhibitors. *In* The Thrombin. R. Machovich, Ed. Vol. II: 1-24. CRC Press Inc. Boca Raton, Florida.
8. LOLLAR, P. & W. G. OWEN. 1980. Clearance of thrombin from circulation in rabbits by high affinity binding sites on endothelium. J. Clin. Invest. **66:** 1222-1230.
9. BAUER, P. I., R. MACHOVICH, P. ARÁNYI, K. BÜKI, E. CSONKA & I. HORVÁTH. 1983. Mechanism of thrombin binding to endothelial cells. Blood **61:** 368-372.
10. MARCUM, J. A., J. B. MCKENNAY & R. D. ROSENBERG. 1984. Acceleration of thrombin-antithrombin complex formation in rat hindquarters via heparin like molecules bound to the endothelium. J. Clin. Invest. **74:** 341-350.
11. ABILDGAARD, U. 1979. Evidence that antithrombin III is the main physiological inhibitor of coagulant enzymes. *In* The Physiological Inhibitors of Blood Coagulation and Fibri-

nolysis. D. Collen, B. Wiman & M. Verstraete, Eds. 31-33. Elsevier/North Holland, Amsterdam.
12. OWEN, W. G. 1982. The control of hemostasis. Role of endothelium in the regulation of inhibitory and catabolic pathways. Arch. Pathol. Lab. Med. **106:** 209-213.
13. MACHOVICH, R. 1985. Blood coagulation-fibrinolytic system and endothelial cells. Acta Biochim. Biophys. Acad. Sci. Hung. **20:** 135-154.
14. COMP, P. C., R. M. JACOCKS, G. L. FERRELL & C. T. ESMON. 1982. Activation of protein C *in vivo*. J. Clin. Invest. **70:** 127-134.
15. GRIFFITH, M. J., H. S. KINGDON & R. L. LUNDBLAD. 1979. Inhibition of heparin-antithrombin III/thrombin reaction by active site blocked-thrombin. Biochem. Biophys. Res. Commun. **87:** 686-692.
16. WHITE, G. C., R. L. LUNDBLAD & M. J. GRIFFITH. 1981. Structure-function relations in platelet-thrombin reactions. Inhibition of platelet-thrombin interactions by lysine modification. J. Biol. Chem. **256:** 1763-1766.
17. AWBREY, B. J., J. C. HOAK & W. G. OWEN. 1979. Binding of human thrombin to cultured human endothelial cells. J. Biol. Chem. **254:** 4092-4095.
18. ROSENBERG, R. D. & P. S. DAMUS. 1973. The purification and mechanism of action of human antithrombin-heparin cofactor. J. Biol. Chem. **248:** 6490-6505.
19. GRIFFITH, M. J. 1979. Covalent modification of human α-thrombin with pyridoxal 5′-phosphate. Effect of phosphopyridoxylation on the interaction of thrombin with heparin. J. Biol. Chem. **254:** 3401-3406.
20. HATTON, M. W. C., L. R. BERRY, R. MACHOVICH & E. REGOECZI. 1980. Tritiation of commercial heparins by reaction with NaB^3H_4: Chemical analysis and biological properties of the product. Anal. Biochem. **106:** 417-426.
21. LI, E. H. H., C. ORTON & R. D. FEINMAN. 1974. The interaction of thrombin and heparin. Proflavine dye binding studies. Biochemistry **13:** 5012-5017.
22. MACHOVICH, R. 1975. Mechanism of action of heparin through thrombin on blood coagulation. Biochim. Biophys. Acta **412:** 13-17.
23. HATTON, M. W. C., E. DEJANA, J. P. CAZENAVE, E. REGOECZI & J. MUSTARD. 1980. Heparin inhibits thrombin binding to rabbit thoracic aorta endothelium. J. Lab. Clin. Med. **96:** 861-870.
24. ARÁNYI, P., J. BATKE & R. MACHOVICH. 1977. Remarks on the interaction of thrombin and heparin. Arch. Biochem. Biophys. **181:** 678-679.
25. OWEN, W. G. 1975. Evidence for the formation of an ester between thrombin and heparin cofactor. Biochim. Biophys. Acta **405:** 380-387.
26. LOLLAR, P., J. C. HOAK & W. G. OWEN. 1980. Binding of thrombin to cultured human endothelial cells: nonequilibrium aspects. J. Biol. Chem. **255:** 10279-10283.
27. SAVION, N., J. D. ISAACS, D. GOSPODAROWICZ & M. A. SCHUMAN. 1981. Internalization and degradation of thrombin and up regulation of thrombin-binding sites in corneal endothelial cells. J. Biol. Chem. **256:** 4514-5419.
28. HATTON, M. W. C., L. B. BERRY & E. REGOECZI. 1978. Inhibition of thrombin by antithrombin III in the presence of certain glycosaminoglycans found in the mammalian aorta. Thromb. Res. **13:** 655-670.
29. COLBURN, P. & V. BUONASSISI. 1982. Anti-clotting activity of endothelial cell cultures and heparan sulfate proteoglycans. Biochem. Biophysics. Res. Commun. **104:** 220-227.
30. HATTON, M. W. C. & S. MOUR. 1984. Uptake and catabolism of ^{125}I-thrombin by the rabbit thoracic aorta *in vitro*: permeability of the endothelium, intima-media and adventitial layers. Thromb. Haemostasis **52:** 105-111.
31. HATTON, M. W. C. & S. L. MOAR. 1985. A role for pericellular proteoglycan in the binding of thrombin or antithrombin III by blood vessel endothelium? The effects of proteoglycan-degrading enzymes and glycosaminoglycan-binding proteins on ^{125}I-thrombin by the rabbit thoracic aorta *in vitro*. Thromb. Haemostasis **53:** 228-234.
32. SHIMADA, K. & T. OZAWA. 1985. Evidence that surface heparan sulfate is involved in the high affinity thrombin binding to cultured porcine aortic endothelial cells. J. Clin. Invest. **75:** 1308-1316.
33. BUSCH, C. & W. G. OWEN. 1982. Identification *in vitro* of an endothelial cell surface cofactor for antithrombin III: Parallel studies with isolated perfused rat hearts and microcarrier cultures of bovine endothelium. J. Clin. Invest. **69:** 726-729.

34. Esmon, C. T. & W. G. Owen. 1981. Identification of an endothelial cell cofactor for thrombin-catalyzed activation of protein C. Proc. Natl. Acad. Sci. USA **78:** 2249-2252.
35. Jakubowski, H. V. & W. G. Owen. 1985. Effect of bovine thrombomodulin on thrombin specificity. Thromb. Haemostasis **54:** 119-123.
36. Esmon, N. L., W. G. Owen & C. T. Esmon. 1982. Isolation of a membrane-bound cofactor for thrombin catalyzed activation of protein C. J. Biol. Chem. **257:** 859-864.
37. Owen, W. G. & C. T. Esmon. 1981. Functional properties of an endothelial cell cofactor for thrombin-catalyzed activation of protein C. J. Biol. Chem. **256:** 5532-5535.
38. Esmon, C. T., N. L. Esmon & K. W. Harris. 1982. Complex formation between thrombin and thrombomodulin inhibits both thrombin-catalyzed fibrin formation and factor V activation. J. Biol. Chem. **257:** 7944-7947.
39. Esmon, N. L., R. C. Carrel & C. T. Esmon. 1983. Thrombomodulin blocks the ability of thrombin to activate platelets. J. Biol. Chem. **258:** 12238-12242.
40. Spolarics, Z., J. Mandl, R. Machovich, P. Lambin, T. Garzó, F. Antoni & I. Horváth. 1985. Association of α_2-macroglobulin-thrombin and α_2-macroglobulin-plasmin complexes with isolated hepatocytes. Biochim. Biophys. Acta **845:** 389-395.
41. Laemmli, U. K. 1970. Cleavage of structural proteins during the assembly of the head of bacteriophage T_4. Nature (London) **277:** 680-685.
42. Bartha, K., T. Kovács, I. Léránt, B. Papp, K. Kolev, É. Csonka & R. Machovich. 1986. Interaction of antithrombin III and thrombin-antithrombin III complex with cultured aortic endothelial cells. Thromb. Haemostasis. Submitted for publication.
43. Barzu, T., P. Molho, G. Tobelem, M. Petitou & J. Caen. 1985. Binding and endocytosis of heparin by human endothelial cells in culture. Biochim. Biophys. Acta **845:** 196-203.
44. Pomerantz, M. W. & W. G. Owen. 1978. A catalytic role for heparin. Evidence for a ternary complex of heparin cofactor, thrombin and heparin. Biochim. Biophys. Acta **535:** 66-77.
45. Machovich, R. & P. Arányi. 1978. Effect of heparin on thrombin inactivation by antithrombin III. Biochem. J. **173:** 869-875.
46. Polgar, F., I. Léránt, L. Muszbek & R. Machovich. 1986. Thrombomodulin inhibits the activation of factor XIII by thrombin. Thromb. Res. **43:** 585-590.
47. Machovich, R., M.-C. Bourin, J. Bombled, D. Barbier & M. C. Boffa. 1983. Effect of thrombomodulin on thrombin activity. Thromb. Haemostasis **50:** 351. (Abstract.)
48. Fischer, A.-M., A. Bros, S. Rafowicz & F. Josso. 1980. Heparin prevents thrombin inhibition by α_2-macroglobulin. Thromb. Res. **19:** 862-867.
49. Léránt, I., B. Papp, T. Kovács, P. Lambin & R. Machovich. 1986. Interaction of thrombin with endothelial cells in the presence of fibrinogen and α_2-macroglobulin: possible role of thrombomodulin and heparin. Thromb. Haemostasis. Submitted for publication.
50. Dejana, E., L. R. Longulno, N. Polentarutti, G. Balconi, J. J. Ryckewaert, M. Larrieu, M. B. Donatti, A. Mantovani & G. Marguerie. 1985. Interaction between fibrinogen and cultured endothelial cells; Induction of migration and specific binding. J. Clin. Invest. **75:** 1-8.

Novel Immunoenzyme Assays for Thrombin-Antithrombin III and Thrombin-α_2-Macroglobulin Complexes in Plasma

PETER C. HARPEL[a] AND JOHN W. FENTON II[b]

[a]*Division of Hematology/Oncology*
Department of Medicine and the Specialized Center of Research in Thrombosis
The New York Hospital-Cornell Medical Center
New York, New York 10021

[b]*Wadsworth Center for Laboratories and Research*
School of Public Health Sciences
New York State Department of Health
Albany, New York 12201

INTRODUCTION

One of the mechanisms by which proteolytic enzymes are modulated in biologic systems is by forming complexes with their naturally occurring inhibitors.[1–3] The formation of these enzyme-inhibitor complexes is a measure of the activation of the protease inasmuch as zymogens do not form such complexes. We have demonstrated that proteolytic enzyme activation may be quantified in plasma by measuring the generation of inhibitor-enzyme complexes using enzyme-linked immunosorbent assays (ELISA). Assays have been developed for complexes that form between α_2-plasmin inhibitor and plasmin,[4] α_1-antitrypsin and leukocyte elastase,[5] antithrombin III (AT III) and coagulation factor Xa,[6] and between $C\bar{1}$ inactivator and the proteases plasma kallikrein,[7] C1s,[8] and Hageman factor.[9] The approach that has been used requires that the antigenic determinants of both protease and inhibitor be expressed following complex formation. In the assay, two different antibodies are used, one against the enzyme and the other directed against the protease inhibitor. The protease-protease inhibitor complex is removed from the fluid-phase and bound to the surface of the ELISA plate with one antibody, and the second reactant in the complex is quantified by the second antibody.

α_2-Macroglobulin (α_2M) forms complexes with a wide variety of proteolytic enzymes.[10,11] In preliminary studies, we have observed that the above method does not recognize the complex that forms between α_2-macroglobulin and plasma kallikrein or thrombin presumably because these enzymes are entrapped by the inhibitor,[12] with the result that their antigenic sites are masked. By contrast, the α_2-macroglobulin-plasmin complex is detectable by the double antibody ELISA.[4] We have used a different approach to measure α_2-macroglobulin-enzyme complexes. This method is based upon the demonstration that the protease bound to α_2-macroglobulin retains hydrolytic activity against low molecular weight substrates and relatively little activity against high molecular weight protein substrates.[13] We have found that α_2-macroglobulin complexes become quantitatively bound to antihuman α_2-macroglobulin antibody that is covalently coupled to an agarose gel matrix and that the catalytic activity of the immunoimmobilized complex can be measured.[14] This method has been used to measure α_2-macroglobulin in complex with trypsin,[14] plasmin,[15] and plasma kallikrein.[16]

The present study details the development of assays for the human α-thrombin-antithrombin III (TAT) complex and the α_2-macroglobulin-thrombin complex that can quantify these complexes in plasma.

METHODS

Plasma was obtained from venous blood collected in plastic containers from normal volunteers and added to 3.8% sodium citrate, 9:1 (vol:vol). The plasma was frozen in plastic tubes at −70°C.

Purification of Human Plasma Proteins

Antithrombin III was a generous gift from Dr. Doris Menache-Aronson, American National Red Cross Laboratories, Bethesda, MD. α_2-Macroglobulin was purified as detailed[17] and labeled with ^{125}I as previously described.[14] Human α-thrombin was purified as described.[18]

Preparation of Antisera and Immunoglobulin Fractions

Rabbits were immunized intradermally three times with 200 μg thrombin, AT III, or α_2-macroglobulin in equal volumes of complete Freund's adjuvant over a six-week period. The IgG fraction of the antisera was isolated by chromatography on DE-52 cellulose (H. Reeve Angel & Co., Inc.) to which cibacron-blue F 3GA (Polysciences, Inc.) was coupled[19] as described.[4] F(ab′)$_2$ fragments were prepared from the rabbit anti-antithrombin III by pepsin digestion followed by immunoaffinity column chromatography using immobilized AT III as described previously for antiplasminogen.[4] The antihuman thrombin F(ab′)$_2$ fragments were labeled with Sigma type VII-S calf mucosa alkaline phosphatase (Sigma) according to the method of Voller *et al.*[20] The IgG fraction of rabbit anti-α_2M antisera was coupled to Bio-Gel A-5m (Bio-Rad) by the cyanogen bromide method as described.[14]

ELISA (Enzyme-Linked Differential Antibody Immunosorbent Assay) of Thrombin-Antithrombin Complexes

This assay was performed with minor modifications of the methods detailed for the assay of C1 inhibitor-kallikrein complexes.[7] Microtitration plates (Linbro, E.I.A. Microtitration Plate, Flow Laboratories) were coated with the IgG fraction of rabbit antihuman thrombin, 0.2 ml containing 5.0 μg of IgG/ml of bicarbonate-coating buffer, and incubated in a humid chamber overnight at 4°C. The wells were washed three times for 3 min each in 0.15 M phosphate-buffered saline, pH 7.4, containing 0.05% Tween 20. Various incubation mixtures, 0.2 ml, containing TAT complexes and diluted in PBS-Tween buffer containing 5 mg/ml bovine serum albumin and 5 mM EDTA were added in duplicate to the antibody-coated wells. The plates were then incubated in a humid chamber for 4 h at room temperature. The washing procedure was repeated, and the alkaline phosphatase-labeled anti-AT III $F(ab')_2$ fragments were added. After an 18-h incubation at 4°C, the wash procedure was repeated and 0.2 ml of the substrate ρ-nitrophenyl phosphate (Sigma), 1 mg/ml in 10% diethanolamine buffer, pH 9.8, was added. The color development at 405 nm was followed in a Titertek Multiskan photometer (Flow Laboratories). The change in absorbance per min was calculated by subtracting the minimum value obtained at 5 min from the maximum value and dividing by the time elapsed between these points. The methods for the generation of TAT complexes in purified systems and in plasma, and for their quantification by ELISA are described in the figure legends.

Assay for α_2-Macroglobulin-Thrombin (α_2M-Thrombin) Complexes

The immunoimmobilization enzyme assay for α_2M-thrombin complexes was performed by minor modifications of the methods detailed for the assay of α_2-macroglobulin-trypsin[14] and α_2-macroglobulin-kallikrein complexes.[16] The gel containing the bound α_2-macroglobulin antibody was diluted twofold with 0.1 M Tris-HCl buffer, pH 8.3, containing 1.25 mM $CaCl_2$. Different amounts of the gel, depending upon the amount of α_2-macroglobulin in the fluid-phase mixtures, were added to filter-centrifuge tubes made as described[21] and the excess buffer removed by centrifugation. Trace quantities of $[^{125}I]\alpha_2M$ were added to various incubations to quantify the binding of α_2-macroglobulin to the immobilized antibody. Varying volumes of the mixtures containing α_2M-thrombin complexes were incubated at room temperature with the immobilized antibody, with end-over-end mixing in a Labquake mixer (Labindustries). The incubation was terminated by centrifugation and washing three times with buffer. The gel was counted for radioactivity in a Searle 1185 dual channel gamma counter and then incubated with end-over-end mixing at room temperature with 0.4 ml of Tris-$CaCl_2$ buffer and 0.2 ml of the substrate tosyl-L-glycyl-L-prolyl-L-arginine-ρ-nitroanilide hydrochloride (Vega Biochemicals) dissolved in distilled water at a concentration of 1.4 mg/ml. Color development was terminated by centrifugation and the addition of 0.2 ml of 30% acetic acid and 0.6 ml of buffer to the supernatant to achieve a final volume of 1.4 ml. The absorbance at 405 nm was measured with a Gilford 240 spectrophotometer. The concentration of ρ-nitroanalide released was determined using a molar absorbancy of 10,500[22] and results expressed following correction for the substrate blank, either as micromoles ρ-nitroanilide released/L/

min, or, when the amount of α_2M bound was determined, as micromoles/L/min/mg α_2M.

Study of the Kinetics of Substrate Hydrolysis

For the derivation of Michaelis-Menten constants, 0.4 μg/ml thrombin, 50 μg/ml α_2M, and a trace quantity of [^{125}I]α_2M were incubated for 30 min in Tris-$CaCl_2$ buffer. The thrombin/α_2M molar ratio of this mixture was 0.16. Portions of 0.2 ml of the α_2M-thrombin incubation mixture were incubated in duplicate with 0.01 ml rabbit anti-α_2M-IgG coupled to Bio-Gel A-5m beads. The gel mixtures were washed four times each with 1.0 ml buffer, and the radioactivity, a measure of α_2M bound to the gel, was determined. The antibody-bound α_2M-thrombin complexes were then assayed for the ability to hydrolyze varying concentrations of Tos-Gly-Pro-Arg-ρNA. Due to the fact that continuous measurements could not be made with the insolubilized α_2M-thrombin complexes, duplicate assays were terminated at time intervals of 10, 20, and 30 min at each substrate concentration.

Portions of the original soluble α_2M-thrombin mixtures, containing an amount of radioactivity equivalent to that bound to the antibody gels described above, were assayed in duplicate at varying substrate concentrations. Hydrolysis of substrate was followed continuously at 405 nm. K_m and V_{max} for the soluble and immobilized α_2M-thrombin complexes were obtained from Lineweaver-Burk linear transformations of the initial reaction velocities and substrate concentrations.

Inhibition of α_2M-Thrombin Complexes by D-Phe-Pro-Arg-CH_2Cl or Hirudin

Ten micrograms α_2M containing a trace quantity of [^{125}I]α_2M was incubated with 2.15 μg thrombin in Tris-$CaCl_2$ buffer, pH 8.0, for 1 h at room temperature. Portions of 0.2 ml of this mixture were incubated with 0.01 ml packed immobilized α_2M antibody. The gel was washed four times with 1.0 ml buffer, and the [^{125}I]α_2M bound to the beads was measured. The immunoimmobilized α_2M-thrombin complexes were incubated in duplicate with varying concentrations of D-Phe-Pro-Arg-CH_2Cl (PPACK, Bio-Rad Labs.) as indicated on the abcissa of FIGURE 5, in a total volume of 0.3 ml in Tris-$CaCl_2$ buffer for 12 min at 25°C. After washing the gel four times as above, and recounting the radioactivity, the gels were assayed for amidolytic activity. The percent activity was calculated as the activity of the inhibited complex divided by the activity in the absence of inhibitor.

The thrombin-inhibiting activity of the hirudin preparation used was established by titration with thrombin; 1.0 ml of the hirudin preparation, as supplied, inhibited the amidolytic activity of 6.4 mg of thrombin. To examine the effect of hirudin on the amidolytic activity of the α_2M-thrombin complex, 79 ng thrombin was preincubated with 20 μg α_2M 30 min at 25°C; then increasing amounts of hirudin, 5-100 μl, diluted 1/5000, was added followed by an additional 5-minute incubation period. The total volume of the reaction mixture was 1.0 ml; 0.2 ml GPA-ρNA, 1.4 mg/ml was added. The reaction was terminated at 15 min by the addition of 0.2 ml 30% acetic acid.

The effect of hirudin on immunoimmobilized α_2M-thrombin complexes was determined. Thrombin, 0.4 μg, was incubated 30 min with 50 μg/ml α_2M that contained a trace quantity of [^{125}I]α_2M; 0.2 ml portions of this mixture were incubated 2 h with 0.01 ml packed immobilized antibody-containing gel. The gel was then washed extensively and the [^{125}I]α_2M bound to the pellet counted in a gamma counter. Varying amounts of hirudin, diluted 1/5000, were added to the immunoimmobilized complexes in a total volume of 0.4 ml Tris-$CaCl_2$ buffer and incubated for 5 minutes. Substrate was added and the amidolytic activity determined as above.

Measurement of α_2M-Thrombin Complexes in Clotting Blood

Venous blood was obtained from normal volunteers through a 19-gauge butterfly needle and was collected directly into a polystyrene tube maintained at 37°C that contained a trace quantity of [^{125}I]-α_2M. The first 2.0 ml collected was discarded. Portions of 0.1 ml were removed at intervals using a plastic pipette and added to Eppendorf tubes containing 0.11 ml 3.8% sodium citrate with 110 units of heparin and 59 μg soybean trypsin inhibitor (Sigma); 0.2 ml plasma, obtained by centrifugation for 2 minutes in an Eppendorf centrifuge, was added to 0.025 ml of packed α_2M antibody-containing gel in Tris-Citrate buffer. The immobilized antibody plasma mixture was incubated for 3 hours at room temperature with end-over-end mixing. The tube was counted in a gamma counter, the gel washed four times in Tris-citrate buffer, and the gel recounted. The amount of α_2M bound was determined by multiplying the counts on the gel/total counts times the concentration of α_2M in the plasma as determined by the Laurell rocket technique. The gel pellet was then assayed for amidolytic activity. After assay, gels with amidolytic activity were incubated 15 minutes with D-Phe-Pro-Arg CH_2Cl, washed and reassayed for amidolytic activity. The amidolytic activity, expressed as micromoles substrate hydrolyzed/L/minute/mg α_2M, was converted to ng thrombin from an activity curve produced by incubating varying concentrations of thrombin with α_2M and determining the amidolytic activity of the mixtures.

Fibrinopeptide A release in the clotting blood was measured by a radioimmunoassay as described[23] and performed by the late Dr. Hymie Nossel, Columbia College of Physicians and Surgeons, Columbia University, New York City.

RESULTS

Detection of Thrombin-Antithrombin III Complexes by ELISA

The capacity of the rabbit anti-AT F(ab')$_2$ antibody labeled with alkaline phosphatase to detect AT III was tested by absorbing the purified inhibitor to the wells of the ELISA microtiter plates. AT III was detected at a concentration of 2 ng/ml with 1/400 dilution of the antibody, and at 4 ng/ml at 1/800 dilution (FIGURE 1). Increasing concentrations of AT produced a linear response to about 62.5 ng/ml inhibitor.

Purified thrombin was added to plasma, and the resulting TAT complexes were quantified by the immunosorbent assay. As shown in FIGURE 2, the addition of increasing amounts of thrombin caused the formation of increasing amounts of complex. At a 1/20 final dilution of the plasma sample, TAT complexes were detected when 12.5 ng thrombin had been added per ml plasma, or a thrombin concentration of 0.35 nM. The development of color was linear to a plasma concentration of 8 nM thrombin. When thrombin was added to plasma immunodepleted of antithrombin III, no increase in signal was found, thus demonstrating that AT III is an obligatory component of this assay.

The effect of plasma on the signal generated by TAT complexes was examined by adding thrombin to a large molar excess of AT III. Either buffer or plasma was then added and the TAT in these mixtures quantified by ELISA (FIGURE 3). The color developed in the presence of plasma was approximately 17% less than that formed in its absence.

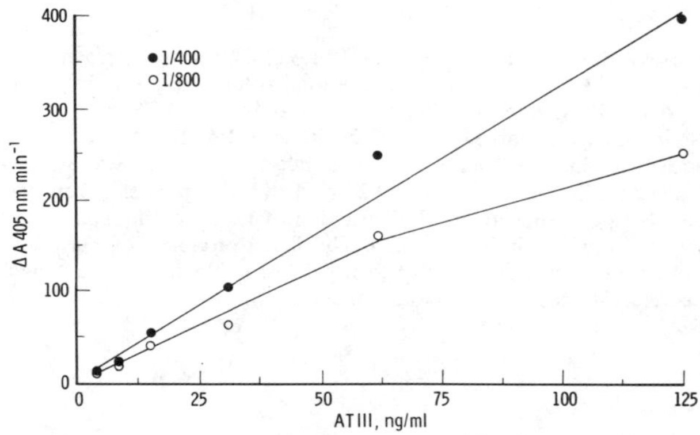

FIGURE 1. Detection of antithrombin III by ELISA. AT III, 1 to 125 ng in carbonate buffer, was absorbed to the wells of an ELISA plate and incubated 18 h at 4°C. Following washing, immunoaffinity purified rabbit $F(ab')_2$ antibodies against AT III labeled with alkaline phosphatase were added at two different dilutions, 1/400 and 1/800. After an 18-h incubation at 4°C and washing, the substrate ρ-nitrophenyl phosphate was added, and color development followed at 405 nm. The ordinate in this figure as well as in FIGURES 2 and 3, indicates the change in absorbance at 405 nm per minute $\times 10^4$.

Immunoimmobilization Enzyme Assay for α_2-Macroglobulin-Thrombin Complexes: Kinetic Studies

α_2M-thrombin complexes were formed by incubating thrombin with a mixture of unlabeled and radiolabled α_2M. These complexes were incubated with the IgG fraction of rabbit anti-human α_2M antiserum covalently coupled to Bio-Gel A5m beads. After extensive washing the gel pellets were found to have bound at least 90% of the radiolabel, indicating that most of the α_2M had been bound to the immobilized antibody. As demonstrated previously for the complexes between trypsin or plasma kallikrein and α_2M, the immobilized α_2M antibody that had been incubated with the α_2M-thrombin complex had gained amidolytic activity against a tripeptide chromo-

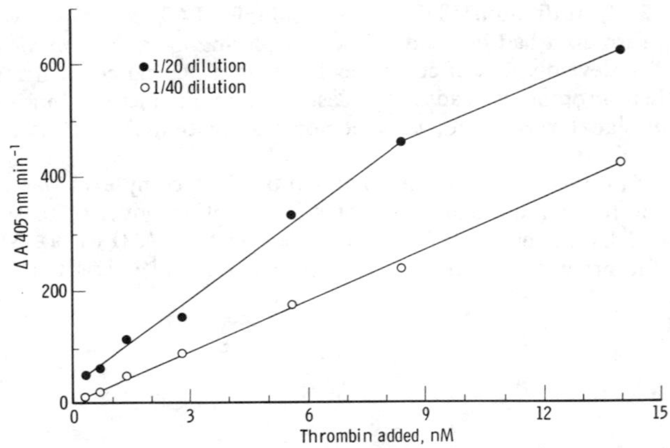

FIGURE 2. ELISA of thrombin-antithrombin III (TAT) complexes in plasma. Human thrombin, 1.25 to 50 ng, was added to 0.1 ml plasma in a total volume of 0.3 ml in phosphate-buffered saline containing 5 mg bovine serum albumin/ml, 0.005 M EDTA, and 0.05% Tween 20. Following a 30-min incubation at 37°C, 5 μl of 10 mM Phe-Pro-Arg-Chloromethyl ketone (PPACK) was added to inhibit residual thrombin activity. The volume was adjusted with buffer so that the final plasma dilution was either 1/20 or 1/40. Samples of 0.2 ml were applied to ELISA microtiter plates coated with the IgG fraction of rabbit antihuman thrombin, and the assay was performed as detailed in METHODS. The signal produced by plasma without added thrombin was subtracted from those samples to which thrombin was added. The concentration of thrombin added is expressed in nanomolar concentration in the figure.

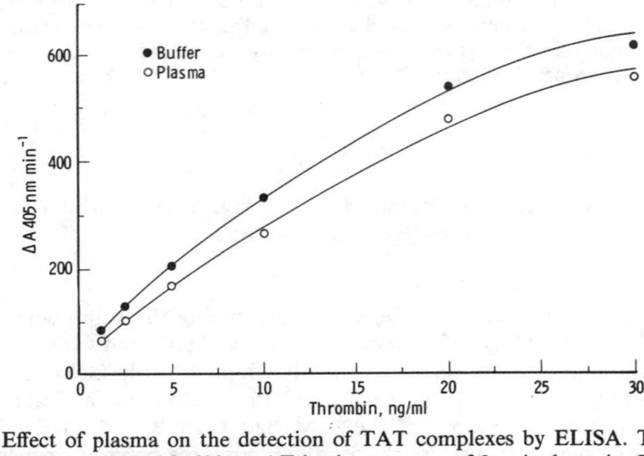

FIGURE 3. Effect of plasma on the detection of TAT complexes by ELISA. Thrombin, 1.25 ng to 30 ng, was incubated with 600 ng AT in the presence of 2 units heparin. Either buffer or 0.1 ml plasma was added, and the volume adjusted to 1.0 ml with PBS-albumin-EDTA-Tween buffer. These mixtures were assayed for TAT activity by ELISA.

genic substrate that was linear with time and proportional to the amount of thrombin in the incubation mixture. The kinetics of substrate hydrolysis in the fluid-phase of α_2M-thrombin complexes as compared to immunoimmobilized complexes demonstrated only slight differences (FIGURE 4). The Michaelis-Menten constants for the fluid-phase complexes as determined by Lineweaver-Burk plots were $K_m = 76\ \mu M$, $V_{max} = 739\ min^{-1}$; for the solid-phase α_2M-thrombin complexes, $K_m = 89\ \mu M$, $V_{max} = 719\ min^{-1}$.

Inhibition of Immunoimmobilized α_2M-Thrombin Complexes by PPACK and Hirudin

The low molecular weight thrombin inhibitor, PPACK, progressively inhibited the amidolytic activity of thrombin and of fluid-phase α_2M-thrombin complexes using

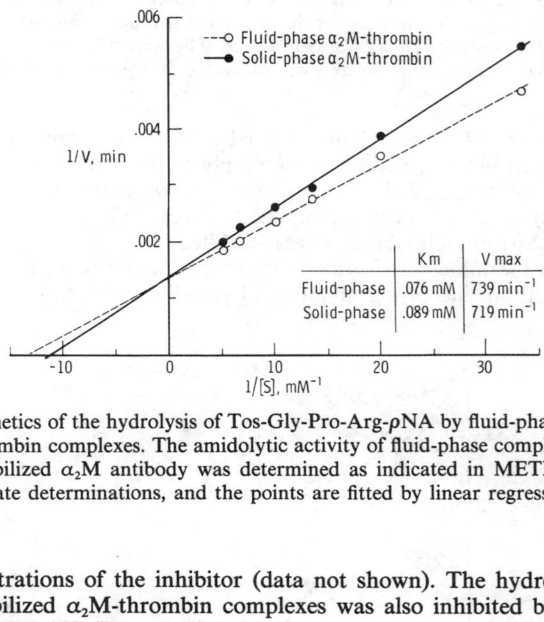

FIGURE 4. Kinetics of the hydrolysis of Tos-Gly-Pro-Arg-ρNA by fluid-phase or by antibody-bound α_2M-thrombin complexes. The amidolytic activity of fluid-phase complexes or complexes bound to immobilized α_2M antibody was determined as indicated in METHODS. All points represent duplicate determinations, and the points are fitted by linear regression analysis.

similar concentrations of the inhibitor (data not shown). The hydrolytic activity of immunoimmobilized α_2M-thrombin complexes was also inhibited by the same concentrations of PPACK (FIGURE 5).

The capacity of hirudin to inhibit the amidolytic activity of thrombin, the fluid-phase α_2M-thrombin complex, and of the immunoimmobilized complex was tested (FIGURE 6). The amount of thrombin used in each of these systems was equivalent. Increasing amounts of hirudin progressively inhibited both free thrombin and fluid-phase α_2M-thrombin complexes. In the case of thrombin, inhibition by hirudin was linear to about 80% inhibition, whereas with the α_2M-thrombin complex, the inhibition curve deviated from linearity at 40% inhibition. Hirudin was less effective in inhibiting the amidolytic activity of the α_2M-thrombin complex than of free thrombin. A straight line was fitted to the initial portion of each inhibition curve by linear regression

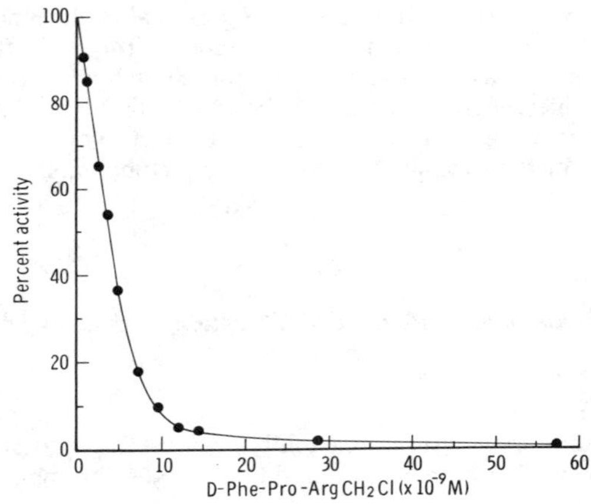

FIGURE 5. Inhibition of the amidolytic activity of immunoimmobilized α_2M-thrombin complexes by D-Phe-Pro-Arg-CH_2Cl. α_2M-thrombin complexes bound to insolubilized antibody were incubated with increasing concentrations of the tripeptide thrombin inhibitor D-Phe-Pro-Arg-CH_2Cl, and residual amidolytic activity was determined. The activity in the presence of inhibitor was compared to that without inhibitor and was expressed as a percent (ordinate).

analysis. The amount of hirudin that achieved a 50% inhibition of thrombin was calculated at 31.0 μl hirudin, and for the fluid-phase complex was 56.9 μl, approximately a twofold difference. At the highest concentration of hirudin used, 94% of the amidolytic activity of thrombin was inhibited, whereas only 57% of the activity of the fluid-phase α_2M-thrombin complex was inhibited.

In contrast to the inhibition of the fluid-phase α_2M-thrombin complex, after an initial small inhibition, increasing amounts of hirudin failed to inhibit further the

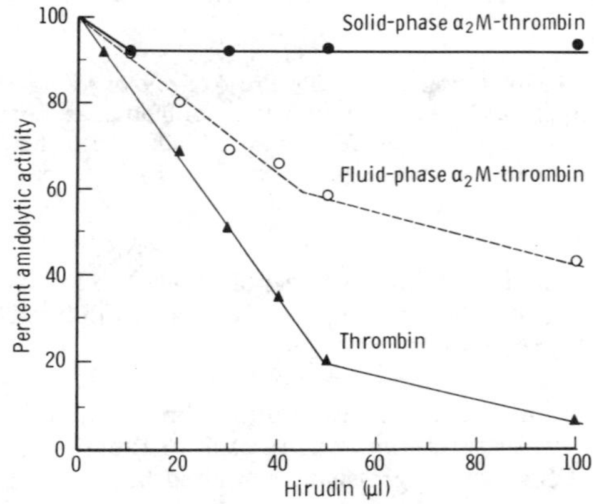

FIGURE 6. Inhibition of α_2M-thrombin complexes by hirudin. Thrombin, fluid-phase α_2M-thrombin complexes or immunoimmobilized α_2M-thrombin complexes were incubated with varying amounts of hirudin as detailed in METHODS and the amidolytic activity was determined. The activity in the presence of inhibitor was compared to that in the absence of hirudin and is expressed as a percent.

amidolytic activity of the solid-phase, antibody-bound α_2M-thrombin complex. At the highest concentration of hirudin used, only 8% of the amidolytic activity of thrombin was inhibited.

Generation of α_2M-Thrombin Complexes by the Addition of Thrombin to Plasma

The demonstration that soluble α_2M-thrombin complexes are bound by solid-phase α_2M antibody and that the hydrolytic activity of the bound thrombin can be measured

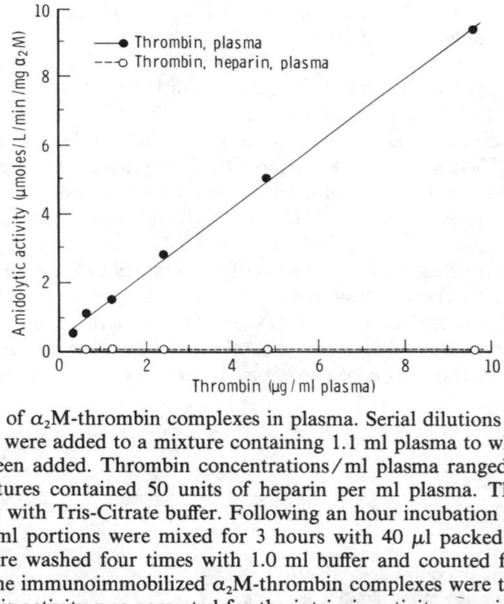

FIGURE 7. Assay of α_2M-thrombin complexes in plasma. Serial dilutions of thrombin, 0.33 to 10.6 μg per system were added to a mixture containing 1.1 ml plasma to which a trace quantity of [^{125}I]α_2M had been added. Thrombin concentrations/ml plasma ranged from 8 to 270 nM. Other plasma mixtures contained 50 units of heparin per ml plasma. The final volume was adjusted to 1.76 ml with Tris-Citrate buffer. Following an hour incubation at 25°C, the clot was removed, and 0.8 ml portions were mixed for 3 hours with 40 μl packed antibody-containing gel. The pellets were washed four times with 1.0 ml buffer and counted for radioactivity in a gamma counter. The immunoimmobilized α_2M-thrombin complexes were then assayed for amidolytic activity. This activity was corrected for the intrinsic activity associated with the plasma to which no thrombin was added. All values represent duplicate determinations.

has made it possible to study the binding of exogenous thrombin to α_2M in plasma. Thrombin was added to plasma to produce thrombin concentrations of 0.3 to 9.6 μg/ml plasma, representing thrombin/α_2M molar ratios of 0.004 to 0.14. The plasma contained a trace amount of [^{125}I]α_2M. Thrombin was also added to plasma that contained heparin. Portions of the plasma were then incubated with the solid-phase α_2M antibody, washed, counted for radioactivity, and the amidolytic activity determined (FIGURE 7). The addition of thrombin or of heparin to plasma did not change the amount of binding of α_2M to the immobilized antibody. The amidolytic activity of the immunoimmobilized α_2M-thrombin complexes derived from plasma was proportional to the initial concentration of thrombin added to the plasma. By contrast, the solid-phase antibody incubated with the samples of plasma that contained heparin prior to the addition of thrombin demonstrated no increase in amidolytic activity as compared to the control plasma to which no thrombin was added.

By using a standard curve produced by incubating various amounts of thrombin with a constant amount of α_2M, and determining the amidolytic activity of the complex, it was possible to quantify that amount of thrombin bound to plasma α_2M. Between 10.5 and 23.1% of the thrombin added to plasma was bound to plasma α_2M (mean of 17.8%).

Formation of α_2M-Thrombin Complexes in Clotting Blood

Using the new assay, the formation of α_2M-thrombin complexes was quantified in freshly obtained human venous blood from four individuals that was allowed to clot by incubation in plastic tubes at 37°C (FIGURE 8). All four samples demonstrated a similar time course of formation of α_2M-thrombin complexes. Three phases were documented. During the interval from the first sample at 2 through 16 min (FIGURE 8, time period A), there was no significant increase in α_2M-thrombin complex-associated amidolytic activity. A slow progressive increase in activity was observed from 20 to 26 minutes (FIGURE 8, time period B). Comparison of the means of each individual blood sample at the two different time periods indicated a significant increase in activity in the second time interval ($p<0.01$). Coincident with visible clot formation was an exponential increase in the formation of α_2M-thrombin complexes.

Other studies demonstrated that the amidolytic activity of the immunoimmobilized α_2M complex isolated from clotting venous blood was inhibited by PPACK at concentrations similar to those used to inhibit purified α_2M-thrombin complexes. This data strongly supports the concept that the observed increase in amidolytic activity was specifically due to the action of thrombin and not caused by a different protease.

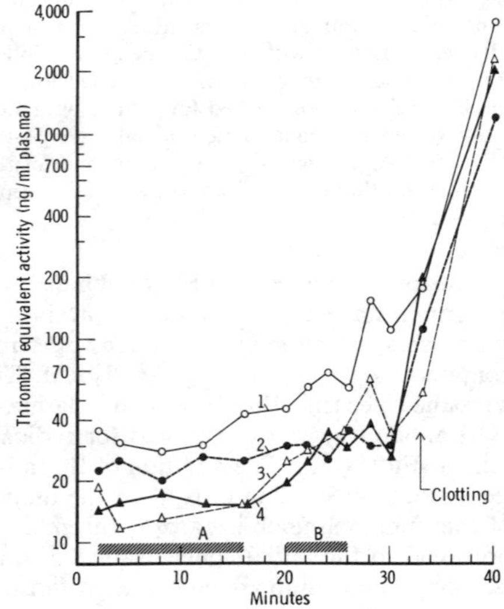

FIGURE 8. α_2M-thrombin complexes in clotting blood. Freshly obtained venous blood from four individuals was collected into polystyrene tubes that contained a trace quantity of $[^{125}I]\alpha_2M$; they were incubated at 37°C. Aliquots were removed at 2-min intervals and added to tubes containing heparin and soybean trypsin inhibitor. The amount of α_2M-thrombin complexes that formed were measured as described in METHODS. The time where clot formation became visible is indicated. The cross-hatched areas A and B indicate two different time intervals designated for comparison of α_2M-thrombin complex formation as discussed in the text.

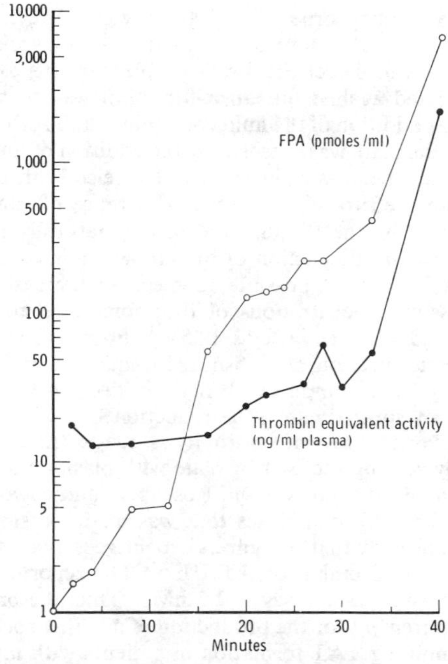

FIGURE 9. Generation of α_2M-thrombin complexes and fibrinopeptide A in clotting blood. α_2M-thrombin complex formation and FPA concentration were determined during the clotting of freshly obtained venous blood from a normal individual as detailed in the legend to FIGURE 8 and in METHODS.

Simultaneous measurement of α_2M-thrombin complexes and fibrinopeptide A (FPA) formation in clotting venous blood was performed (FIGURE 9). FPA generation occurred progressively during the incubation period, whereas α_2M-thrombin complex formation showed no change during the first 16 minutes. Visible clot formation was associated with an explosive increase in FPA concentration that paralleled α_2M-thrombin complex formation.

DISCUSSION

The plasma protease inhibitors antithrombin III, α_2-macroglobulin, heparin cofactor II, and α_1-antitrypsin are thrombin inhibitors in purified incubation mixtures.[1,24,25] *In vivo,* antithrombin III is considered to be the most important inhibitor of the blood coagulation mechanism.[26] Several previous studies have demonstrated that when exogenous thrombin is added to plasma, a portion of the thrombin forms a complex with α_2-macroglobulin; direct quantitation of the complex, however, was not performed.[27,28] In the present study, two new methods have been developed to directly quantify the complex that forms between thrombin and either antithrombin III or α_2-macroglobulin in plasma.

The enzyme-linked immunosorbent assays that we have previously used to measure proteases in complex with $\overline{C1}$ inactivator or with α_1-antitrypsin have been applied with minor modifications to detect the TAT complex. In this assay the IgG fraction of rabbit antisera directed against human α-thrombin was coated onto the wells of the ELISA plates. After addition of the fluid containing the TAT complex and washing, the complex bound to the plate was detected by the addition of immunoaffinity purified $F(ab')_2$ fragments of rabbit anti-antithrombin III labeled with alkaline phosphatase. $F(ab')_2$ fragments were used to minimize the occurrence of spurious high values in the immunoassay caused by the Rheumatoid factor, naturally occurring human antibodies directed against the Fc portion of immunoglobulin molecules.[29]

With this ELISA, it proved possible to measure increasing amounts of TAT complexes as progressive concentrations of thrombin were added to plasma. TAT complexes were detected when as little as 12.5 ng thrombin/ml plasma were added, representing a final concentration of 0.35 nM. Plasma had an inhibitory effect upon the signal produced by TAT complexes. When purified TAT complexes were added to plasma, there was an approximate 17% reduction in TAT concentration as compared to buffer. Whether this loss of sensitivity is due to trace cross-reactivity of the antithrombin antibody coating the ELISA plate with plasma prothrombin or whether some other factor is involved is not known. Rosenberg and coworkers have developed a radioimmunoassay for TAT complexes that was made possible by the production of a rabbit polyclonal antibody that recognizes neoantigens associated with the complex but not present on either thrombin or AT III.[30,31] The reported mean level of TAT in normal individuals using their assay is 2.3 nM.[31] Thus the present ELISA, which dispenses with the requirement for the production of a highly specific antibody, should prove suitable for examining TAT formation in patients with intravascular thrombin production. A similar assay for TAT complexes has been recently reported.[32]

Our approach to measuring the α_2M-thrombin complex involves immunoabsorption of the complex onto solid-phase anti-α_2-macroglobulin antibody. The immunoimmobilized α_2M-thrombin complex is then incubated with a relatively thrombin-specific tripeptide chromogenic substrate. Similar to previously reported data for the α_2M-trypsin complex,[14] the Michaelis-Menten constants for fluid-phase and solid-phase α_2M-thrombin complexes were found to be similar. This indicates that the α_2M-thrombin complex bound to antibody that is coupled to dextran beads is as effective in catalyzing the hydrolysis of the substrate as is the free complex. PPACK, the low molecular weight chloromethyl ketone thrombin inhibitor described by Kettner and Shaw,[33] inhibited the amidolytic activity of thrombin, the free α_2M-thrombin complex, and the insoluble complexes at similar concentrations. Thus the capacity of PPACK to inhibit thrombin's catalytic activity is apparently not effected by complexing with α_2M or by the binding of the α_2M-thrombin complex to the insoluble antibody.

By contrast, a different pattern of inhibition was demonstrated with hirudin, the protein with a molecular weight of 7400, derived from leech salivary glands that is a specific thrombin inhibitor.[34] Hirudin inhibited free thrombin more effectively than a similar concentration of thrombin bound to α_2M. At the highest concentration of hirudin used, 94% of the amidolytic activity of free thrombin was inhibited, whereas 57% of the activity of the α_2M-thrombin complex was inhibited. Hirudin was ineffective in inhibiting the catalytic activity of the immunoimmobilized α_2M-thrombin complex, because only 8% of the thrombin activity was inhibited. Hirudin forms a stoichiometric complex with thrombin and inhibits fibrinogen clotting and small molecular weight substrate hydrolysis.[35] Hirudin also displaces proflavine from the catalytic site of thrombin and immobilizes sulfonating spin label probes conjugated at the active site serine.[35] Inasmuch as hirudin binds with active-site inhibited thrombin,[35,36] it is apparent that hirudin binds to a recognition binding site on α-thrombin.[37]

Our data suggest that complex formation with α_2M partially masks this binding site on the thrombin molecule. Further, the dramatic resistence of the α_2M-thrombin complex to inhibition by hirudin when bound to immobilized antibody suggests that the size of the active site-pocket in the α_2M-thrombin complex must be further restricted when the complex is bound to antibody.

The assay for α_2M-thrombin complexes was found to be applicable to plasma systems. The addition of progressive amounts of thrombin to plasma resulted in a linear increase in amidolytic activity associated with the immunoimmobilized α_2M-thrombin complex. Approximately 18% of the added thrombin became bound to the α_2M. In the presence of heparin, however, there was no increase in α_2M-thrombin complexes, as thrombin was added to plasma. The lack of binding of thrombin to α_2M in plasma presumably reflects the essentially instantaneous binding of thrombin to antithrombin III and heparin cofactor II as catalyzed by heparin.[25,38] These results also confirm in plasma the findings of Fischer *et al.*, that when thrombin was added to a purified mixture of α_2M, AT III, and heparin, all of the added thrombin was bound to AT III.[28] Further, these authors demonstrated that heparin itself inhibited the binding of thrombin to α_2M.[39]

Our new methodology has made it possible to quantify α_2M-thrombin complex formation in clotting blood. These complexes were measured at two-minute intervals during the clotting of blood in plastic tubes at 37°C. A progressive, slow increase in α_2M-thrombin complex formation began at about 20 min of incubation, followed by a rapid 40- to 60-fold increase during visible clotting. The amount of thrombin bound to α_2M during the coagulation process appears to be in great excess of the 40 to 50 ng thrombin/ml generated as measured by a radioimmunoassay for thrombin.[40] This discrepancy may be explained by the inability of this assay to measure thrombin in complex with its plasma inhibitors.[40] We have also studied the relationship between the formation of α_2M-thrombin complexes and the generation of FPA in clotting blood. The concentration of FPA was found to increase progressively from the first sample at 2 min of incubation, confirming earlier results.[41] Although the levels of peptide increased during the first 18 min of incubation of blood, thereby indicating thrombin activation, no change in α_2M-thrombin complex concentration was measured. The failure of α_2M-thrombin complex formation to reflect thrombin generation during early events in the coagulation cascade may be due to the relative insensitivity of the α_2M-thrombin complex assay, or may be due in part to the formation of thrombin on the platelet surface[41] where the enzyme may be protected from plasma inhibitors. With clot formation, both FPA and α_2M-thrombin complex levels increase logarithmically.

In conclusion, we have developed sensitive and specific assays for thrombin in complex with two of its plasma inhibitors, antithrombin III and α_2-macroglobulin, that are applicable to both purified system and to plasma. These assays may serve to further define thrombin activation in both *in vitro* and *in vivo* studies.

REFERENCES

1. Harpel, P. C. 1986. *In* Hemostasis and Thrombosis. Basic Principles and Clinical Practice. R. W. Colman, J. Hirsh, V. J. Marder & E. W. Salzman, Eds. 2nd Edition. J. B. Lippincott Co. Philadelphia, PA.
2. Travis, J. & G. S. Salvesen. 1983. Annu. Rev. Biochem. **52:** 655-709.

3. Aoki, N. & P. C. Harpel. 1984. Semin. Thromb. Hemostasis **10:** 24-41.
4. Harpel, P. C. 1981. J. Clin. Invest. **68:** 46-55.
5. Brower, M. S. & P. C. Harpel. 1983. Blood **59:** 842-849.
6. Jesty, J., S. A. Morrison & P. C. Harpel. 1984. Anal. Biochem. **139:** 158-167.
7. Lewin, M. F., A. P. Kaplan & P. C. Harpel. 1983. J. Biol. Chem. **258:** 6415-6421.
8. Harpel, P. C. & N. R. Cooper. 1982. Clin. Res. **20:** 563(abst).
9. Kaplan, A. P., B. Gruber & P. C. Harpel. 1985. Blood **66:** 636-641.
10. Harpel, P. C. & R. D. Rosenberg. 1976. Progress in Hemostasis and Thrombosis. T. H. Spaet, Ed.: 145-189. 3rd Edition. Grune & Stratton. New York.
11. Barrett, A. J. 1981. Methods Enzymol. **80:** 737-754.
12. Feldman, S. R., S. L. Gonias & S. V. Pizzo. 1985. Proc. Natl. Acad. Sci. USA **82:** 5700-5704.
13. Harpel, P. C. & M. W. Mosesson. 1973. J. Clin. Invest. **52:** 2175-2184.
14. Harpel, P. C. & M. B. Hayes. 1980. Anal. Biochem. **108:** 166-175.
15. Harpel, P. C. 1983. Ann. N. Y. Acad. Sci. **421:** 134-142.
16. Harpel, P. C., M. F. Lewin & A. P. Kaplan. 1985. J. Biol. Chem. **260:** 4257-4263.
17. Harpel, P. C. 1976. Methods Enzymol. **45:** 639-652.
18. Fenton, J. W., M. J. Fasco, A. B. Stackrow, D. L. Aronson, A. M. Young & J. S. Finlayson. 1977. J. Biol. Chem. **252:** 3587-3598.
19. Travis, J., J. Bowen, D. Tewksbury, D. A. Johnson & R. N. Pannell. 1976. Biochem. J. **157:** 301-306.
20. Voller, A., D. E. Bidwell & A. Bartlett. 1976. *In* Manual of Clinical Immunology. N. R. Rose & H. Freedman, Eds.: 506-512. American Society of Microbiology. Washington, D.C.
21. Harpel, P. C., T-S. Chang & E. Verderber. 1985. J. Biol. Chem. **260:** 4432-4440.
22. Aurell, L., P. Friberger, G. Karlsson & G. Claeson. 1977. Thromb. Res. **11:** 595-609.
23. Nossel, H. L., I. Yudelman, R. E. Canfield, V. P. Butler, K. Spanondis, G. D. Wilner & G. D. Qureshi. 1974. J. Clin. Invest. **54:** 43-53.
24. Downing, M. R., J. W. Bloom & K. G. Mann. 1978. Biochemistry **17:** 2649-2653.
25. Tollefsen, D. M., D. W. Majerus & M. K. Blank. 1982. J. Biol. Chem. **257:** 2162-2169.
26. Rosenberg, R. D. & J. S. Rosenberg. 1984. J. Clin. Invest. **74:** 1-6.
27. Shapiro, S. S. & D. B. Anderson. 1977. *In* Chemistry and Biology of Thrombin. R. L. Lundblad, J. W. Fenton & K. G. Mann, Eds.: 361-374. Ann Arbor Science Publishing. Ann Arbor, Michigan.
28. Fischer, A-M., J. Tapon-Bretaudiere, A. Bros & F. Josso. 1981. Thromb. Haemostasis **45:** 51-54.
29. Johnson, P. M. & W. P. Faulk. 1976. Clin. Immunol. Immunopathol. **6:** 414-430.
30. Lau, H. K. & R. D. Rosenberg. 1980. J. Biol. Chem. **255:** 5885-5893.
31. Teitel, J. M., K. A. Bauer, H. K. Lau & R. D. Rosenberg. 1982. Blood **59:** 1086-1097.
32. Pelzer, H., P. Fuhge, H. Bleyl & N. Heimburger. 1985. Thromb. Haemostasis **54:** 24A.
33. Kettner, C. & E. Shaw. 1979. Thromb. Res. **14:** 969-973.
34. Bagdy, D., E. Barabas, L. Graf, T. E. Petersen & S. Magnusson. 1976. Methods Enzymol. **45:** 669-678.
35. Fenton II, J. W., B. H. Landis, D. A. Walz, D. H. Bing, R. D. Feinman, M. P. Zabinski, S. A. Sonder, L. J. Berliner & J. S. Finlayson. 1979. *In* The Chemistry and Physiology of the Human Plasma Proteins. D. H. Bing, Ed.: 151-183. Pergamon Press. New York.
36. Markwardt, F. 1960. Methods Enzymol. **19:** 924-932.
37. Tam, S. W., J. W. Fenton & T. C. Detwiler. 1979. J. Biol. Chem. **254:** 8723-8725.
38. Rosenberg, R. D. & P. S. Damus. 1973. J. Biol. Chem. **248:** 6490-6505.
39. Fischer, A-M., A. Bros, S. Rafowicz & F. Josso. 1980. Thromb. Res. **18:** 567-571.
40. Shuman, M. A. & P. W. Majerus. 1976. J. Clin. Invest. **58:** 1249-1258.
41. Kaplan, K. L., M. Drillings & G. Lesznik. 1981. J. Clin. Invest. **67:** 1561-1568.

Nontoxic Irreversible Inhibitors of Factors IX_a, X_a, and Thrombin: Potential Therapeutic Agents for the *in Vivo* Regulation of Thrombin Generation and Activity[a]

SALVATORE V. PIZZO,[b,c] A. DENISE TURNER,[d]
STEVEN L. GONIAS,[b] DOUGALD M. MONROE,[e]
HAROLD R. ROBERTS,[e] AND NED A. PORTER[d]

The Departments of[b] Pathology,[c] Biochemistry, and[d] Chemistry
Duke University and Duke University Medical Center,
Durham, North Carolina 27710

[e]The Department of Medicine
Center for Thrombosis and Hemostasis
University of North Carolina School of Medicine
Chapel Hill, North Carolina 27514

INTRODUCTION

Antithrombotic agents function by altering different elements of the hemostatic response. Some drugs affect platelet function (*e.g.* aspirin or dipyridamole). Others inhibit synthesis of functional vitamin-K dependent factors (dicumarol) or serve to activate antithrombin III (heparin). More recently, a class of agents has been developed that reversibily inhibits α-thrombin (*e.g.* MD-805). These compounds are of particular interest because they can be administered orally, show a low degree of toxicity, and act rapidly. Unfortunately, endothelial-bound thrombin activity soon reappears unless drug levels are maintained, because inhibition is reversible, and the drug clears rapidly from the circulation ($t\frac{1}{2} \sim 5$ min).[1] A more viable strategy for anticoagulation might involve irreversible inhibition of enzymes earlier in the cascade so that the amplification mechanism is aborted and less prothrombin is activated.

We now describe the use of three *p*-amidino esters as irreversible inhibitors of factors IX_a, X_a, and thrombin. These agents exhibit low toxicity and profoundly suppress the generation of thrombin activity. Of these compounds, the *p*-amidinophenyl esters of benzoic acid and cinnamic acid were originally developed to produce acyl-streptokinase-plasmin complexes,[2] whereas the third, the *p*-amidinophenyl ester of α-

[a]This study was supported by Grants from the National Heart, Lung, and Blood Institute (HL-24066, HL-31932, HL-6350, HL-07255, and HL-17921).

methylcinnamic acid, is described for the first time. These compounds will be designated as BENZ, CINN, and MECINN in the remainder of this report.

MATERIAL AND METHODS

The synthesis and chemical characterization of these compounds is described elsewhere.[2,3] Factors IX_a and X_a were prepared and characterized as previously described.[4,5] Human and bovine α-thrombin were purified and characterized as described[4,5] or were kind gifts of Dr. Frank C. Church and Dr. Herbert C. Whinna. Standard coagulation tests were performed in a General Diagnostics Coag-a-Mate X2. Radioiodinated proteins, including factors IX_a, X_a, thrombin, diisopropyl phosphoryl (DIP)-factor X_a, DIP-thrombin, BENZ-factor IX_a, BENZ-factor X_a, and BENZ-thrombin were cleared from the circulation of CD-1 mice as previously reported.[4,5] Drug clearance and toxicity experiments were also performed in mice. In the toxicity experiments, groups of at least four animals were injected with different concentrations of MECINN (dissolved in phosphate-buffered saline (PBS) containing up to 15% ethanol) to achieve plasma levels of 0.1 to 1.0 mM. Concentrations of MECINN above 1.0 mM were not studied in toxicity experiments because the concentration of alcohol necessary to dissolve the drug was lethal to the mice. Toxicity studies of BENZ and CINN have been previously reported.[2] Second-order rate constants for the inhibition of thrombin and factor X_a (human and bovine) and human factor IX_a by BENZ, CINN, and MECINN were obtained by a displacement assay employing the fluorescent probe *p*-aminobenzamidine.[6] A complete analysis of the kinetic data is presented elsewhere.[3]

RESULTS AND DISCUSSION

At a two to fourfold excess, BENZ was a potent α-thrombin inhibitor. The second-order rate constants for the inhibition of human and bovine thrombin by BENZ were 1.08×10^6 and 1.92×10^6 M^{-1} min^{-1}, respectively.[3] For comparison, the second-order rate constant for the inhibition of α-thrombin by antithrombin III (in the absence of heparin) is 3.5×10^5 M^{-1} min^{-1}.[7] Significant deacylation of BENZ-α-thrombin or BENZ-factor X_a complexes did not occur for at least 53 hours at 23°C. BENZ also inhibited human factors X_a and IX_a with rate constants of 7.8×10^5 and 4.8×10^4 M^{-1} min^{-1}, respectively.

The rate constants for the inhibition of human and bovine α-thrombin and factor X_a by CINN were comparable to those of BENZ. CINN was also a potent inhibitor of human factor IX_a with a second-order rate constant of 6.1×10^5 M^{-1} min^{-1}. This contrasts with the second order rate constant of 2.2×10^4 M^{-1} min^{-1} for the inhibition of porcine factor IX_a by dansyl-Glu-Gly-Arg chloromethyl ketone (DEGER).[8] Preliminary studies in our laboratory suggest a similar rate constant for inhibition of human IX_a by DEGER. CINN-α-thrombin deacylated at a relatively rapid rate (complete reactivation in less than one hour). Factor X_a complex was stable for at least four hours. Deacylation of CINN-factor IX_a has not been studied.

MECINN inhibited human α-thrombin with a second-order rate constant of 2.2

$\times 10^5 M^{-1} min^{-1}$. It inhibited human and bovine factor X_a at a rate approximately tenfold less than CINN or BENZ. The inhibition rate constant for factor IX_a was eightfold greater than that of DEGER. MECINN-thrombin and MECINN-factor X_a complexes did not reactivate during more than 50 hours at room temperature.

Animal studies have shown that CINN and BENZ are relatively nontoxic.[2] CINN-acyl-streptokinase-plasmin is in human trials as a fibrinolytic agent. Because MECINN is previously unreported, preliminary toxicity experiments were performed in a murine model. No acute or chronic toxicity was observed in mice injected daily with 500 μl (intraperitoneal) of up to 3.5 mM MECINN for one week. The calculated maximum plasma drug level achieved with this dose schedule is 1 mM, and it is suggested that the LD_{50} exceeds this concentration.

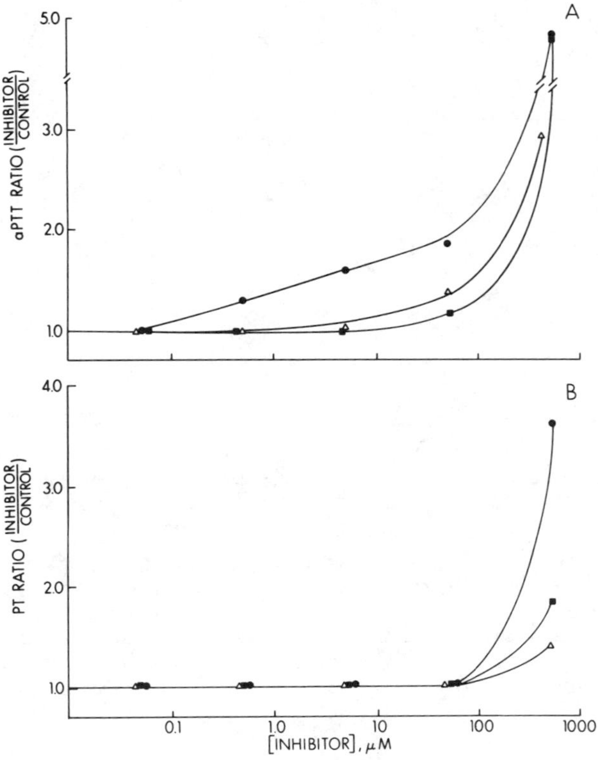

FIGURE 1. The effect of BENZ (■), CINN (●), and MECINN (△) on the aPTT and PT of human plasma. Data are expressed as the ratio of the test sample to the control plasma. Each point is the average of duplicate determinations.

Fresh frozen human plasma was incubated with the three drugs at concentrations between 5 nM and 0.5 mM (well below the LD_{50}). Inhibition of coagulation was studied by performing activated partial thromboplastin times (aPTT) and prothrombin times (PT) (FIGURE 1). BENZ and CINN, at 500 μM, increased the aPTT to greater than 150 seconds (offscale for the instrument). This represents at least a fivefold increase in the aPTT compared to a threefold increase measured with a similar concentration of MECINN. At the same concentration (500 μM), the PT increased 3.6-, 1.85-, and 1.4-fold for CINN, BENZ, and MECINN, respectively. The increases in the aPTT and PT, demonstrated at 500 μM, are greater than those achieved during clinical use of heparin and dicumarol.

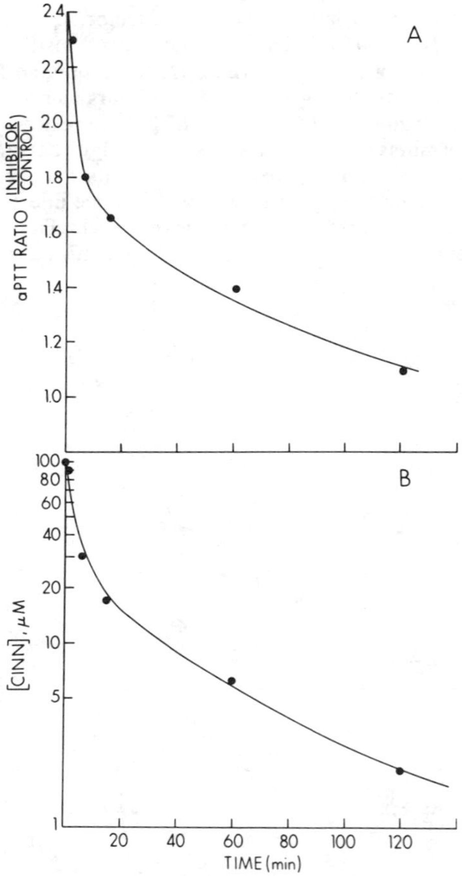

FIGURE 2. The clearance of CINN administered as a single intravenous injection in mice. CINN was injected into the lateral tail vein of CD-1 female mice. Panel **A** shows the change in the aPTT ratio with time. Panel **B** is the calculated drug level based on the standard curve of aPTT versus drug concentration as shown in FIGURE 1. Blood was collected into a syringe containing sodium citrate (final concentration of 0.35%) by cardiac puncture. Each puncture provided enough blood to perform two aPTT assays. Each point represents the average of three animals.

At every concentration tested, CINN was the most effective drug in prolonging the aPTT. Higher concentrations of CINN (> 50 μM) were required to prolong the PT. This effect is consistent with the potent activity of CINN as a IX_a inhibitor in experiments with the purified protein described above. CINN may suppress coagulation by way of the intrinsic pathway by inhibiting factor IX_a as well as factor X_a and thrombin. MECINN was more effective than BENZ at prolonging the aPTT when both were studied at low concentration. This result may also reflect the relative efficacy of MECINN compared with BENZ as a factor IX_a inhibitor.

The clearance of CINN in mice was studied after introduction of a single intravenous bolus of drug (300 μl, 1 mM). The aPTT was used to monitor approximate drug concentration (FIGURE 2A). The aPTT ratio was 2.3 at the earliest blood sampling, 1 minute. When the curve was extrapolated to 0 time, the predicted aPTT ratio was 2.4, in good agreement with the *in vitro* studies with human plasma. The therapeutic half life was about 100 minutes.

Each aPTT value from FIGURE 2A was correlated with the CINN concentration from FIGURE 1. These data are shown in FIGURE 2B. Clearance is at least biphasic initially and nearly linear after 15 minutes. The initial rapid phase probably represents distribution into the extravascular space. From the present data, it would be difficult to calculate accurate half lives even if one assumes only a two-compartment model. It must again be emphasized, however, that the aPTT ratio remained at or above therapeutic indices for at least 60 to 100 minutes.

The final series of experiments examined the clearances of the procoagulant proteinases. α-Thrombin, DIP-thrombin, factor X_a, DIP-factor X_a, and factor IX_a cleared rapidly from the circulation of mice reflecting binding to specific cell-surface receptors on endothelium as previously described (see reference 5 for review). These studies demonstrate that the active sites of α-thrombin and factor X_a are not required for binding. Inactivated factor IX_a was not studied previously because no inhibitor of this proteinase was available at the time of the original study.[5] By using the *p*-amidino esters, it was possible to form inactive factor IX_a and study it in clearance experiments. Active-site acylated factor IX_a cleared rapidly and at the same rate as the active proteinase. This study suggests equivalent receptor recognition of active and inactive factor IX_a. Thus, endothelial binding of thrombin, factor X_a, and factor IX_a are all independent of enzymatic activity.

In summary, we have characterized three inhibitors of factor IX_a that have second-order inhibition rate constants 2-30-fold higher than that of DEGER. These compounds are also inhibitors of thrombin and factor X_a and have the added advantages of ease of synthesis[3] and very low toxicity. Given their ability to abort the cascade mechanism for thrombin generation, these agents are potentially important as antithrombotic drugs.

REFERENCES

1. SHIFMAN, M. A. & S. V. PIZZO. 1983. *In vivo* metabolism of reversibly inhibited thrombin. Biochem. Pharmacol. **32:** 739-741.
2. SMITH, R. A. G. 1981. Enzyme derivatives for use in the treatment of venous thrombosis. U.S. Patent #4, 285, 932.
3. TURNER, A. D., D. M. MONROE, H. R. ROBERTS, N. A. PORTER & S. V. PIZZO. 1986. Biochemistry **25:** 4929-4935.
4. FUCHS, H. E. & S. V. PIZZO. 1983. The regulation of factor X_a *in vitro* in human and mouse plasma and *in vivo* in mouse. J. Clin. Invest. **72:** 2041-2049.
5. FUCHS, H. E., H. G. TRAPP, M. J. GRIFFITH, H. R. ROBERTS & S. V. PIZZO. 1984. Regulation of factor IX_a *in vitro* in human and mouse plasma and *in vivo* in the mouse. J. Clin. Invest. **73:** 1696-1703.
6. MONROE, D. M., H. R. ROBERTS & M. J. GRIFFITH. 1985. The effect of calcium on the interaction of p-aminobenzamidine and human factor IX_a. Thromb. Haemostasis **54:** 149. Abst #879.
7. CHURCH, F. C., C. M. NOYES & M. J. GRIFFITH. 1985. Inhibition of chymotrypsin by heparin cofactor II. Proc. Natl. Acad. Sci. USA **82:** 6431-6434.
8. LOLLAR, P. & D. N. FASS. 1984. Inhibition of activated porcine factor IX by dansyl-glutamyl-glycyl-arginyl-chloromethylketone. Arch. Biochem. Biophys. **233:** 438-446.

Pharmacological Approaches to Thrombin Regulation

F. MARKWARDT

Institute of Pharmacology and Toxicology
Medical Academy Erfurt
Erfurt, German Democratic Republic

INTRODUCTION

The clotting enzyme thrombin takes a central position in the blood coagulation system. This is especially evident when one takes into account that thrombin catalyzes not only the formation of insoluble fibrin, but also initiates further reactions that are of decisive importance in hemostasis and thrombosis. It activates the clotting factors V and VIII required for prothrombin conversion and factor XIII, which stabilizes the fibrin clot formed. Moreover, it causes drastic changes in the permeability of the platelet membrane followed by aggregation of platelets and the release of biologically active components. Furthermore, thrombin has been shown to have direct effects on vascular endothelium and to mediate other nonhemostatic cellular events. Therefore, the inhibition of thrombin represents an effective interference in the coagulation process and modulates the multiple bioregulatory effects of the enzyme.

At present, the pharmacological control of thrombin activity *in vivo* is possible only with the aid of the sulfated glycosaminoglycan heparin, which has certain properties that influence its use as an antithrombotic agent. Apart from the necessity of parenteral administration, heparin exerts its inhibitory effect on the clotting enzyme indirectly by way of a potentiation of the inhibitory function of the endogenous antithrombin III and heparin cofactor II. Therefore, its inhibitory activity depends on the blood level of these plasma proteins. Furthermore, heparin interacts with other blood constituents such as platelets, fibrinolytic components, and lipoprotein lipases. Finally, heparin can be neutralized by antiheparins such as platelet factor 4.

The lack of other means for *in vivo* control of thrombin activity and effects is a challenge for chemists, biochemists, and pharmacologists to develop directly acting selective inhibitors of thrombin. We attempted initially to solve this problem by isolation and pharmacological characterization of naturally occurring inhibitors from blood sucking animals.[1] The analysis of these substances revealed that a number of them are proteins with strong specific thrombin-neutralizing potencies. It is, however, very difficult to obtain the starting material for isolation of the inhibitors. In the late 1950s we succeeded in isolating the anticoagulant substance produced by the salivary glands of medicinal leeches.[2] It was characterized as a selective thrombin inhibitor with polypeptide structure and was named hirudin.[3]

Due to its pronounced and specific anticoagulant effect, hirudin preparations are employed for diagnostic and scientific uses. It is estimated that about 50 000 leeches are required annually to obtain adequate amounts of hirudin for these purposes.

Medicinal leeches are available in a limited number only, and they have been recently placed on the list of endangered species. Therefore, hirudin is not available in adequate amounts for therapeutic uses. Hirudin, however, has been brought into the focus of interest again since advanced methods of gene technology will allow us to obtain pure hirudin in sufficient yield. This prompted us to reconsider our biochemical-pharmacological investigations in this subject and to review the present state of development.[4]

The development of synthetic, low molecular weight inhibitors of the clotting enzyme presents an alternative approach in the search for selective and highly effective thrombin inhibitors.[5] The design of such inhibitors is based on the knowledge of the catalytic functionality of the clotting enzyme and particularly on the findings on the structure of its active site, which is the receptor for the inhibitory drugs. Systematic investigations of the structure-activity relationships have resulted not only in the development of potent agents with antithrombin activity, but also in remarkable increase in the specificity of the inhibitory effect.[6] Estimating the different types of inhibitors under the aspect of a pharmacological control of the clotting enzyme, it could be shown that only few of them could find potential use as an anticoagulant.[7,8] Therefore, the presentation is limited on the most potent synthetic reversible inhibitors of the benzamidine type, which can serve as a model for selective tight-binding thrombin inhibitors.[9]

The aim of this communication is to draw attention to the pharmacological problems in connection with these inhibitors, although the goals behind our investigations have been several. The inhibitors are also of importance in biochemical research into blood coagulation and are particularly suited in chromogenic clotting factor assays to remove thrombin specifically. They are also used in affinity chromatography for enzyme isolation and are especially employed as probes of topographical differences in the active sites of clotting enzymes.[6]

BIOCHEMISTRY OF THROMBIN INHIBITORS

The naturally occurring inhibitor, hirudin, is extracted from homogenized whole leeches or their head parts and enriched by various methods. Recently, we developed a chromatographic procedure for isolation of the anticoagulant agent from crude material using affinity chromatography on matrix-bound thrombin.[10] The analysis of the pure substance, which we isolated, showed a one-chain carbohydrate-free polypeptide stabilized by three intramolecular disulfide bridges. Of special interest is the proportion of basic to acidic amino acid residues. Besides only three lysins, it contains large amounts of glutamic and aspartic acid that account for the low isoelectric point. The preliminary establishment of the primary structure showed that the polypeptide chain contains 65 amino acids from which a molecular weight of about 7500 was calculated (FIGURE 1). The results obtained in complete sequencing of highly purified hirudin preparations varied with several investigators.[11–13] Different N-terminal amino acids and certain differences in the amino acid sequence are suggestive of the existence of isoinhibitors.

The analysis of the anticoagulant effect of hirudin showed that it possesses special affinity for the clotting enzyme thrombin. Hirudin forms with thrombin, an inactive enzyme-inhibitor complex with a very low dissociation, whereby the active center of the enzyme is blocked (K_i = 50 pmol/l).

The fast and specific reaction of hirudin with thrombin can be used for quantitative determination of the tight-binding inhibitor. One μg of pure hirudin inhibits about 5

μg of pure human α-thrombin. The antithrombin activity corresponds to a 1 : 1 reaction calculated on the basis of the molecular weight.[14] The catalytic serine of the active site of thrombin does not contribute considerably to complex formation, because hirudin forms a complex with thrombin, in which the active center serine is acylated as well. Hirudin occupies the apolar binding site near the specificity pocket inasmuch as it displaces proflavin from thrombin. Interaction between secondary binding sites, particularly with those responsible for the binding of fibrinogen, are believed to account for the tight binding. Accordingly, esterase thrombin, which is unable to bind fibrinogen, has only slight affinity for hirudin.

The question arises as to which structural features the specific and pronounced affinity of hirudin for thrombin is due. It is most likely that the secondary and tertiary

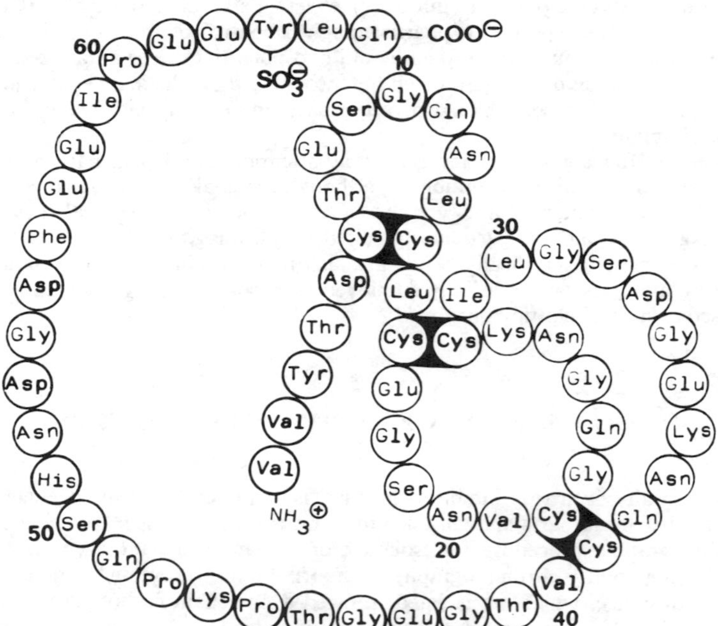

FIGURE 1. Proposed structure of hirudin.

structure of hirudin is of decisive importance for its antithrombin activity, which is lost during oxidation or reduction of the disulfide bridges or proteolytic degradation of the molecule.

Hirudin contains a highly acidic C-terminal portion. There are clusters of acidic amino acids and one Tyr-SO_3H within this segment. It is concluded that this segment of hirudin binds to the region of the fibrinopeptide site and associates with the apolar binding sites neighboring the arginine side-chain pocket of the active center of thrombin.[15] The compact N-terminal portion of hirudin stabilized by disulfide bridges can be attached to the fibrin binding site of the enzyme. Among the three lysine residues, two are buried in the N-terminal segment and one, which is possibly the active site of the inhibitor, is flanked by two prolines. That is why the lysine bonds are not accessible to digestion by serine proteinases.

Modification of substrates is a common principle for designing synthetic inhibitors. These inhibitors are assumed to be fixed at the active site of the enzyme on grounds of their structural relationship to the substrate.

Several peptide substrates and inhibitors have been modeled after the amino acid sequence in fibrinogen that immediately precedes the thrombin scissile bond. The most useful skeleton in designing thrombin inhibitors was the sequence Phe-Pro-Arg, especially when L-Phe is replaced by D-Phe.[16] The peptide aldehyde H-D-Phe-Pro-ArgH[17] and the chloromethyl ketone H-D-Phe-Pro-ArgCH_2Cl[18] have been found to be potent irreversible inhibitors of thrombin. They are, in principle, peptide substrates of the clotting enzyme with a reactive group that forms a stable covalent bond with the enzyme. It must be noted that irreversible inhibitors react not only with the target enzyme, but also with other constituents of blood and tissue containing amino or thiol groups, because they possess usually a reactive alkylating or acylating function. This property makes the compounds unsuited as thromboprophylactic drugs.[19]

First efforts for designing reversible thrombin inhibitors were directed towards imitating the acylating portion of the synthetic thrombin substrate *N*α-tosyl-L-arginine methylester (TAME). Extensive variation of the *N*α-substituent and of the residue substituted on the carboxyl group of arginine yielded interesting structure-activity relationships.[20] Besides the L-configuration, structural elements of the compounds such as the guanidinoalkyl moiety, the carbonamide or ester structure, and the substituted α-amino group are of equal importance for optimum binding of the *N*α-arylsulfonyl-L-arginine derivatives to thrombin. Tight-binding inhibitors were found among the respective cyclic amides. Particularly, the *N*α-dansyl-L-arginine 4-ethylpiperidide (K_i = 0.037 μmol/l) and the (2 R, 4 R)-4-methyl-1-[N^2-(3-methyl-1,2,3,4-tetrahydro-8-quinoline sulfonyl)-L-arginyl]-2-piperidine carboxylic acid (K_i = 0.011 μmol/l) are potent thrombin inhibitors with favorable pharmacological properties.[21,22]

Besides guanidino compounds structurally related to arginine, compounds with other cationic groups have been tested for antithrombin activity. An amidino side chain on benzene causes higher antithrombin activity than an aminomethyl or guanidino group.[23] Thus extensive substitutions have been carried out to maximize the affinity of benzamidines for thrombin. Quantitative structure-activity relationships have shown that especially hydrophobic interactions and inductive effects of the substituents influence the enzyme-inhibitor binding. Besides the hydrophobic interaction, a carbonyl group seems to account for the strong inhibitory effect produced by formation of a tetrahedral arrangement at the active center serine hydroxyl.[24]

Selective thrombin inhibitors of the benzamidine type have been found among the *N*α-substituted cyclic amides of amidinophenylalanine.[25] These compounds can be considered amino acid derivatives with an amidinophenyl moiety. An essential prerequisite for strong inhibition of thrombin is the secondary amide structure. Replacement of the tosyl residue at the α-amino group for a naphthylsulfonyl residue increased the inhibitory activity slightly. Introduction of amino acids, particularly of glycine, in the *N*α-position caused a marked increase in inhibitors of thrombin with K_i values in the range of 10^{-8} mol/liter. A representative of this group of inhibitors is βNas-Gly-(pAm)Phe-Pip (FIGURE 2). This compound possesses the highest affinity for thrombin that has ever been reported for a synthetic inhibitor (K_i = 0.006 μmol/l).[26] Obviously, the high antithrombin activity of this compound is due to its affinity for the substrate binding sites of thrombin. The benzamidine moiety occupies the specificity pocket to which the protonated side chain of arginine of the substrate is attracted. The *N*α-substituent and the carbonyl substituent of the inhibitor interact with secondary binding sites at both sides of the specificity pocket that, during substrate

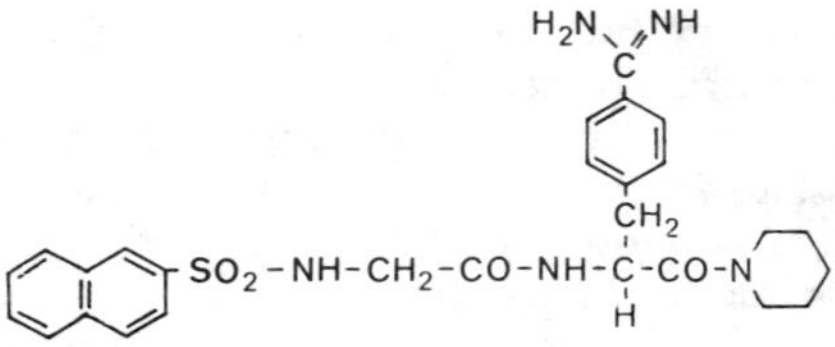

FIGURE 2. *Nα*-(2-Naphthylsulfonyl-glycyl)-4-amidinophenylalanine piperidide (α-NAPAP, βNas-Gly-(pAm)Phe-Pip).

binding, accept the leaving group and the amino acids bound to the α-nitrogen of arginine. Additionally, the carbonyl function is involved in the enzyme-inhibitor binding. A tetrahedral arrangement between the electrophilic carbonyl carbon and the Ser 195 alkoxyde seems to account for the tight binding of the inhibitor.

ANTITHROMBIN EFFECTS IN BLOOD

The highly effective naturally occurring inhibitor, hirudin, and the most potent synthetic inhibitor, βNas-Gly-(pAm)Phe-Pip, can serve as pharmacological tools and allow an estimate of the anticoagulant effect of thrombin inhibitors. Due to the high affinity for thrombin, relatively low concentrations of the representative inhibitors are necessary to neutralize the clotting enzyme. The inhibition of fibrin formation corresponded to the blockade of thrombin, either added to or generated in plasma.

By instantaneous inhibition of the small amount of thrombin generated after activation of the clotting system, the autocatalytic reaction is prevented that otherwise would lead to accelerated generation of further thrombin. Thus, dependent on the inhibitor concentration in blood, coagulation is retarded or completely inhibited. The clotting variables, such as thrombin time, partial thromboplastin time, and prothrombin time, vary with different inhibitor concentrations. Despite differences in the mechanism of antithrombin action, the highly potent thrombin inhibitors may be compared to heparin as regards the concentrations for prolonging *in vitro* clotting times (FIGURE 3).

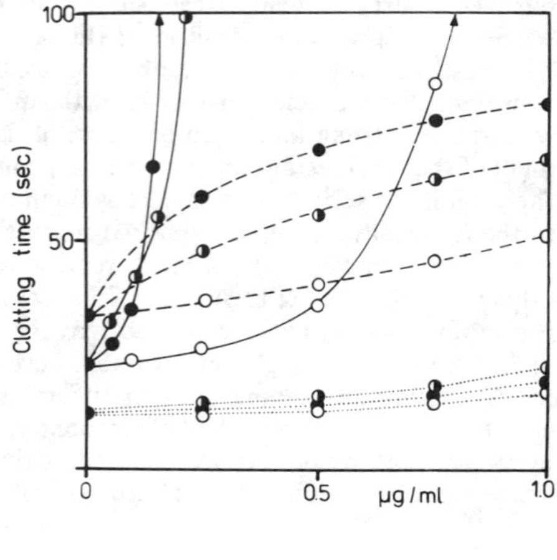

FIGURE 3. Relationships between the concentration of hirudin (●), βNas-Gly-(pAm)Phe-Pip (◑), and heparin (○) in human citrated plasma and thrombin time (——), partial thromboplastin time (— —), and prothrombin time (· · · ·).

The blockade of thrombin prevents not only fibrinogen clotting but also further thrombin-catalyzed reactions such as activation of blood platelets. We carried out detailed studies on the influence of the inhibitors on the thrombin-platelet reaction.[27,28] This reaction plays a major role in thrombus formation, and the interaction of thrombin with platelets may be regarded as an example of the effect of the clotting enzyme in other cellular events.

In this context, it has to be taken into consideration that the kinetics of the thrombin-platelet reaction and its inhibition deviate in several aspects from the kinetics valid for common enzymatic reactions. In contrast to the action of thrombin on the soluble substrate fibrinogen, the thrombin-platelet reaction proceeds in a heterogeneous system. The soluble enzyme reacts with the substrate fixed on the platelet surface. The first step in these reactions is the binding of thrombin to receptors on the platelet surface that differ in affinity for the enzyme as well as in number. Therefore, the interaction of thrombin with platelets may be regarded both as an agonist-receptor reaction and an enzyme-substrate reaction.

The effects of competitive inhibitors on the thrombin-induced release reaction correspond to their affinity for thrombin and, in principle, to their effect on the

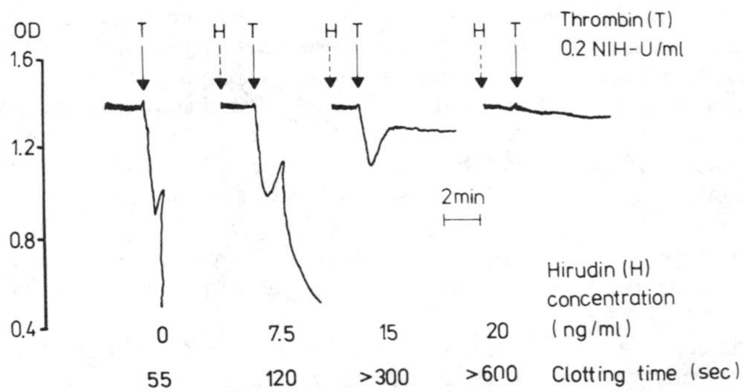

FIGURE 4. Inhibitory effect of hirudin on thrombin-induced platelet aggregation (first wave) and coagulation (second phase) in human citrated plasma.

thrombin-fibrinogen reaction. Comparison of the inhibitory effects in the two test systems, however, showed some differences. In the presence of equimolar enzyme and inhibitor concentrations, the inhibitory effect on the thrombin-platelet reaction was less pronounced than that on fibrinogen conversion. Under these circumstances fibrinogen clotting is inhibited without complete suppression of the platelet reaction (FIGURE 4).

A possible explanation for this difference would be the special kinetics that characterize the interaction between the inhibitor, the enzyme, and the glycoproteins of the platelet membrane. The rate of formation of the enzyme-inhibitor complex is important for interruption of the rapid thrombin-platelet reaction, which, in general, is terminated after 5-30 seconds. When the concentrations of both enzyme and inhibitor are very low, the association reaction may be extraordinarily slow and does not suffice for blocking platelet activation. On the other hand, the platelet reaction induced by submaximal thrombin concentrations can be interrupted when the velocity of complex formation is sufficiently enhanced by addition of the inhibitor in large excess.

PHARMACOKINETICS

Inasmuch as the anticoagulant action of the thrombin inhibitors depends directly on their concentration in the blood, the concentration-time course of the inhibitors was studied in experimental animals and in humans using various routes of administration. To study the pharmacokinetics of the inhibitors, methods are required that assess the inhibitor content in body fluids. The assay of the inhibitors is based on the complexing with thrombin and determination of the residual thrombin activity.[29] Low inhibitor concentrations in plasma are best detected by measuring thrombin times. Furthermore, for pharmacokinetic studies, radiolabeled inhibitors were used.[30,31]

Hirudin, given intravenously to experimental animals (dog, rabbit, rat) and human volunteers, is relatively rapidly eliminated. After the initial disappearance, which was interpreted as a distribution phenomenon, first-order elimination kinetics followed. The decline in plasma hirudin concentration was most adequately expressed by an equation describing a two-compartment model. An elimination half-life of 50-60 min and a volume of distribution of 0.25 1/kg were calculated, indicating extracellular distribution (TABLE 1).

The results of the clotting tests obtained at different times after administration varied with the hirudin level in plasma. Following subcutaneous application or intravenous infusion of hirudin, plateau values were reached within 30 minutes. It must be emphasized that a large percentage of the acidic polypeptide is excreted through the kidneys in unchanged form and is obviously not metabolized or bound in the organism.[32,33]

The pharmacokinetics of the synthetic inhibitor corresponds in principle with that of the naturally occurring inhibitor. Accordingly, after intravenous injection, the plasma concentration of βNas-Gly-(pAm)Phe-Pip declined rapidly. The time course of the inhibitor plasma level may be described by an open two-compartment model. The half-life of distribution amounted to 2.1 min and the elimination half-life to 9.0 min (see TABLE 1).

Intravenous infusion of the thrombin inhibitor led to a rapid increase in concentrations in plasma with a plateau phase being reached after 15-20 minutes. After cessation of infusion, the plasma level rapidly declined. According to these pharmacokinetic characteristics, the inhibitor plasma level may be easily controlled by the rate of infusion. Subcutaneous administration of the inhibitor yielded maximum plasma levels after 20-45 minutes. In contrast to intravenous administration, the longer-lasting inhibitor plasma level is obviously caused by slow absorption from the injection site.[34,35]

TABLE 1. Pharmacokinetic Parameters of Naturally Occurring and Synthetic Thrombin Inhibitors after Intravenous Injection of 1 mg/kg in Rabbits

		Hirudin	βNas-Gly-(pAm)Phe-Pip
$t_{1/2\alpha}$	[min]	10.0	2.0
$t_{1/2\beta}$	[min]	62.0	9.0
V^a	[1/kg]	0.25	0.8
Cl_{tot}^b	[ml/min]	230	530

[a] Apparent volume of distribution.
[b] Total body clearance.

TABLE 2. Comparison of Antithrombotically Effective Plasma Concentrations of Hirudin, βNas-Gly-(pAm)Phe-Pip, and Heparin in Experimental Disseminated Intravascular Coagulation (I), Venous Thrombosis (II), Arterial Thrombosis (III), and Arterio-Venous Shunt Thrombosis (IV) in Rats

	Plasma concentration [μg/ml]				
Inhibitor	I	II	III	IV	V[a]
Hirudin	0.05	0.6	1.8	2.3	1.1
βNas-Gly-(pAm)Phe-Pip	0.05	0.7	5.5	6.5	1.7
Heparin	2.5	11.5	4.0	5.7	5.5

[a] Plasma concentration for prolongation (doubling) of bleeding time.

ANTITHROMBOTIC EFFECTS

The ultimate criterion for therapeutic effectiveness of thrombin inhibitors as antithrombotic agents must be the prevention of thrombosis. Although there are various factors inducing formation of intravascular thrombi, the underlying process is coagulation caused by thrombin. Therefore, the thrombin inhibitors are expected to prevent thrombosis or its progression.

The antithrombotic action was studied in comparison with heparin in various animal models that largely correspond to the pathogenetic mechanisms of venous and arterial thrombosis or disseminated intravascular coagulation in humans.[36–40] The inhibitors have been extensively tested in stasis-induced venous thrombosis, in arterial thrombosis after electrically induced damage of the vessel wall, and in extracorporeal arteriovenous shunt thrombosis. A suitable method to demonstrate the effectiveness of the inhibitors in preventing microthrombosis proved to be the continuous measurement of ^{125}I-fibrin deposition after administration of ^{125}I-fibrinogen.

In order to exclude species differences, all investigations on the antithrombotic action of the thrombin inhibitors were carried out in rats. Because the plasma level of the inhibitors rapidly declined after intravenous injection, the thrombin inhibitors were infused intravenously in order to maintain constant blood levels over a defined period of time.

The results summarized in TABLE 2 show the antithrombotic effectiveness of the inhibitors in various models of localized thrombi, microthrombosis, and extracorporeal shunt thrombosis. In dependence on the dose and blood level, the inhibitors are effective in reducing the size of thrombosis or preventing its formation as well as in prolonging the period of patency of an extracorporeal shunt. The efficacy of the inhibitors in thrombin-induced microthrombosis corresponded to their affinity for thrombin.

Antithrombotic effects are produced at doses that markedly prolong clotting times in *ex vivo* blood samples. In contrast to heparin, inhibitor plasma levels preventing thrombus formation do not significantly prolong the bleeding time. The extent of anticoagulation necessary to prevent thrombus formation in a given animal model is dependent on the model and the strength of the thrombogenic stimulus. Therefore, the doses and plasma concentrations of the inhibitors required for the antithrombotic effect varied according to the different experimental models used in this study. In the course of venous thrombus formation, predominantly plasmatic coagulation factors are activated leading to generation of the coagulation enzyme thrombin. According to their high antithrombin activity, the inhibitors were antithrombotically most effective in stasis-induced venous thrombosis; that is, at relatively low plasma concentrations, the occurrence of venous thrombi could be completely prevented. Heparin, at the same concentration, used for comparison, was less effective.

In preventing microthrombosis, the synthetic inhibitor tested surpassed the effectiveness of heparin and approached that of the naturally occurring inhibitor hirudin. In higher dosages than in venous thrombosis, the thrombin inhibitors were effective in experimental models of thrombotic occlusion of the carotid artery and of an extracorporeal arteriovenous shunt.

Blood platelets seem to play an important role in thrombus formation on damaged endothelium or on foreign surfaces such as in electrically induced arterial thrombosis or in shunt thrombosis. Such conditions stimulate the initial adherence of platelets and subsequently the activation of the plasmatic coagulation system leading to fibrin formation. Therefore, a possible explanation would be that higher inhibitor concentrations are necessary for the inhibition of the thrombin-platelet reaction than for the thrombin-fibrinogen reaction.

CONCLUDING REMARKS

Investigations of the selected inhibitors have demonstrated that, based on their high affinity for thrombin, they are potent anticoagulants. They are antithrombotically effective provided that there is an adequate inhibitor level in blood.

The naturally occurring thrombin inhibitor hirudin, from medicinal leeches, is an anticoagulant of high quality. The rapid development in the field of biotechnology and peptide research will allow us to obtain this interesting polypeptide in sufficient yield in the near future. For this reason, the possibility for its clinical use is taken into consideration at present, and there is renewed interest in the pharmacology of hirudin.

The goal-oriented development of synthetic inhibitors has led to selective, highly effective inhibitors of thrombin anticoagulantly active *in vitro* and *in vivo.* Animal experiments on models of localized thrombi and disseminated microthrombosis demonstrated the antithrombotic effectiveness of the novel anticoagulants. It is assumed that these drugs could improve the possibilities of antithrombotic treatment.

The objective of the development of selective tight binding thrombin inhibitors is to obtain alternatives to other anticoagulants such as heparin. Due to their different mode of action, it is difficult to balance the benefits of the naturally occurring and synthetic thrombin inhibitors against that of heparin. Compared to heparin, the thrombin inhibitors are advantageous in that they are not inactivated by heparin-neutralizing factors and are able to exert anticoagulant activity independent of plasmatic antithrombins and, moreover, do not affect other enzyme systems in blood. At doses equieffective in preventing thrombosis, they had fewer hemorrhagic side effects than heparin. Furthermore, the selective thrombin inhibitors are superior to oral anticoagulants because they do not interfere with the biosynthesis of clotting factors.

Due to their special pharmacological properties, the naturally occurring and synthetic thrombin inhibitors may have some advantages over the established anticoagulants, and their introduction into clinical medicine would be a definate improvement in the therapeutic management of thromboembolic disorders.

REFERENCES

1. MARKWARDT, F. 1983. Blutgerinnungshemmende Wirkstoffe aus blutsaugenden Tieren. Fischer, Jena.
2. MARKWARDT, F. 1957. Die Isolierung und chemische Charakterisierung des Hirudins. Hoppe-Seyler's Z. Physiol. Chem. **308:** 147-156.
3. MARKWARDT, F. 1970. Hirudin as an inhibitor of thrombin. *In* Methods in Enzymology. S. P. Colowick & N. O. Kaplan, Eds.: Vol. 19: 924-932. Academic Press. New York.
4. MARKWARDT, F. 1985. Pharmacology of hirudin: One hundred years after the first report of the anticoagulant agent. Biomed. Biochim. Acta **44:** 1007-103.
5. MARKWARDT, F. 1981. Pharmacologic control of blood coagulation by synthetic, low molecular weight inhibitors of clotting enzymes. Ann. N. Y. Acad. Sci. **370:** 757-764.
6. STÜRZEBECHER, J. 1984. Inhibitors of thrombin. *In* The Thrombin. R. Machovich, Ed.: Vol. 1: 131-160. CRC Press. Inc. Boca Raton, Florida.
7. MARKWARDT, F. 1974. Synthetic, low molecular thrombin inhibitors. A new concept of anticoagulants? Haemostasis **3:** 185-202.
8. GERATZ, J. D. & R. R. TIDWELL. 1978. Current concepts on action of synthetic thrombin inhibitors. Haemostasis **7:** 170-176.
9. MARKWARDT, F. 1982. Approaches for designing synthetic, low molecular weight inhibitors of clotting enzymes. Folia Haematol. (Leipzig) **109:** 7-15.
10. WALSMANN, P. & F. MARKWARDT. 1985. On the isolation of the thrombin inhibitor hirudin. Thromb. Res. **40:** 563-570.
11. MARKWARDT, F. & P. WALSMANN. 1967. Reindarstellung und Analyse des Thrombininhibitors Hirudin. Hoppe-Seyler's Z. Physiol. Chem. **348:** 1381-1386.
12. BAGDY, D., E. BARABAS, L. GRAF, T. E. PETERSON & S. MAGNUSSION. 1976. Hirudin. *In* Methods in Enzymology. L. Lorand, Ed.: Vol. 45B: 669-678. Academic Press. New York.
13. DODT, J., U. SEEMÜLLER, R. MASCHLER & H. FRITZ. 1985. The complete covalent structure of hirudin. Biol. Chem. Hoppe-Seyler **366:** 379-385.
14. WALSMANN, P. & F. MARKWARDT. 1981. Biochemische und pharmakologische Aspekte des Thrombininhibitors Hirudin. Pharmazie **36:** 653-660.
15. CHANG, J.-Y. 1983. The function of hirudin, a thrombin-specific inhibitor. FEBS Lett. **164:** 307-313.
16. KETTNER, C. & E. SHAW. 1979. D-Phe-Pro-ArgCH_2Cl - a selective affinity label for thrombin. Thromb. Res. **14:** 9696-973.
17. BAJUSZ, S., E. BARABAS, P. TOLNAY, E. SZELL & D. BAGDY. 1978. Inhibition of thrombin and trypsin by tripeptide aldehyde. Int. J. Pept. Protein Res. **12:** 217-221.
18. COLLEN, D., O. MASUO, J. M. STASSEN, C. KETTNER & E. SHAW. 1982. *In vivo* studies of a synthetic inhibitor of thrombin. J. Lab. Clin. Med. **99:** 76-83.
19. HAUPTMANN, J. & F. MARKWARDT. 1980. Studies in the anticoagulant and antithrombotic action of an irreversible thrombin inhibitor. Thromb. Res. **20:** 347-351.
20. TONOMURA, S., R. KIKUMOTO, Y. TAMAO, K. OHKUBO, S. OKAMOTO, K. KINJO & A. HIJIKATA. 1980. A novel series of synthetic thrombin-inhibitors. II. Relationships between structure of modified OM-inhibitors and thrombin inhibitory effect. Kobe J. Med. Sci. **26:** 1-9.
21. OKAMOTO, S., A. HIJIKATA, R. KIKUMOTO & Y. TAMAO. 1979. A synthetic thrombin inhibitor taking extremely active stereo-structure. Thromb. Haemostasis **42:** 205.
22. KIKUMOTO, R., Y. TAMAO, T. TEZUKA, S. TONOMURA, H. HARA, K. NINOMIYA, A. HIJIKATA & S. OKAMOTO. 1984. Selective inhibition of thrombin by (2R,4R)-4-methyl-1-[N^2-[(3-methyl-1,2,3,4-tetrahydro-8-quinolinyl)sulfonyl]-L-arginyl]-2-piperidine-carboxylic acid. Biochemistry **23:** 85-90.
23. MARKWARDT, F., H. LANDMANN & P. WALSMANN. 1986. Comparative studies on the inhibition of trypsin, plasmin and thrombin by derivatives of benzylamine and benzamidine. Eur. J. Biochem. **6:** 502-506.
24. STÜRZEBECHER, J., F. MARKWARDT, G. WAGNER & P. WALSMANN. 1976. Synthetische Hemmstoffe der Serinproteinasen. 13. Quantitative Struktur-Wirkungs-Beziehungen

beider Hemmung von Trypsin, Plasmin und Thrombin durch 4-Amidino-phenylverbindungen mit Ketonstruktur. Acta Biol. Med. Ger. **35:** 1665-1676.

25. Markwardt, F., G. Wagner, J. Stürzebecher & P. Walsmann. 1980. *N*α-Arylsulfonyl-ω-(4-amidinophenyl)-α-aminoalkyl-carboxylic acid amides—novel selective inhibitors of thrombin. Thromb. Res. **17:** 425-431.
26. Stürzebecher, J., F. Markwardt, B. Voigt, G. Wagner & P. Walsmann. 1983. Cyclic amides of *N*α-arylsulfonamino-acylated 4-amidinophenylalanine-tight binding inhibitors of thrombin. Thromb. Res. **29:** 635-642.
27. Markwardt, F., A. Hoffmann & J. Stürzebecher. 1983. Influence of thrombin inhibitors on the thrombin-induced activation of human platelets. Haemostasis **13:** 227-233.
28. Hoffmann, A. & F. Markwardt. 1984. Inhibition of the thrombin-platelet reaction by hirudin. Haemostasis **14:** 164-169.
29. Griessbach, U., J. Stürzebecher & F. Markwardt. 1985. Assay of hirudin in plasma using a chromogenic thrombin substrate. **39:** 771-775.
30. Markwardt, F., J. Hauptmann, M. Richter & P. Richter. 1979. Tierexperimentelle Untersuchungen zur Pharmakokinetik von 4-Amidinophenylbrenztraubensäure (APPA). Pharmazie **34:** 178-181.
31. Hauptmann, J., F. Markwardt & M. Richter. 1982. Tierexperimentelle Untersuchungen zur Pharmakokinetik von Nα-Tosyl-3-amidinophenylalaninpiperidid (TAPAP), einem neuen Thrombininhibitor. Pharmazie **37:** 430-433.
32. Markwardt, F., J. Hauptmann, G. Nowak, Ch. Klessen & P. Walsmann. 1982. Pharmacological studies on the antithrombotic action of hirudin in experimental animals. Thromb. Haemostasis **47:** 226-229.
33. Markwardt, F., G. Nowak, J. Stürzebecher, U. Griessbach, P. Walsmann & G. Vogel. 1984. Pharmacokinetics and anticoagulant effect of hirudin in man. Thromb. Res. **52:** 160-163.
34. Kaiser, B., J. Hauptmann, A. Weiss & F. Markwardt. 1985. Pharmacological characterization of a new highly effective synthetic thrombin inhibitor. Biomed. Biochim. Acta **44:** 1201-1210.
35. Hauptmann, J., B. Kaiser & F. Markwardt. 1985. Anticoagulant action of synthetic tight binding inhibitors of thrombin *in vitro* and *in vivo.* Thromb. Res. **39:** 771-775.
36. Hauptmann, J., A. Barth, F.-P.-Schönberger & F. Markwardt. 1983. Comparative study on the antithrombotic effects of a synthetic thrombin inhibitor and of heparin in animal models. Biomed. Biochim. Acta **42:** 959-965.
37. Hauptmann, J., B. Kaiser, F. Markwardt & G. Nowak. 1980. Anticoagulant and antithrombotic action of novel specific inhibitors of thrombin. Thromb. Haemostasis **43:** 118-123.
38. Markwardt, F., G. Nowak & J. Hoffmann. 1983. Comparative study on thrombin inhibitors in experimental microthrombosis. Thromb. Haemostasis **49:** 235-237.
39. Nowak, G. & F. Markwardt. 1980. Influence of hirudin on endotoxin-induced disseminated intravascular coagulation (DIC) in weaned pigs. Exp. Pathol. (Jena) **18:** 438-443.
40. Kaiser, B. & F. Markwardt. 1986. Experimental studies on the antithrombotic action of a highly effective synthetic thrombin inhibitor. Thromb. Haemostasis. **55:** 194-196.

Interaction of Thrombin with Thrombomodulin

C. T. ESMON,[a] N. L. ESMON,[a] S. KUROSAWA,[a] AND A. E. JOHNSON[b]

[a] *Thrombosis/Hematology Research Program*
Oklahoma Medical Research Foundation
Oklahoma City, Oklahoma 73104

[b] *Department of Chemistry*
University of Oklahoma
Norman, Oklahoma 73069

Product regulation of complex pathways is well established in metabolism. The role of product regulation, however, in protease cascades is less well established. Although thrombin has long been recognized as a positive feedback activator of coagulation,[1] its potential for serving as a negative regulator is only recently becoming understood. Protein C activation and the subsequent expression of the activated protein C anticoagulant function provides one mechanism by which thrombin can serve as a negative regulator of coagulation. Thrombin's critical role in this pathway is as the protein C activating enzyme.[2–4] Once thrombin participates in the protein C anticoagulant pathway, its function is transformed from a procoagulant to an anticoagulant. The mechanisms by which this transformation occurs constitute the central theme of this paper.

One of the major problems of a product feedback system using proteolysis involves how to regulate rather than destroy the system. In the protein C pathway, this is accomplished at a minimum of two levels. First, activated protein C demonstrates remarkable specificity for activated factors V and VIII as compared to their precursor forms.[5,6]

A second feature of the pathway that imparts unique properties is that protein C activation occurs in response to formation of a complex between thrombin and thrombomodulin,[7] an endothelial cell-specific protein.[7–9] This feature implies that protein C activation probably occurs primarily in the microcirculation where, because of the high surface to volume ratio, the concentration of thrombomodulin is relatively high.[7,10] Activation probably occurs downstream from the site of injury and hence prevents propagation of coagulation reactions downstream. In addition to catalyzing protein C activation, the complex between thrombin and thrombomodulin has significantly reduced coagulant activity in terms of fibrinogen clotting activity, factor V activation, and platelet activation.[11–13] At least two models could account for this change in macromolecular specificity. First, as we have proposed, complex formation could alter either the substrate binding sites and/or the active site. Alternatively, complex formation could result in steric hindrance, preventing the interaction of thrombin with fibrinogen, platelets, or factor V. Such a model would predict that the substrates like fibrinogen might compete with thrombomodulin for interaction with thrombin. Such

TABLE 1. Ca^{2+} Influence on Protein C Activation[15]

Substrate	Activator	Effect of Ca^{2+}	One-Half Maximal Concentration	K_m (No Ca^{2+})	K_m (3 mM Ca^{2+})
Protein C	Thrombin	Inhibition	250 μM	1.2 μM	≈60 μM
GD-PC	Thrombin	Inhibition	50 μM	—	—
Protein C	T-TM[a] Complex	Acceleration	250 μM	> 100 μM	8 μM
GD-PC	T-TM Complex	Acceleration	50 μM	> 50 μM	8 μM

[a] T-TM, thrombin-thrombomodulin.

a model is favored by Jakubowsky and Owen.[14] Indeed, they find that fibrinogen does inhibit thrombin's interaction with thrombomodulin and does so competitively. During the development of this paper, I would like to indicate, however, why we feel these two models are kinetically similar.

To probe how thrombomodulin functions, it is useful to examine first the requirements for protein C activation by thrombin alone and the thrombin-thrombomodulin complex. We reported previously that whereas Ca^{2+} inhibits activation of protein C by thrombin, Ca^{2+} is required for activation by the thrombin-thrombomodulin complex (TABLE 1). One of the intriguing, but potentially coincidental, features is that both events are one-half maximal at 250 μM Ca^{2+}. Similar results are obtained with selected other metals such as Mn^{2+} or Cd^{2+} (FIGURE 1). In general, ions that fail to inhibit

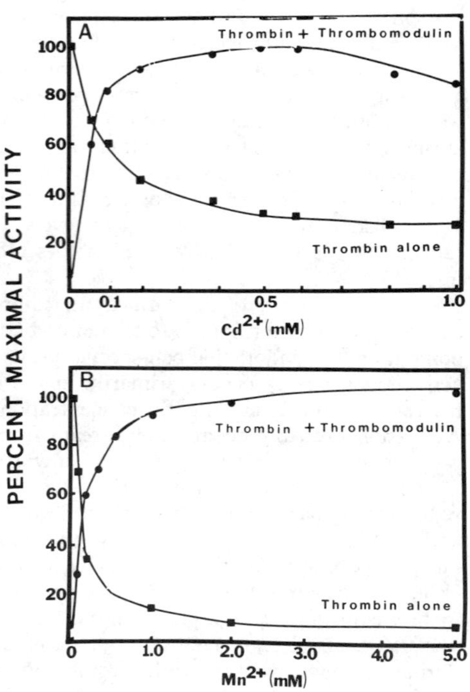

FIGURE 1. The effect of Cd^{2+} and Mn^{2+} on protein C activation by thrombin and the thrombin-thrombomodulin complex. Protein C (1 μM) was activated with thrombin (17 nM) (■) or thrombin-thrombomodulin complex (1.6 nM thrombin, 15 nM thrombomodulin) (●) at 37°C in 0.1 M NaCl, 0.02 M Tris HCl, pH 7.5 containing the cation concentrations indicated. Activated protein C was monitored as reported previously.[15]

protein C activation by thrombin fail to support activation by the thrombin-thrombomodulin complex.[15] Because no detectable Ca^{2+} binding to thrombin is observed at these concentrations,[16] and because Ca^{2+} is not required for thrombin-thrombomodulin interaction,[11] we felt that these effects were likely mediated through the substrate. Additional evidence for substrate participation came from studies with a modified form of protein C from which residues 1-44 were removed proteolytically from the light chain. This form of bovine protein C, referred to as Gla domainless protein C, and abbreviated GD-PC, activates completely with either thrombin alone or the thrombin-thrombomodulin complex.[15] The Ca^{2+} dependence for both reactions is shifted to 50 ± 10 μM Ca^{2+}. Thus, modification of the substrate alters Ca^{2+} dependence. With either activator, the major influence of Ca^{2+} is on the K_m of the reaction, increasing the K_m of the reaction with thrombin and decreasing the K_m with thrombin-thrombomodulin. Evidence for a Ca^{2+}-dependent change in the substrate

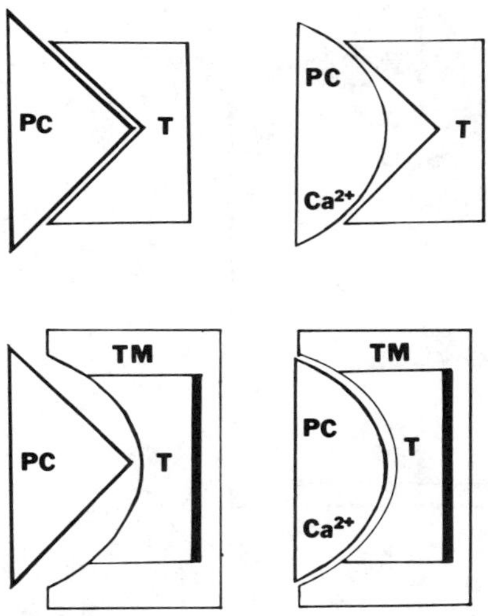

FIGURE 2. A plausible mechanism for thrombomodulin function.[16] See text for a discussion of the model. Abbreviations: PC, protein C; T, thrombin; TM, thrombomodulin.

that would correlate with the activation requirements was obtained by measuring fluorescence quenching and circular dichroism.[16] Given these observations, we postulated a mechanism illustrated diagrammatically in FIGURE 2. Basically, the model proposes that thrombin interacts well with protein C in the absence of Ca^{2+}, but when bound to thrombomodulin, thrombin cannot effectively bind protein C. Ca^{2+} induces a structural change in protein C that prevents optimal interaction of thrombin with the substrate. In this model, thrombomodulin interaction with thrombin results in a change in the binding site, resulting in a form of the enzyme capable of binding the Ca^{2+}-stabilized conformation of protein C.

From a physiological point of view, the essential question is whether this change in specificity, implied by the above model, is manifest by an inhibition of the functions free thrombin is known to catalyze. Among the substrates for thrombin generally considered important in the propagation of the coagulant response are fibrinogen, factor V, and platelets. Complex formation with thrombomodulin blocks all of these activation events.[11,12] Recently, studies with human thrombomodulin demonstrated that the human protein was much less effective than the rabbit protein.[13] Nonetheless, human thrombomodulin did inhibit these reactions. Although thrombin combines stoichiometrically with both proteins and although inhibition is achieved in both cases, it appears likely that the human thrombin-thrombomodulin complex is also ineffective in catalyzing coagulant reactions and that the difference observed is related to the affinity of human thrombin for thrombomodulin under the conditions of the experiments. On the cell surface the affinity of human thrombomodulin for thrombin is comparable to that of the rabbit protein,[17] suggesting that some of the differences could either arise during isolation or that the human protein may have an increased requirement for membranes to function optimally.

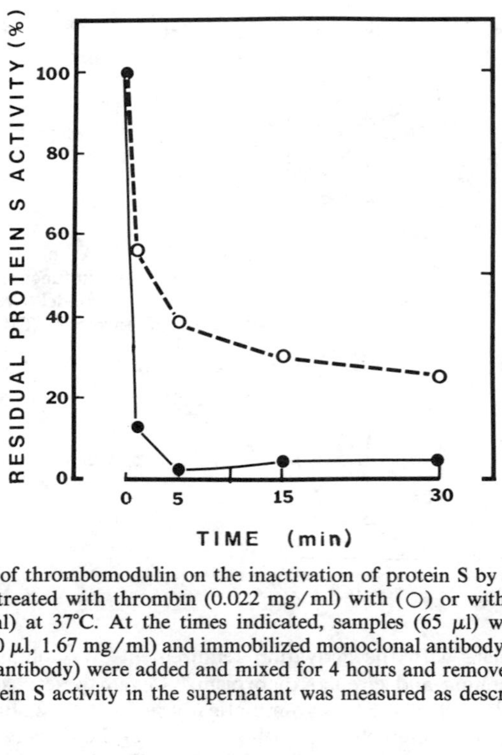

FIGURE 3. Effect of thrombomodulin on the inactivation of protein S by thrombin. Protein S (0.14 mg/ml) was treated with thrombin (0.022 mg/ml) with (○) or without (●) thrombomodulin (0.04 mg/ml) at 37°C. At the times indicated, samples (65 μl) were withdrawn, and antithrombin III (30 μl, 1.67 mg/ml) and immobilized monoclonal antibody to thrombomodulin (30 μl, 2.5 mg/ml antibody) were added and mixed for 4 hours and removed by centrifugation. The remaining protein S activity in the supernatant was measured as described.[19]

The changes observed in macromolecular specificity all occur with high molecular weight substrates and, as would be suggested by FIGURE 2, occur with or without Ca^{2+}. To study the influence of thrombomodulin on thrombin specificity, we decided to examine also the influence on the inactivation of protein S. Protein S, a cofactor for activated protein C, is inactivated by limited proteolysis with thrombin. Protein S has a molecular weight of approximately 64 000, and cleavage occurs near the N terminal.[18] Thus, this protein differs significantly in size from those previously studied. To examine the influence of thrombomodulin on thrombin-catalyzed protein S inactivation, thrombin was incubated with protein S either with or without thrombomodulin (FIGURE 3). Even under conditions where thrombomodulin and thrombin are roughly equimolar, the inactivation of protein S is markedly inhibited. Because protein S inactivation results in a loss of anticoagulant activity, cleavage of protein S by thrombin could be considered as a procoagulant event. Thus, as with the other substrates so far studied, the general theme beginning to emerge is that thrombomodulin blocks reactions that facilitate clotting and in general promotes the anticoagulant nature of the endothelium. This anticoagulant property can be mediated either directly by protein C activation or indirectly by neutralizing procoagulant properties. The change in macromolecular specificity discussed above provides further support for the concept of a change in the substrate binding site of thrombin, but as mentioned previously, whether the change involves alteration of the enzyme conformation or is simply steric remains to be determined. To approach this question, we thought it useful to develop a probe that might sense alterations in and around the active site of thrombin brought on by complex formation with thrombomodulin. We examined two probes, the reversible complex between dansylarginine-*N*-(3-ethyl-1,5-pentanediyl)amide (DAPA) and dansyl covalently attached to thrombin. This second derivative is formed by incubating human thrombin with dansyl fluoride to block the active site.[20] Although a small change in the DAPA signal occurred upon complex formation with thrombomodulin, the change ($\approx$10%) was insufficient to accurately monitor association. The dansyl thrombin, however, proved a very useful probe. Complex formation was accompanied by a 45% decrease in the fluorescence emission. This occurred in the presence or absence of Ca^{2+}. We feel these data are consistent with the concept of an alteration of thrombin's conformation near the active site upon complex formation with thrombomodulin and provide the first evidence not involving macromolecular substrates for the type of conformational modification illustrated in FIGURE 2. Two additional features strongly suggest that this change in fluorescence emission monitors complex formation. First, the maximum decrease in fluorescence emission occurs at a 1 $\pm$ 0.1 molar ratio of thrombin to thrombomodulin. Second, the dissociation constant calculated from the fluorescence decrease ($\approx$0.2-0.5 nM) agrees favorably with that obtained with kinetics ($\approx$0.2-0.5 nM).

The above arguments demonstrate that protein substrates differ markedly in their ability to interact with the thrombin-thrombomodulin complex versus free thrombin. The Ca^{2+} dependence data suggest that this change in specificity occurs upon complex formation and does not require Ca^{2+}. The Ca^{2+} requirement then evolves, due to a requirement for the substrate, to adopt a conformation recognized by the thrombin-thrombomodulin complex. Direct evidence for the alteration of the active site of thrombin by complex formation with thrombomodulin comes from the dansyl thrombin studies. Unfortunately, although this strongly suggests alteration of the environment around the active site, it does not prove that this alteration is responsible for the observed change in macromolecular specificity. Perhaps arguing in favor of the steric proposal is the observation that the hydrolysis of small *p*-nitroanilide peptides and arginine esters is altered little by complex formation of thrombin with thrombomodulin.[15] This may, however, reflect flexibility in these substrates and/or reduced stringency in the requirements for interaction with thrombin. The competitive aspect of the interaction of thrombin with either thrombomodulin or fibrinogen could be taken as additional evidence supporting steric hinderance. This kinetic behavior, however, could also be explained if one assumes that thrombin is in equilibrium between at least two conformational states, one that catalyzes fibrinogen clotting, and the other that catalyzes protein C activation. A function of thrombomodulin could then be to stabilize the second conformation. Inherent in this hypothesis is the concept that thrombin in the conformation required to activate protein C is a small percentage of the possible thrombin structures and that fibrinogen stabilizes the conformer that does not interact with thrombomodulin. Clearly, additional work is required to differentiate these models. The properties of the system, however, suggest that this may be an ideal model to use in gaining new insights into how complex formation enhances zymogen activation.

REFERENCES

1. JACKSON, C. M. & Y. NEMERSON. 1980. Blood coagulation. Annu. Rev. Biochem. **49:** 765-811.
2. SEEGERS, W. H. 1981. Protein C and autoprothrombin II-A. Semin. Thromb. Hemostasis **7:** 257-261.
3. ESMON, C. T. 1984. Protein C. *In* Progress in Hemostasis and Thrombosis. T. H. Spaet, Ed. Vol. **7:** 25-54. Grune & Stratton, Inc. Orlando, FL.
4. KISIEL, W. 1979. Human plasma protein C: Isolation, characterization and mechanism of activation by α-thrombin. J. Clin. Invest. **64:** 761-769.
5. WALKER, F. J., P. W. SEXTON & C. T. ESMON. 1979. The inhibition of blood coagulation by activated protein C through the selective inactivation of activated factor V. Biochim. Biophys. Acta **571:** 333-342.
6. MARLAR, R. A., A. J. KLEISS & J. H. GRIFFIN. 1982. Mechanism of action of human activated protein C, a thrombin-dependent anticoagulant enzyme. Blood **59:** 1067-1072.
7. ESMON, C. T. & W. G. OWEN. 1981. Identification of an endothelial cell cofactor for thrombin-catalyzed activation of protein C. Proc. Natl. Acad. Sci. USA **78:** 2249-2252.
8. MARUYAMA, I., C. E. BELL & P. W. MAJERUS. 1985. Thrombomodulin is found on endothelium of arteries, veins, capillaries and lymphatics and on syncytiotrophoblasts of human placenta. J. Cell Biol. **101:** 363-371.
9. DEBAULT, L. E., N. L. ESMON, J. R. OLSON & C. T. ESMON. 1986. Distribution of the thrombomodulin antigen in the rabbit vasculature. Lab. Invest. **54:** 172-178.
10. BUSCH, C., P. CANCILLA, L. E. DEBAULT, J. C. GOLDSMITH & W. G. OWEN. 1982. Use of endothelium cultured on microcarriers as a model for the microcirculation. Lab. Invest. **47:** 498-504.
11. ESMON, C. T., N. L. ESMON & K. W. HARRIS. 1982. Complex formation between thrombin and thrombomodulin inhibits both thrombin-catalyzed fibrin formation and factor V activation. J. Biol. Chem. **257:** 7944-7947.
12. ESMON, N. L., R. C. CARROLL & C. T. ESMON. 1983.Thrombomodulin blocks the ability of thrombin to activate platelets. J. Biol. Chem. **258:** 12238-12242.
13. MARUYAMA, I., H. H. SALEM, H. ISHII & P. W. MAJERUS. 1985. Human thrombomodulin is not an efficient inhibitor of the procoagulant activity of thrombin. J. Clin. Invest. **75:** 987-991.
14. JAKUBOWSKI, H. V., M. D. KLINE & W. G. OWEN. 1986. The effect of bovine thrombomodulin on the specificity of bovine thrombin. J. Biol. Chem. **261:** 3876-3882.
15. ESMON, N. L., L. E. DEBAULT & C. T. ESMON. 1983. Proteolytic formation and properties of Gla-domainless protein C. J. Biol. Chem. **258:** 5548-5553.
16. JOHNSON, A. E., N. L. ESMON, T. M. LAUE & C. T. ESMON. 1983. Structural changes required for activation of protein C are induced by Ca^{2+} binding to a high affinity site that does not contain γ-carboxyglutamic acid. J. Biol. Chem. **258:** 5554-5560.
17. OWEN, W. G. & C. T. ESMON. 1981. Functional properties of an endothelial cell cofactor for thrombin-catalyzed activation of protein C. J. Biol. Chem. **256:** 5532-5535.
18. DAHLBACK, B. 1983. Purification of human vitamin K-dependent protein S and its limited proteolysis by thrombin. Biochem. **209:** 837-846.
19. COMP, P. C., R. R. NIXON, M. R. COOPER & C. T. ESMON. 1984. Familial protein S deficiency is associated with recurrent thrombosis. J. Clin. Invest. **74:** 2082-2088.
20. BERLINER, L. J. & Y. Y. L. SHEN. 1977. Active site fluorescent labeled dansyl and anthraniloyl human thrombin. Thromb. Res. **12:** 15-25.

Complex Interaction between Factor V_a-Light Chain and Thrombomodulin in the Regulation of Protein C Activation[a]

HATEM H. SALEM,[b] NAOMI L. ESMON,[c]
CHARLES T. ESMON,[c] AND PHILIP W. MAJERUS[d]

[b]*Department of Medicine*
Monash Medical School
Prahran, Victoria, 3168, Australia

[c]*Thrombosis/Hematology Research Laboratory*
Oklahoma Medical Research Foundation
Oklahoma City, Oklahoma 73104

[d]*Division of Hematology-Oncology*
Washington University School of Medicine
St. Louis, Missouri 63110

INTRODUCTION

The presence of an anticoagulant in prothrombinex preparations treated with thrombin was first recognized in Seeger's laboratories in 1960.[1] This activity was purified in 1972, and it was demonstrated that the purified protein retarded coagulation *in vitro* as well as *in vivo* and induced fibrinolysis.[2] The protein was named autoprothrombin II_a and was believed to be derived from prothrombin.

In 1976, Stenflo purified a vitamin K-dependent protein from bovine plasma, which he named protein C.[3] It was soon realized that this newly identified protein was identical to the previously recognized autoprothrombin II_a.[4] Since then, progress has been rapid in the understanding of the structure and function of protein C and its role as an anticoagulant.

The human protein is a glycoprotein with a molecular weight of 62 000. It is synthesized by the liver as a single chain polypeptide, which is cleaved posttranslationally into a heavy and a light chain linked by disulphide bonds.[5] The protein circulates in plasma as a zymogen and can be activated to a serine protease with potent anticoagulant properties. These are mediated through the proteolysis of the procoagulant cofactors, V_a and VIII_a.[6,7]

[a]This work was supported by Grants HLBI 14147 (Specialized Center for Research in Thrombosis) and HL 16634 from the National Institutes of Health (to P. W. Majerus) and by Grants HL 29807 and HL 30340 from the National Institutes of Health (to C. T. Esmon).

THE ACTIVATION OF PROTEIN C

A number of proteases such as thrombin, trypsin, and Russel viper venom have been reported to convert protein C to the active form referred to as activated protein C (APC). Among these, thrombin, is the only candidate as a potential circulating pathophysiological activator of the protein in the circulation. In this regard thrombin is rather inefficient, with an activation rate of 0.01 mole of APC/mole of thrombin/ml/min.[8] This activity of thrombin is enhanced at least 1000-fold by the endothelial cell-surface protein, thrombomodulin, which binds thrombin with high affinity and converts it to a potent protein C activator.[9]

The existence of a circulating cofactor for protein C activation was suspected with the observation that factor V_a, the substrate for APC, was rapidly inactivated after blood clotting *in vitro.* This was associated with the loss of the heavy chain of the molecule, similar to the effects of APC on factor V_a.

The possibility that the circulating cofactor could be related to factor V_a was born out with the demonstration that APC was generated when factor V_a was incubated with protein C in the presence of trace concentrations of thrombin.[10] In this system, the formation of APC was detected by the rapid inactivation of the factor V_a, when phospholipid was added to the reaction mixture. (Phospholipid is required for rapid inactivation of factor V_a by APC.) In the absence of thrombin or protein C, factor V_a remained stable. Similarly, under the experimental conditions used, the incubation of protein C and thrombin in the absence of factor V_a was not associated with generation of significant amounts of APC. In more detailed studies, it was established that factor V_a acted as a thrombin cofactor for protein C activation. The K_m of factor V_a in this reaction was 30 nM, which is considerably higher than its K_m for prothrombin activation.[10]

The factor V_a molecule consists of three major polypeptide chains, an activation peptide (molecular mass, 150 kDa), a heavy chain (molecular mass 110 kDa), and a light chain of 78 kDa. The heavy and light chains of the molecule are linked by Ca^{++} bonds and are both required for the expression of factor V_a procoagulant activity. The three chains of the molecule could be separated by chromatography on QAE sephadex in the presence of EDTA (FIGURE 1 and 2). Although this fractionation does not totally resolve the components, early eluting fractions contained essentially homogeneous light chains. When the column fractions were tested for their ability to support protein C activation, as seen in FIGURE 3, only the light chains containing fractions demonstrated this activity.[11]

Comparison of Thrombomodulin and Factor V_a-Light Chain (FV_a-LC) as Thrombin Cofactors for Protein C Activation

Studies on the kinetics of protein C activation by thrombin in the presence of thrombomodulin and FV_a-LC revealed that thrombomodulin was 20-fold more efficient as a cofactor in the reaction (FIGURE 4). The activation of protein C lacking the γ-carboxyglutamic acid domain (herewith referred to as gla-less protein C) by both cofactors was also examined.[8] Gla-less protein C was prepared by limited proteolysis of the intact molecule with chymotrypsin. Thrombomodulin (0.25-1 nM) in the presence of 10 nM thrombin, activated intact and gla-less protein C at an indistinguishable rate (FIGURE 5). When human FV_a-LC was used as the cofactor instead of thrombomodulin, gla-less protein C was activated at only 5% of the rate of the intact protein (FIGURE 6).

THE EFFECT OF FV_a-LC ON THE COFACTOR ACTIVITY OF THROMBOMODULIN

The observation that thrombomodulin was 20-fold more efficient than FV_a-LC allowed the study of the effects of FV_a-LC on the thrombin-thrombomodulin catalyzed protein C activation. Thrombin was used at concentrations where FV_a-LC contributed

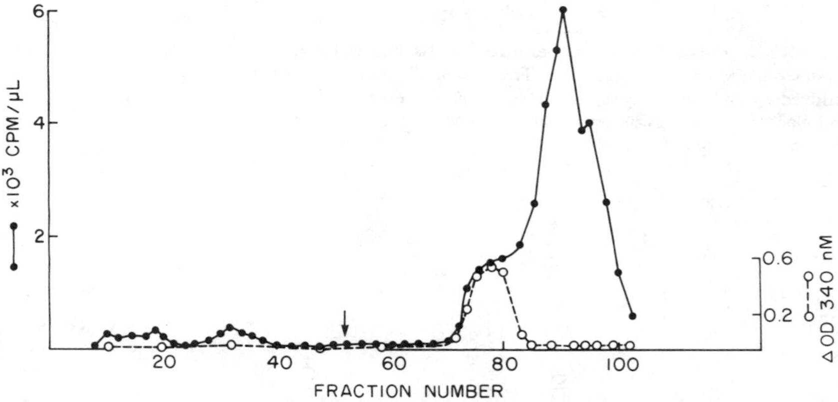

FIGURE 1. Chromatography of ^{125}I-factor V_a on QAE-sephadex in the presence of 1 mM EDTA. The column was eluted with 20 mM Tris-Hepes, pH 7.8 containing 1 mM EDTA. The arrow indicates start of 0.05-0.5 M NaCl linear gradient. One ml fractions were collected. The solid line is the profile of radioactivity. The dotted line represents protein C cofactor activity. (H. H. Salem *et al.*[11] With permission from the *Journal of Biological Chemistry.*)

minimally to the overall rate of protein C activation. At a concentration of 30 nM FV_a-LC, protein C activation by 1 nM thrombin and 2 nM thrombomodulin was significantly inhibited. Increasing FV_a-LC to 90 nM resulted in complete inhibition of the reaction (FIGURE 7). Interestingly, although FV_a-LC by itself did not stimulate the activation of gla-less protein C, it still inhibited the ability of the thrombin-thrombomodulin complex to activate this protein.

The inhibitory activity of 90 nM FV_a-LC could not be overcome by increasing the concentration of protein C up to 3 μM, suggesting that the effect of FV_a-LC is unlikely to be mediated through binding to the protein C. Thrombomodulin in concentrations up to 128 nM did not reverse the effects of 90 nM FV_a-LC. Increasing the concentration of both thrombin and thrombomodulin resulted in a linear increase in the rate of the reaction, but the inhibition was not completely overcome even at 400 nM thrombin-thrombomodulin complex.

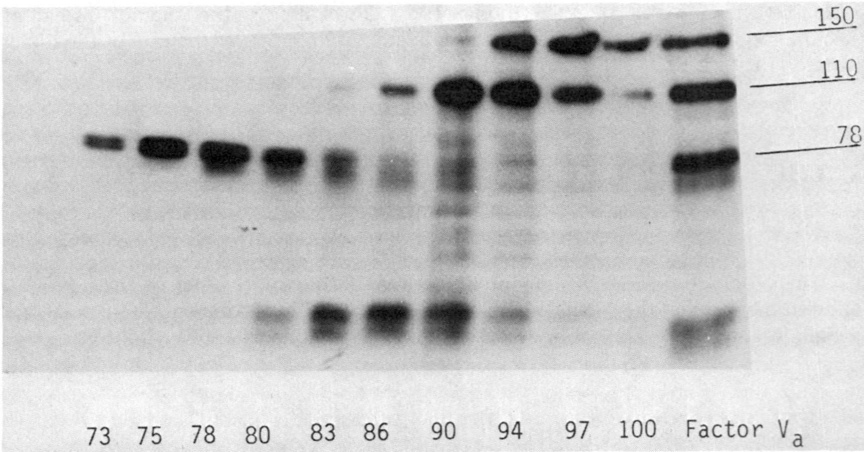

FIGURE 2. Polyacrylamide gel electrophoresis and autoradiography of samples from QAE-sepharose fractions in FIGURE 1. The indicated fractions (corresponding to FIGURE 1) were reduced by boiling in the presence of 0.5% β-mercaptoethanol and sodium dodecyl sulphate, and electrophoresed as described in reference 11. (H.H. Salem *et al.*[11] With permission from the *Journal of Biological Chemistry.*)

FIGURE 3. Protein C activation by factor V_a-light chain. Factor V_a-light chain at the indicated concentrations was incubated with protein C at the three different concentrations shown in the presence of 10 nM thrombin. The reaction was for 15 min and was terminated using hirudin. The amount of activated protein C formed was measured as detailed in reference 11. (H. H. Salem *et al.*[11] With permission from the *Journal of Biological Chemistry.*)

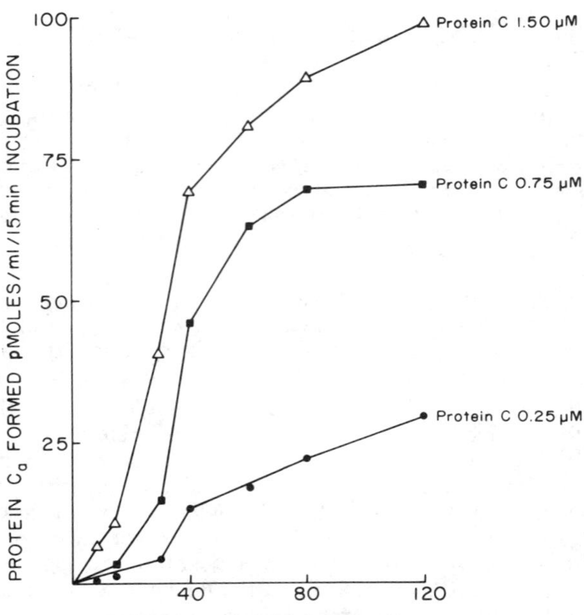

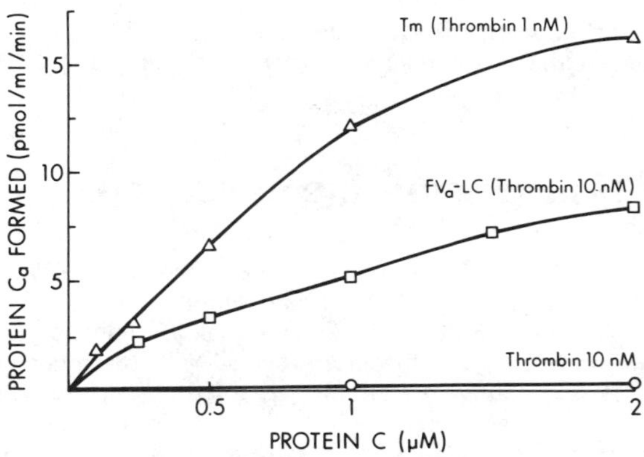

FIGURE 4. Comparison of thrombomodulin and Factor V_a-light chain as cofactors for protein C activation by thrombin. Reaction mixtures contained the indicated concentrations of protein C in the presence of 10 nM thrombin alone (0), 10 nM thrombin and 75 nM factor V_a-light chain (□), or 1 nM thrombin and 2 nM thrombomodulin (△). The assay for activated protein C was performed as detailed in reference 8. (H. H. Salem *et al.*:[8] With permission from the *Journal of Clinical Investigation.)*

THE EFFECT OF THROMBOMODULIN ON THE THROMBIN-COFACTOR ACTIVITY OF FV_a-LC

The observation that high concentration of FV_a-LC inhibited the activity of thrombomodulin facilitated the design of experiments to study the effects of thrombomodulin on the ability of FV_a-LC to activate protein C. In these experiments, FV_a-LC was used at 125 nM, a concentration that readily activates protein C and also completely inhibits the activity of thrombomodulin. Thrombomodulin, in concentrations from 2 nM-1 μM, did not inhibit protein C activation by 120 nM FV_a-LC in the presence of 5-20 nM thrombin. In fact, as the concentration of thrombomodulin was increased,

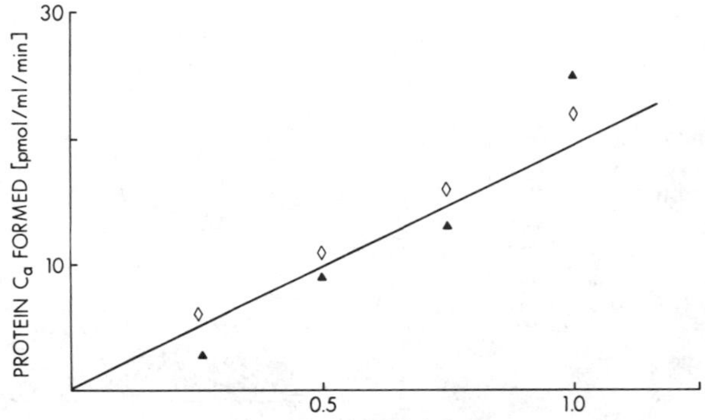

FIGURE 5. The activation of native and gla-less bovine protein C by thrombin in the presence of thrombomodulin. Assay mixtures contained the indicated concentrations of thrombomodulin in the presence of 10 nM thrombin and 1 μM native (▲) or gla-less (◇) protein C. Details of the experimental conditions used are in reference 8. (H. H. Salem *et al.*[8] With permission from *The Journal of Clinical Investigation.*)

the rate of protein C activation slowly accelerated from 2.7 to 6.7 pmol/ml/minute. These results suggest that thrombomodulin does not inhibit the cofactor activity of FV_a-LC.

DISCUSSION AND CONCLUSION

These studies have resolved a number of issues. First, the activation of protein C by thrombomodulin or FV_a-LC involves the recognition of different structural features on the protein C molecule. Specifically, FV_a-LC has an obligatory requirement for the gla domain of protein C, a feature not observed with thrombomodulin. In blood clotting, the γ-carboxyglutamyl residues are regarded as calcium binding sites. It is thus of interest that whereas protein C activation by thrombomodulin demonstrates calcium dependence, both the intact and the gla-less forms of the proteins are activated at identical rates, suggesting that the calcium site involved in protein C activation by the thrombin-thrombomdulin complex is distinct from the gla domain. By contrast, the region in protein C containing the gla domain is involved in substrate recognition by the light chain, and this involvement does not depend on calcium. Indeed, high concentrations of calcium are inhibitory.

The physiological importance of FV_a-LC as a thrombin cofactor for protein C activation is not clear. Studies in patients with congenital factor V deficiency are difficult to interpret because these patients not only lack the protein C-activating potential of factor V_a, but are also deficient in thrombin generation. It is, however, of interest to note that despite marked impairment in thrombin generation, thrombosis has been reported in three patients with factor V deficiency.[12,13] All three individuals presented with deep venous thrombosis, and in one case this was complicated by pulmonary embolism.

In the microvasculature where endothelial cell density is greatest, thrombomodulin is probably the major determinant of protein C activation. At these sites, FV_a-LC may play a role in modulating protein C activation by its ability to inhibit the thrombin-thrombomodulin catalyzed reaction. In the vessel lumen, where the concentration of thrombomodulin is very low, FV_a-LC may play a more important role as thrombin cofactor for protein C activation. Further studies on the physiological role of FV_a-LC in the regulation of protein C activation will have to be addressed in animal model experiments.

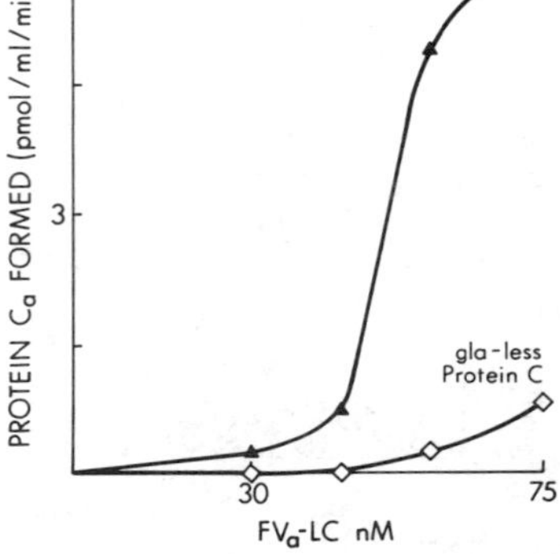

FIGURE 6. The activation of native and gla-less bovine protein C by thrombin in the presence of factor V_a-light chain. Experimental conditions were identical to FIGURE 4, except that factor V_a-light chain at the indicated concentrations was used as the thrombomodulin cofactor instead of thrombomodulin. (H. H. Salem *et al.*[8] With permission from the *Journal of Clinical Investigation.*)

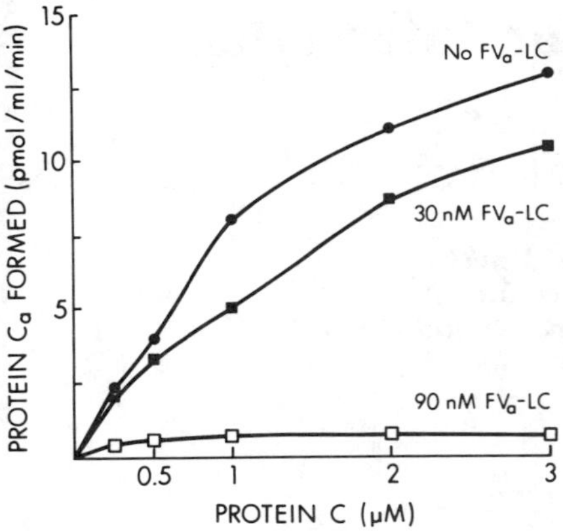

FIGURE 7. The inhibition of thrombin-thrombomodulin-catalyzed protein C activation by factor V_a-light chain. Reaction mixtures contained 1 μM human protein C, 1 nM thrombin, and 2 nM thrombomodulin in the presence of no factor V_a-light (no FV_a-LC) or the indicated concentrations of that cofactor. Experimental details are in reference 8. (H. H. Salem *et al.*[8] With permission from the *Journal of Clinical Investigation.*)

REFERENCES

1. Mammen, E. F., W. R. Thomas & W. H. Seegers. 1960. Activation of purified prothrombin to autoprothrombin I or autoprothrombin II (Platelet cofactor II) or autoprothrombin II_a. Thromb. Diath. Haemorrh. **5:** 218.
2. Seegers, W. H., L. E. McCoy & H. D. Groben. 1972. Purification and some properties of autoprothrombin II_a — an anticoagulant perhaps related to fibrinolysis. Thromb. Res. **1:** 443-460.
3. Stenflo, J. 1976. A new vitamin K dependent protein: purification from bovine plasma and preliminary characterization. J. Biol. Chem. **251:** 355-363.
4. Seegers, W. H., E. Novoa & R. L. Henry. 1976. Relationship of "new" vitamin K dependent protein C and "old" autoprothrombin II_a. Thromb. Res. **8:** 543-552.
5. Foster, D. & E. W. Davie. 1984. Characterization of cDNA coding for human protein C. Proc. Natl. Acad. Sci. USA **81:** 4766-4770.
6. Walker, F. J., P. W. Sexton & C. T. Esmon. 1979. The inhibition of blood coagulation by activated protein C through the selective inactivation of activated factor V. Biochim. Biophs. Acta **571:** 333-342.
7. Fulcher, C. A., J. E. Gardiner & J. H. Griffith. 1984. Proteolytic inactivation of human factor VIII procoagulant protein by activated protein C and its analogy with factor V. Blood **63:** 486-489.
8. Salem, H. H., N. L. Esmon, C. T. Esmon & P. W. Majerus. 1984. Effects of thrombomodulin and coagulation factor V_a-light chain on protein C activation *in vitro.* J. Clin. Invest. **73:** 968-972.
9. Esmon, N. L., W.G. Owen & C. T. Esmon. 1982. Isolation of a membrane bound cofactor for thrombin catalyzed activation of protein C. J. Biol. Chem. **257:** 859-64.
10. Salem, H. H., G. J. Broze, J. P. Miletich & P. W. Majerus. 1983. Human coagulation factor V_a is a cofactor for the activation of Protein C. Proc. Natl. Acad. Sci. USA **80:** 1584-88.
11. Salem, H. H., G. J. Broze, J. P. Miletich & P. W. Majerus. 1983. The light chain of factor V_a contains the activity of factor V_a that accelerates protein C activation by thrombin. J. Biol. Chem. **258:** 8531-8533.
12. Miller, S. P. 1965. Coagulation dynamics in factor V deficiency: A family study, with note on the occurence of thrombophlebitis. Thromb. Diath. Haemorrh. **13:** 500.
13. Reich, N. E., G. C. Hoffman, V. G. deWolfe & H. S. Van Ordstrand. 1976. Reccurrent thrombophlebitis and pulmonary emboli in factor 5 deficiency. Chest **69:** 113.

Thrombin-Cellular Interactions

MARC A. SHUMAN

Department of Medicine
Cancer Research Institute
University of California Medical Center
San Francisco, California

INTRODUCTION

Although the principal function of thrombin is to clot blood, it is an agonist for a diverse number of cellular activities in many types of cells and tissues (TABLE 1). The concentrations of thrombin at which these effects occur are within the range observed during blood clotting,[1] suggesting their potential physiologic significance. Furthermore, the effects of thrombin are relatively specific: Other serine proteinases involved in blood clotting do not exert these effects. It is likely that most types of cells, with the exception of erythrocytes, are responsive to thrombin and that a number of other effects will be demonstrated in the future. Caution, however, must be exercised in interpreting the results of these experiments, because their ultimate significance is dependent on demonstrating that the reactions occur *in vivo.* Thus it is possible that some of the *in vitro* effects of thrombin on cells and tissues mimic physiologic events, whereas others are secondary to thrombin's resemblance to other serine proteinases or hormones that mediate these effects *in vivo.* Whether or not thrombin is the physiologic mediator of these responses, important information has and will be obtained on the mechanism by which thrombin and similar proteins exert their effects on cells and tissues.

Although thrombin is internalized by some cells,[2] current evidence favors the hypothesis that the effects of thrombin are mediated directly by its interaction with cell-surface proteins. Initial experiments analyzing the interaction of thrombin with the cell surface involved kinetic measurement of thrombin receptors on platelets.[3,4] In these studies, it was assumed that this receptor mediated thrombin activation of platelets, although this has not been directly demonstrated. Subsequent studies have described multiple different cellular proteins that bind thrombin, some of which may be classical receptors, whereas the function of others has not been determined. Furthermore, cellular substrates for thrombin have also been identified. Thus, thrombin reacts both as a hormone and an enzyme with cell surfaces. The following discussion is focused on delineating the different types of reactions of thrombin with cells and the consequences on cell function.

BINDING OF THROMBIN TO CELL-SURFACE RECEPTORS

Initial experiments describing binding of [^{125}I]thrombin to cells involved platelets[3,4] (articles by Berndt *et al.* and Jamieson, this volume). Previous investigators had shown that thrombin is the only clotting factor that activates platelets.[5] Thrombin stimulates platelet secretion and aggregation in blood at physiologic concentrations (2-5 nM),[5] although an absolute requirement for thrombin in normal platelet function has not been demonstrated. The mechanism by which thrombin activates platelets has not been determined, but there is evidence to suggest that it differs from that of other agonists. Activation is not a simple enzyme-substrate reaction. At low thrombin concentrations, the extent of platelet secretion is proportional to the thrombin concentration. When thrombin is reacted with platelets, most of the thrombin remains free and active in solution, but a small amount is bound to the platelet.[3] On the other hand, the serine active site on thrombin is required for platelet activation.[6] Although the active serine site of thrombin is required for clotting of fibrinogen and activation of platelets, there appear to be separate and distinct fibrinogen and platelet binding sites on thrombin.[7] Furthermore, the mechanisms by which thrombin activates platelets appear to differ depending upon the particular function that is analyzed. When platelets are briefly incubated with thrombin followed by hirudin, platelet aggregation and

TABLE 1. Cell and Tissue Functions Modulated by Thrombin

Proliferation
Fibroblasts
Splenocytes
Secretion
Platelets
Endothelial cells
Prostaglandin Synthesis
Platelets
Endothelial cells
Fibroblasts
Neuronal cells
Chemotaxis
Monocytes
Contractility
Smooth muscle

secretion of dense granule contents continue to completion.[8] Secretion of acid hydrolases and liberation of arachidonate from phospholipids, however, are inhibited. Therefore, it appears that continuous exposure of platelets to thrombin is required for these latter reactions.

Active-site-independent thrombin binding to platelets has been proposed as the first step in activation (TABLE 2). Binding of [^{125}I]thrombin is rapid, specific, saturable, and reversible.[3] There is an excellent correlation between the number of molecules bound to platelets and the extent of platelet secretion.[9] Furthermore, thrombin is unaltered in its reaction with platelets.[10] Equilibrium binding of thrombin to a limited number of platelet receptors has been proposed as the explanation for the observation that the extent of platelet secretion is dependent on the thrombin concentration. Evidence that the receptor described by these kinetics studies may not be involved in activation of platelets comes from experiments in which active site-inhibited thrombin, which binds equally as well as native thrombin, completely inhibits binding of the active enzyme, yet has no effect on platelet secretion induced by the latter.[3] This evidence seems to indicate that the receptor characterized by these binding studies is not responsible for activation of platelets. On the other hand, as will be described in succeeding sections, receptors that bind active-site-independent thrombin have important physiologic functions in endothelium and monocytes.

Subsequently, thrombin has been shown to bind to virtually all types of cells with the exception of erythrocytes. Active-site-independent binding of thrombin to endothelial cells and fibroblasts similar to platelets has been described.[11,12] Thrombin rapidly stimulates prostacyclin and prostaglandin synthesis in endothelial cells at physiologic concentrations.[13] Thrombin also stimulates synthesis of platelet-activating factor,[14] as well as release of von Willebrand factor,[15] tissue plasminogen activator, and inhibitor[16] by vascular endothelium. It is likely that many other biological effects of thrombin on endothelium will be discovered. Binding of thrombin to human umbilical vein endothelium is rapid: maximal within one minute.[11] Like platelets, there are high and low affinity receptors for active-site-inhibited and native thrombin.

An additional type of thrombin binding to endothelium has been described, which occurs only with native and not active-site-inhibited enzyme[17] (TABLE 3). Binding also differs from active-site-independent thrombin binding in that it occurs more slowly. Thrombin forms an M_r = 77 000 complex that appears to be covalent and very similar to the thrombin-antithrombin III complex. The endothelial cell component of the complex has an M_r of approximately 40 000. This type of binding appears to have as its primary function inhibition of excessive protease activity at the cell surface. The receptor that is present on many types of cells, and is not specific for thrombin, will be discussed in greater detail in succeeding sections.

TABLE 2. Active-Site-Independent Thrombin Binding

Rapid
Native and active-site-inhibited enzyme bind equally well
Saturable
Reversible
Specific
High and low affinity receptors
Thrombin unaltered by reaction

IDENTITY OF THROMBIN RECEPTORS (TABLE 4)

There is considerably more information about the identity of thrombin receptors on endothelium than platelets. Initial studies showed that vascular endothelium enhanced the activation of protein C by thrombin.[18] Subsequently, it was shown that rabbit endothelial cells contain an M_r = 74 000 protein, thrombomodulin, on their surface, which binds native and serine-inactive thrombin[19] (Esmon *et al.* and Salem *et al.*, this volume). Binding of thrombin to thrombomodulin is high affinity (K_D = 0.48 nM). Thrombin binds stoichiometrically to this cell-surface protein forming a 1:1 noncovalent complex. Thrombomodulin stimulates activation of protein C by thrombin approximately 1000-fold, and this appears to be its primary physiologic function. Thrombin, however, is also inhibited once it is bound to thrombomodulin. Thus the ability of thrombin to clot fibrinogen, and activate factor V and platelets,

TABLE 3. Active-Site-Dependent Thrombin Binding

Slow
Temperature-dependent
Irreversible component
Two steps
Formation of thrombin-cell protein complex
Binding of complex to cell-surface receptor
Single class of high-affinity receptors

is inhibited once it is bound to thrombomodulin.[20,21] This is presumably due to a conformational change because thrombin dissociated from thrombomodulin has normal activity. The extent of inhibition appears to vary considerably, however, depending on the species from which thrombomodulin is derived. Inhibition is at least 10-fold greater with rabbit, compared to human thrombomodulin.[22] Thrombomodulin appears to be specific for endothelial cells as it has not been detected in other types of cells. It is unknown at this time as to whether thrombomodulin is the receptor on endothelium by which thrombin activates these cells.

Thrombin has also been shown to bind to cell-surface heparan sulfate on vascular endothelium[23] (see Machovich, this volume). When cultured porcine aortic endothelial cells were treated with heparitinase, the amount of high-affinity, active-site-independent thrombin binding was reduced approximately 50 percent. Neither the rate nor affinity of binding was altered. The significance of thrombin binding to heparan sulfate-containing molecules on the cell surface is unclear. Previous studies have suggested that vascular endothelium can accelerate binding of thrombin to antithrombin III.[24] In addition, antithrombin III has been shown to bind specifically to cultured vascular endothelial cells.[25] Thus it has been proposed that thrombin binding to heparan on vascular endothelium accelerates its inactivation by antithrombin III.[24] By contrast, evidence that thrombin binding to endothelium has no affect on its reaction with antithrombin III has also been presented.[26] In addition, once thrombin is bound to thrombomodulin, its ability to bind to antithrombin III is unaltered. The relative contribution of thrombomodulin and glycosaminoglycans to the interaction of thrombin with antithrombin III is unclear. The extent to which either of these cellular compounds is involved in inactivation of thrombin by antithrombin III is unknown.

The specific identity of the receptor-mediating activation of platelets by thrombin has been sought by several groups. Affinity labeling using [^{125}I]thrombin has been one

TABLE 4. Cellular Proteins that Bind Thrombin

Platelets
GP Ib
Thrombospondin
76-kDa protein
200-kDa complex
900-kDa complex
Endothelial Cells
Thrombomodulin
Heparan proteoglycans 77-kDa complex

of the approaches used to study this problem. A 200 000-dalton complex formed between serine-inactive [^{125}I]thrombin and platelets at enzyme concentrations associated with high-affinity binding has been observed using glutaraldehyde as a cross-linking reagent[27] or photo-reactive thrombin.[28] When native enzyme was used, a 120 000-dalton complex was observed.[28] At concentrations of thrombin associated with low-affinity binding, additional complexes were identified of 400 000 and 46 000 daltons.[28] The nature of the platelet component of these complexes has not been determined.

It has also been shown that purified glycocalicin, a platelet membrane glycoprotein, is a competitive inhibitor of thrombin binding to platelets.[29] Moreover, in patients with the Bernard-Soulier syndrome, a disorder characterized by a deficiency of glycoprotein I (GP I) from which glycocalicin is derived, thrombin binding to platelets is reduced.[30] The role of GP I in platelet activation is discussed in greater detail in subsequent chapters (see articles by Berndt *et al.* and Jamieson, this volume).

Thrombin also forms a complex with a secreted platelet protein[31,32] identified as thrombospondin.[33] Thrombospondin is a 420 000-dalton glycoprotein present in platelet α-granules[34] and cultured cells.[35] Based on the inhibitory effect of antithrombospondin antibodies,[36] it is likely that this protein plays a role in platelet aggregation. The consequences of thrombin binding to thrombospondin are unknown. It is known that thrombin and plasmin cleave thrombospondin;[39] thus they have the potential to modify its physiologic activity, although this has not been shown. Many other proteins have also been shown to bind to thrombospondin,[37,38] but their relative affinity versus thrombin for thrombospondin has not been determined. Thus, more information is necessary to assess the significance of thrombin binding to thrombospondin.

Thrombin has also been shown to bind to a 900 000-dalton platelet binding site with a dissociation constant of 0.3 nM.[40] In these experiments, radiation inactivation of platelets at −135°C was used to determine the size of the platelet binding site. Thus the physiologic significance of thrombin binding to platelets first exposed to this temperature is unknown. The large size of the platelet binding site was interpreted as possibly reflecting the interaction of peptides involved in binding.

Additional platelet proteins have been shown to react with thrombin. An M_r = 74 000 protein, purified from a 1% Triton extract of platelets using affinity chromatography with wheat germ agglutinin, was shown to inhibit platelet aggregation by thrombin but not adenosine diphosphate or trypsin.[47] A smaller protein, M_r = 55 000, which copurified with the M_r = 74 000 protein, also inhibited platelet aggregation by thrombin. When, however, the M_r = 74 000 and M_r = 55 000 proteins were incubated together with platelets, there was no inhibition of thrombin-induced aggregation. An antibody against the M_r = 74 000 protein cross-reacted with the M_r = 55 000 protein as well as additional copurifying proteins. Whether the lower molecular mass proteins are degradation products of the M_r = 74 000 protein was not determined. Because the cellular location of these proteins was not determined, it is unknown whether they are on the surface of intact platelets and therefore exposed to thrombin. Furthermore, the relationship of these proteins to glycocalicin, which has also been shown to have thrombin inhibitory activity, was not determined.

REACTIONS FOLLOWING THROMBIN BINDING TO CELL RECEPTORS

Reactions preceding platelet aggregation or secretion triggered by thrombin but not other agonists have not been well characterized. Although thrombin stimulates a variety of metabolic changes in platelets, these reactions occur in response to most agonists. Platelets incubated with chymotrypsin do not respond normally to thrombin.[41] The principal abnormality is a lag period between the time platelets are first incubated with thrombin and secretion. This abnormality occurs in spite of the fact that equilibrium binding of thrombin to chymotrypsin-treated platelets is normal. These experiments indicate a specific event following thrombin binding to platelets that does not occur with other agonists. This event may be cleavage of a cell-surface protein by chymotrypsin; this protein, however, has not been identified.

When platelets are pretreated with thrombin under conditions in which secretion is inhibited, then reexposed to fresh thrombin, there is diminished secretion of serotonin compared to platelets not pretreated with thrombin.[42] Refractoriness to thrombin is dependent on the initial thrombin concentration during pretreatment. The higher the thrombin concentration, the greater the degree of inhibition of secretion on subsequent exposure to thrombin. The inhibitory effect of preincubation with thrombin is not reversible. Inhibition of secretion is specific for thrombin inasmuch as secretion induced by other agonists is unaffected by preincubation of the platelets with thrombin.

Platelets pretreated with thrombin bind thrombin normally. Equilibrium binding of ^{125}I-labeled thrombin to platelets preincubated with unlabeled thrombin that are then washed give virtually identical results to control platelets. Thus the effect of thrombin preincubation does not appear to be due to inhibition of binding. These results differ from those obtained in similar studies on the effect of repeated exposure of a fibrosarcoma cell line to thrombin on prostaglandin synthesis.[43] Refractoriness to thrombin stimulation appears to be due to continued occupancy of thrombin receptors on the surface of the cells after washing because addition of antithrombin III reverses the inhibitory effect.

A likely explanation for the observation that platelets preincubated with thrombin demonstrate a diminished response on subsequent exposure to thrombin is that there are additional thrombin-mediated events following thrombin binding to platelets that are necessary for platelet activation. Evidence for modification of the platelet binding site for thrombin once the thrombin-receptor complex has formed has been presented.[44] When hirudin was added to a thrombin-platelet incubation mixture, initially a rapid and then a slower dissociation rate of thrombin was observed. The longer the interval between preincubation of thrombin with platelets and addition of hirudin, the greater the fraction of bound thrombin that dissociated at the slower rate. The transition to the slower dissociation rate of thrombin was interpreted as representing processing of the platelet receptor.

CELLULAR SUBSTRATES FOR THROMBIN (TABLE 5)

One platelet membrane protein clearly shown to be a substrate for thrombin is glycoprotein V (GP V), M_r = 89 000 (see Berndt *et al,* this volume). When platelets are incubated with physiologic concentrations of thrombin, GP V disappears from the platelet membrane; in addition, a 70 000-M_r glycoprotein appears in the platelet supernatant.[45] The 70 000-M_r glycoprotein has been shown to be the cleavage product of hydrolysis of GP V by thrombin. GP V is a peripheral membrane protein that is cleaved by thrombin and other proteases with similar cleavage specificity. Using an antibody to GP V, immunologically similar material has been found in plasma and serum. Evidence that GP V may be a physiologic substrate for thrombin involved in platelet activation is indicated by the fact that cleavage of GP V occurs several seconds before platelet aggregation at thrombin concentrations as low as 0.01 U/ml. In addition, proteases with similar cleavage specificity cleave GP V and induce platelet aggregation.

McGowan *et al.*[46] reported studies indicating that cleavage of GP V by thrombin may not directly result in platelet activation. These experiments differed from those described above, however, in that hydrolysis of GP V was indirectly measured. Platelet surface glycoproteins were first radiolabeled with tritium. The platelets were then thrombin-activated and the supernatant assayed for the [^{3}H]-labeled cleavage product of GP V. Using this experimental approach, the investigators found that when platelets were pretreated with thrombin, there was decreased reactivity on subsequent exposure to thrombin, although the extent of hydrolysis of GP V was the same in the thrombin-pretreated and control platelets. Thus cleavage of GP V appears to be insufficient by itself to activate platelets. Similarly, when platelets were pretreated with chymotrypsin, the rate of platelet activation by thrombin was unchanged, although the rate of hydrolysis of GP V was markedly diminished. Thrombin-induced secretion of dense granule adenosine triphosphate by platelets occurred when less than 1% of GP V was hydrolyzed. Platelet secretion correlated with the rate of hydrolysis of GP V but not the extent. In any case, the mechanism by which cleavage of GP V results in platelet activation has not yet been defined.

Several groups have studied the effects of thrombin on cell-surface proteins in relation to mitogenesis (see articles by Cunningham and Farrell, Carney *et al.*, and

TABLE 5. Cell Membrane Substrates for Thrombin

Platelet GP V
Endothelial cell coagulation factor V
205-kDa chick embryo fibroblast protein?
43-kDa–45-kDa protein? (mouse splenocytes, fibroblasts)

Wilner and Bar-Shavit, this volume). In 1970, two groups showed that small amounts of trypsin stimulated proliferation of contact-inhibited 3T3 mouse fibroblast or chick embryo fibroblasts.[48,49] The mitogenic effect was dependent on proteolytic activity. Subsequently, thrombin was shown to be mitogenic for chick embryo fibroblasts.[50] Mitogenesis of fibroblasts by thrombin also requires an intact active site. The mechanism by which serine proteases induce cell division appears to involve a reaction on the cell surface, because immobilized trypsin is mitogenic.[51] Trypsin, but not thrombin, cleaves a 250 000-dalton protein as well as two other proteins on chick embryo fibroblasts.[52] Although cleavage of the 250 000-dalton protein was originally assumed to be involved in regulation of cell growth, the absence of an effect of thrombin on this protein has dampened enthusiasm for this concept. A 205 000-dalton protein on chick embryo fibroblasts is not detected after these cells are treated with thrombin or trypsin.[53] The identity of this protein and its function in mitogenesis has not been determined.

Thrombin is mitogenic for mouse splenocytes.[54] Mitogenesis is accompanied by the loss of a 45 000-dalton cell-surface protein. Although it was assumed that thrombin cleaved the 45 000-dalton protein, this was not directly shown. Similar observations have been made with fibroblasts derived from embyronic and foreskin tissue.[55] A 43 000-dalton cell-surface protein is found to decrease when mitogenesis is induced by thrombin. Disappearance of the 43 000-dalton protein was assumed to be due to cleavage by thrombin, although this has not been demonstrated. It was concluded that the 43 000-dalton protein was the cellular receptor for thrombin-induced mitogenesis. A sodium dodecyl sulfate (SDS)-stable 79 000-dalton complex between thrombin and the cell was also found, and it was concluded that the 43 000-dalton cellular membrane protein, which decreased with exposure to thrombin, was actually involved in formation of this complex with thrombin. It was hypothesized that this protein was the receptor for thrombin-induced mitogenesis. This is discussed in greater detail in the article by Cunningham (this volume).

The thrombin-binding protein termed protease nexin[56] is released normally into the culture medium by a variety of cells. The plasminogen activator, urokinase, as well as thrombin also binds to this protein.[57] The resulting complex binds to the cell surface. Some cells then internalize the complex (bovine corneal endothelium and human fibroblast) resulting in degradation of the proteinase by lysosomal enzymes.[2,56]

It is highly unlikely that this protease-binding protein is the mitogenic receptor. The group that originally proposed this concept later proposed that protease nexin served as a negative regulator of mitogenesis by thrombin.[58] It is quite possible, however, that protease nexin actually serves as a cellular inhibitor for endogenous urokinase, which is not mitogenic.[57] It is also possible that the disappearance of the ^{125}I-labeled surface protein is not due to cleavage by thrombin as originally proposed, but rather due to internalization following complex formation with thrombin. The receptor for the protease nexin-enzyme complex has not been identified, but may be a glycosaminoglycan, inasmuch as heparin inhibits binding and protease nexin has a heparin binding site.[59] As cited in the section on endothelial cell receptors, a protein very similar to protease nexin has been described in these cells.[17]

In contrast to thrombin-induced mitogenesis of fibroblasts and splenocytes, induction of proliferation of macrophage-derived cells does not require an intact active site (see Wilner and Bar-Shavit, this volume). Thus, there are at least two different mechanisms by which thrombin is mitogenic.

Plasma coagulation factor V is cleaved by thrombin resulting in its activation.[60] Vascular endothelial cells synthesize factor V[61] and express it on their surface.[62] Previously, we showed that factor V on the endothelial cell surface is activated when prothrombin and factor X_a are incubated with these cells.[62] Factor V activation is due to thrombin generated on the cell surface. By contrast, when thrombin is added directly to endothelial cells, factor V does not appear to be activated.[62] Thus there is a clear-cut difference between the effects of thrombin on cell-surface proteins when it is added to cells compared to when it is generated on the cell surface. This could be due to a difference in receptor binding: endogenous thrombin binding to an inhibitory protein such as thrombomodulin, whereas thrombin generated on the cell surface may bind to a noninhibitory receptor. An alternative possibility is that the receptors for thrombin that are generated on the cell surface are in proximity to factor V, whereas receptors for exogenously added thrombin are not. This aspect of the interaction of thrombin with cell surfaces has not been taken into consideration in previous studies.

SUMMARY

It is clear that there are a number of different types of reactions between thrombin and the cell surface (TABLE 6). In one type, thrombin binds to cell-surface receptors resulting in cellular activation. In other types of reactions, there are at least two components to the thrombin-specific pathway of cellular activation: a classical receptor to which thrombin binds, and a protein that is cleaved. In both types of reactions, thrombin binding and/or proteolysis is linked to changes in GTP-binding proteins, protein kinase C, or other pathways.[63] In most cases, the receptor and membrane substrates involved in cellular activation are not well characterized.

In another type of reaction, the interaction between thrombin and proteins in the extracellular fluid is regulated by cell-surface receptors. Binding of thrombin to these receptors can result in acceleration or inhibition of the reactions with the soluble proteins. In the fourth type of reaction, thrombin cleaves a cell-membrane protein that is involved in reactions with plasma proteins. Recognition of the different types of interactions between thrombin and the cell surface is necessary for the correct interpretation of experimental observations. Although the term receptor has classically referred to a cell-surface component to which an agonist binds, it is now clear that there are additional membrane components that specifically bind potential agonists not leading to cellular activation.

TABLE 6. Thrombin Receptors

Signal Transduction
Binding receptor
+/− Proteolytic Substrate
Inhibition/internalization of thrombin
Modulation of interaction between thrombin and plasma coagulation factors
Acceleration
Inhibition
Substrate for extracellular reactions following cleavage by thrombin

REFERENCES

1. SHUMAN, M. A. & P. W. MAJERUS. 1976. The measurement of thrombin in clotting blood by radioimmunoassay. J. Clin. Invest. **58:** 2249-1258.
2. SAVION, N., J. D. ISAACS, D. GOSPODAROWICZ & M. A. SHUMAN. 1981. Internalization and degradation of thrombin and up-regulation of thrombin binding sites in corenal endothelial cells. J. Biol. Chem. **256:** 4514-4519.
3. TOLLEFSEN, D. M., J. R. FEAGLER & P. W. MAJERUS. 1974. The binding of thrombin to the surface of human platelets. J. Biol. Chem. **249:** 2646-2651.
4. GANGULY, P. 1974. Binding of thrombin to human platelets. Nature (London) **247:** 306-307.
5. SHUMAN, M. A. & S. P. LEVINE. 1978. Thrombin generation and secretion of platelet factor 4 during blood clotting. J. Clin. Invest. **61:** 1102-1106.
6. DAVEY, M. G. & E. F. LUSCHER. 1967. Actions of thrombin and other coagulant and proteolytic enzymes on blood platelets. Nature (London) **216:** 857-858.
7. CHARO, I. F., R. D. FEINMAN & T. C. DETWILER. 1977. Interrelations of platelet aggregation and secretion. J. Clin. Invest. **60:** 866-873.
8. HOLMSEN, H., C. A. DANGELMAIER & H.-K. HOLMSEN. 1981. Thrombin-induced platelet responses differ in requirement for receptor occupancy. J. Biol. Chem. **256:** 9393-9396.

9. SHUMAN, M. A. & P. W. MAJERUS. 1975. The perturbation of thrombin binding to human platelets by anions. J. Clin. Invest. **56:** 945-950.
10. MARTIN, B. M., W. W. WASIEWSKI, J. W. FENTON II & T. C. DETWILER. 1976. Equilibrium binding of thrombin to platelets. Biochemistry **15:** 4886-4893.
11. AWBREY, B. J., J. C. HOAK & W. G. OWEN. 1979. Binding of human thrombin to cultured human endothelial cells. J. Biol. Chem. **254:** 4092-4095.
12. CARNEY, D. H. & D. D. CUNNINGHAM. 1978. Role of specific cell surface receptors in thrombin-stimulated cell division. Cell **15:** 1341-1349.
13. WEKSLER, B. B., C. W. LEY & E. A. JAFFE. 1978. Stimulation of endothelial cell prostacyclin production by thrombin, trypsin, and the ionophore A23187. J. Clin. Invest. **62:** 923-930.
14. PRESCOTT, S. M., G. A. ZIMMERMAN & T. M. MCINTYRE. 1984. Human endothelial cells in culture produce platelet-activating factor (1-alkyl-2-acetyl-sn-glycoro-3-phosphocholine) when stimulated by thrombin. Proc. Natl. Acad. Sci. USA **81:** 3534-3538.
15. DE GROOT, P. G., M. D. GONSALVES, C. LOESBERG, M. F. VAN BUUL-WORTELBOER, W. G. VAN AKEN & J. A. VAN MOURIK. 1984. Thrombin-induced release of von Willebrand factor from endothelial cells is mediated by phospholipid methylation. J. Biol. Chem. **259:** 13329-13333.
16. GELEHRTER, T. D. & R. SZNYCER-LASZYK. 1986. Thrombin induction of plasminogen activator-inhibitor in cultured human endothelial cells. J. Clin. Invest. **77:** 165-169.
17. ISAACS, J., N. SAVION, D. GOSPODAROWICZ & M. A. SHUMAN. 1981. Effect of cell density on thrombin binding to a specific site on bovine vascular endothelial cells. J. Cell Biol. **90:** 670-674.
18. ESMON, C. T. & W. G. OWEN. 1981. Identification of an endothelial cell cofactor for thrombin-catalyzed activation of protein C. Proc. Natl. Acad. Sci. USA **78:** 2249-2252.
19. ESMON, N. L., W. G. OWEN & C. T. ESMON. 1982. Isolation of a membrane-bound cofactor for thrombin-catalyzed activation of protein C. J. Biol. Chem. **257:** 859-864.
20. ESMON, C. T., N. L. ESMON & K. W. HARRIS. 1982. Complex formation between thrombin and thrombomodulin inhibits both thrombin-catalyzed fibrin formation and factor V activation. J. Biol. Chem. **257:** 7994-7947.
21. ESMON, N. L., R. C. CARROLL & C. T. ESMON. 1983. Thrombomodulin blocks the ability of thrombin to activate platelets. J. Biol. Chem. **258:** 12238-12242.
22. MARUYAMA, I., H. H. SALEM, H. I. SHII & P. W. MAJERUS. 1985. Human thrombomodulin is not an efficient inhibitor of the procoagulant activity of thrombin. J. Clin. Invest. **75:** 987-991.
23. SHIMADA, K. & T. OZAWA. 1985. Evidence that cell surface heparan sulfate is involved in the high affinity thrombin binding to cultured porcine aortic endothelial cells. J. Clin. Invest. **75:** 1308-1316.
24. MARCUM, J. A., J. B. MCKENNEY & R. D. ROSENBERG. 1984. Acceleration of thrombin-antithrombin complex formation in rat hindquarters via heparin-like molecules bound to the endothelium. J. Clin. Invest. **74:** 341-350.
25. STERN, D., P. NAWROTH, J. MARCUM, D. HANDLEY, W. KISIEL, R. ROSENBERG & K. STERN. 1985. Interaction of antithrombin III with bovine aortic segments. Role of heparin in binding and enhanced anticoagulant activity. J. Clin. Invest. **75:** 272-279.
26. LOLLAR, P., S. C. MACINTOSH & W. G. OWEN. 1984. Reaction of antithrombin III with thrombin bound to the vascular endothelium. Analysis in a recirculating perfused rabbit heart preparation. J. Biol. Chem. **259:** 4335-4338.
27. TOLLEFSEN, D. M. & P. W. MAJERUS. 1976. Evidence for a single class of thrombin-binding sites on human platelets. Biochemistry **15:** 2144-2149.
28. LARSEN, N. E. & E. R. SIMON. 1981. Preparation and application of a photoreactive thrombin analogue: Binding to human platelets. Biochemistry **20:** 4141-4147.
29. OKUMURA, T., M. HASITZ & G. A. JAMIESON. 1978. Platelet glycocalicin. Interaction with thrombin and role as thrombin receptor of the platelet surface. J. Biol. Chem. **253:** 3435-3443.
30. JAMIESON, G. A. & T. OKUMURA. 1978. Reduced thrombin binding and aggregation in Bernard-Soulier platelets. J. Clin. Invest. **61:** 861-864.
31. MAEROWITZ, T., M. BOTNEY, K. GLENN, D. CUNNINGHAM, L. JOHNSON, J. W. FENTON II & M. SHUMAN. 1981. A new type of thrombin binding to human platelets. Clin. Res. **29:** 339a.

32. SHUMAN, M. A., J. D. ISAACS, T. MAEROWITZ, N. SAVION, D. GOSPODAROWICZ, K. GLENN, D. CUNNINGHAM & J. W. FENTON II. 1981. Endothelial cell and platelet binding sites for thrombin. Ann. N.Y. Acad. Sci. **370:** 57-66.
33. DANISHEFSKY, K. J., R. J. ALEXANDER & T. C. DETWILER. 1984. Formation of a stable complex of thrombin and the secreted platelet glycoprotein G (thrombin-sensitive protein, thrombospondin) by thiol-disulfide exchange. Biochemistry **23:** 4984-4990.
34. BAENZIGER, N. L., G. N. BRODIE & P. W. MAJERUS. 1972. Isolation and properties of a thrombin-sensitive protein of human platelets. J. Biol. Chem. **247:** 2723-2731.
35. JAFFE, E. A., J. T. RUGGIERO, L. K. LEUNG, M. J. DOYLE, P. J. MCKEOWN & D. F. MOSHER. 1983. Cultured human fibroblasts synthesize and secrete thrombospondin and incorporate it into extracellular matrix. Proc. Natl. Acad. Sci. USA **80:** 998-1002.
36. LEUNG, L. L. K. 1984. The role of thrombospondin in platelet aggregation. J. Clin. Invest. **74:** 1764-1772.
37. LEUNG, L. L. K. & R. L. NACHMAN. 1982. Complex formation of platelet thrombospondin with fibrinogen. J. Clin. Invest. **70:** 542-549.
38. SILVERSTEIN, R. L., L. L. K. LEUNG, P. C. HARPEL & R. L. NACHMAN. 1985. Platelet thrombospondin forms a trimolecular complex with plasminogen and histidine-rich glycoprotein. J. Clin. Invest. **75:** 2065-2073.
39. LAWLER, J. W. & H. S. SLAYTER. 1981. The release of heparin binding peptides from platelet thrombospondin by the proteolytic action of thrombin, plasmin and trypsin. Thromb. Res. **22:** 267-279.
40. HARMON, J. T. & G. A. JAMIESON. 1985. Thrombin binds to a high-affinity $\simeq$ 900,000-dalton site on human platelets. Biochemistry **24:** 58-64.
41. TAM, S. W., J. W. FENTON II & T. C. DETWILER. 1980. Platelet thrombin receptors. Binding of α-thrombin is coupled to signal generation by a chymotrypsin-sensitive mechanism. J. Biol. Chem. **255:** 6626-6632.
42. SHUMAN, M. A., M. BOTNEY & J. W. FENTON II. 1979. Thrombin-induced platelet secretion. Further evidence for a specific pathway. J. Clin. Invest. **63:** 1211-1218.
43. BECHERER, P. R., L. F. MERTZ & N. L. BAENZIGER. 1982. Regulation of prostaglandin synthesis mediated by thrombin and B_2 bradykinin receptors in a fibrosarcoma cell line. Cell **30:** 243-251.
44. TAM, S. W., J. W. FENTON II & T. C. DETWILER. 1979. Dissociation of thrombin from platelets by hirudin. J. Biol. Chem. **254:** 8723-8725.
45. BERNDT, M. D. & D. R. PHILLIPS. 1981. Purification and preliminary physicochemical characterization of human platelet membrane glycoprotein V. J. Biol. Chem. **256:** 59-65.
46. MCGOWAN, E. B., A.-H. DING & T. C. DETWILER. 1983. Correlation of thrombin-induced glycoprotein V hydrolysis and platelet activation. J. Biol. Chem. **258:** 11243-11248.
47. CHELLADURAI, M., N. G. FOSSETT & P. GANGULY. 1983. A novel thrombin-reactive protein complex in human platelets. J. Biol. Chem. **258:** 1407-1410.
48. BURGER, M. M. 1970. Proteolytic enzymes initiating cell division and escape from contact inhibition of growth. Nature (London) **227:** 170-171.
49. SEFTON, B. M. & H. RUBIN. 1970. Release from density-dependent growth inhibition by proteolytic enzymes. Nature (London) **227:** 843-845.
50. CHEN, L. B. & J. M. BUCHANAN. 1975. Mitogenic activity of blood components. I. Thrombin and prothrombin. Proc. Natl. Acad. Sci. USA **72:** 131-135.
51. CARNEY, D. H. & D. D. CUNNINGHAM. 1977. Initiation of chick cell division by trypsin action at the cell surface. Nature (London) **268:** 602-606.
52. NELSON, N., H. TENG & L. B. CHEN. 1975. The role of surface proteins in cell proliferation as studied with thrombin and other proteases. Proc. Natl. Acad. Sci USA **72:** 413-417.
53. TENG, N. N. H. & L. B. CHEN. 1976. Thrombin-sensitive surface protein of cultured chick embryo cells. Nature (London) **259:** 578-580.
54. CHEN, L. B., N. N. H. TENG & J. M. BUCHANAN. 1976. Mitogenicity of thrombin and surface alterations on mouse splenocytes. Exp. Cell Res. **101:** 41-46.
55. GLENN, K. C. & D. D. CUNNINGHAM. 1979. Thrombin-stimulated cell division involves proteolysis of its cell surface receptor. Nature (London) **278:** 711-714.
56. LOW, D. A., J. B. BAKER, W. C. KOONCE & D. D. CUNNINGHAM. 1981. Released protease-nexin regulates cellular binding internalization and degradation of serine proteinases. Proc. Natl. Acad. Sci. USA **78:** 2340-2344.

57. Eaton, D. L., R. W. Scott & J. B. Baker. 1984. Purification of human fibroblast urokinase proenzyme and analyses of its regulation by proteases and protease nexin. J. Biol. Chem. **259:** 6241-6247.
58. Low, D. A., R. W. Scott, J. B. Baker & D. D. Cunningham. 1982. Cells regulate their mitogenic response to thrombin through release of protease nexin. Nature (London) **298:** 476-478.
59. Baker, J. B., D. A. Low, D. L. Eaton & D. D. Cunningham. 1982. Thrombin-mediated mitogenesis: The role of secreted protease nexin. J. Cell. Physiol. **112:** 291-297.
60. Papahadjopoulous, D., C. Hougie & D. J. Hanahan. 1964. Purification and properties of bovine factor V: A change of molecular size during blood coagulation. Biochemistry **3:** 264-270.
61. Cerveny, T. J., D. N. Fass & K. G. Mann. 1984. Synthesis of coagulation factor V by cultured aortic endothelium. Blood **63:** 1467-1474.
62. Rodgers, G. M. & M. A. Shuman. 1983. Prothrombin is activated on vascular endothelial cells by factor Xa and calcium. Proc. Natl. Acad. Sci. USA **80:** 7001-7005.
63. Zavdico, G. B., S. P. Halenda, R. I. Sha'afi & M. B. Feinstein. 1985. Phorbol myristate acetate inhibits thrombin-stimulated Ca^{2+} mobilization and phosphatidylinosotiol 4,5 bisphosphate hydrolysis in human platelets. Proc. Natl. Acad. Sci. USA **82:** 3859-3862.

Thrombin Interactions with Cultured Fibroblasts: Relationship to Mitogenic Stimulation[a]

DENNIS D. CUNNINGHAM AND
DAVID H. FARRELL

Department of Microbiology and Molecular Genetics
College of Medicine
University of California
Irvine, California 92717

INTRODUCTION

The mitogenic action of thrombin was first described by Chen and Buchanan in studies on cultured chick embryo fibroblasts.[1] Since then, several investigators have shown that thrombin can stimulate the division of a variety of cultured early passage fibroblast-like cells.[2,3] This response to thrombin is frequently lost as cells are serially subcultured;[3] in fact, many established cell lines are not responsive to its mitogenic action.[4] Although it is difficult to design experiments to directly test the physiological functions of thrombin-stimulated cell division, it is usually assumed that it plays a role in tissue repair because thrombin is produced at sites of tissue injury. Studies on the mitogenic mechanism of thrombin have been facilitated by the ability of highly purified thrombin to stimulate cells in serum-free medium, permitting studies under chemically defined conditions.

Early studies to probe the requirements for thrombin-stimulated cell division revealed that cellular internalization of thrombin is not necessary.[5] In addition, the proteolytic activity of thrombin is required for cell activation inasmuch as thrombin derivatized at the catalytic site serine with a diisopropylphospho-group (DIP)-thrombin is not mitogenic.[6] Together, these results lead to the conclusion that cleavage of one or more cell-surface proteins is necessary for thrombin-stimulated cell division.

The finding that cell-surface action of thrombin is sufficient for mitogenic stimulation[5] has prompted detailed studies on the mechanisms by which it interacts with responsive cells. These studies, summarized below, have revealed that the binding of thrombin differs significantly from the binding of other transmembrane signaling polypeptides.

[a] This work was supported by Grants CA-12306 and GM-31609 from the National Institutes of Health.

THROMBIN BINDS TO CELLS BY WAY OF TWO PATHWAYS

FIGURE 1 diagramatically summarizes our studies on the binding of thrombin to several kinds of cultured fibroblast-like cells. One pathway for thrombin binding involves a protein called protease nexin (PN) that is synthesized and released by a variety of cultured cells.[7–11] PN can form complexes with thrombin as well as several other proteases including urokinase and plasmin. These thrombin:PN complexes then bind back to the cells that release the PN and are rapidly internalized and degraded.

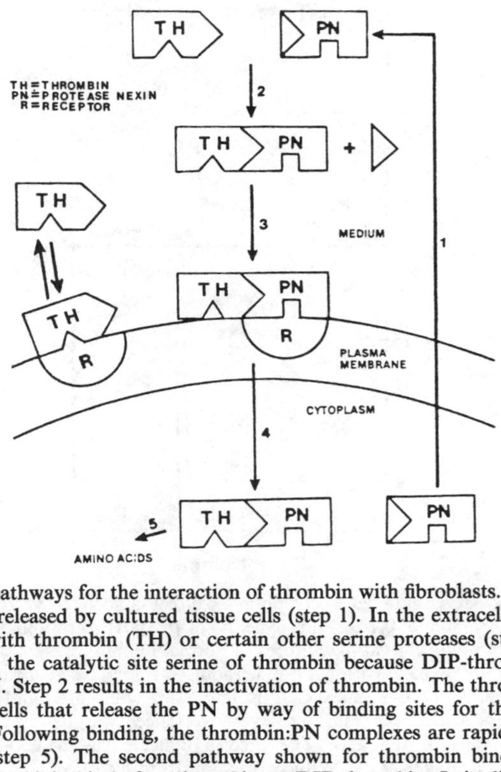

FIGURE 1. Two pathways for the interaction of thrombin with fibroblasts. Protease nexin (PN) is synthesized and released by cultured tissue cells (step 1). In the extracellular environment, it forms complexes with thrombin (TH) or certain other serine proteases (step 2). Formation of complexes involves the catalytic site serine of thrombin because DIP-thrombin does not form complexes with PN. Step 2 results in the inactivation of thrombin. The thrombin:PN complexes bind back to the cells that release the PN by way of binding sites for the PN moiety of the complex (step 3). Following binding, the thrombin:PN complexes are rapidly internalized (step 4) and degraded (step 5). The second pathway shown for thrombin binding involves a cell-surface site that reversibly binds free thrombin or DIP-thrombin. It is different from the site that binds thrombin-PN complexes (summarized from references 6-8).

The thrombin:PN complexes bind to the cells by way of sites for the PN moiety of the complex. FIGURE 1 also shows the second pathway for thrombin binding to cells. This involves another binding site, distinct from the thrombin:PN binding site, to which unlinked thrombin reversibly binds.[6]

The data in FIGURE 2 show how PN was first detected.[7] In this experiment, human foreskin fibroblasts were incubated at 23°C with [^{125}I]thrombin (panel A) or [^{125}I]DIP-thrombin (panel B) with (open symbols) or without (closed symbols) a large excess of unlabeled thrombin. After rinsing away unbound thrombin, the cells were solubilized by boiling in sodium dodecyl sulfate (SDS), and cellular proteins were electrophoresed on SDS polyacrylamide gels. The arrows in each panel show the position of the [^{125}I]thrombin:PN complexes; the lower molecular weight peak comigrated with free thrombin. Remembering that the specific binding of [^{125}I]thrombin is obtained by subtracting the open symbols from the closed symbols, it can be seen from panel A that the [^{125}I]thrombin:PN complexes account for most of the [^{125}I]thrombin binding to these cells. This is because these human fibroblasts have few of the binding sites for unlinked thrombin described above. The data in panel B lead to the important

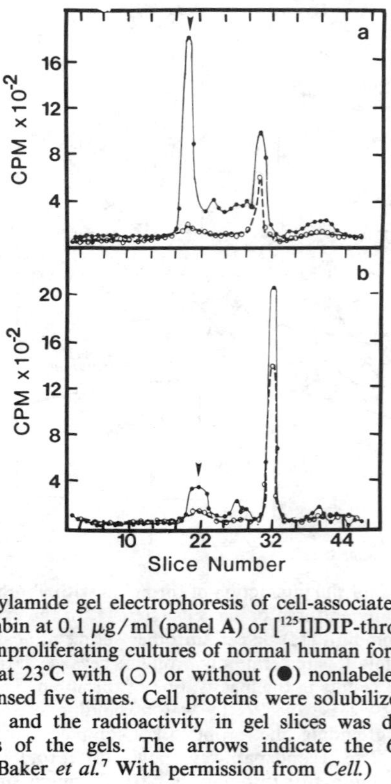

FIGURE 2. SDS-polyacrylamide gel electrophoresis of cell-associated [^{125}I]thrombin and [^{125}I] DIP-thrombin. [^{125}I]thrombin at 0.1 μg/ml (panel A) or [^{125}I]DIP-thrombin at 0.1 μg/ml (panel B) was incubated with nonproliferating cultures of normal human foreskin fibroblasts in serum-free medium for 2 hours at 23°C with (○) or without (●) nonlabeled thrombin at 10 μg/ml. The cultures were then rinsed five times. Cell proteins were solubilized and electrophoresed on SDS-polyacrylamide gels, and the radioactivity in gel slices was determined. Gel slices are numbered from the tops of the gels. The arrows indicate the 68 000-dalton complex of [^{125}I]thrombin:PN. (J. B. Baker *et al.*[7] With permission from *Cell.*)

conclusion that DIP-thrombin cannot bind to cells by way of PN. The small amount of ^{125}I-radioactivity present at the thrombin:PN position was due to a small amount of active thrombin in this DIP-thrombin preparation. The inability of [^{125}I]DIP-thrombin to bind to cells by way of complexes with PN occurs because DIP-thrombin does not form complexes with PN.

The cell-surface binding site for unlinked thrombin can readily be detected using [^{125}I]DIP-thrombin.[6] This binding site is easily measured on chick embryo and mouse embryo fibroblasts as well as a line of Chinese hamster lung fibroblasts; it is much less abundant, however, on human foreskin fibroblasts, as noted above, and not detectable on a subclone of Chinese hamster embryonic fibroblasts. Studies on the binding of [^{125}I]thrombin and [^{125}I]DIP-thrombin to mouse embryo fibroblasts have shown that both thrombin forms bind with about the same affinity; competition experiments indicate that they bind to the same site.[6] Thus, [^{125}I] DIP-thrombin can be used to measure binding to the cell-surface site for unlinked thrombin, and to distinguish the two binding pathways shown in FIGURE 1.

ROLE OF PN IN THROMBIN-STIMULATED CELL DIVISION

To determine if the binding of thrombin:PN complexes to cells was involved in transmitting the mitogenic signal, we took advantage of the finding that added heparin inhibits the cellular binding of the complexes by about 95 percent. In experiments on both human foreskin fibroblasts and mouse embryo fibroblasts, concentrations of heparin that almost completely blocked the binding of thrombin:PN complexes did not significantly affect the thrombin dose-response curve for mitogenic stimulation.[12] Thus, the binding of these complexes appeared not to be involved in activation of the cells by thrombin.

In view of the ability of PN to inhibit the proteolytic activity of thrombin, it seemed likely that PN might modulate the mitogenic response of the cells to thrombin.[13] This was tested directly by the experiment shown in FIGURE 3. Here, purified PN was added along with either epidermal growth factor or thrombin to determine if it affected the mitogenic response. A subclone of Chinese hamster embryonic fibroblasts was used for this experiment that released little PN. The closed symbols show the mitogenic response when the medium was changed to fresh serum-free medium just prior to adding the growth factors; the closed circles show the response in the absence of added PN, and the closed triangles show the response in the presence of added PN. As can be seen, the PN inhibited the mitogenic response to thrombin but not to epidermal growth factor.[13] (The open circles in FIGURE 3 show the mitogenic response to these factors in the presence of serum-free "conditioned" medium; as shown, the response to both thrombin and epidermal growth factor was increased.)

ACCELERATION BY THE FIBROBLAST SURFACE OF THE REACTION BETWEEN THROMBIN AND PN

Another dimension to the complex interactions of thrombin with cultured fibroblasts was unraveled in experiments to determine if the cell surface itself affected the formation of complexes between PN and thrombin. In these studies, [^{125}I]thrombin was incubated with PN in the presence or absence of cells, and the formation of thrombin:PN complexes was monitored by electrophoresing the reaction mixtures on SDS-polyacrylamide gels, cutting out the bands containing [^{125}I]thrombin:PN complexes and assaying radioactivity in a gamma counter. The human foreskin fibroblasts used in these experiments had been rinsed and cultured in serum-free medium for two days to remove residual serum components. They were then fixed in 2.0% paraformaldehyde to prevent release or uptake of materials during the assay.

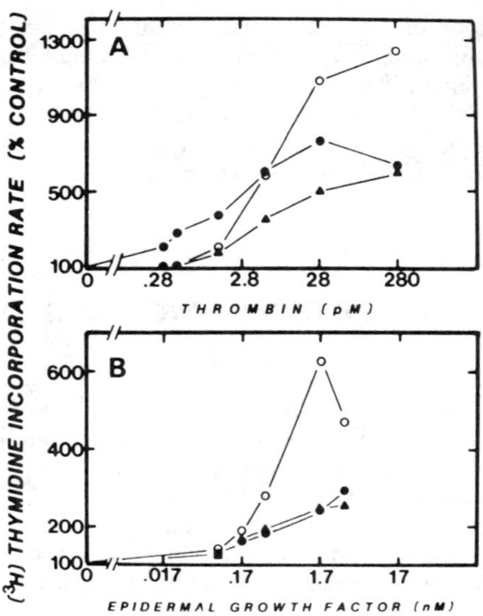

FIGURE 3. Effects of partially purified PN and conditioned medium on the mitogenic response of Chinese hamster embryonic fibroblasts to thrombin and epidermal growth factor. Confluent cultures of cells in medium containing 5% fetal calf serum were rinsed and switched to serum-free medium containing human transferrin (5 μg/ml), bovine insulin (10 μg/ml), fibroblast growth factor (10 ng/ml), and ovalbumin (0.1%). The indicated amounts of thrombin and epidermal growth factor were either added immediately (fresh medium) or after one day of incubation (conditioned medium). Eighteen hours after growth factor addition, the medium was withdrawn and replaced with fresh medium containing [^{3}H]thymidine (1 μC/ml). After two hours of incubation, cell cultures were processed to measure [^{3}H]thymidine incorporated into an acid-insoluble product. Values are expressed relative to control dishes that did not receive growth factor. Additionally, medium that had first been incubated with mitogenic concentrations of thrombin and then with hirudin to inactivate thrombin did not stimulate DNA synthesis (data not shown). These results showed that thrombin must interact with the cells to stimulate them mitogenically. Panel **A**, thrombin. Panel **B**, epidermal growth factor addition to cells in fresh medium (●) or fresh medium with addition of a partially purified fraction of PN (▲), or to cells in conditioned medium (○). (D. A. Low *et al.*[13] With permission from *Nature*.)

The data in FIGURE 4 show that the reaction between PN and thrombin was significantly accelerated by the fixed cells, and was even more accelerated by a membrane fraction prepared from unfixed cells. In view of previous studies which have suggested that PN is well suited for controlling protease activity in interstitial fluid, in contrast to plasma protease inhibitors which likely function in the vascular compartment of the body, we determined if the reaction between thrombin and plasma antithrombin III was similarly accelerated by fibroblasts. The data in FIGURE 4 show that there was no significant acceleration of this reaction by either fixed human foreskin fibroblasts or by membranes prepared from unfixed cells. Together, these results support the hypothesis that the physiological site of PN action is in interstitial fluid at or near the surface of tissue cells. They also indicate that fibroblasts, and perhaps other tissue cells, possess components that enable them to modulate thrombin activity in the extracellular environment.

ROLE OF CELL-SURFACE BINDING SITES FOR FREE THROMBIN IN MITOGENIC STIMULATION

Early experiments on the binding of [^{125}I]thrombin to mouse embryo fibroblasts indicated that this binding was related to mitogenic stimulation.[14] With the information gained from the above studies, however, it was possible to design experiments to more directly test the role in mitogenic stimulation of the cell-surface site that binds both thrombin and DIP-thrombin. From the beginning of these studies, it was clear that simple occupancy of this site is not sufficient for mitogenic stimulation, for DIP-thrombin is not mitogenic.[6]

In view of the finding that thrombin and DIP-thrombin bind to the site for unlinked thrombin with the same apparent affinity,[6] it was possible to add DIP-thrombin under conditions that it competed for the binding of thrombin to these sites and ask if it also competed for mitogenic stimulation.[15] If the mitogenic effect of thrombin occurred by way of these sites, then DIP-thrombin should compete with thrombin for mitogenic

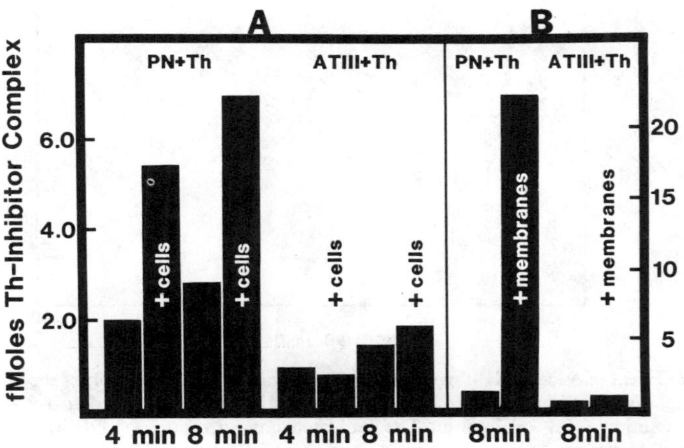

FIGURE 4. Acceleration by human foreskin fibroblasts of complex formation between PN and thrombin. In panel **A**, confluent cultures of cells in medium containing 10% calf serum were changed to serum-free medium for two days. The cells were rinsed three times in phosphate-buffered saline (PBS), fixed for 15 minutes in 2% paraformaldehyde in PBS, and rinsed five times in PBS before use. PN or antithrombin III was added at a final concentration of 2.7 nM to serum-free medium containing 0.1 mg/ml bovine serum albumin; the medium was then added to the cells or to empty culture dishes and warmed to 37°C. [^{125}I]thrombin was added to the cultures at a final concentration of .27 nM and incubated for 4 or 8 minutes. The reaction was stopped by adding an equal volume of SDS electrophoresis sample buffer to the medium. Aliquots were electrophoresed on SDS-polyacrylamide gels, and the gels were dried. The radioactive bands corresponding to [^{125}I]thrombin:PN complexes or [^{125}I]thrombin:antithrombin III complexes were excised, and the radioactivity was determined.

In panel **B**, 500 μg/ml of purified plasma membranes from unfixed human foreskin fibroblasts were incubated in imidazole-buffered saline containing 0.1 mg/ml bovine serum albumin. PN or antithrombin III was added at a final concentration of 14 nM or 140 nM, respectively, and warmed to 37°C. [^{125}I]thrombin was then added at a final concentration of 1.4 nM and incubated for 8 minutes. The reaction was stopped by adding an equal volume of SDS sample buffer; the samples were electrophoresed as described above.

stimulation. This experiment was conducted with mouse embryo fibroblasts as shown in FIGURE 5. The closed circles show the mitogenic response, measured by the increase in cell number, as a function of added thrombin. The closed triangles show the increase in cell number as a function of added DIP-thrombin. It is important to emphasize that the DIP-thrombin is not mitogenic; the increase in cell number seen at 100-fold higher concentrations of DIP-thrombin than thrombin can be accounted for by the fact that this preparation of DIP-thrombin contained 1% active thrombin. The open circles in FIGURE 4 show the mitogenic response when 14 nM DIP-thrombin was added along with the indicated concentrations of active thrombin. Although this concentration of DIP-thrombin occupied over 80% of the binding sites for free throm-

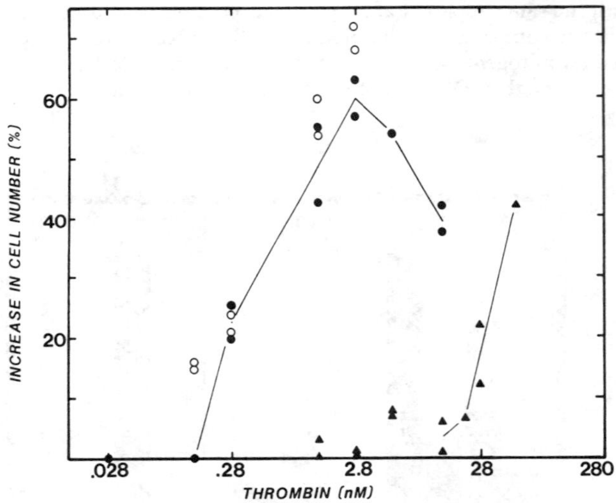

FIGURE 5. Effect of added DIP-thrombin on thrombin-stimulated division of secondary mouse embryo cells. Nonproliferating cells in serum-free medium were switched to fresh serum-free medium containing 0.5% ovalbumin. The indicated concentrations of DIP-thrombin (▲) or thrombin in the absence (●) or presence (○) of 14 nM DIP-thrombin were then added. (The DIP-thrombin employed contained 1% active thrombin.) Cell number was determined using a Coulter particle counter 48 hours after additions were made. Cultures that received no additions contained 7.0×10^{-4} cells/cm^2. (D. A. Low *et al.*[15] With permission from the Cold Spring Harbor Laboratory.)

bin, it can be seen that it did not inhibit thrombin-stimulated cell division. Thus, even though DIP-thrombin competed for most of the thrombin binding, it did not compete for mitogenic stimulation.[15] Studies on a subclone of Chinese hamster embryonic fibroblasts also indicated that the major mitogenic action of thrombin was not mediated by cell-surface binding sites for free thrombin. These cells have only barely detectable levels of these sites, but are the most responsive cell we have found to the mitogenic action of thrombin. Together, these studies do not rule out a role for these thrombin binding sites in mitogenic stimulation, but they indicate that other cellular components mediate the major mitogenic effect of thrombin.[15]

CONCLUSIONS AND FUTURE DIRECTIONS

Our studies on the mechanism by which thrombin interacts with cultured fibroblast-like cells have revealed new information about ways that they control thrombin in their extracellular environment. This occurs mainly by way of PN as summarized in FIGURE 1. Although PN can inhibit several different serine proteases, it inhibits thrombin most rapidly,[11] suggesting that thrombin is a physiological target of it *in vivo.* The finding that the surface of fibroblasts can accelerate this reaction supports the hypothesis that the control of thrombin by PN in the extracellular environment is likely of physiological importance. This control is undoubtedly related to thrombin-stimulated cell division, inasmuch as cultured tissue cells show few other responses to thrombin.

The function of the cell-surface site that binds free thrombin and DIP-thrombin with equal affinity is not clear at this time. The results summarized above have failed to reveal a role for it in thrombin-stimulated cell division.[15] It appears not to be necessary for the mitogenic action of thrombin, because a line of cells that is very responsive to thrombin virtually lacks these sites. These studies do not, of course, rule out a role of these sites in thrombin-stimulated cell division, but they do indicate that other cellular components mediate most of the mitogenic action of thrombin. Of course, thrombin must interact with these components to activate the cells, but the interaction required appears not to be the relative high-affinity binding detected by the usual receptor binding assays.

All evidence to date points to a requirement for cleavage of one or more cell-surface proteins as the primary event in thrombin-stimulated cell division. Other events, such as hydrolysis of polyphosphoinositides to produce diacylglycerol and inositol phosphates,[16,17] may also be required, but they undoubtedly are a consequence of cell-surface proteolysis by thrombin. Efforts to identify cell-surface substrates of thrombin have been limited by available techniques to label and resolve membrane proteins. Accordingly, we have been developing techniques that permit identification of membrane proteins. One technique involves labeling surface proteins to a high specific activity with a sulfated form of the ^{125}I-labeled Bolton-Hunter reagent.[18] Studies with erythrocytes show that surface proteins can be labeled to a very high specific activity by this reagent without labeling hemoglobin and thus cytoplasmic proteins. Another technique to improve identification of membrane proteins involves differential detergent extraction of membrane proteins into four groups that can be separately resolved on long one-dimensional SDS polyacrylamide gels.[19] In our hands, this provides better resolution of membrane proteins than separations on two-dimensional polyacrylamide gels. We are now using these techniques to identify and examine cell-surface substrates of thrombin.

ACKNOWLEDGMENT

We thank John W. Fenton II for gifts of highly purified thrombin.

REFERENCES

1. CHEN, L. B. & J. M. BUCHANAN. 1975. Proc. Natl. Acad. Sci. USA. **72:** 131-135.
2. POHJANPELTO, P. 1977. J. Cell. Physiol. **91:** 387-392.
3. CARNEY, D. H., K. C. GLENN & D. D. CUNNINGHAM. 1978. J. Cell. Physiol. **95:** 13-22.
4. BUCHANAN, J. M., L. B. CHEN & B. R. ZETTER. 1976. Protease-related effects in normal and transformed cells. *In* Cancer Enzymology. J. Schultz & F. Ahmad, Eds.: 1. Academic Press. New York.
5. CARNEY, D. H. & D. D. CUNNINGHAM. 1978. Cell. **14:** 811-823.
6. GLENN, K. C., D. H. CARNEY, J. W. FENTON II & D. D. CUNNINGHAM. 1980. J. Biol. Chem. **255:** 6609-6616.
7. BAKER, J. B., D. A. LOW, R. SIMMER & D. D. CUNNINGHAM. 1980. Cell **21:** 37-45.
8. LOW, D. A., J. B. BAKER, W. KOONCE & D. D. CUNNINGHAM. 1981. Proc. Natl. Acad. Sci. USA **78:** 2340-2344.
9. KNAUER, D. J. & D. D. CUNNINGHAM. 1984. Trends Biochem. Sci. **9:** 231-233.
10. SCOTT, R. W. & J. B. BAKER. 1983. J. Biol. Chem. **258:** 10439-10444.
11. SCOTT, R. W., B. L. BERGMAN, A. BAJPAI, R. T. HERSH, H. RODRIGUEZ, B. N. JONES, C. BARREDA, S. WATTS & J. B. BAKER. 1985. J. Biol. Chem. **260:** 7029-7034.
12. BAKER, J. B., D. A. LOW, D. L. EATON & D. D. CUNNINGHAM. 1982. J. Cell Physiol. **112:** 291-297.
13. LOW, D. A., R. W. SCOTT, J. B. BAKER & D. D. CUNNINGHAM. 1982. Nature **298:** 476-478.
14. CARNEY, D. H. & D. D. CUNNINGHAM. 1978. Cell. **15:** 1341-1349.
15. LOW, D. A., H. S. WILEY & D. D. CUNNINGHAM. 1985. Role of cell-surface thrombin-binding sites in mitogenesis. *In* Growth Factors and Transformation. J. Feramisco, B. Ozanne & C. Stiles, Eds. **3:** 401-408. Cold Spring Harbor Laboratory. New York.
16. CARNEY, D. H., D. L. SCOTT, E. A. GORDON & E. F. LABELLE. 1985. Cell **42:** 479-488.
17. RABEN, D. M. & D. D. CUNNINGHAM. 1985. J. Cell. Physiol. **125:** 582-590.
18. THOMPSON, J. A., A. LAU & D. D. CUNNINGHAM. 1986. Biochemistry. In press.
19. THOMPSON, J. A. & D. D. CUNNINGHAM. 1986. Methods Enzymol. In press.

Thrombin-Receptor Occupancy Initiates a Transient Increase in cAMP Levels in Mitogenically Responsive Hamster (NIL) Fibroblasts[a]

ERIC A GORDON,[b] JOHN W. FENTON II,[c] AND DARRELL H. CARNEY[b]

[b] *Department of Human Biological Chemistry and Genetics*
The University of Texas Medical Branch
Galveston, Texas 77550

[c] *Center for Laboratories and Research*
New York Department of Health
Albany, New York 12201

INTRODUCTION

Highly purified human alpha-thrombin stimulates proliferation of fibroblasts and other cells in serum-free medium.[1–5] Thrombin also stimulates mitogenic responses in mixed lymphocyte cultures[6] and acts synergistically with other growth factors to stimulate certain lines of fibroblasts and endothelial cells.[7,8] There appear to be several similarities in the response of these cells to thrombin and the responses elicited by thrombin interaction with platelets.[9] Yet it is not clear which of these responses are directly related to initiation of cell proliferation.

At least part of the thrombin interaction with fibroblastic cells involves binding to high-affinity receptors that have been characterized by [^{125}I]thrombin binding,[10–12] by a hirudin binding assay,[13] and by immunofluorescent visualization.[14] [^{125}I]thrombin cross-linking studies[15,16] and preliminary immunocharacterization[17] indicate that these receptors are cell-surface proteins with an apparent molecular mass of approximately 150 000 daltons (for review, see ref. 18). These receptors are clustered on the surface of cells prior to thrombin binding[12,14] but are not associated with coated pits or receptor-mediated endocytosis.[12,19] Internalization and degradation of thrombin occurs through a different pathway requiring protease-nexin (PN)-thrombin complex formation,[20] but this pathway does not initiate cell proliferation.[21] Early studies indicated that high-affinity binding of thrombin to its receptors on these cells was involved in initiating

[a] This work was supported by NIH Grants AM-25807 to D. H. Carney and HL-13160 to J. W. Fenton. E. A. Gordon received graduate support from the University of Texas. D. H. Carney is the recipient of a Research Career Development Award (CA-00805) from the NCI.

proliferative events.[10,11] Binding of proteolytically inhibited diisopropylfluorophosphate (DIP)-thrombin to these receptors, however, does not by itself initiate a complete mitogenic response,[22–25] nor does it inhibit initiation by active alpha-thrombin.[24,25] This data has suggested that enzymic activity of thrombin with the receptor or with additional cell-surface substrates is also involved and may be as important as receptor occupancy.

To assess the separate roles of receptor binding and enzymic activity in initiation of cell proliferation, we have examined the effects of proteolytically inhibited DIP-thrombin that binds to high-affinity receptors,[22,23,25] and proteolytically active gamma-thrombin that through limited proteolysis[26] has lost its ability to bind receptors with high affinity.[22,23,25] In previous studies, we have shown that neither the receptor occupancy of DIP-thrombin nor the enzymic activity of gamma-thrombin alone initiate a complete mitogenic signal.[22,23] In combination, however, DIP-thrombin and gamma-thrombin initiate mouse embryo fibroblast cell proliferation to levels approaching the maximal stimulation observed with intact alpha-thrombin.[23,25] This synergistic stimulation is observed when the derivatives are either added at the same time or up to six hours apart.[23] Thus, initiation appears to involve two types of signals: one generated by receptor occupancy, and the other generated by enzymic activity (for reviews, see references 18,25). We, and others, have shown that thrombin stimulates ion fluxes,[27–29] turnover of phosphoinositides,[30,31] and Ca^{++} mobilization (manuscript in preparation) in fibroblasts. In all cases these effects are not stimulated by DIP-thrombin. Thus, these signals appear to be related to the enzymic activity of thrombin rather than to receptor occupancy.

In the present studies, we have discovered that thrombin interaction with fibroblasts stimulates a transient increase in intracellular cyclic adenosine monophosphate (cAMP). Unlike previous signals, this increase in cAMP is caused by addition of DIP-thrombin alone, suggesting that this signal is caused by receptor occupancy-related events. Thus, it appears that the observed requirement for receptor occupany in thrombin mitogenesis may involve regulation of cAMP levels within these cells.

METHODS

Cell Culture

NIL cells are an established strain of hamster fibroblasts provided by Frank Solomon. NIL cells were subcultured and plated onto 60-mm culture dishes or 24-well plates (Falcon Plastics, Becton-Dickson, Oxnard, CA) at a density of 6.0×10^4 cells/cm^2 in a 50:50 mixture of Dulbecco Modified Eagles Medium (DV) and Ham's F12 Nutrient Mixture containing 10% calf serum (Hyclone, Logan, UT). Serum-containing medium was replaced, after 24 hours, with serum-free DV-F12 medium. As described previously, these cultures were then incubated at 37°C for 48 hours in serum-free medium to bring the cells to a quiescent nonproliferative state prior to growth binding or cAMP studies.

^{125}I-Thrombin Binding

Growth-arrested NIL cultures were rinsed with serum-free Dulbecco Vogt (DV)-medium buffered with 15 mM *N*-2-hydroxyethylpiperazine-*N*′2-ethane sulfonic acid

(HEPES), and then equilibrated with DV-HEPES medium containing 0.5% bovine serum albumin (BSA) for 30 minutes. The binding mixtures were added to the culture dishes and incubated for 2 hours as previously described.[10] The dishes were then rinsed in phosphate-buffered saline (PBS), and 0.5 N NaOH was added to solubilize the cells. The total [^{125}I]thrombin bound to the cells was measured by a gamma counter.

cAMP Assay

cAMP levels were determined by radioimmunoassay using a commercially prepared kit (New England Nuclear, DuPont, Boston, MA). Cultures of quiescent fibroblasts in 60-mm dishes were treated with thrombin or various thrombin derivatives at 37°C without changing their serum free medium. After treatments, the medium was removed and cells were rinsed twice with ice cold 5% trichloroacetic acid (TCA). The cells were then freeze-thawed in a dry ice-methanol bath. Later, cells were scraped off the surface of the dish with a rubber policeman, and the cell material was collected in test tubes. The TCA-precipitated cell material was centrifuged out of suspension, and the aqueous supernatent fluid containing the cAMP was collected. Lipid contaminants were extracted with ethyl ether, and the remaining aqueous phase was lyophilized to dryness. This material was resuspended in citrate buffer and used in the radioimmunoassay procedure described by Steiner *et al.*[32]

Thymidine Incorporation

Quiescent cultures of NIL cells, as described above, were treated with the indicated experimental agents. After a 20-hour incubation [^{3}H]thymidine (1 μCi/well) was added to the cultures for 2 hours. After this incubation, the plates were rinsed in cold 10% TCA. Acid precipitable material was solubilized in 0.5 N KOH, and radioactivity was measured by liquid scintillation.

RESULTS

Characteristics of Thrombin Derivatives

Previous studies have described the enzymic properties of alpha-thrombin, gamma-thrombin, and proteolytically inactivated DIP-thrombin.[22,23,33] As shown in TABLE 1, the preparation of highly purified alpha-thrombin used for these studies exhibited approximately 2700 NIH fibrinogen clotting units per mg of protein and was judged to be nearly 100% esterolytically active by active-site titration with *p*-nitrophenyl-*p*-guanidinoate hydrochloride (NPGP). The DIP-inactivated thrombin, prepared by repeated treatment with diisopropylfluorophosphate (DIP) under controlled conditions, exhibited negligible clotting or esterase activity.[33] Gamma-thrombin, prepared by limited autolytic cleavage of the B chain (see Fenton II, this volume), exhibited nearly 50% of its esterolytic activity but less than 1 NIH clotting unit per mg or less than 0.1% of its original fibrinolytic activity. Thus, consistent with previous data, this preparation of gamma thrombin appears to retain enzymic activity, but has totally lost the ability to cleave fibrinogen.

As shown in FIGURE 1, DIP-thrombin and alpha-thrombin compete equally with [^{125}I]alpha-thrombin for binding sites on NIL cells. Because PN-thrombin binding requires formation of aminoacyl complexes between active thrombin and PN, DIP-thrombin, which has no active esterase activity, would not be able to competitively inhibit alpha-thrombin-PN complex formation. Under our binding conditions thrombin and DIP-thrombin compete equally for high-affinity sites on NIL cells. Thus, both alpha and DIP-thrombin bind to high-affinity thrombin receptors with little or no contribution of PN. In contrast to the results with DIP-thrombin, gamma-thrombin addition at concentrations up to 2000 ng/ml shows little, if any, ability to compete with alpha-thrombin for these binding sites. Thus, the affinity of gamma-thrombin interaction with these sites is at least two orders of magnitude lower than that of alpha-thrombin. This suggests that the initial proteolysis of alpha-thrombin that converts it to gamma-thrombin may directly alter the high-affinity binding domain or its molecular conformation. Therefore, as described previously,[23,25] DIP- and gamma-thrombin can be used to distinguish between high-affinity receptor-occupancy generated events (those stimulated by alpha and DIP-thrombin) and events triggered by low-affinity interactions with enzymically active gamma-thrombin.

TABLE 1. Enzymic Activities of Thrombin Preparations[a]

Preparation	Specific clotting activity (Units/mg)	Active-site titration with NPGP (percent active enzyme)
Alpha-thrombin	2747	100
Gamma-thrombin	0.376	48
DIP-thrombin	0.379	(<1%)

[a] Specific clotting activity was determined by measuring fibrin clot formation in a purified fibrinogen solution, and esterase activity measured by active-site titration with *p*-nitrophenyl-*p*-guanidinoate hydrochloride (NPGP) as previously described.[33]

Thrombin Stimulates a Transient Increase in Intracellular cAMP

A number of recent studies have begun to reexamine the possible role of intracellular cAMP in stimulation of cellular proliferation by epidermal growth factor (EGF), platelet derived growth factor (PDGF), and insulin.[34-36] Therefore, in our efforts to define the types of signals that might be involved in initiation of cellular proliferation by thrombin, we examined the effects of thrombin on intracellular cAMP levels in nonproliferating fibroblasts that are mitogenically responsive to alpha-thrombin.

Addition of 250 ng/ml alpha-thrombin to growth-arrested serum-free NIL cell cultures caused an early, transient, increase in the amount of intracellular cAMP

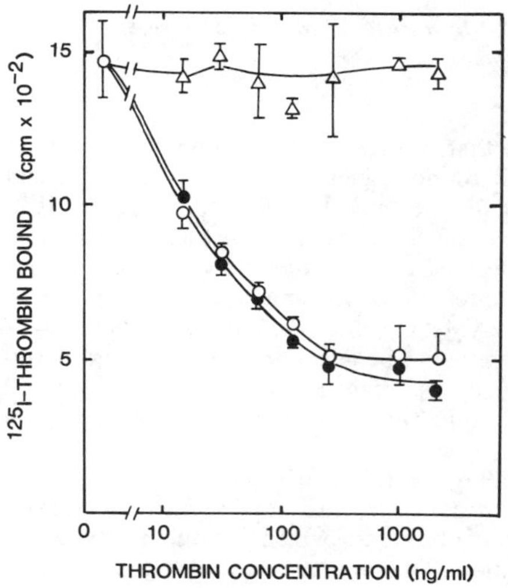

FIGURE 1. [^{125}I]thrombin binding: competition with unlabeled alpha-thrombin or thrombin derivatives. [^{125}I]alpha-thrombin (20 ng/ml) was incubated with quiescent monolayers of NIL cells in the presence of the indicated concentrations of unlabeled alpha-thrombin (●), DIP-alpha-thrombin (○), or gamma-thrombin (△). After 90 minutes, plates were rinsed in phosphate-buffered saline (PBS), and total cell-associated radioactivity was measured as described in METHODS. Error bars indicate +/− one standard deviation from the mean of triplicate determinations.

(FIGURE 2). In four separate experiments we observed a similar temporal increase in cAMP levels, with stimulation ranging from 50 to 200% over controls within 10 minutes of thrombin addition. Shortly after the peak of stimulation, the cAMP levels dropped below resting levels. Interestingly, this transient increase in intracellular cAMP was only demonstrated with thrombin doses that give approximately half-maximal stimulation of cell proliferation in these same cultures. Thus, there may be a link between this transient increase and initiation of cell proliferation.

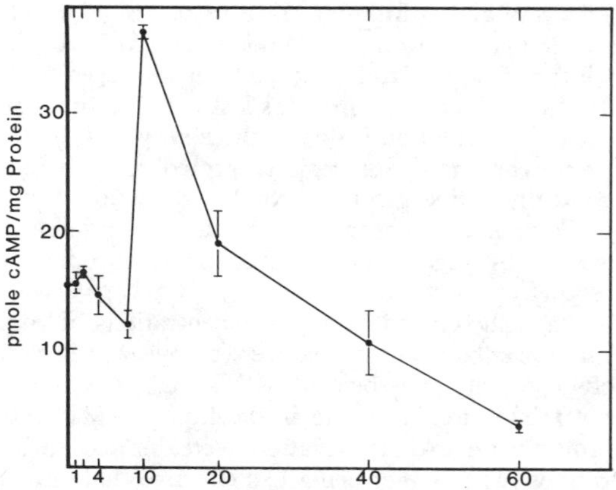

FIGURE 2. Stimulation of transient increase of intracellular cAMP levels initiated by the addition of 60 ng/ml alpha-thrombin. Cells were incubated for the indicated length of time and immediately rinsed and frozen in a dry-ice/methanol bath. cAMP was isolated from freeze-fractured cells and measured as described in METHODS. The error bars represent +/− one standard deviation from the mean of duplicate data points.

Measurement of Intracellular cAMP following Thrombin Derivative Treatment

Our earlier studies have demonstrated that mitogenic stimulation requires both receptor occupancy and enzymic activity.[23] As described above, these activities can be examined separately by using proteolytically inhibited DIP-thrombin that binds to the thrombin receptor with high affinity, and proteolytically active gamma-thrombin that appears to interact with the receptor or other molecules only with an affinity approaching that of an enzyme-substrate interaction. Inasmuch as alpha-thrombin caused a transient increase in intracellular cAMP at mitogenic concentrations, it was important to determine whether this increase could be generated by individual derivatives retaining either receptor occupancy or enzymic activity or whether cAMP increases only resulted from treatment with alpha-thrombin that generated both types of signals.

As shown in FIGURE 3, 30 minutes after treatment of NIL cells with alpha-thrombin, there was a dose-dependent increase in cAMP levels. This increase is maximal at 30 to 60 ng/ml concentrations of thrombin, which stimulate from 30 to 60% of maximal initiation of cell proliferation. The observation that higher concentrations of thrombin did not cause cAMP increases could indicate either that the increase and subsequent decrease in cAMP levels occurs more rapidly at higher concentrations, or that the higher concentrations of thrombin produce other signals that attenuate the increase in cAMP. In additional experiments, where cAMP levels were measured following 5- or 10-minute incubations with thrombin, we observed that the peak of cAMP stimulation occurred with similar doses of thrombin. Thus, at least at these early times, the high concentrations of thrombin do not increase intracellular cAMP. Therefore, the higher concentrations of thrombin may produce other signals that attenuate the increase in cAMP. It is perhaps noteworthy that the thrombin concentration that stimulates increase in cAMP corresponds to the amount of thrombin that approximately half saturates the thrombin receptors on these cells.[10,28]

Similar to the effects of alpha-thrombin, DIP-thrombin addition at concentrations of 30 and 60 ng/ml stimulated a transient increase in cAMP accumulation. As shown in FIGURE 3, this increase was slightly higher than that seen with alpha-thrombin. Because this DIP-thrombin preparation retains less that 1% of its proteolytic activity, it would appear that this stimulation is due to the ability of DIP-thrombin to occupy high-affinity binding sites and not to any residual proteolytic activity. Indeed, as shown in FIGURE 3, enzymically active gamma-thrombin does not stimulate the transient increase in cAMP. Therefore, it appears that the increase in cAMP is caused not by proteolytic cleavage but by high-affinity interaction of thrombin or DIP-thrombin with thrombin receptors.

Previous studies have shown that similar concentrations of gamma-thrombin activate ion fluxes[28] and phosphoinositide turnover (manuscript in preparation) in these cells. Thus, proteolytic activity is associated with signal generation in these cells, but these signals are not related to the rise in intracellular cAMP. As noted above, the effects of alpha-thrombin on cAMP elevation were limited to a narrow range of thrombin concentrations, with higher being less effective than low mitogenic concentrations. This raised the possibility that thrombin might generate both positive and negative signals that regulate intracellular cAMP.

Interestingly, the highest stimulation of cAMP was observed following addition of DIP-thrombin, which does not activate phosphoinositide turnover. Alpha-thrombin stimulation was somewhat lower than that of DIP-thrombin and more rapidly attenuated at higher concentrations, whereas gamma-thrombin did not stimulate at all.

This may suggest that there is some type of feed-back regulation between the signals generated by receptor occupancy and proteolysis. Because initiation of cell proliferation by thrombin requires both types of signals, it is possible that both the early stimulation and rapid attenuation of the cAMP response represents important steps in completing the proliferative signal.

Effects of Artificial Elevation of Intracellular cAMP

To further evaluate the possible role of cAMP in initiation of cell proliferation, we tried several experiments to artificially increase intracellular cAMP levels to determine if such increases could augment thrombin-stimulated mitogensis. Consistent

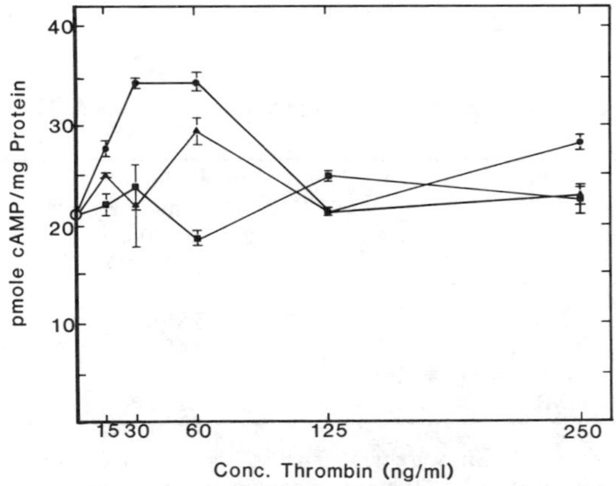

FIGURE 3. Effect of thrombin derivatives on intracellular cAMP levels over indicated concentration of thrombin at 30 minutes after thrombin addition. Alpha-thrombin (▲) and DIP-alpha-thrombin (●) both stimulate an increase in cAMP levels, whereas gamma-thrombin (■) was ineffective at stimulating cAMP levels. Error bars represent +/− standard deviation from the mean of duplicate data points.

with the findings of other investigators,[37] long-term exposure to drugs elevating cAMP appeared to have inhibitory rather than stimulatory effects. Addition and continuous exposure to cholera toxin, at 100 ng/ml, to activate adenylate cyclase, completely inhibited alpha-thrombin-dependent stimulation of thymidine incorporation (data not shown). Long-term exposure of cells to inhibitors of phosphodiesterase (*e.g.,* theophylline and 3-isobutyl-1-methylxanthine (IBMX)) also caused a decrease in thrombin-stimulated DNA synthesis. Finally, the addition of cAMP analogue such as dibutyryl cAMP, 8′-Br cAMP, and monobutyryl cAMP, all seem to attenuate thymidine incorporation in a dose-dependent manner when left on the cells for the duration of the experiment (TABLE 2). In all cases thrombin stimulation was inhibited approximately 60% by addition of cAMP analogues at 1 mM. Thus, exposure of cells to drugs that increase intracellular cAMP for extended periods blocks the ability of thrombin to stimulate DNA synthesis. This suggests that both elevation and attenuation of the cAMP signal may be important factors in initiating cell proliferative events.

To more nearly simulate a transient rise in intracellular cAMP, we carried out additional experiments in which cells were exposed to cAMP derivatives or IBMX for a brief period and then switched to medium containing alpha-thrombin or gamma-thrombin. Under these conditions, elevation of cAMP appeared to cause a slight enhancement of initiation by either low concentrations of alpha-thrombin or gamma-thrombin (data not shown). If one assumes the most simplistic model of two signals stimulating cell proliferation (one, a receptor occupancy-related increase in cAMP and the second, a proteolytically activated increase in phosphoinositide turnover), it might be expected that this experiment should duplicate the synergistic stimulation observed in previous studies, when DIP-thrombin and gamma-thrombin are added to cells. That we only see a slight enhancement by artificially elevating cAMP may indicate that we cannot manipulate cAMP levels well enough to simulate natural cell regulation or that additional signals generated by receptor occupancy are also required for cell proliferation.

TABLE 2. Effect of cAMP Analogues on Thrombin-Stimulated Thymidine Incorporation[a]

	Stimulation of [^{3}H]thymidine incorporation ($\times 10^{-3}$ CPM)	Inhibition by cAMP (percent)
Alpha-thrombin (250 ng/ml)	5.96	—
Dibutyryl cAMP (1 mM) + Thr[b]	2.45	59%
Monobutyryl cAMP (1 mM) + Thr	2.35	61%
8′-Br cAMP (1 mM) + Thr	2.15	64%

[a] Quiescent cultures of NIL cells were treated with thrombin alone or thrombin in the presence of various cAMP derivatives. After 20 hours of continuous exposure, [^{3}H]thymidine was added to cultures, and incorporation into acid-precipitable material was measured as described in METHODS. [^{3}H]thymidine incorporation is expressed as thrombin-stimulated incorporation above control levels (1600 CPM).

[b] Thr = thrombin.

DISCUSSION

Initiation of fibroblastic cell proliferation by human alpha-thrombin appears to require two types of cellular interactions, one involving high-affinity binding with thrombin receptors, and the other involving enzymic activity. In previous studies, we have shown that a complete mitogenic signal can be generated by the addition of both proteolytically inhibited DIP-thrombin, which exhibits high-affinity binding, and gamma-thrombin, which retains esterase activity but not high-affinity binding.[23,25] Thus, whereas neither of the derivatives alone are mitogenic in combination they can stimulate cell proliferation to levels similar to alpha-thrombin. We have used these derivatives to study the nature of the two types of required signals and to establish which signal events are necessary or sufficient to commit cells to enter a proliferative cycle. We now report that alpha-thrombin and DIP-inhibited thrombin both cause a transient increase in intracellular cAMP shortly after their addition to NIL fibroblasts. Gamma-thrombin, however, does not increase cAMP. This indicates that high-affinity binding, and not proteolysis generates this early increase in cAMP.

Double-Signal Hypothesis

Because both binding and proteolytic activity of the thrombin molecule seem to be necessary for the stimulation of cell division, we have proposed a double-signal hypothesis model for thrombin mitogenesis,[25] and have used this model to further study the nature of these signals. This model is shown in FIGURE 4. Previously we have reported that alpha-thrombin stimulates the turnover of phosphoinositides as a necessary part of its mitogenic stimulation.[30] More recently we have discovered that gamma-thrombin also stimulates phosphoinositide turnover, whereas DIP-thrombin does not (manuscript in preparation). Similarly, both alpha-thrombin and gamma-thrombin stimulate Ca^{++} mobilization from intracellular stores, whereas DIP-thrombin does not. Therefore, interaction of alpha-thrombin or gamma-thrombin with cells may cleave part of the receptor or an adjacent substrate, thereby activating phosphoinositide turnover. This causes both release of diacyl glycerol (DAG) and inositol trisphosphate (IP_3). DAG can activate protein kinase C, and IP_3 may cause mobilization of intracellular stores of Ca^{++}.[38] Recent studies have indicated that phorbol esters that stimulate protein kinase C activate the Na^+/H^+ antiport.[39]

Previous studies in our laboratory have shown that amiloride, which blocks Na^+/H^+ antiport, inhibits progression of cells into a proliferative cycle.[27] Other studies have also shown that in the absence of a chloride/bicarbonate exchange, amiloride-sensitive Na^+/H^+ antiport is necessary to increase intracellular pH and allow cell progression.[40] Thus, it would appear that stimulation of Na^+/H^+ antiport is necessary for initiation. We have also found that both alpha-thrombin and gamma-thrombin both stimulate Na^+/H^+ antiport-dependent activation of Na^+/K^+-ATPase, whereas DIP-thrombin does not.[28] Thus, these studies suggest that this part of the signal is also generated by the proteolytic activity of thrombin.

That all of these earlier-identified signals appeared to be generated by potential proteolytic cleavage led us to question the role of high-affinity binding in completion of the mitogenic signal. As described above, stimulation of cell proliferation in our system requires both receptor occupancy and enzymic activity. To further test the requirement for high-affinity receptor interaction, we have recently prepared monoclonal antibodies to the thrombin receptor[17] and synthesized peptides, based on the prothrombin amino acid sequence, that contain the high-affinity binding domain of thrombin (manuscript submitted). Both of these molecules compete with alpha-thrombin for receptor binding and, like DIP-thrombin, are not by themselves mitogenic. In combination with gamma-thrombin, however, both the monoclonal antibody and the peptide produce a synergistic stimulation of DNA synthesis and cell proliferation (manuscript in preparation). Thus, these experiments also demonstrate a requirement in this system for both proteolytic activation and high-affinity receptor interaction. The present results demonstrating that high-affinity interactions of alpha- or DIP-thrombin with receptors causes an increase in intracellular cAMP indicate that this stimulation may be at least part of the required high-affinity occupancy-dependent signal (see FIGURE 4).

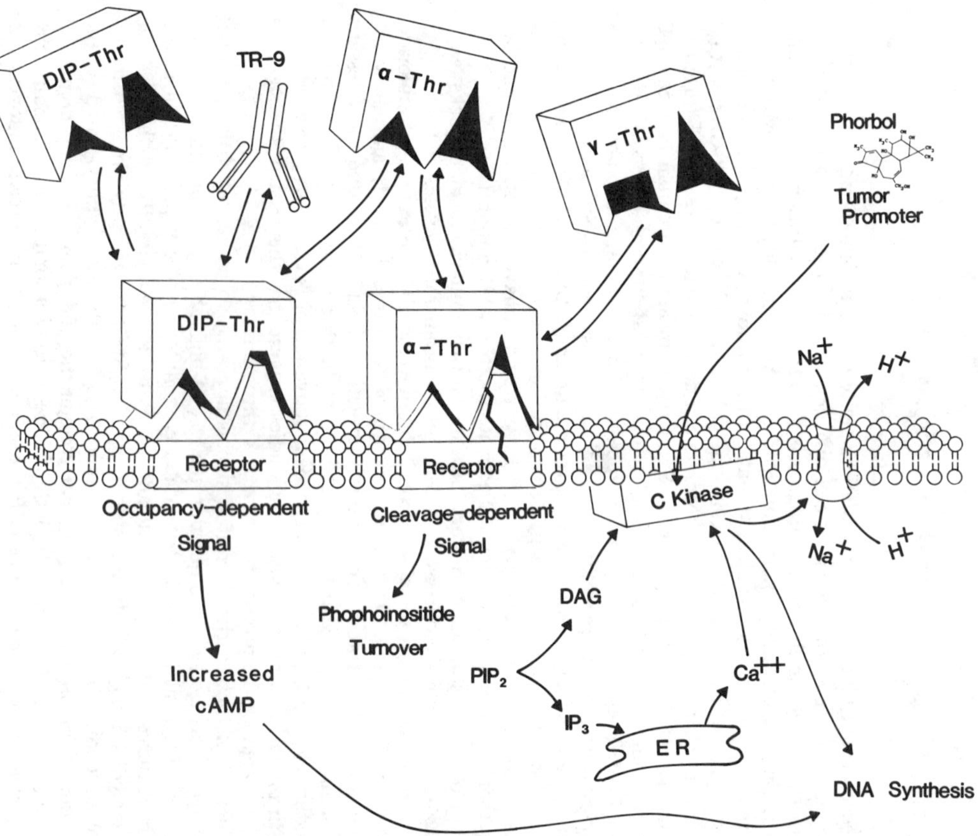

FIGURE 4. Model of double-signal hypothesis of thrombin-stimulated initiation of cell proliferation. Our investigations indicate that both high-affinity receptor occupancy as well as enzymic activity are involved in thrombin initiation of cell proliferation (see text for details).

Other investigators have suggested that high-affinity binding of thrombin is not required for mitogenesis.[16,24] Part of their conclusions are based on the inability of inactive thrombin to block stimulation of cell proliferation by alpha-thrombin. We recently have shown that there is a rapid on-off exchange between alpha and DIP-thrombin.[25] Thus, active thrombin could transiently occupy the receptors, cleaving the receptor or a nearby substrate. Therefore, this type of experiment does not fully address the requirements of receptor occupancy. Another line of evidence against the requirement for receptor occupancy comes from studies with a selected line of hamster Chef IIC9 cells, which are extremely responsive to thrombin yet appear to express very few high-affinity binding sites.[24] Because these cells were initially selected for thrombin responsiveness, it is possible that they have altered thrombin receptors, which may only bind thrombin with low affinity, or have altered downstream signals that mimic or bypass the need for high-affinity receptor occupancy. Thus, in these selected cells receptor occupancy may play a minor role relative to the proteolytic activation of phosphoinositide turnover and other related signals.

Role of cAMP in Thrombin Mitogenesis

The involvement of cAMP in the regulation of cell growth has been investigated for several years. Initially, cAMP was described as an inhibitor of cell division. Otten *et al.*[41] and Pardee[37] described mouse 3T3 cells with low cAMP levels during logarithmic growth, but the concentration of cAMP increased with cessation of growth at confluency. Furthermore, transformed cell lines show lower basal cAMP concentration[42] when compared to their untransformed parents. There was also an early indication that cAMP acts in combination with cyclic guanosine monophosphate (cGMP) to form a dualistic control of cell growth. Quiescent cells express high cAMP concentration and low cGMP, but upon initiation this situation reverses, yielding low cAMP and high cGMP levels.[43,44] This theory, also known as the Yin-Yang hypothesis, suggests that cAMP and cGMP act in opposition to each other for a more precise control of mitogenesis. Snider *et al.*[45] have recently shown that thrombin interaction with neuroblastoma cells stimulates an increase in cGMP. Therefore, it is possible that cGMP effects may also play a role in thrombin mitogenesis in these cells.

More recent findings suggest that cAMP may play a stimulatory role at certain stages of the cell cycle, but at other times may be inhibitory, especially at high concentrations. Rozengurt has shown that increasing intracellular cAMP acts synergistically with an array of growth factors and drugs to stimulate cell growth in mouse 3T3 cells.[34,35] Similarly, Wharton *et al.*[36] have indicated that the elevation of intracellular cAMP in BALB/c-3T3 cells enhances the competence-forming activity of PDGF, making the cells more sensitive to the mitogenic stimulation of EGF. In this same system, cholera toxin, effectively an irreversible activator of adenylate cyclase, or long-term exposure to monobutyryl cAMP, inhibits EGF stimulation. If monobutyryl cAMP is exposed to the cells for only a short period, however, EGF effectively stimulates growth.[46] Thus, some event in the G_0/G_1 phase of the cell cycle may require high cAMP levels for commitment and progression of cells into the S phase, whereas prolonged high levels of cAMP may be inhibitory.

Our results show that thrombin addition to quiescent fibroblasts stimulates an early transient increase in intracellular cAMP for these cells. We also found that long-term exposure of cells to cAMP derivatives, cholera toxin, or IBMX blocked the ability of thrombin to stimulate DNA synthesis. Thus, it is possible that increased cAMP plays both stimulatory and inhibitory roles depending upon the duration or timing of the increase. Consistent with this hypothesis, Bar-Shavit and Wilner have found that a one-hour treatment of quiescent cells with dibutyryl cAMP enhanced the ability of thrombin to stimulate thymidine incorporation (R. Bar-Shavit, personal communication). We have attempted to reconstitute a complete mitogenic signal using alpha-thrombin and a short exposure to cAMP derivatives or agents such as IBMX to transiently increase intracellular cAMP. In these experiments, we see an additive stimulatory effect on thymidine incorporation, but not the full synergistic stimulation that can be achieved by the addition of DIP- and gamma-thrombin. These results, therefore, suggest either that additional signals or metabolic events may be involved in completion of the occupancy-dependent portion of the mitogenic signal, or that the natural increase in cAMP stimulated by receptor occupancy are more precisely controlled.

It has been suggested that cAMP inhibits mitogenic stimulation in growth-arrested cells by blocking necessary increases in intracellular Ca^{++}, but that growth factors can overcome this blockade by alternate mechanisms.[47] This follows from the findings of Pardee[37] and Otten[41] that cAMP inhibits progression of cells from G_1 to S phase. Growth factors may introduce the required Ca^{++} by other mechanisms such as mobilization of Ca^{++} from intracellular stores. Furthermore, the elevated level of Ca^{++} may cause a drop in cAMP by inhibiting adenylate cyclase or activating phosphodiesterase. Interestingly, we have shown that proteolytically active alpha- or gamma-thrombin stimulate Ca^{++} mobilization, but DIP-thrombin does not (manuscript in preparation). It is therefore possible that this rise in Ca^{++} may explain the inability of gamma-thrombin to stimulate increases in intracellular cAMP.

It is interesting that in our analysis of the effects of thrombin derivatives on intracellular cAMP, DIP-thrombin-stimulated cells had higher levels of cAMP than cells stimulated with alpha-thrombin, whereas gamma-thrombin-treated cells had cAMP levels slightly lower than controls. Inasmuch as both alpha- and gamma-thrombin stimulate Ca^{++} mobilization, it is possible that this increase in Ca^{++} acts to attenuate the increase in intracellular cAMP caused by receptor occupancy-related events. Because GTP binding proteins appear to be involved in both activation of adenylate cyclase and growth-factor stimulation of phospholipase C,[48] it has been suggested that there may be a more direct feedback regulation of these two signals.[49]

Our discovery that thrombin-receptor occupancy by DIP-thrombin or alpha-thrombin stimulates an early transient increase in intracellular cAMP, linked to earlier studies showing a need for both receptor occupancy and proteolytic activity, suggests that this increase in cAMP may be necessary for thrombin stimulation of cell proliferation. Our inability to reconstitute a complete mitogenic signal with gamma-thrombin and artificially elevated intracellular cAMP suggests that additional signal events may be required to allow progression of cells towards entry into a proliferative cycle.

SUMMARY

Previous studies from our laboratory have shown that thrombin mitogensis requires both high-affinity receptor occupancy and enzymic activity. Combined addition of DIP-inactivated-thrombin, which retains the ability to bind to thrombin receptors, and enzymically active gamma-thrombin generates a complete set of signals sufficient to initiate cell proliferation. Several possible signals, including stimulation of ion fluxes and phosphoinositide turnover, appear to be stimulated by thrombin's enzymic activity, but not by receptor occupancy. We now report that alpha-thrombin and DIP-thrombin stimulate an early, transient increase of 60 to 200% in intracellular levels of cAMP. This stimulation occurs at low mitogenic concentrations of alpha-thrombin where less than half the receptors are occupied. Enzymically active gamma-thrombin, which stimulates other types of signals, has no stimulatory effects on cAMP. Thus, this effect appears to be generated by high-affinity interaction of thrombin with its cell-surface receptors. Artificially increasing cAMP levels within these cells, however, cannot replace the requirement for thrombin-receptor occupancy in completing the mitogenic stimulation. Therefore, thrombin-receptor occupancy may generate additional, as yet unidentified, required signals.

REFERENCES

1. CHEN, L. B. & J. M. BUCHANAN. 1975. Mitogenic activity of blood components. I. Thrombin and prothrombin. Proc. Natl. Acad. Sci. USA **72:** 131-135.
2. CARNEY, D. H., K. C. GLENN & D. D. CUNNINGHAM. 1978. Conditions which affect initiation of animal cell division by trypsin and thrombin. J. Cell. Physiol. **95:** 13-22.
3. POHJANPELTO, P. 1978. Stimulation of DNA synthesis in human fibroblasts by thrombin. J. Cell. Physiol. **95:** 189-194.
4. ZETTER, B. R., L. P. CHEN & J. M. BUCHANAN. 1977. Binding and internalization of thrombin by normal and transformed chick cells. Proc. Natl. Acad. Sci. USA **74:** 596-600.
5. PEREZ-RODRIQUEZ, R., A. FRANCHI & J. POUYSSEGUR. 1981. Growth factor requirements of Chinese hamster fibroblasts in serum-free media: High mitogenic action of thrombin. Cell Biol. Int. Rep. **5:** 347-357.
6. CHEN, L. B., N. N. H. TENG & J. M. BUCHANAN. 1976. Mitogenicity of thrombin and surface alterations on mouse splenocytes. Exp. Cell Res. **101:** 41-46.
7. ZETTER, B. R. & H. N. ANTONIANDES. 1979. Stimulation of human vascular endothelial cell growth by platelet-derived growth factor and thrombin. J. Supramol. Struct. **11:** 361-370.
8. CHERINGTON, P. V. & A. B. PARDEE. 1980. Synergistic effects of epidermal growth factor and thrombin on the growth stimulation of diploid Chinese hamster fibroblasts. J. Cell. Physiol. **105:** 25-32.
9. CHAMBARD, J-C. & J. POUYSSEGUR. 1983. Thrombin-induced protein phosphorylation in resting platelets and fibroblasts: Evidence for common post-receptor molecular events. Biochem. Biophysics Res. Comm. **111:** 1034-1044.
10. CARNEY, D.H. & D. D. CUNNINGHAM. 1978. Role of specific cell surface receptors in thrombin-stimulated cell division. Cell **15:** 1341-1349.
11. PERDUE, J. F., W. LUBENSKYI, E. KIVITY, S. A. SONDER & J. W. FENTON II. 1981. Protease mitogenic response of chick embryo fibroblasts and receptor binding/processing of human alpha-thrombin. J. Biol. Chem. **256:** 2767-2776.
12. CARNEY, D. H. & J. S. BERGMANN. 1982. ^{125}I-Thrombin binds to clustered receptors on noncoated regions of mouse embryo cell surfaces. J. Cell Biol. **95:** 697-703.
13. LOW, D. A. & D. D. CUNNINGHAM. 1982. A novel method for measuring cell surface-bound thrombin. J. Biol. Chem. **257:** 850-858.
14. CARNEY, D. H. 1983. Immunofluorescent visualization of specifically bound thrombin reveals cellular heterogeneity in number and density of preclustered receptors. J. Cell. Physiol. **117:** 297-307.
15. MOSS, M., S. H. WILEY, J. W. FENTON II & D. D. CUNNINGHAM. 1983. Photoaffinity labeling of specific alpha thrombin binding sites on Chinese hamster lung cells. J. Biol. Chem. **258:** 3996-4002.

16. VAN OBBERGHEN-SHILLING, E., J. POUYSSEGUR. 1985. Affinity labeling of high-affinity alpha-thrombin binding sites on the surface of hamster fibroblasts. Biochim. Biophys. Acta **847:** 335-343.
17. HERBOSA, G., W. C. THOMPSON & D. H. CARNEY. 1984. Thrombin receptor characterization by monoclonal antibodies. J. Cell. Biochem. **8A:** 237.
18. CARNEY, D. H. 1987. Characterization of the thrombin receptor and its involvement in initiation of cell proliferation. *In* Control of Animal Cell Proliferation, Vol. 2. Boyton and Leffert, Eds.: **10:** 265-296. Academic Press. In press.
19. BERGMANN, J. S. & D. H. CARNEY. 1982. Receptor bound thrombin is not internalized through coated pits in mouse embryo cells. J. Cell. Biochem. **20:** 247-258.
20. KNAUER, D. J. & D. D. CUNNINGHAM. 1984. Protease nexin: Cell-secreted proteins which regulate extracellular serine proteases. Trends Biol. Sci. **149:** 231-233.
21. LOW, D. A., J. B. BAKER, W. C. KOONCE & D. D. CUNNINGHAM. 1981. Released protease-nexin regulates cellular binding, internalization, and degradation of serine proteases. Proc. Natl. Acad. Sci. USA **78:** 2340-2344.
22. GLENN, K. C., D. H. CARNEY, J. W. FENTON II & D. D. CUNNINGHAM. 1980. Thrombin active site regions required for fibroblast receptor binding and initiation of cell division. J. Biol. Chem. **255:** 6609-6616.
23. CARNEY, D. H., J. STIERNBERG & J. W. FENTON II. 1984. Initiation of proliferative events by human thrombin requires both receptor binding and enzymic activity. J. Cell. Biochem. **26:** 181-195.
24. LOW, D. A., H. S. WILEY & D. D. CUNNINGHAM. 1985. Role of cell-surface thrombin-binding sites in mitogenesis. *In* Cancer Cells 3/ Growth factors and transformations. pp. 401-408. Cold Spring Harbor Laboratory. New York.
25. CARNEY, D. H., G. J. HERBOSA, J. STIERNBERG, J. S. BERGMANN, E. A GORDON, D. L. SCOTT & J. W. FENTON II. 1986. Double signal hypothesis for thrombin initiation of cell proliferation. *In* Seminars in Thrombosis Research. **12:** 231-240.
26. SONDER, S. A. & J. W. FENTON II. 1984. Proflavin binding within the fibrinopeptide groove adjacent to the catalytic site of human alpha-thrombin. Biochemistry **23:** 1818-1823.
27. STIERNBERG, J., E. F. LABELLE & D. H. CARNEY. 1983. Demonstration of a late amiloride-sensitive event as a necessary step in initiation of DNA synthesis by thrombin. J. Cell. Physiol. **117:** 272-281.
28. STIERNBERG, J., D. H. CARNEY, J. W. FENTON II & E. F. LABELLE. 1984. Initiation of DNA synthesis by human thrombin: Relationship between receptor binding, enzymic activity and stimulation of $^{86}Rb^+$ influx. J. Cell. Physiol. **120:** 289-295.
29. POUYSSEGUR, J., J. C. CHAMBARD, A. FRANCHI, S. PARIS & E. VAN-OBBERGHEN-SHILLING. 1982. Growth factor activation of an amiloride-sensitive Na^+/H^+ exchange system in quiescent fibroblasts: Coupling to ribosomal protein S6 phosphorylation. Proc. Natl. Acad. Sci. USA **79:** 4492-4495.
30. CARNEY, D. H., D. L. SCOTT, E. A GORDON & E. F. LABELLE. 1985. Phosphoinositides in mitogenesis: Neomycin inhibits thrombin-stimulated phosphoinositide turnover and initiation of cell proliferation. Cell **42:** 479-488.
31. RABEN, D. M. & D. D. CUNNINGHAM. 1985. Effects of EGF and thrombin on inositol-containing phospholipids of cultured fibroblasts: Stimulation of phosphatidylinositol synthesis by thrombin but not EGF. J. Cell. Physiol. **125:** 582-590.
32. STEINER, A. L., C. W. PARKER & D. M. KIPNIS. 1972. Radioimmunoassay for cyclic nucleotides: I. Preparation of antibodies and iodinated cyclic nucleotides. J. Biol. Chem. **247:** 1106-1113.
33. FENTON II, J. W., M. J. FASCO, A. B. STACKROW, D. L. ARONSON, A. M. YOUNG & J. S. FINLAYSON. 1977. Human thrombins. Production, evaluation, and properties of alpha-thrombin. J. Biol. Chem. **252:** 3587-3598.
34. ROZENGURT, E., A. LEGG, G. STRANG & N. COURTENAY-LUCK. 1981. Cyclic AMP: A mitogenic signal for Swiss 3T3 cells. Proc. Natl. Acad. USA **78:** 4392-4396.
35. ROZENGURT, E. 1982. Synergistic stimulation of DNA synthesis by cyclic AMP derivatives and growth factors in mouse 3T3 cells. J. Cell. Phys. **112:** 243-250.
36. WHARTON, W., E. B. LOEF, N. OLASHAW, H. S. EARP & W. J. PLEDGER. 1982. Increase in cyclic AMP potentiate competence formation in BALB/c-3T3 Cells. J. Cell. Physiol. **111:** 201-206.

37. PARDEE, A. B., L. JIMENEZ DE ASUA & E. ROZENGURT. 1974. Functional membrane changes and cell growth: Significance and mechanism. *In* Control of Proliferation in Animal Cells. B. Clarkson & R. Baserga, Eds.: Vol. 1. Cold Spring Harbor Conference on Cell Proliferation.
38. MARX, J. L. 1984: A new view of receptor action. Research on the calcium ion linked receptors features the identification of a new second messenger and a possible connection to oncogene action. Science **224:** 271-274.
39. BESTERMAN, J. M. & P. CUATRECASAS. 1984. Phorbol esters rapidly stimulate amiloride-sensitive Na^+/H^+ exchange in human leukemic cell line. J. Cell Biol. **99:** 340-343.
40. POUYSSEGUR, J., C. SARDET, A. FRANCHI, G. L'ALLEMAIN & S. PARIS. 1984. A specific mutation abolishing Na^+/H^+ antiport activity in hamster fibroblasts precludes growth at neutral and acidic pH. Proc. Natl. Acad. Sci. USA **81:** 4833-4837.
41. OTTEN, J., G. S. JOHNSON & I. PASTAN. 1972. Regulation of cell growth by cyclic adenosine 3′,5′-monophosphate: Effect of cell density and agents which alter cell growth on cyclic adenosine 3′,5′-monophosphate levels in fibroblasts. J. Biol. Chem. **247:** 7082-7087.
42. PASTAN, I., W. B. ANDERSON, R. A. CARCHMAN, M. C. WILLINGHAM, T. R. RUSSELL & G. S. JOHNSON. 1974. Cyclic AMP and malignant transformation. *In* Control of Proliferation in Animal Cells. B. Clarkson & R. Baserga, Eds.: Vol. 1. Cold Spring Harbor Conference on Cell Proliferation.
43. GOLDBERG, N. D., M. K. HADDOX, E. DUNHAM, C. LOPEZ & J. W. HADDEN. 1974. The Yin Yang hypothesis of biological control: Opposing influences on cyclic GMP and cyclic AMP in the regulation of cell proliferation and other biological processes. *In* Control of Proliferation in Animal Cells. B. Clarkson & R. Baserga, Eds.: Vol. 1. Cold Spring Harbor Conference on Cell Proliferation.
44. SEIFERT, W. E. & P. S. RUDLAND. 1974. Possible involvement of cyclic GMP in growth control of cultured mouse cells. Nature (London) **248:** 138-140.
45. SNIDER, R. M., M. MCKINNEY, J. W. FENTON II & E. RICHELSON. 1984. Activation of cyclic nucleotide formation in murine neuroblastoma NIE-115 cells by modified human thrombin. J. Cell. Physiol. **117:** 272-281.
46. OLASHAW, N. E., E. B. LEOF, E. J. O'KEEFE & W. J. PLEDGER. 1984. Differential sensitivity of fibroblasts to epidermal growth factor is related to cyclic AMP concentration. J. Cell. Phys. **118:** 291-297.
47. RALPH, R. K. 1983. Cyclic AMP, calcium and control of cell growth. FEBS Let. **161:** 1-8.
48. COCKCROFT, S. & B. D. GOMPERTS. 1985. Role of guanine nucleotide binding protein in the activation of polyphosphoinositide phosphodiesterase. Nature (London) **314:** 534-536.
49. NISHIZUKA, Y. 1983. Phospholipid degradation and signal translation for protein phosphorylation. Trends. Biol. Sci. **8:** 13-16.

Effects of Thrombin on the Fibronectin-Containing Extracellular Matrix

DEANE F. MOSHER AND ELIZABETH D. THOMPSON

Departments of Medicine and Physiological Chemistry
University of Wisconsin
Madison, Wisconsin 53706

INTRODUCTION

One of the biologic actions of thrombin is growth stimulation of fibroblasts.[1-6] In early studies of how thrombin causes fibroblasts to proliferate, particular attention was paid to cleavage or release of extracellular fibronectin as a possible mechanism of growth stimulation. Such experiments were prompted by the observation that transformed cells with altered growth control were deficient in the fibronectin-containing matrix.[7] Thrombin, unlike a number of other proteases, did not cause changes in the amount of extracellular fibronectin in chick fibroblast cultures.[2,3] Thrombin, however, did cause an increased turnover of extracellular fibronectin in the chick cultures.[8] In human fibroblast cultures, active alpha-thrombin caused loss of extracellular fibronectin accompanied by increased synthesis and secretion of fibronectin.[8]

Subsequent studies established that the bulk of extracellular fibronectin in confluent cultures is in a pericellular fibrillar network, which also contains procollagens and glycosaminoglycans.[9] This matrix can be isolated from confluent cultures by extraction with sodium deoxycholate in hypotonic buffer. When isolated matrix from human lung fibroblast cultures metabolically labeled with [^{14}C]glycine was treated with thrombin, there was massive release of fibronectin and procollagen into the medium and cleavage of a 66 kDa polypeptide to a 62 kDa polypeptide that remained in the matrix.[10] Procollagen and fibronectin were also cleaved. The observation that matrix fibronectin was cleaved is consistent with previous reports that soluble fibronectin is a substrate for thrombin.[11,12]

In the present experiments, we studied the effects of thrombin on the incorporation of exogenous fibronectin into the extracellular matrix. Exogenous fibronectin, as well as endogenous fibronectin, synthesized by cultured cells, is incorporated into the extracellular matrix.[13-15] The dominant reaction is not binding of fibronectin directly to the fibrils; rather, the fibrils seem to be elaborated at the cell surface.[15] Human plasma fibronectin binds rapidly and reversibly to 100-400 000 sites per fibroblast; binding is half saturated when the concentration of fibronectin is 10-15 μg/ml.[15] Over the subsequent hour, binding becomes irreversible.[15] Irreversible binding is associated with the appearance of labeled fibronectin in the deoxycholate-insoluble fraction of the cell layer.[15] The same is true for metabolically labeled endogenous fibronectin.[16] Irreversibility of binding is also associated with formation of disulfide-bonded multimers due to disulfide exchange[15–17] and accumulation of labeled fibronectin in fibrillar structures.[15,18] Thus, fibronectin seems to be incorporated into the extracellular matrix by a pathway that involves reversible binding to a cell-surface receptor followed by transfer and translocation of bound molecules to the extracellular matrix. Binding to the cell-surface matrix-assembly receptor is not mediated by the cell-adhesion domain of fibronectin, but rather by the disulfide-bonded type I homology units, especially those in the amino-terminal region.[18] Thrombin, therefore, could cause loss of the fibronectin matrix by down-regulation of the matrix-assembly receptor, by cleavage of fibronectin in the region of the disulfide-bonded homology units so that fibronectin could not interact with the receptor, by cleavage or down-regulation of molecules responsible for transfer and/or translocation of bound fibronectin to the extracellular matrix, or by proteolysis of fibronectin already in the matrix.

MATERIAL AND METHODS

Material and methods for culture of human skin fibroblasts, purification and iodination of human plasma fibronectin, and quantitation of fibronectin binding to pools I and II (the reversible and irreversible binding pools described above) of monolayer cultures have been described previously.[15]

Human alpha-thrombin was a kind gift from Dr. John Fenton II, New York State Department of Health, Albany, NY. It was frozen at −70° C at a concentration of >2000 U/ml. Prior to a series of experiments, a portion was thawed and diluted in medium containing 0.2% albumin, activity was assayed by clotting activity towards citrated human plasma, and medium was added so the final concentration was 100 U/ml. This stock was refrozen in portions at −70° C, thawed prior to individual experiments, and diluted in albumin-containing medium to the final concentrations specified in individual experiments.

Binding experiments were done on newly confluent cell layers containing about 2 000 000 cells per replicate 35-mm diameter culture dish. The cells were washed with medium containing 0.2% bovine albumin to remove the serum proteins in growth medium and then subjected to the various incubations, washes, and extractions described in the RESULTS. In some experiments, cell layers and media were prepared for polyacrylamide gel electrophoresis in sodium dodecyl sulfate in the absence of a reducing agent in order to assess whether [^{125}I]fibronectin was disulfide-bonded into multimers[15] or degraded.[12]

RESULTS

Preincubation of confluent cell layers with thrombin, 0.01-10 U/ml (approximately 0.005-5 μg/ml or 0.14-140 nM), had no effect on the subsequent binding of fibronectin to the reversible (pool I) binding site (FIGURE 1). By contrast and as evidence that the pool I binding site is labile, treatment of confluent cell layers for 1 to 3 hr with cholera toxin over the same concentration range resulted in a 60 to 70% decrease in subsequent pool I binding.[19]

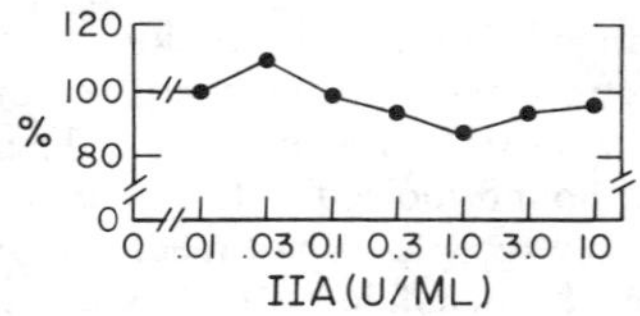

FIGURE 1. Effect of thrombin on the binding of [^{125}I]fibronectin to pool I. Cultures of freshly confluent fibroblasts were incubated for 4 hr with the indicated concentrations of thrombin in serum-free medium, washed, and incubated for an additional 15 min with 1 ml of medium containing 1000 ng of [^{125}I]fibronectin. Unbound fibronectin was removed by washing, and bound fibronectin was determined in a gamma counter after extraction with 0.1 N sodium hydroxide. Nonspecific binding was defined as [^{125}I]fibronectin bound in the presence of 300 μg/ml unlabeled fibronectin and was subtracted to give specific binding. For each thrombin concentration, 6 cultures, 3 without and 3 with excess unlabeled fibronectin, were analyzed. Specifically bound fibronectin for the cultures incubated with thrombin is expressed as the percent of the value for the cultures incubated without thrombin. This value was 9.8 ng per dish.

When [^{125}I]fibronectin was incubated with cell layers for 3 hr, (so that there were approximately equal amounts of labeled fibronectin bound in pools I and II), and the cell layers were then incubated with thrombin, there was a marked decrease in the amounts of fibronectin remaining in pools I and II of the cultures exposed to the higher thrombin concentrations (FIGURE 2). Electrophoresis of media at the end of the second incubations revealed that labeled fibronectin released from cell layers exposed to <0.3 U/ml thrombin was in the form of a disulfide-bonded dimer, that is, the form originally added to the cultures (FIGURE 3). Fibronectin released from cell layers exposed to higher thrombin concentrations was degraded and consisted of large fragments only slightly smaller than the fibronectin subunit and a smaller fragment of 30 kDa.

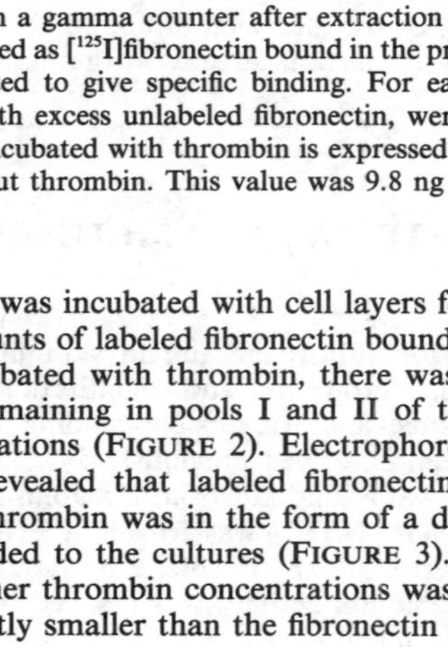

FIGURE 2. Effect of thrombin on [^{125}I]fibronectin bound to pool I or pool II. Cultures of freshly confluent fibroblasts were incubated for 3 hr with 1 ml of serum-free medium containing 1000 ng of [^{125}I]fibronectin and washed. After this first incubation, there were 19.6 ng fibronectin in pool I (soluble in 1% deoxycholate) and 6.0 ng fibronectin in pool II (insoluble in 1% deoxycholate). Cultures were incubated an additional 3 hr with the indicated concentrations of thrombin. After the second incubation, medium was removed for analysis of radioactivity and electrophoresis (see FIGURE 3), the cultures were washed, and bound fibronectin in pools I and II was determined in a gamma counter after separation of the two fractions by centrifugation. Fibronectin associated nonspecifically with cells was subtracted for each point. Results are expressed as the percent of the value for cells incubated without thrombin during the second incubation, as described in the legend of FIGURE 1. At the end of the second incubation, there were 8.1 ng fibronectin in the medium, 8.2 fibronectin in pool I, and 7.1 ng fibronectin in pool II of the cultures incubated without thrombin. Closed and open circles: fibronectin in pools I and II, respectively (left ordinate); closed squares: fibronectin in the medium (right ordinate).

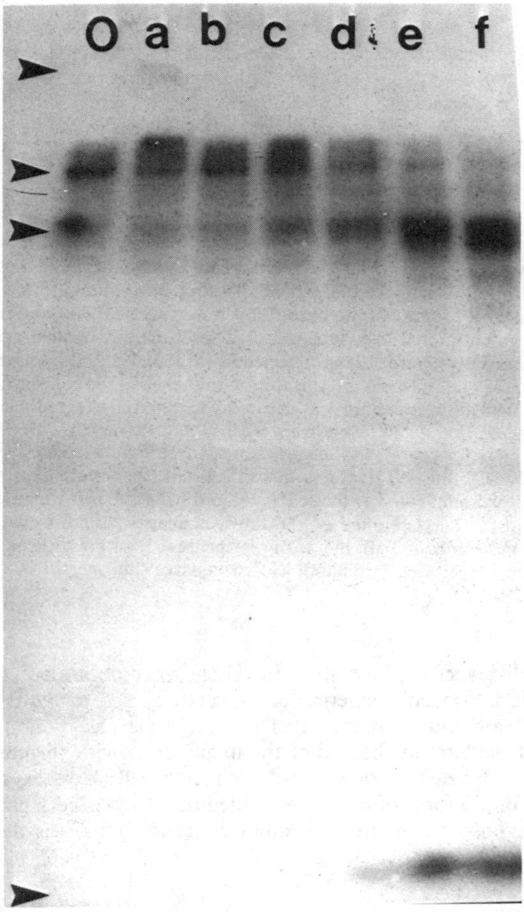

FIGURE 3. Electrophoretic analysis of [^{125}I]fibronectin released into the medium during the 3-hr second incubation shown in FIGURE 2. Medium was mixed with one-tenth volume of 10% sodium dodecyl sulfate and dialyzed extensively against 0.1% sodium dodecyl sulfate. Proteins were concentrated by lyophilization, dissolved in one-fifth the original volume of medium, and analyzed on an 8% polyacrylamide gel. Samples were not reduced prior to electrophoresis. Shown are the autoradiographic patterns of media from cultures incubated with no thrombin (0) and 0.01, 0.03,. . .10 U/ml thrombin (a, b,. . .f). Arrowheads, from top to bottom, point to the top of the stacking gel, the position of the fibronectin dimer (500 kDa), the position of the fibronectin monomer (250 kDa), and the tracking dye (<30 kDa).

When [^{125}I]fibronectin was incubated with cell layers for 22 hr and chased for 4 hr (so that >94% of bound labeled fibronectin was in pool II), and the cell layers were then incubated with thrombin, there was a decrease in the amount of fibronectin remaining in the cell layers of cultures exposed to the higher thrombin concentrations (FIGURE 4). Electrophoresis of the cell layers after the incubations with thrombin revealed that most of the fibronectin remaining in all of the cell layers was in the form of disulfide-bonded multimers characteristic of pool II, matrix fibronectin[15,18]

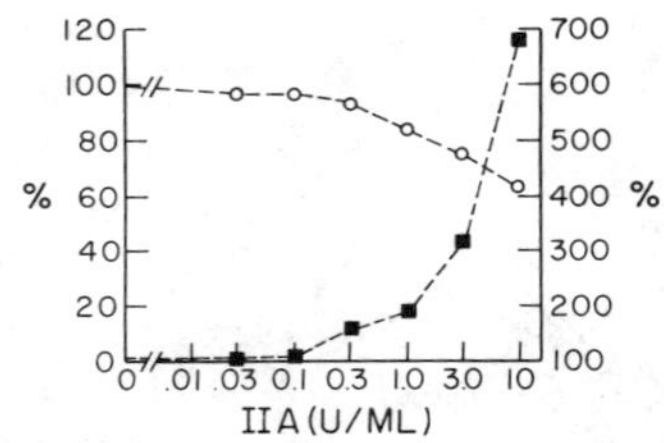

FIGURE 4. Effect of thrombin on [^{125}]fibronectin bound largely to pool II. Cultures of freshly confluent fibroblasts were incubated for 22 hr with 1 ml of serum-free medium containing 1000 ng fibronectin and then washed. At the end of this first incubation, 15.7 ng fibronectin were specifically bound in pool I, and 24.0 ng fibronectin were specifically bound in pool II. Cultures were incubated for an additional 4 hr in serum-free medium and washed again. At the end of the second incubation, there were 7.2 ng fibronectin in pool I and 28.7 ng fibronectin in pool II. Cultures were incubated for 3 more hr, this time with the indicated concentrations of thrombin. At the end of the incubation, medium was removed for analysis of radioactivity and electrophoresis (see FIGURE 5B), and cell layers were washed and extracted with 3% sodium dodecyl sulfate for analysis of radioactivity and electrophoresis (see FIGURE 5A). [^{125}I]fibronectin associated nonspecifically with the cell fractions was subtracted. Values are expressed as the percent of the values for cultures incubated without thrombin during the third incubation, as described in the legend in FIGURE 1. At the end of the third incubation, there were 39.4 ng in the cell layer and 2.4 ng in the medium of the cultures incubated without thrombin. Open circles: fibronectin in the cell layer (left ordinate); closed squares: fibronectin in the medium (right ordinate).

(FIGURE 5A). Cell layers exposed to <1.0 U/ml thrombin also contained a small amount of dimeric fibronectin, whereas cell layers exposed to >1.0 U/ml thrombin contained a small amount of material of the same size as monomeric fibronectin. Electrophoresis of medium at the end of the incubations with thrombin revealed that the small amount of labeled fibronectin released from cell layers exposed to <1.0 U/ml thrombin was in the form of disulfide-bonded dimers, whereas fibronectin released from cell layers exposed to higher thrombin concentrations was degraded (FIGURE 5B).

DISCUSSION

Plasma fibronectin is a substrate for thrombin.[11,12] Furie and Rifkin[12] characterized two cleavage sites, one near the carboxyl terminus of the molecule to release the intrachain disulfide bridge(s) and render the remainder of the molecule monomeric, and the second near the amino terminus to cleave the monomer into fragments of 30 kDa and 220/225 kDa. Sequence data reported subsequently[20–22] suggest that the bonds cleaved in human fibronectin by thrombin are $Arg_{259}-Ala_{260}$ and $Arg_{2239}-Thr_{2240}$[1].[a] These bonds are also highly susceptible to cleavage by plasmin.[20]

[a] The numbering is based on the sequence of bovine plasma fibronectin[22] and is for a molecule with no extra domain (ED) and a full connecting segment between the carboxyl terminals of the type III homology units (IIICS). In the sequence reported for human fibronectin containing the ED and a truncated IIICS,[21] the carboxyl terminal thrombin cleavage site is at Arg_{2299}-Thr_{2300}.

The $Arg_{259}-Ala_{260}$ bond is in a 32-residue connecting strand, which separates the fifth and sixth units of type I homology. Just beyond the bond is a stretch of 14 residues that contains six prolines. It has been hypothesized that the prolyl residues cause the connecting strand to assume a conformation that is particularly susceptible to proteolytic cleavage.[23] The $Arg_{2239}-Thr_{2240}$ bond is in the connecting strand between the twelfth (last) unit of type I homology and a pair of interchain cystines. Arg_{2239} is seven residues from the first of the cystines.

The results of the present study indicate that thrombin solubilizes fibronectin that already has been assembled into the extracellular matrix. The data also suggest that fibronectin released from the cell layer binds less well to cells and fails to be assembled into the extracellular matrix.

FIGURE 5A and **B**. Electrophoretic analysis of fibronectin associated with cell layer (**A**) and released into the medium (**B**) during the third 3-hr incubation shown in FIGURE 4. Cell layers were extracted directly into sodium dodecyl sulfate as described in the legend in FIGURE 4. Medium samples were concentrated by lyophilization as described in the legend FIGURE 3. Electrophoretic conditions were the same as in FIGURE 3, and labeling of the figures is the same except that the stacking gel, which contained no radioactive bands, is omitted from FIGURE 5B, along with the uppermost arrowhead.

The apparent failure of thrombin-digested fibronectin to be assembled into the matrix is compatible with recent studies of the assembly process.[15,17,18] In order for assembly to proceed, fibronectin must be intact or nearly intact. Thus, the 70 kDa cathepsin D-derived amino terminal fragment, which contains nine units of type I homology, binds tightly to the receptor, but cannot be assembled into the matrix.[18]

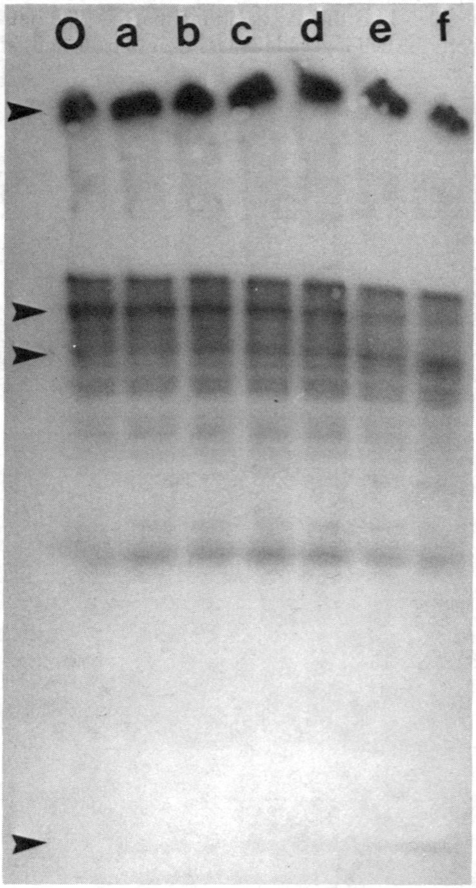

FIGURE 5B. See legend on page 269.

Cleavage of the 70 kDa fragment with trypsin at $Arg_{259}-Ala_{260}$ results in significant loss of binding, although the two subfragments do bind.[18] Cleavage of intact fibronectin with trypsin at $Arg_{259}-Ala_{260}$ and $Arg_{2239}-Thr_{2240}$ results in loss of binding to the receptor, although, again, the fragments do bind.[18] The tryptic fragments, like the 70 kDa fragment, cannot be assembled into the matrix.[18] In the present experiments, the thrombin cleavages presumably had an effect similar to the limited trypsin cleavages.

The mechanism of solubilization of fibronectin from pool II is less clear. The fibronectin fragments solubilized by thrombin were monomeric, whereas fibronectin remaining in matrix was disulfide-bonded into multimers. These multimers appear to be held together by exchanged disulfides somewhere within the 70 kDa amino terminal region.[17] Despite multiple attempts, we have been unable to detect multimers of the major trypsin or thrombin fragments, that is, multimers of the 30 or 220/225 kDa fragments. If thrombin cleaved only at the $Arg^{259}-Ala_{260}$ bond in the middle of the 70 kDa region, one of the fragments should be multimeric. There are several possible explanations for this observation. The first is that the solubilization, which in the case of thrombin was not quantitative (FIGURE 4), selectively leaves behind multimeric fibronectin. The second is that the disulfide exchange is accompanied by a conformational change that renders new bonds susceptible to cleavage. Further experiments are needed to decide among these and other possibilities.

Proteolytic fragments of fibronectin have effects on cells that are not shared by the intact molecule. Cathepsin D digests of fibronectin have been shown to stimulate DNA synthesis in quiescent fibroblast cultures.[24] Fragments of plasmin- or cathepsin G-treated fibronectin enhance morphological cell transformation of Rous sarcoma virus-infected fibroblasts.[25] Trypsin and plasmin digests of fibronectin accelerate the formation of tubular structures in endothelial cell cultures,[26] and heparin-binding fragments of fibronectin are inhibitors of endothelial cell growth.[27] Binding of such fragments to the matrix-assembly receptor is one way that fragments can interact with cells in a manner that is different from intact fibronectin, that is, the fragments can bind to the presumptive receptor but are not assembled into the extracellular matrix.

Is fibronectin, therefore, in any way related to the growth-stimulatory effects of thrombin on fibroblasts? The concentrations of thrombin required to digest fibronectin are somewhat greater than the concentrations that stimulate growth, but are only a fraction of the concentrations generated during blood coagulation. Thus, if thrombin were to be somehow protected from antithrombins, nearby fibronectin would be susceptible to fragmentation by thrombin. This would be particularly true if thrombin at the same time stimulated local production of fibronectin.[8] Such fragmentation would result in loss of occupancy of the matrix-assembly receptor by intact fibronectin and occupancy of the receptor by fragments that cannot be assembled into the matrix. In addition, loss of fibronectin from the extracellular matrix might make the matrix less adhesive for cells. It seems unlikely that fibronectin is the mediator of the growth-stimulatory effects of thrombin in the way that the epidermal growth factor (EGF) receptor mediates the growth-stimulatory effects of EGF. It does seem possible, however, that cleavage products of fibronectin could modulate the effects of thrombin in a more complex manner, for example, the way that transforming growth factor (TGF)-beta modulates the effects of EGF.[28]

SUMMARY

The effects of human alpha-thrombin on the incorporation of exogenous human fibronectin into the extracellular matrix of cultured human skin fibroblasts were studied. Thrombin had no effect on the saturable cell-surface receptor for soluble fibronectin. Thrombin, however, did digest fibronectin bound reversibly to the cell surface and fibronectin incorporated irreversibly into the extracellular matrix. The products of thrombin digestion of cell surface and matrix-bound fibronectin were similar to the products of thrombin digestion of soluble fibronectin. These results indicate that fibronectin can potentially modulate some of the effects of thrombin on cells.

REFERENCES

1. CHEN, L. B. & J. M. BUCHANAN. 1975. Proc. Natl. Acad. Sci. USA **72:** 131-135.
2. TENG, N. N. H. & L. B. CHEN. 1975. Proc. Natl. Acad. Sci. USA **72:** 413-417.
3. BLUMBERG, P. M. & P. W. ROBBINS. 1975. Cell **6:** 137-147.
4. POHJANPELTO, P. 1977. J. Cell. Physiol. **91:** 387-395.
5. ZETTER, B. R., T.-T. SUN, L. B. CHEN & J. M. BUCHANAN. 1977. J. Cell. Physiol. **92:** 233-240.
6. BAKER, J. B., R. L. SIMMER, K. C. GLEN & D. D. CUNNINGHAM. 1979. Nature (London) **278:** 743-745.
7. VAHERI, A. & D. F. MOSHER. 1978. Biochim. Biophys. Acta **516:** 1-25.
8. MOSHER, D. F. & A. VAHERI. 1978. Exp. Cell Res. **112:** 323-334.
9. HEDMAN, K., A. VAHERI & J. WARTIOVAARA. 1978. J. Cell Biol. **76:** 748-760.
10. KESKI-OJA, J., G. J. TODARO & A. VAHERI. 1981. Biochim. Biophys. Acta **673:** 323-331.
11. MOSHER, D. F. 1975. J. Biol. Chem. **250:** 6614-6621.
12. FURIE, M. B. & D. B. RIFKIN. 1980. J. Biol. Chem. **255:** 3134-3140.
13. HAYMAN, E. G. & E. RUOSLAHTI. 1979. J. Cell Biol. **83:** 255-259.
14. RENNARD, S. I., M. L. WIND, A. T. HEWITT & H. K. KLEINMAN. 1981. Arch. Biochem. Biophys. **206:** 205-212.
15. MCKEOWN-LONGO, P. J. & D. F. MOSHER. 1983. J. Cell Biol. **97:** 466-472.
16. CHOI, M. G. & R. O. HYNES. 1979. J. Biol. Chem. **254:** 12050-12057.
17. MCKEOWN-LONGO, P. J. & D. F. MOSHER. 1984. J. Biol. Chem. **259:** 12210-12215.
18. MCKEOWN-LONGO, P. J. & D. F. MOSHER. 1985. J. Cell Biol. **100:** 364-374.
19. ALLEN-HOFFMANN, B. L. & D. F. MOSHER. 1985. J. Cell Biol. **101:** 9a.
20. PETERSEN, T. E., H. C. THOGERSEN, K. SKORSTENGAARD, K. VIBE-PEDERSEN, P. SAHL, L. SOTTRUP-JENSEN & S. MAGNUSSON. 1983. Proc. Natl. Acad. Sci. USA **80:** 137-141.
21. KORNBLIHTT, A. R., K. UMEZAWA, K. VIBE-PEDERSEN & F. E. BARALLE. 1985. EMBO J. **4:** 1755-1759.
22. SKORSTENGAARD, K., M. S. JENSEN, P. SAHL, T. E. PETERSEN & S. MAGNUSSON. 1986. Eur. J. Biochem. In press.
23. GOLD, L. I., A. GARCIA-PARDO, B. FRANGIONE, E. C. FRANKLIN & E. PEARLSTEIN. 1979. Proc. Natl. Acad. Sci. USA **76:** 4803-4807.
24. HUMPHRIES, M. J. & S. R. AYAD. 1983. Nature (London) **305:** 811-813.
25. DEPETRO, G., S. BARLATI, T. VARTIO & A. VAHERI. 1981. Proc. Natl. Acad. Sci. USA **78:** 4965-4969.
26. MACIAG, T., J. KADISH, L. WILKINS, M. B. STEMERMAN & R. WEINSTEIN. 1982. J. Cell Biol. **94:** 511-520.
27. HOMANDBERG, G. A., J. E. WILLIAMS, D. GRANT, B. SCHUMACHER & R. EISENSTEIN. 1985. Am. J. Pathol. **120:** 327-332.
28. ASSOIAN, R. K. 1985. J. Biol. Chem. **260:** 9613-9617.

Thrombin and Chymotrypsin Interactions with Thrombospondin[a]

JACK LAWLER,[b] JOSEPH E. CONNOLLY,
PAULA FERRO, AND LAURA H. DERICK

Departments of Biomedical Research and Medicine
Division of Hematology/Oncology
St. Elizabeth's Hospital of Boston and
Tufts University School of Medicine
Boston, Massachusetts 02135

Thrombospodin is a high molecular weight glycoprotein with the ability to bind to heparin,[1,2] fibronectin,[3,4] fibrinogen,[4,5] plasminogen,[6] histidine-rich glycoprotein,[7] type V collagen,[8] laminin,[8] calcium,[9] and sulfated glycolipids.[10] Although the functional significance of these interactions is not known, some of them probably result in the incorporation of thrombospondin into extracellular matrices.[11–15] Thrombospondin has been shown to be present in the extracellular matrices produced by endothelial cells, smooth muscle cells, and fibroblasts in culture.[11–15] McKeown-Longo *et al.*[13] have shown that some of the radiolabeled thrombospondin that is added to human embryonic lung fibroblasts in culture is incorporated into the extracellular matrix. In contrast to fibronectin, the matrix-bound thrombospondin is slowly degraded over a period of hours.[13] Recent studies indicate that thrombospondin biosynthesis by cells in culture is proportional to cell density and is modulated by platelet-derived growth factor and glycosaminoglycans.[14,16] In addition, the incorporation of thrombospondin into the extracellular matrix can be detected in cultures of human endothelial cells from neonatal skin, but not from adult skin.[15] These data suggest that thrombospondin may have a specific role in the formation of the extracellular matrix and may be affected by variations in biosynthetic phenotype.

The developing fibrin clot may represent a specialized example of an extracellular matrix. The incorporation of thrombospondin into fibrin and plasma clots can be demonstrated by determining the amount of radiolabeled thrombospondin that is associated with these clots and by immunofluorescence.[17,18] Studies of thrombospondin distribution in the clot as a function of time suggest that the majority of thrombospondin is only transiently associated with the clot.[17] Bale *et al.*[18] have reported that thrombospondin is incorporated into the clot while the fibrin is forming. Tuszynski *et al.*[19] have reported that more thrombospondin is incorporated into fibrin clots if cross-linking by factor XIII_a is inhibited. Thrombospondin is covalently incorporated into high molecular weight complexes in the presence of factor XIII_a, suggesting that

[a] We acknowledge the Robert J. Kleberg Jr. and Helen C. Kleberg Foundation for its generous donation of equipment funds to the Electron Microscopy Facility at St. Elizabeth's Hospital of Boston.

[b] Recipient of National Institutes of Health Research Grant HL 28749 from the National Heart, Lung, and Blood Institute.

thrombospondin is a substrate for factor XIII_a.[18] In the presence of thrombospondin, the clots are composed of more numerous, thinner fibers than in the absence of thrombospondin. In addition to affecting the structure of the clot, thrombospondin may modulate fibrinolysis through its interactions with plasminogen and histidine-rich glycoprotein.[6,7,20]

Exposure of thrombospondin to α-thrombin in the presence of calcium results in the selective removal of a 30 000-dalton heparin-binding fragment from the NH_2-terminal of each chain.[1,21–23] Additional sites for α-thrombin proteolysis are exposed when calcium is removed from the molecule with EDTA.[22,23] Cleavages at these sites result in the production of fragments of 130 000, 95 000, 65 000, and 25 000 daltons.[22,23] These fragments are produced, at least in part, by removal of mass from the COOH-terminal.[22] Takahashi and coworkers[23] have reported that thrombospondin is not a substrate for γ-thrombin.

A complex of thrombospondin and radiolabeled thrombin has recently been identified.[24,25] Crossed immunoelectrophoresis of the proteins released from platelets, which had been incubated with [^{125}I]thrombin, revealed the radiolabeling of immunoprecipitates representing thrombospondin, albumin, and the "line" form of platelet factor 4.[24] Danishefsky and coworkers[25] have identified the mechanism for the formation of the thrombospondin-thrombin complex. They report that thrombospondin contains a free thiol group that is capable of reacting with a disulfide bond of thrombin. This thiol-disulfide exchange results in the formation of a covalent bond between thrombospondin and thrombin. This complex forms within 30 minutes after the addition of [^{125}I]α-thrombin to washed platelets and is found associated with the platelets and in the supernatant from the thrombin-treated platelets.[26]

In this paper the properties of thrombospondin fragments produced by thrombin and chymotrypsin are compared by electron microscopy, and by monoclonal antibody and Lens culinaris lectin-binding studies. In addition, the binding of a high molecular weight chymotryptic fragment, designated Chy-1 (the 210 000-dalton chymotryptic fragment of thrombospondin) to fibronectin, laminin, type V collagen, fibrinogen, and plasminogen is compared with that of the intact molecule. These data permit the formation of a model for the structural and functional organization of the thrombospondin molecule.

MATERIAL AND METHODS

Proteolytic Digestion

Thrombospondin was isolated from human blood platelets by the method described previously.[22] Digestion with human α-thrombin was obtained from Dr. J. Fenton II, division of Laboratories and Research, New York State Department of Health, Albany, NY. TPCK-trypsin (L-1-tosylamido-2-phenylethyl chloromethyl ketone-treated trypsin) (Worthington, Malvern, PA) or chymotrypsin (Worthington) was performed on thrombospondin samples in Tris-buffered saline (TBS, containing 15 mM Tris-HCl (pH 7.6), 0.14 M NaCl, and 0.02% NaN_3) containing 2 mM $CaCl_2$, both with and without prior treatment with 5 mM EDTA. Samples received 4 U/ml of thrombin and were incubated for 1-16 hours, as indicated. Limited tryptic or chymotryptic digestion was carried out at 0° C for 16 hours at enzyme-to-substrate ratios of 1:10 000,

1:1 000, 1:100, and 1:10 (w/w). Digestion was terminated by the addition of 1 mM diisopropyl fluorophosphate (DFP) or a one-fourth volume of sample buffer (pH 7.5) containing 0.25 M Tris, 5% sodium dodecyl sulfate (SDS), 1.25 M sucrose, .01 M EDTA, both with and without 0.1 M dithiothreitol, and heated to 100° C for 60 seconds.[27]

SDS-Polyacrylamide Gel Electrophoresis - (SDS-PAGE) and Protein Blotting

SDS-PAGE was carried out on the discontinuous system of Laemmli[27] as described previously.[22] After SDS-PAGE, the proteins were electrophoretically transferred to nitrocellulose paper (BioRad, Richmond, CA) at 50 volts for 24-72 hours in pH 8.3 buffer containing 25 mM Tris, 192 mM glycine, and 20% methanol. For monoclonal antibody binding studies, the nitrocellulose paper containing a replica of the gel was washed briefly in 0.15 M NaCl and incubated with TBS containing 20 mM Tris-HCl (pH 7.6), 0.14 M NaCl, and 5% bovine serum albumin (BSA) for 1 hour at 22°C. The protein blot was washed with five changes of 0.15 M NaCl within a 30-minute interval and incubated with TBS-BSA containing monoclonal anti-thrombospondin antibodies (10-20 μl/10 ml TBS-BSA) for 16 hours at 22° C. The production and epitope mapping of the monoclonal antibodies has been described previously.[22] The protein blots were washed again and incubated with goat antimouse IgG conjugated with horseradish peroxidase (10 μl/10 ml TBS-BSA: N.L. Cappel Laboratories Inc, Cochranville, PA) for 1 hour at 22° C. After the final incubation, the protein blots were washed and placed in a substrate solution containing 40 mM Tris-HCl (pH 7.6), 0.16 M NaCl, 0.015% H_2O_2, 20% (v/v) methanol, and 3.36 mM 4-chloro-1-naphthol for 1-5 minutes for the detection of horseradish peroxidase-conjugated antimouse IgG. For Lens culinaris lectin- (Polysciences, Warrington, PA) binding studies, the nitrocellulose paper containing a replica of the gel was washed briefly in 0.15 M NaCl and incubated in 15 mM Tris-HCl (pH 7.6), 0.14 M NaCl, 2 mM $CaCl_2$, and 3% periodic acid-treated BSA (TBS-P-BSA) for 1 hour at 22° C.[28] The protein blots were washed as described above and incubated with TBS-P-BSA containing horseradish peroxidase conjugated Lens culinaris lectin (150 μl/30 ml TBS-P-BSA) for 16 hours at 22°C. The blots were washed and incubated with the substrate solution described above.

Isolation of Thrombospondin Fragments

A sample of thrombospondin in TBS containing 2 mM $CaCl_2$ was treated with 5 mM EDTA prior to digestion with chymotrypsin at an enzyme-to-substrate ratio of 1:100 (w/w) for 20 hours at 0°C. Digestion was terminated by the addition of DFP to 1 mM and the sample was incubated at 0°C for 2 hours. The sample was then chromatographed on a column (0.8×3.2 cm) of immobilized soybean trypsin inhibitor (Pierce, Rockford, IL) to remove the chymotrypsin. The nonaffinity peak was applied to a column (0.8×3.0 cm) of heparin-Sepharose CL-6B (Pharmacia, Piscataway, NJ) equilibrated in TBS at 4° C. Stepwise elution was carried out with 15 mM Tris-HCl (pH 7.6) and 0.02% NaN_3 containing 0.15, 0.25, 0.55, and 2.0 M NaCl. Elution of the column with 0.55 M NaCl produces a peak that contains the 25 000-dalton fragment, indicating that this fragment contains the heparin-binding site. This peak was concentrated by pressure dialysis (Amicon) and dialyzed for iodination. The nonaffinity peak contains the 70 000-dalton fragment and some minor low molecular weight bands. The nonaffinity peak was concentrated by pressure dialysis and applied to a column (1.3×29 cm) of Sephadex G-200 (Pharmacia) equilibrated in TBS at 4°C. The Chy-1 fragment was eluted as a high molecular weight peak near the void volume of the column. Calibration of the column with molecular weight standards indicates that the high molecular weight peak is eluted at a molecular weight of approximately 200 000. This peak electrophoreses as a single band with a molecular weight of 70 000 in the presence of reducing agent. In the absence of reducing agent, the protein electrophoreses near the origin of a 10% gel and at a molecular weight of approximately 220 000 on a 3-10% gradient gel.

Protein Iodination

Samples for iodination were dialyzed into 0.1 M borate buffer (pH 7.6) containing 0.14 M NaCl with or without 2 mM $CaCl_2$ for intact thrombospondin or the proteolytic fragments (Chy-1 and 25 000-dalton heparin-binding peptide), respectively. The polypeptides were incubated with [^{125}I]Bolton-Hunter reagent (New England Nuclear, Boston, MA) at 0° C overnight, followed by extensive dialysis against TBS both with and without 2 mM $CaCl_2$. The specific activity of the proteins was $0.2-1.0 \times 10^6$ cpm/ug.

Solid-Phase Binding Assay

The binding of thrombospondin to purified fibrinogen,[4,5] plasminogen,[6] histidine-rich glycoprotein,[7] fibronectin,[3,4] type V collagen,[8] and laminin[8] can be demonstrated using solid-phase binding assays. These interactions have been shown to be concentration-dependent and saturable. The interaction of thrombospondin with these various ligands, with the exception of laminin, has been corroborated by additional methods. Thus, the solid-phase binding assay represents a system for investigating the macromolecular association that may be involved in extracellular matrix formation with relatively small amounts of matrix proteins. The binding of the Chy-1 fragment, the 25 000-dalton heparin-binding peptide, and the intact thrombospondin molecule to human fibrinogen (IMCO Corp., Stockholm, Sweden), human plasminogen (Worthington), human type V collagen (Calbiochem, San Diego, CA), human plasma fibronectin (Calbiochem or Sigma, St. Louis, MO), or murine laminin (Bethesda Research Laboratories, Gaithersburg, MD) was quantitated by a solid-phase binding assay.[4,6] All binding assays were performed in plastic wells (Immulon 2 Removawell Strips, Dynatech Laboratories, Alexandria, VA). Plasminogen was treated with 1 mM DFP, to inhibit possible plasmin contamination, prior to use in coating the wells. The wells were incubated overnight at 4° C with 200 μl of the above protein solutions at 10 μg/ml dissolved in coating buffer (pH 9.6) containing 15 mM Na_2CO_3, 35 mM Na HCO_3, and 0.02% NaN_3.[6] The wells were washed three times with 300 μl of assay buffer (pH 7.6) containing 10 mM Tris, 0.14 M NaCl, 0.02% NaN_3, and 0.05% Tween 20 both with and without 500 μM $CaCl_2$. Equal amounts of radiolabeled thrombospondin or proteolytic fragment (Chy-1 or the 25 000-dalton heparin-binding peptide) were added to dilutions of unlabeled thrombospondin or proteolytic fragment prepared in the assay buffer.[4,29] One hundred microliters of these protein solutions were added to each well, and they were incubated overnight at 4° C. Each concentration of thrombospondin or proteolytic fragment was prepared in duplicate. The wells were washed twice with assay buffer, and the bound radioactivity was determined.

Electron Microscopy

Samples of thrombospondin or its proteolytic fragments in TBS were diluted 1:10 with 70% glycerol and 0.15 M ammonium acetate just prior to spraying. The samples were sprayed and rotary shadowed with platinum from an angle of 6° to the horizontal by the method of Tyler and Branton.[30] A shadow thickness of approximately 12 Å was used. Replicas were coated with a 100 Å thick supporting film of carbon from an angle of 90°.

RESULTS

Thrombin Digestion of Thrombospondin

Exposure of thrombospondin to α-thrombin (4 U/ml) at 37°C in the presence of calcium results in a time-dependent decrease in the staining intensity of the 185 000-dalton band and the concomitant appearance of major bands at 160 000 and 30 000 daltons. The 30 000-dalton fragment contains the epitope for the monoclonal antibody MA-II and a carbohydrate group that binds the lentil lectin Lens culinaris (FIGURE 1). The fragment also contains the heparin-binding site.[1,21–23] The 160 000-dalton fragment also binds Lens culinaris. When α-thrombin digestion of thrombospondin is performed in the absence of calcium, a second cleavage site is expressed.[22] Proteolysis at this site results in the removal of a 25 000-dalton fragment from the COOH-terminal of each chain. The mass of the residual high molecular weight fragment is 130 000 daltons. Whereas the 130 000-dalton fragment contains a carbohydrate group that binds Lens culinaris, the 25 000-dalton fragment does not (FIGURE 1). Reduction of the samples results in a considerable decrease in the 25 000-dalton fragment, as compared to nonreduced samples. Thus, a third site for thrombin digestion exists in this fragment and an undetermined number of disulfide bonds connect the two regions of polypeptide on either side of the cleavage site.

Chymotryptic Digestion of Thrombospondin

Limited chymotryptic digestion of thrombospondin at a low enzyme-to-substrate ratio (1:10 000 w/w) in the absence of calcium produces a broad spectrum of polypeptides ranging in molecular weight from 25 000 to 185 000 (FIGURE 2). When the enzyme-to-substrate ratio is increased to 1:1000 or 1:100 (w/w), the principal species

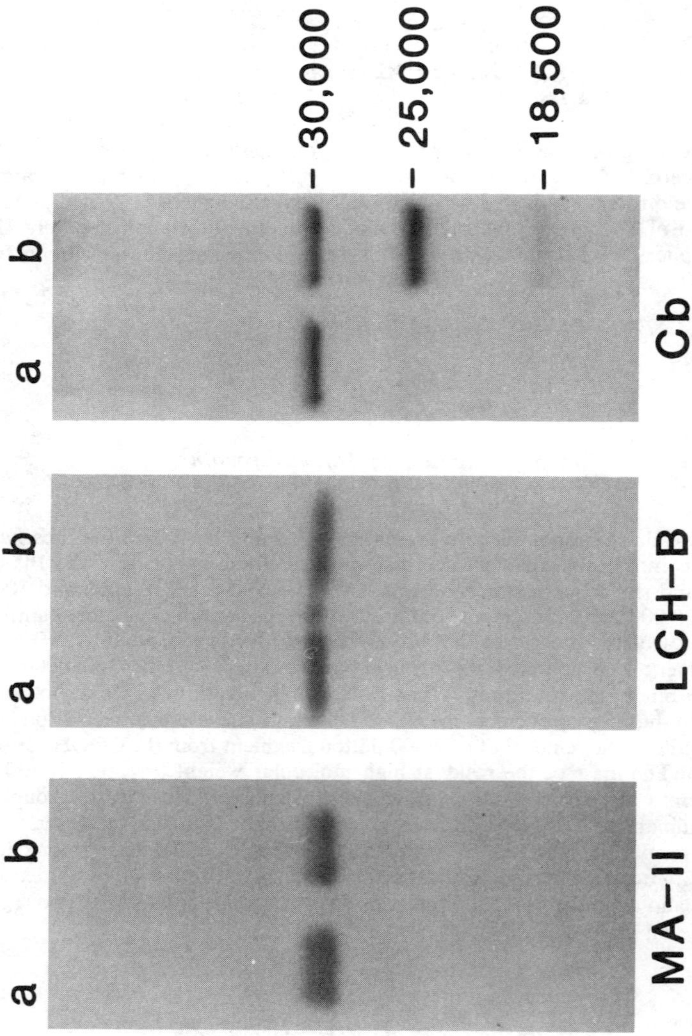

FIGURE 1. Electrophoresis of the low molecular weight fragments of thrombospondin produced by thrombin digestion in the presence (a) and absence (b) of calcium. After electrophoresis, the gels were stained with Coomassie blue (Cb) or electrophoretically transferred to nitrocellulose paper. The blots were probed with MA-II or Lens culinaris (LCH-B). The molecular masses for the principal bands are indicated on the right.

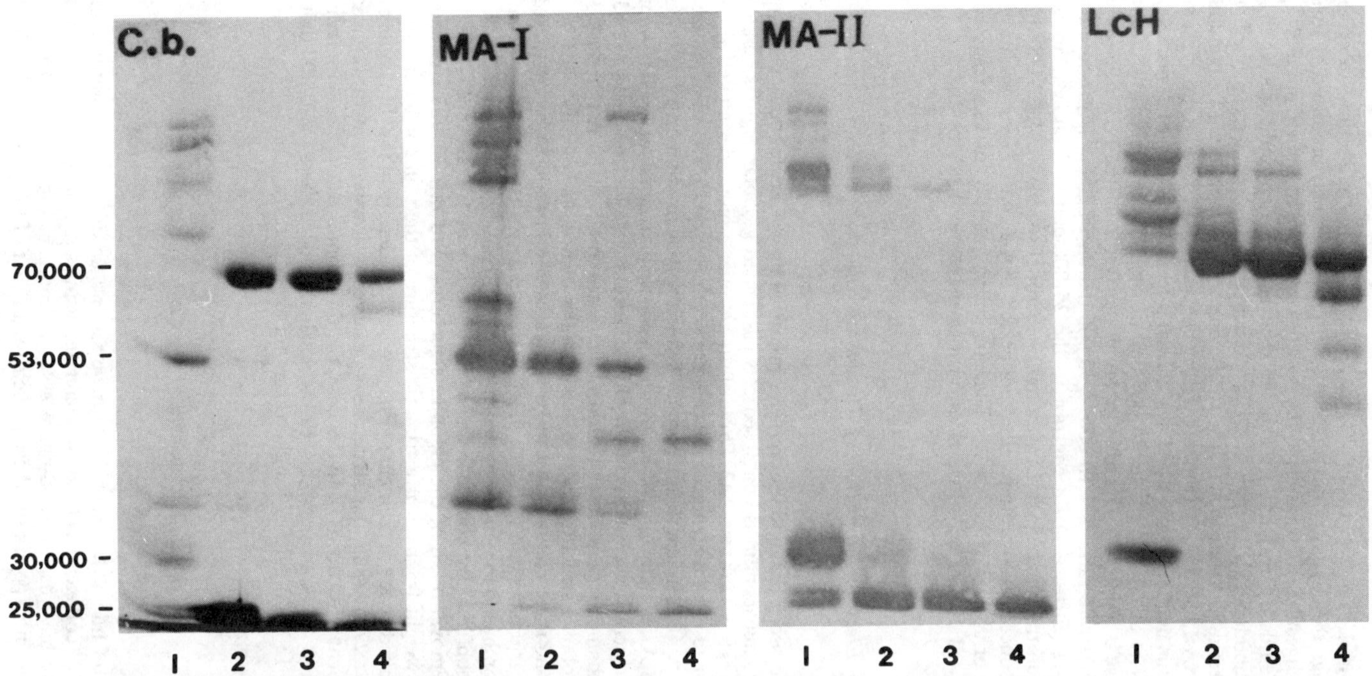

FIGURE 2. Limited chymotryptic digestion of thrombospondin. Thrombospondin was treated with chymotrypsin at enzyme-to-substrate ratios (w/w) of 1:10 000 (lanes 1), 1:1000 (lanes 2), 1:100 (lanes 3), or 1:10 (lanes 4) for 20 hours at 0°C in the absence of calcium. The digests were electrophoresed on 10% polyacrylamide gels and stained with Coomassie blue (C.b.) or electrophoretically transferred to nitrocellulose paper. The blots were probed with MA-I, MA-II, or Lens culinaris lectin (LcH). The masses of some of the principal bands are indicated on the left.

produced have molecular weights of 70 000 and 25 000 after reduction. In order to compare and align the chymotryptic fragments with the fragments produced by thrombin and trypsin digestion, we transferred the peptides produced by limited chymotryptic digest to nitrocellulose paper and probed the replicas with Lens culinaris lectin and monoclonal antibodies (MA-I and MA-II).[22] When these digests were probed with Lens culinaris lectin, MA-I or MA-II, the 70 000-dalton fragment bound Lens culinaris lectin but not MA-I nor MA-II (FIGURE 2). By contrast, the 25 000-dalton fragment bound MA-II but neither MA-I nor Lens culinaris lectin (FIGURE 2). This 25 000-dalton fragment is distinct from the 25 000-dalton fragment produced by thrombin digestion because it binds MA-II and is therefore derived from the NH_2-terminal. At an enzyme-to-substrate ratio of 1:10 000, a 30 000-dalton fragment is produced that also binds MA-II (FIGURE 2). In contrast to the 25 000-dalton fragment, however, the 30 000-dalton fragment binds Lens culinaris lectin (FIGURE 2). A 53 000-dalton fragment is produced that contains the epitope for MA-I, but does not bind Lens culinaris lectin or MA-II (FIGURE 2). The maximum quantity of this fragment is produced at low (1:10 000 w/w) enzyme-to-substrate ratios (FIGURE 2).

Electron Microscopy of Thrombospondin Fragments

Electron microscopy of platinum replicas produced by low angle rotary shadowing reveals that thrombospondin is composed of well-defined globular regions connected by thin flexible regions (FIGURE 3A). Three of the globular regions, designated globular region C, appear to be at the ends of the thin connecting regions. The thin connecting regions are 291 ± 46 Å in length and adopt a wide variety of orientations.[22,31] Globular region C is 118 Å in diameter. When thrombospondin is treated with EDTA prior to electron microscopy, the length of the thin connecting region increases to 383 ± 30 Å, and the diameter of globular region C decreases to 80 ± 7.4 Å (FIGURE 3B).

A fourth globular structure, designated globular region N, appears close to the intersection of the three chains and can be seen, in some images, to be composed of three spherical structures that are 70 ± 7.1 Å in diameter (FIGURE 3A).[22,31] Thrombin digestion of thrombospondin in the presence of calcium results in the selective removal of globular region N.[22] By contrast, thrombin digestion in the absence of calcium results in the removal of all of the globular structures (FIGURE 3C). The remaining high molecular weight fragment is a trimeric structure of the thin connecting regions that are cross-linked at one of their ends (FIGURE 3C). The length of the thin connecting regions is 402 ± 27 Å. A similar structure is observed in low-angle metal replicas of the Chy-1 fragment (FIGURE 3D). In this case, the thin-connecting regions are reduced in length to 314 ± 55 Å, consistent with the smaller reduced mass of 70 000 daltons as compared to 130 000 daltons for the thrombin-generated fragment.

The Binding Properties of the Chy-1 Fragment

The binding of intact thrombospondin to plasminogen, fibrinogen, laminin, fibronectin, and type V collagen has been characterized using solid-phase binding assays.[4-8] In this study, we have used a solid-phase assay to compare the binding of the Chy-1 fragment of thrombospondin to these proteins with that of the intact molecule. The dissociation constants were determined from linear regressions of the double-reciprocal plots (TABLE 1). The Chy-1 fragment of thrombospondin bound to the various solid-phase proteins with comparable affinities. The dissociation constants for these interactions were between 5.9×10^{-8} M and 6.9×10^{-8} M. With the exception of laminin (correlation coefficient of .886), the data could be fit to a straight line. The laminin data points had a slight concaved curvature (FIGURE 4). The binding of the Chy-1 fragment to all five ligands was not significantly affected by the presence or absence of 0.5 mM $CaCl_2$. The dissociation constants for the binding of the Chy-1 fragment to laminin, type V collagen, or fibronectin were comparable to the dissociation constants for the binding of intact thrombospondin to these ligands (TABLE 1). By contrast, the dissociation constant for the binding of the Chy-1 fragment to fibrinogen or plasminogen was approximately twofold higher than the dissociation constant for the binding of intact thrombospondin to these ligands (TABLE 1, FIGURE 5). The binding of the 25 000-dalton heparin-binding peptide produced by chymotryptic digestion to the various ligands was comparable to the very low level of nonspecific binding observed when no protein was adsorbed to the plastic wells.

TABLE 1. The Binding of Thrombospondin and the Chy-1 Fragment to Solid-Phase Proteins

	Thrombospondin			Chy-1		
solid-phase protein	$K_d \times 10^8$ M[a]	N(n)[b]	r[c]	$K_d \times 10^8$ M[a]	N(n)[b]	r[c]
laminin	4.37 ± 1.35	6(46)	.9551	6.54 ± 2.83	4(32)	.8860
collagen	5.38 ± 1.03	5(40)	.9467	6.22 ± 1.71	4(32)	.9476
fibronectin	5.27 ± 3.46	5(38)	.9432	6.59 ± 2.20	4(31)	.9546
fibrinogen	15.56 ± 4.21	5(40)	.9649	6.88 ± 2.23	4(32)	.9700
plasminogen	11.71 ± 3.71	7(60)	.9839	5.94 ± 1.32	4(32)	.9806

[a] The dissociation constant (K_d) is expressed as the mean ± the standard deviation.

[b] The values are the average of N different experiments in each of which a line was fit through n points by linear regression when the data was plotted as a double reciprocal plot.[4]

[c] r is the average correlation coefficient for the N experiments.

DISCUSSION

The interaction of thrombospondin with thrombin has provided a mechanism for the elucidation of several aspects of thrombospondin structure. The differences between the peptide pattern produced by thrombin digestion in the presence or absence of calcium was the first indication that thrombospondin binds calcium by a conformation-dependent mechanism.[9] Application of thrombin digests of thrombospondin to heparin-Sepharose resulted in the first identification and localization of the structural domain that contains the heparin-binding site. The correlation of the peptide patterns produced by thrombin digestion with electron microscopic data has provided the first clues to the overall structural organization of the molecule.[22] These data will form the basis for interpretation of functional data on a structural level, eventually leading to an understanding of structure-function relationships in thrombospondin.

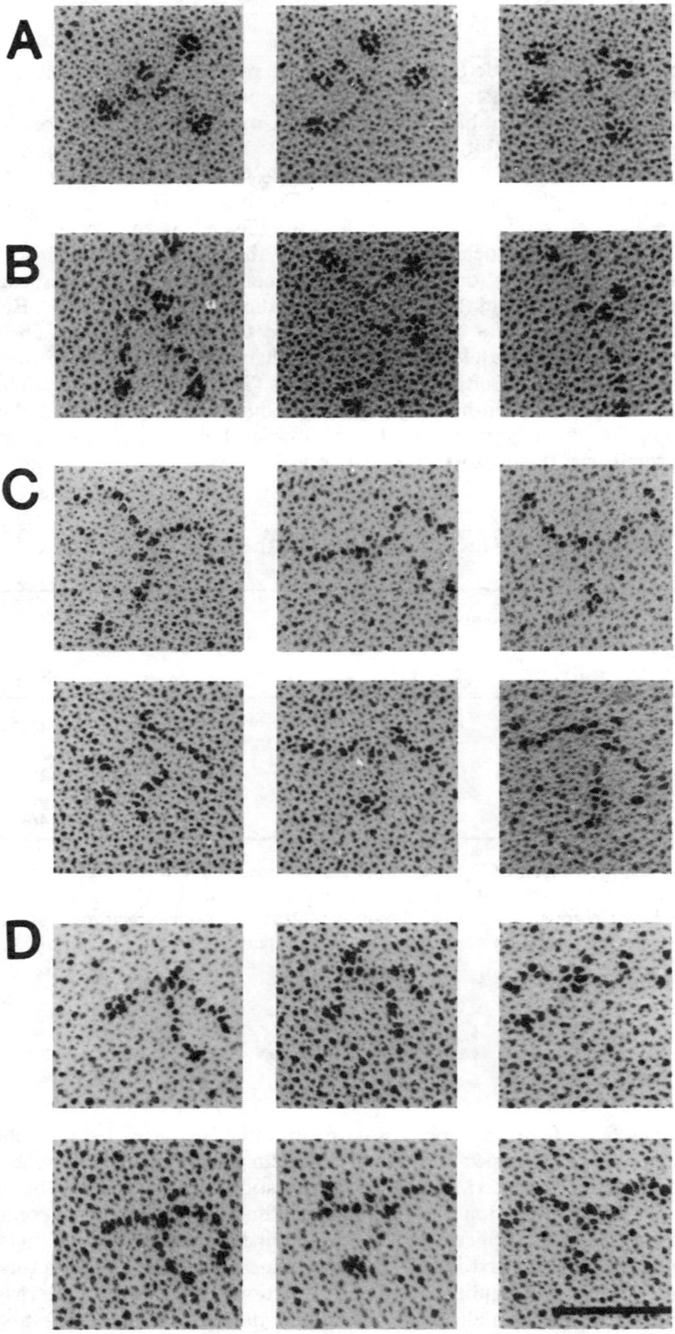

FIGURE 3. Electron microscopy of the high molecular weight fragments of thrombospondin produced by thrombin and chymotrypsin digestion. **A**, intact thrombospondin in the presence of calcium; **B**, intact thrombospondin in the absence of calcium; **C**, the high molecular weight

The properties of the Chy-1 fragment indicate that it is a timeric structure and that its constituent 70 000-dalton polypeptides are derived from the segment II portion of the native thrombospondin polypeptide (FIGURE 6).[22] The 70 000-dalton polypeptides are similar to the 130 000-dalton fragment produced by thrombin digestion and the 85 000-dalton tryptic fragment that comprises segment II in that (1) they are produced in the absence of calcium, (2) they contain the interchain disulfide bonds, (3) they have similar electron microscopic appearance, and (4) they bind Lens culinaris lectin. The 70 000-dalton Chy-1 fragment is similar to the 85 000-dalton tryptic

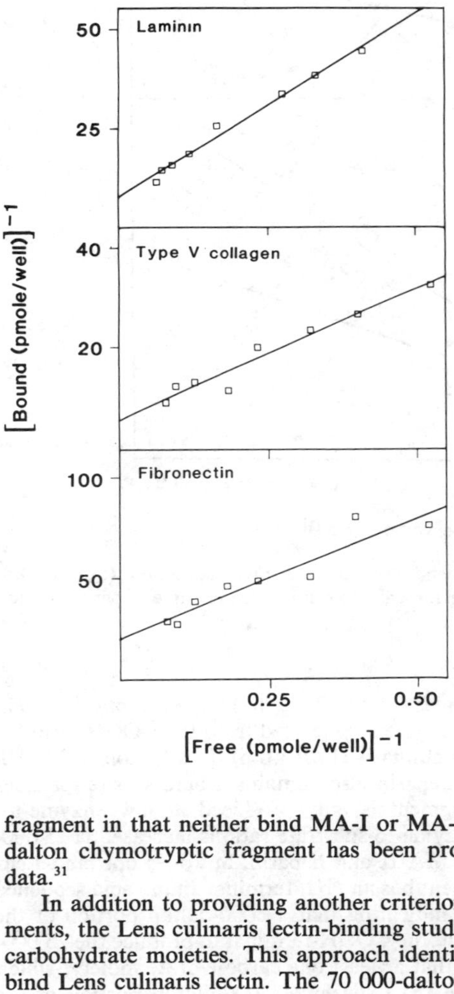

FIGURE 4. The binding of the Chy-1 fragment to solid-phase laminin, type V collagen, or fibronectin. Double-reciprocal plots for representative experiments are shown.

fragment in that neither bind MA-I or MA-II.[22] A similar alignment for the 70 000-dalton chymotryptic fragment has been proposed based on amino acid sequencing data.[31]

In addition to providing another criterion for comparison of the proteolytic fragments, the Lens culinaris lectin-binding studies permit the localization of some of the carbohydrate moieties. This approach identifies only those carbohydrate groups that bind Lens culinaris lectin. The 70 000-dalton polypeptides that constitute the Chy-1

---

fragment of thrombospondin produced by thrombin digestion in the absence of calcium; **D**, the high molecular weight fragment (Chy 1) of thrombospondin produced by chymotryptic digestion; bar=500Å.

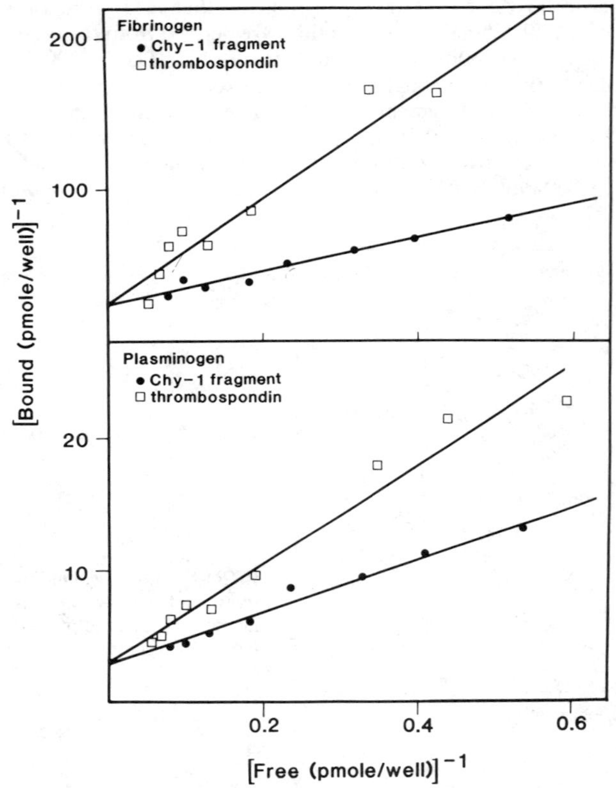

FIGURE 5. The binding of the Chy-1 fragment (●) and intact thrombospondin (□) to solid-phase fibrinogen or plasminogen. Double-reciprocal plots for representative experiments are shown.

fragment bind Lens culinaris lectin, whereas the 53 000-dalton chymotryptic fragment that binds MA-I and the 25 000-dalton fragment generated from the COOH-terminal by thrombin digestion do not bind Lens culinaris (FIGURE 6). In addition, a 30 000-dalton fragment that binds MA-II and heparin also contains a binding site for Lens culinaris lectin. The 30 000-dalton fragment is only produced at low enzyme-to-substrate ratios (1:10 000). When the enzyme-to-substrate ratio is increased, a 25 000-dalton fragment is produced that binds MA-II and heparin, but does not bind Lens culinaris lectin. The 25 000-dalton fragment has an NH_2-terminal amino acid sequence that is identical to the intact molecule, indicating that a 5000-dalton portion of the 30 000-dalton fragment was removed from the COOH-terminal to produce the 25 000-dalton fragment.[31,32] These data suggest that at least one carbohydrate moiety, which binds Lens culinaris lectin, is located in the C-terminal 5000-dalton portion of the 30 000-dalton fragment (FIGURE 6).

The data presented here indicate that the binding site for laminin, type V collagen, fibronectin, fibrinogen, and plasminogen is located in the Chy-1 fragment of thrombospondin. Because we have only assayed the Chy-1 fragment, and the 25 000-dalton heparin-binding fragment, we cannot preclude the possibility that additional binding sites exist for these ligands in other portions of the thrombospondin molecule. The dissociation constants for the binding of the Chy-1 fragment to laminin, type V collagen, and fibronectin are comparable to the dissociation constants for the binding of intact thrombospondin to these ligands. These data support the hypothesis that the Chy-1 binding site is functional in the intact molecule. Mumby *et al.*[8] have shown that the Chy-1 fragment is selectively bound when entire chymotryptic digests of thrombospondin are applied to affinity columns of type V collagen-Sepharose.

The dissociation constants for the Chy-1 fragment of thrombospondin to plasminogen and fibrinogen are approximately twofold higher than the dissociation constants for the binding of intact thrombospondin to these ligands. The decreased affinity that is observed in the binding of the native molecule to these ligands may be due to a partial or complete masking of the Chy-1 binding site by another portion of the molecule. Alternatively, the Chy-1 binding site may be completely masked, and a distinct binding site, which remains to be identified, may account for the binding activity of the native molecule. A third possibility is that the proteolytic removal of the other portions of the molecule has modified the conformation of the Chy-1 fragment. Galvin *et al.*[31] have reported that the binding of monoclonal antibodies to the NH_2-terminal, heparin-binding peptides affects the conformation of the entire thrombospondin molecule.

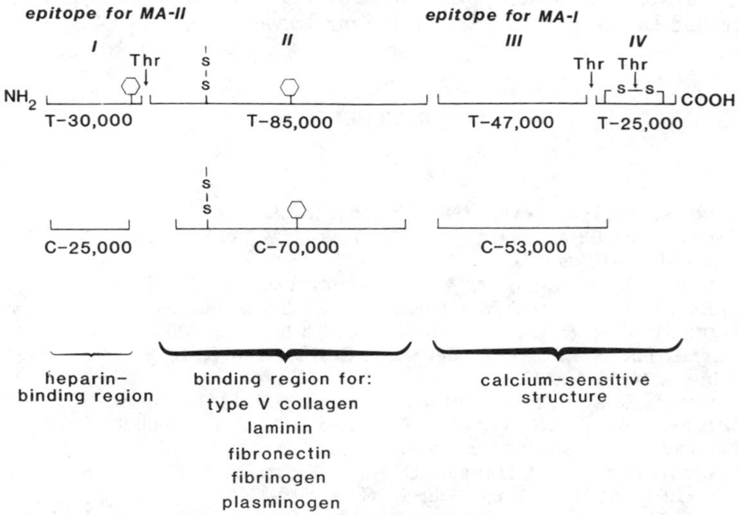

FIGURE 6. Alignment of the chymotryptic fragments and binding regions of thrombospondin. The segments are identified by Roman numerals starting at the NH_2 terminus.[22] The sites for thrombin (Thr) cleavage are indicated by arrows. The masses of the fragments produced by trypsin (T) and chymotrypsin (C) are indicated underneath each fragment. Those fragments that contain carbohydrate moieties (⬡) that bind Lens culinaris lectin are indicated. The position and number of Lens culinaris lectin-binding sites within segment II are not known. The number of Lens culinaris lectin-binding sites within segment I is not known, and the rationale for the localization near the COOH-terminal of segment I is given in the text (see DISCUSSION). The locations of the binding regions and the calcium-sensitive structure are given at the bottom of the diagram. Note that the binding studies were performed on the Chy-1 fragment, which is a trimeric structure of the 70 000-dalton fragment.

The localization of the fibrinogen binding site to the Chy-1 region is consistent with results from other laboratories.[18,31,33] Dixit *et al.*[33] have identified a 120 000-dalton thermolysin-derived fragment of thrombospondin that binds to fibrinogen. Comparison of the properties of this fragment with our data on the chymotryptic and tryptic fragments suggests that this 120 000-dalton fragment most closely overlaps with segments II and III.[22,31,33] In addition, Bale *et al.*[18] have shown that the Chy-1 region contains the site where thrombospondin can become cross-linked to fibrin by factor XIII_a. Finally, Lahav[34] has shown that fibrinogen and fibronectin compete with each other for binding to intact thrombospondin. Localization of the thrombospondin binding sites for laminin, type V collagen, fibronectin, fibrinogen, and plasminogen to the Chy-1 fragment does not mean that they have a common binding site. This fragment is large enough to accommodate multiple distinct binding sites. In this case, competition between the various ligands might occur as a result of steric hinderance. We are presently investigating the substructure of the Chy-1 fragment.

ACKNOWLEDGMENTS

The artwork was done by Mia Thurlow. The manuscript was typed by Loretta Wencis and Lucille Paul, and edited by Sami Lawler.

REFERENCES

1. Lawler, J. & H. Slayter. 1981. Thromb. Res. **22:** 267-279.
2. Dixit, V. M., G. A. Grant, S. A. Santoro & W. A. Frazier. 1984. J. Biol. Chem. **259:** 10100-10105.
3. Lahav, J., M. A. Schwartz & R. O. Hynes. 1982. Cell **31:** 253-262.
4. Lahav, J., J. Lawler & M. Gimbrone. 1984. Eur. J. Biochem. **145:** 151-156.
5. Leung, L. L. K. & R. L. Nachman. 1982. J. Clin. Invest. **70:** 542-549.
6. Silverstein, R. L., L. L. K. Leung, P. C. Harpel & R. L. Nachman. 1984. J. Clin. Invest. **74:** 1625-1633.
7. Leung, L. L. K., R. Nachman & P. Harpel. 1984. J. Clin. Invest. **73:** 5-12.
8. Mumby, S. M., G. J. Raugi & P. Bornstein. 1984. J. Cell Biol. **98:** 646-652.
9. Lawler, J. & E. Simons. 1983. J. Biol. Chem. **258:** 12098-12101.
10. Roberts, D. D., D. M. Haverstick, V. M. Dixit, W. A. Frazier, S. A. Santoro & V. Ginsburg. 1985. J. Biol. Chem. **260:** 9405-9411.
11. Raugi, G. J., S. M. Mumby, D. Abbott-Brown & P. Bornstein. 1982. J. Cell Biol. **95:** 351-354.
12. Jaffe, E. A., J. T. Ruggiero, L. L. K. Leung, M. J. Doyle, P. J. McKeown-Longo & D. F. Mosher. 1983. Proc. Natl. Acad. Sci. USA **80:** 998-1002.
13. McKeown-Longo, P. J., R. Hanning & D. F. Mosher. 1984. J. Cell Biol. **98:** 22-28.
14. Mumby, S. M., D. Abbott-Brown, G. J. Raugi & P. Bornstein. 1984. Cell. Physiol. **120:** 280-288.
15. Kramer, R. H., G. M. Fuh, K. G. Bensch & M. A. Karasek. 1985. J. Cell. Physiol. **123:** 1-9.
16. Majack, R. A., S. C. Cook & P. Bornstein. 1985. J. Cell Biol. **101:** 1059-1070.
17. Murphy-Ullrich, J. E. & D. F. Mosher. 1985. Blood **66:** 1098-1104.
18. Bale, M. D., L. G. Westrick & D. F. Mosher. 1985. J. Biol. Chem. **260:** 7502-7508.

19. TUSZYNSKI, G. P., S. SRIVASTAVA, H. I. SWITALSKA, J. C. HOLT, G. S. CIERNIEWSKI & S. NIEWIAROWSKI. 1985. J. Biol. Chem. **260:** 12240-12245.
20. SILVERSTEIN, R. L., L. L. K. LEUNG, P. C. HARPEL & R. L. NACHMAN. 1985. J. Clin. Invest. **75:** 2065-2073.
21. LAWLER J., F. C. CHAO & C. M. COHEN. 1982. J. Biol. Chem. **257:** 12257-12265.
22. LAWLER, J., L. H. DERICK, J. E. CONNOLLY, J. H. CHEN & F. C. CHAO. 1985. J. Biol. Chem. **260:** 3762-3772.
23. TAKAHASHI, K., M. AIKEN, J. W. FENTON & D. A. WALZ. 1984. Biochem. J. **224:** 673-676.
24. HAGEN, I., G. O. GOGSTAD, F. BROSSTAD & N. O. SOLUM. 1983. Biochim. Biophys. Acta **732:** 600-606.
25. DANISHEFSKY, K. J., R. J. ALEXANDER & T. C. DETWILER. 1984. Biochemistry **23:** 4984-4990.
26. YEO, K-T & T. C. DETWILER. 1985. Archives Biochem. Biophys. **236:** 299-410.
27. LAEMMLI, U. K. 1970. Nature (London) **227:** 680-685.
28. GLASS II, W. F., R. C. BRIGGS & L. S. HNILICA. 1981. Anal. Biochem. **115:** 219-224.
29. ALMEDA, S., R. D. ROSENBERG & D. H. BING. 1983. J. Biol. Chem. **258:** 785-791.
30. TYLER, J. M. & D. BRANTON. 1980. J. Ultrastruct. Res. **71:** 95-102.
31. GALVIN, N. J., V. M. DIXIT, K. M. O'ROURKE, S. A. SANTORO, G. A. GRANT & W. A. FRAZIER. 1985. J. Cell Biol. **101:** 1434-1441.
32. RAUGI, G. J., S. M. MUMBY, D. A. READY & P. BORNSTEIN. 1984. Thromb. Res. **36:** 165-175.
33. DIXIT, V. M., G. A. GRANT, W. A. FRAZIER & S. A. SANTORO. 1984. Biochem. Biophysics Res. Comm. **119:** 1075-1081.
34. LAHAV, J. 1985. Thromb. Haemostasis **54:** 63.

Thrombin Cleavage of Extracellular Matrix Proteins

RONALD H. GOLDFARB[a,c] AND LANCE A. LIOTTA[b]

[a]*Cancer Metastasis Research Group*
Pfizer Central Research Division
Groton, Connecticut 06340

[b]*Laboratory of Pathology*
National Cancer Institute
National Institutes of Health
Bethesda, Maryland 20892

PROTEOLYTIC ENZYMES AND CANCER METASTASIS

Proteolytic enzymes appear to play important roles in the degradation of a number of host extracellular matrices.[1–10] The investigation of the role of proteolytic enzymes in degradation of extracellular matrices has largely contributed to our understanding of biochemical mechanisms involved in tumor invasion and metastasis. Cancer metastases are the major cause of treatment failure, morbidity, and death for patients with solid malignant tumors.[11] At the time of diagnosis of the primary tumor, most patients presenting with primary tumors already have occult subclinical secondary micrometastases to which the patient ultimately succumbs.[11,12] The dispersed anatomic location of metastases and their heterogeneous cell composition often prevents surgical removal and responsiveness to radiotherapy and systemic anticancer agents that are currently available. There is therefore a critical need for the development of new methods to predict the aggressive metastatic properties of a patient's individual tumor, to identify clinically occult micrometastases, and to prevent and treat local tumor invasion and established metastatic disease.[11,12] Our research approach towards achieving these goals is the study of the biochemical mechanisms involved in tumor invasion and metastasis.[1,2,7,12] The exploration of invasive tumor cells and their proteolytic enzymes has been an important component in unraveling these biochemical mechanisms, because they contribute to the degradation of host matrices including the basement membrane.[1,2,12,17]

The process of cancer metastasis is dependent upon a complex and dynamic interaction between host factors, such as antitumor immune reactivity, and the biochemical properties of invasive, metastatic cells.[11] In addition, the process of metastasis is highly selective and only a few cells comprising a subpopulation within the heterogeneous primary neoplasm can survive and complete all the steps required for the establishment of distant secondary metastatic tumor colonies.[11] Local tumor invasion

[c]Current address: Pittsburgh Cancer Institute and Department of Pathology, University of Pittsburgh, School of Medicine, Pittsburgh, PA 15213-2592.

is an early step in the complex process that leads to metastasis. After invasion of host tissue barriers adjacent to the borders of primary tumors, tumor cells must invade the vascular wall or lymphatic channels in order to disseminate. Tumor cells in the circulation must be able to evade host defenses such as natural killer cells, survive the mechanical trauma of blood flow, and stop in the venous or capillary bed of the target organ.[7,11] Mechanisms of vascular arrest include mechanical wedging, entrapment with platelets and fibrin, attachment to endothelium, and interaction with exposed subendothelial basement membrane. Once arrested, the tumor cells must again invade through the vascular wall to enter organ parenchyma. This process can be repeated to give rise to metastases from metastases.

Metastasizing tumor cells encounter a number of host extracellular barriers as they disseminate from the primary tumor and establish metastatic colonies.[7,12] Such matrices may be composed of a dense meshwork of proteoglycans, glycoproteins, and collagenous components. The basement membrane is one type of extracellular matrix that invasive tumor cells encounter at more than one step in the metastatic cascade as they cross from one tissue to another or as they enter and exit blood vessels.[7,12] The basement membrane, which includes type IV collagen, laminin, and heparan sulfate proteoglycan as components, forms a scaffolding support for organ parenchymal cells and also delineates the boundaries between organ parenchyma and interstitial stroma.[7,12] In adult normal tissues, the extracellular basement membrane is a stable structure with a slow turnover rate. During certain disease states, such as malignant cancer, histological studies have shown the rapid dissolution of the basement membrane.[7,12] Penetration of the basement membrane appears to involve a battery of proteolytic enzymes directly or indirectly associated with tumor cells.[1–10]

A three-step hypothesis describes the sequence of biochemical events during tumor cell invasion of the extracellular matrix.[12] The first step is tumor-cell attachment, which appears to be mediated through specific glycoproteins such as laminin or fibronectin through cell membrane receptors.[7,12] The second step is local degradation of the matrix by tumor-cell-associated proteases.[1,2] Such proteases may degrade both the attachment proteins as well as locally degrade the collagenous and noncollagenous components of the matrix. Proteolysis may be localized at the tumor-cell surface where the amount of active enzymes outbalances the natural inhibitors of proteolytic enzymes present in serum or extracellular matrices. The third step is tumor-cell locomotion into the region of the matrix modified by proteolysis. The direction of locomotion may be influenced by chemotactic factors. Continued invasion of the extracellular matrix may take place by a cyclic repetition of these three steps.[12]

It is clear that invasive tumor cells produce a number of separate and distinct degradative enzymes that contribute to tumor invasion, including plasminogen activator, plasmin, type IV collagenase, cathepsin B, and an endoglycosidase (heparanase).[1,2,13,16,17] We have examined the effect of a number of highly purified degradative and regulatory, neutral serine proteases, including alpha thrombin, for their effects on isolated basement membranes or purified basement membrane components, as described below.[7,13–15]

THROMBIN DEGRADATION OF MATRIX PROTEINS

For the studies to be described below, purified enzymes were employed.[13–15] Electrophoretic analysis indicated that the alpha thrombin employed, generously supplied by Dr. John Fenton, had a M_r of 39 000.[13] The M_r of the pure human plasminogen used was 90 000, and the M_r forms of purified plasminogen activator (urokinase) were 53 000 and 34 000.[13] In studies directed towards evaluating the capacity of neutral serine proteases to cleave type IV collagen and type V collagen, purified type IV collagenase and purified type V collagenase were employed as positive controls under conditions that yielded reproducible cleavage products.

We observed that at either physiological levels, or at levels 1000-fold in excess of physiological levels, urokinase failed to significantly degrade the plasma form of fibronectin under partial or complete reducing conditions.[13,14] The activity of the urokinase employed was verified before and after the incubation with fibronectin.[14] By contrast, fibronectin was cleaved by plasmin and alpha thrombin, in agreement with other studies in the literature.[18]

The effect of these proteases on degradation of laminin, type IV collagen, and type V collagen was also examined.[13,14] We observed that plasmin degraded both the alpha and beta chains of native laminin at 25 degrees centigrade. By contrast, alpha-thrombin was found to degrade the 400 kDa beta chain of laminin but failed to degrade the 200 kDa alpha chain. Rotary shadowing electron microscopy studies indicated that alpha-thrombin selectively cleaved the long arm of laminin embodied within the beta subunit.[7,15] Alpha-thrombin selectively digested the beta subunit of laminin without digesting the alpha subunit. Digestion of laminin by alpha-thrombin, therefore, constitutes a method for the isolation of the alpha subunit of laminin in native form. Additional studies, employing a variety of different proteases, have identified a number of laminin fragments.[15] We have subsequently identified domains of the laminin molecule involved in distinct biological functions.[7,19] Our studies have indicated that laminin is involved in the attachment of highly invasive tumor cells to basement membrane type IV collagen through laminin receptors.[19] It is noteworthy that the alpha-thrombin-generated alpha subunit is as effective as native laminin in mediating this attachment. By contrast, additional protease-derived fragments of laminin, such as those isolated following treatment with cathepsin G, prevent this attachment event *in vitro* and inhibits tumor metastasis formation *in vivo*.[7,15,19]

In addition to the studies dealing with glycoprotein degradation, we also examined whether the neutral serine proteases described above could also cleave type IV collagen or type V collagen. We observed that thrombin failed to degrade acid-extracted type IV collagen and pepsinized type IV collagen.[13,14] At high concentrations, however, plasmin produced a small reduction in the lower of the two type IV collagen chains, consistent with nonspecific removal of a part of the nonhelical telopeptide region.[13,14]

Type V collagen, when incubated at 25° C with alpha-thrombin, was not significantly degraded. With incubation as high as 33° C and prolonged digestion times, type V collagen was not cleaved by alpha-thrombin.[13,14] At 35° C, however, alpha-thrombin did produce specific cleavage products of type V collagen; plasmin also showed a temperature-dependent cleavage of type V collagen.[13,14]

Because plasmin degraded two noncollagenous components associated with the basement membrane zone, that is, fibronectin and laminin, and had a small effect on acid-extracted type IV collagen, we also examined the effect of plasmin on whole, isolated amnion basement membrane.[14] The effects of plasmin treatment on the immunofluorescent localization of antitype IV collagen and antilaminin antibodies for intact basement membrane were examined. It was found that plasmin removed the laminin, but not the type IV collagen immunoreactivity, from the intact basement membrane.[14] Even though the basement membrane lamina densa was not completely destroyed by treatment with plasmin, immunoreactivity was lost for antilaminin and antifibronectin antibodies.[14] By contrast, immunoreactivity for antitype IV collagen antibodies was preserved after plasmin treatment of the intact basement membrane.

CONCLUDING STATEMENTS

In summary, our findings have suggested that basement membrane components are poor substrates for urokinase alone. In addition, plasmin alone is not sufficient to completely degrade the basement membrane. Plasmin, generated by plasminogen activation, may play a key role in degradation of noncollagenous components of the basement membrane, and in activation of latent collagenases.

Alpha-thrombin has the capacity to cleave fibronectin and laminin into distinct fragments. In the case of laminin, alpha-thrombin selectively cleaves the beta chain of this glycoprotein. In addition, alpha-thrombin does not appear to have the capacity to cleave basement membrane type IV collagen. Type V collagen can be cleaved by alpha-thrombin at 35° C, but not at temperatures below 33° C. Because type V collagen can be denatured at 35° C, the physiological significance of type V collagen cleavage by alpha-thrombin at thirty-five degrees Centigrade remains an open question. By contrast, the action of alpha-thrombin on subendothelial basement membrane laminin may be an important regulatory effect of this protease. For example, degradation of laminin by alpha-thrombin may play a role in endothelial migration during wound healing or vascularization because migration may involve a sequential series of binding events.

The degradation of laminin by neutral serine proteases, and the generation of distinct laminin fragments, may facilitate the passage of immune cells and tumor cells through various extracellular matrices including basement membranes.[20] The protease-derived fragments of laminin that we have observed should continue to be useful probes in the study of the functional and immunologic properties of the molecule.

REFERENCES

1. GOLDFARB, R. H. & L. A. LIOTTA. 1986. Proteolytic enzymes in cancer invasion and metastasis. Semin. Thromb. Hemostasis. **12:** 294-307.
2. GOLDFARB, R. H. 1986. Proteolytic enzymes in tumor invasion and degradation of host extracellular matrices. *In* Mechanisms of Cancer Metastasis. Potential Therapeutic Implications. K. V. Honn, W. E. Powers & B. F. Sloane, Eds.: 341-375. Martinus Nijhoff. Boston, MA.
3. JONES, P. A., E. BOGENMANN, Y. A. DE CLERCK, W. E. LAUG, M. HEISEL, H. B. NEUSTEIN & H. ISAACS. 1984. Degradation of artificial tissue substrates. *In* Cancer Invasion and Metastasis: Biologic and Therapeutic Aspects. G. L. Nicolson & L. Milas, Eds.: 177-186. Raven Press. New York.
4. NICOLSON, G. L., M. NAKAJIMA & T. IRIMURA. 1986. Invasion of vascular endothelium and organ tissue *in vitro* by B16 melanoma variants. *In:* Mechanisms of Cancer Metastasis. Potential Therapeutic Implications. K. V. Honn, W. E. Powers & B. F. Sloane, Eds.: 275-298. Martinus Nijhoff. Boston, MA.
5. QUIGLEY, J. P., R. H. GOLDFARB, C. J. SCHEINER, J. O'DONNEL-TORMEY & T. YEO. 1980. Plasminogen activator and the membrane of transformed cells. *In* Prog. Clin. Biol. Res. (Tumor Cell Surfaces and Malignancy) **41:** 773-796.
6. QUIGLEY, J. P., E. CRAMER, S. FAIRBAIRN, R. GILBERT, J. LACOVARA, G. OJAKIAN & R. SCHWIMMER. 1986. *In* Mechanisms of Cancer Metastasis. Potential Therapeutic Implications. K. V. Honn, W. E. Powers & B. F. Sloane, Eds.: 309-340. Martinus Nijhoff. Boston, MA.

7. LIOTTA, L. A. & R. H. GOLDFARB. 1984. Interaction of tumor cells with the basement membrane of endothelium. *In* Hemostatic Mechanisms and Metastasis. K. V. Honn & B. F. Sloane, Eds.: 319-336. Martinus Nijhoff. Boston, MA.
8. SLOANE, B. F., J. ROZHIN, R. E. RYAN, T. T. LAH, N. A. DAY, J. D. CRISSMAN & K. V. HONN. 1986. Cathepsin B-like cysteine proteinases and metastasis. *In* Mechanisms of Cancer Metastasis. Potential Therapeutic Implications. 377-398. Martinus Nijhoff. Boston, MA.
9. STRAULI, P., A. J. BARRETT & A. J. BAICI, Eds. 1980. Proteinases and Tumor Invasion. Raven Press. New York.
10. PAULI, B. U., E. E. SCHWARTZ, E. J-M. THONAR & K. E. KUETTNER. 1983. Tumor invasion and host extracellular matrix. Cancer Met. Rev. **2:** 129-152.
11. GOLDFARB, R. H., K. W. BRUNSON & H. E. KAISER. 1987. Overview of current understanding of tumor spread. *In* Progressive Stages of Malignant Neoplastic Growth. H. E. Kaiser, Ed. Martinus. In Press.
12. LIOTTA, L. A. 1986. Tumor invasion and metastasis—Role of the extracellular matrix: Rhoads memorial award lecture. Cancer Res. **46:** 1-7.
13. LIOTTA, L. A., R. H. GOLDFARB & V. P. TERRANOVA. 1981. Cleavage of laminin by thrombin and plasmin: Alpha thrombin selectively cleaves the beta chain of laminin. Thromb. Res. **21:** 663-673.
14. LIOTTA, L. A., R. H. GOLDFARB, R. BRUNDAGE, G. P. SIEGAL, V. TERRANOVA & S. GARBISA. 1981. Effect of plasminogen activator (urokinase), plasmin, and thrombin on glycoprotein and collagenous components of basement membrane. Cancer Res. **41:** 4629-4636.
15. RAO, C. N., I. M. K. MARGULIES, R. H. GOLDFARB, J. A. MADRI, D. T. WOODLEY & L. A. LIOTTA. 1982. Differential proteolytic susceptibility of laminin alpha and beta subunits. Arch. Biochem. Biophys. **219:** 65-70.
16. GOLDFARB, R. H. & J. P. QUIGLEY. 1978. Synergistic effect of tumor virus transformation and tumor promoter treatment on the production of plasminogen activator by chick embryo fibroblasts. Cancer Res. **38:** 4601-4609.
17. GOLDFARB, R. H. & J. P. QUIGLEY. 1980. Purification of plasminogen activator from Rous sarcoma virus transformed chick embryo fibroblasts treated with the tumor promoter phorbol 12-myristate 13-acetate. Biochemistry **19:** 5463-5471.
18. FURIE, M. B. & D. B. RIFKIN. 1980. Proteolytically derived fragments of human plasma fibronectin and their localization within the intact molecule. J. Biol. Chem. **255:** 3134-3140.
19. LIOTTA, L. A., N. C. RAO, S. H. BARSKY & T. M. TURPEENIEMI-HUJANEN. 1986. Domains of laminin and basement membrane collagen which play a role in metastases. *In* Mechanisms of Cancer Metastasis. Potential Therapeutic Implications. K. V. Honn, W. E. Powers & B. F. Sloane, Eds.: 299-308. Martinus Nijhoff. Boston, MA.
20. GOLDFARB, R. H. 1986. Cell-mediated cytotoxic reactions. Hum. Pathol. **17:** 138-145.

Thrombin-Induced Alterations in Endothelial Permeability[a]

ASRAR B. MALIK, SIU K. LO, AND RENA BIZIOS

Department of Physiology
Albany Medical College of Union University
Albany, New York 12208

INTRODUCTION

The primary function of thrombin is the inducement of the clotting of fibrinogen.[1] Distinct fibrinogen recognition and catalytic sites are found on the B chain of the molecule.[1] The thrombin molecule also has other potentially important physiological functions that are closely related to the specific domains on the molecule[1] (FIGURE 1). Recently, it has been recognized that there is a chemotactic domain on the B chain, which allows the thrombin molecule to produce alterations in the function of leukocytes, in particular, chemotaxis of monocytes[2,3] and neutrophils.[4] The finding that there is a chemotactic domain raises the interesting implication that thrombin is an important mediator of the inflammatory response, in which leukocyte migration is an essential feature of the response. This review addresses the potential role of thrombin as an inflammatory mediator.

Because vascular permeability alterations are an important aspect of the inflammatory response, we have examined the effects of thrombin on microvascular permeability. FIGURE 2 defines endothelial permeability, as the term is applied to the pulmonary microcirculation. With a few modifications, it is also applicable to other vascular beds. FIGURE 2 shows a semipermeable vessel surrounded by a perivascular interstitial space. The interstitial space is connected to the lymphatic drainage (FIGURE 2).

By cannulation of a main efferent lymphatic vessel, it is possible to assess the changes in lymph flow and lymph protein clearance, and thereby make inferences about transvascular fluid and protein fluxes occurring at the level of the vessel wall.[5] The factors governing the transvascular fluid exchange are represented by the four pressures in the Starling equation: $J_v = K_f[P_c - P_i) - \sigma_d(\pi_p - \pi_i)]$, where P_c is the capillary pressure acting outwardly, that is, P_c drives fluid into the interstitial spaces; P_i is the interstitial hydrostatic pressure acting inwards; π_i is the interstitial oncotic pressure resulting from the interstitial protein concentration (generated by the semipermeable endothelial barrier), and this pressure acts outwards; π_p is the plasma oncotic pressure resulting from the fact that endothelium is poorly permeable to plasma proteins, and this pressure acts inwards, that is, π_p draws fluid into the capillary. These pressures are summated in the Starling equation: the net transvascular volume

[a] This work was supported by HL-32418 (program project) from the National Institutes of Health.

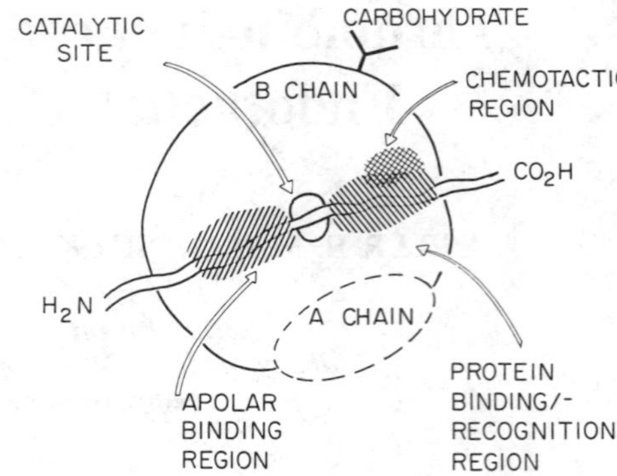

FIGURE 1. A schematic representation of the thrombin molecule. Note that there are distinct domains on the B chain of the molecule.

flow (J_v) in steady-state is equal to the lymph flow (Qlym), which in turn is equal to a constant (K_f, the capillary filtration coefficient) times the summation of these four pressures. The important point of the Starling equation is that it is possible to estimate the net transvascular volume flow or the net fluid filtration rate across the microvascular barrier by the measurement of lymph flow.[5,6] The vessel wall protein reflection coefficient (σ_d) (a constant in the Starling equation) is a measure of the vessel permeability to proteins ($\sigma_d = 1$ indicates that the microvascular barrier is impermeable

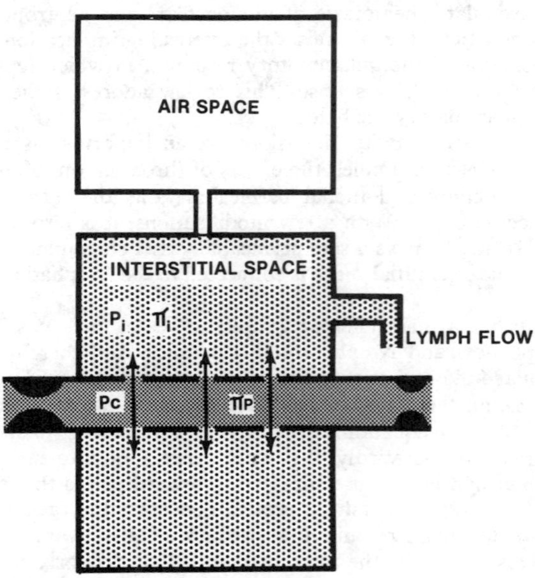

$$J_V = J_L = K_F[(P_c - P_i) - \sigma(\pi_P - \pi_i)]$$

FIGURE 2. Diagram depicts a microvessel passing through the interstitial space. The net fluid filtered across the microvessel forms the lymph, and rate of fluid filtration is governed by the Starling equation (described in the text). During pulmonary edema, excess interstitial fluid can flow into the alveolar space.

to proteins, whereas $\sigma_d = 0$ indicates complete permeability to proteins). The σ_d determines the effective colloid osmotic pressure gradient acting across the capillary wall, and thus the degree to which the oncotic pressure gradient influences the transcapillary fluid filtration rate. In the unanesthetized sheep, the normal pulmonary vasculature σ_d averages 0.70.[7]

EFFECTS OF THROMBIN ON TRANSVASCULAR FLUID AND PROTEIN EXCHANGE

What happens to the transvascular fluid filtration and protein exchange when intravascular coagulation in the pulmonary microvessels is induced by an intravenous injection of thrombin? FIGURE 3 shows the effects of such an experiment in which thrombin (1 U/ml blood volume) is infused. There is a large increase in pulmonary lymph flow, indicating an increase in the pulmonary transvascular filtration rate. The response is rapid, reaching a maximum within 30 minutes after the thrombin challenge. Another important feature of the response is the marked increase in plasma-lymph protein transport as measured by transvascular protein clearance (Qlym $\times$ lymph/plasma protein concentration ratio). A large increase in protein clearance is a good measure of an increased permeability of the microvasculature to proteins.[8,9] At a high pulmonary lymph flow, such as that observed after thrombin, the lymph-to-plasma protein ratio should decrease as a result of ultra filtration, and the transvascular protein clearance would not increase markedly.[10] This is a characteristic response if the increase in transvascular fluid filtration occurs as a result of a rise in the capillary hydrostatic pressure.[10] The response after thrombin, however, was quite different, because it was not associated with a decrease in the lymph-to-plasma protein concentration ratio. In addition, the pulmonary vascular protein reflection coefficient decreased from 0.70 to 0.59[7] following thrombin challenge, indicating that thrombin resulted in an increase in lung vascular permeability to proteins.

Another characteristic feature of the response is the rapid decrease in the peripheral blood leukocyte count and a delayed decrease in the platelet count (FIGURE 4). Platelet aggregation is a well-known function of thrombin,[11–13] and may explain the thrombocytopenia observed with thrombin. Because the decrease in platelet count occurred after the neutropenia, neutrophil sequestration may have contributed to the platelet response. Fibrin microemboli were present in the pulmonary microvessels (FIGURE 5). Neutrophils were present in both the vascular and interstitial spaces. In the vascular space, neutrophils were often observed trapped in the fibrin matrix. Neutrophils in the microvessels were also observed actively phagocytosing fibrin fibrils (FIGURE 5a). There was evidence of endothelial injury at sites close to the fibrin deposition (FIGURE 5b), which could account for the increase of lung vascular permeability to protein.

ROLE OF NEUTROPHILS IN MEDIATING VASCULAR INJURY

Fibrin accumulation appears to be an important factor in the pulmonary neutrophil sequestration observed after thrombin. Studies were made in which fibrin entrapment was prolonged by inhibition of the fibrinolytic system using tranexamic acid. Neu-

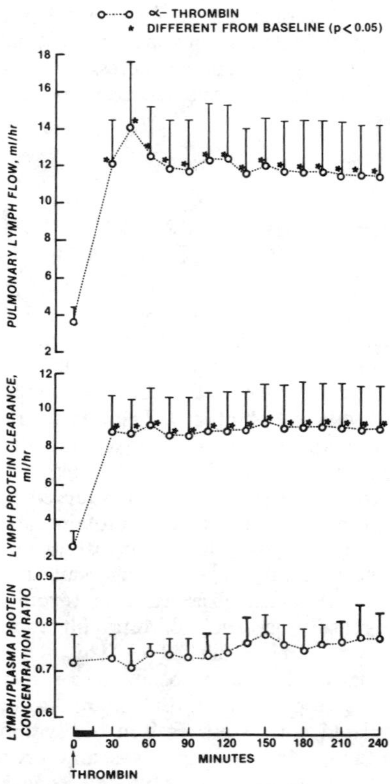

FIGURE 3. Effects of infusion of α-thrombin (1 U/ml blood volume) on pulmonary lymph flow, lymph protein clearance, and lymph-to-plasma protein concentration ratio in halothane-anesthetized sheep. Note the marked and immediate increase in pulmonary lymph flow following thrombin. The increase is associated with no change in lymph-to-plasma protein concentration ratio, suggesting an increase in pulmonary vascular permeability.

trophil uptake in lung was followed by injecting Indium oxine (^{111}In)-labeled neutrophils. The labeled neutrophil activity over the lung increased following thrombin infusion, and the increase paralleled the uptake of fibrin (FIGURE 6a). In the presence of normal fibrinolysis, however, the uptake of neutrophils following thrombin was short-lived (FIGURE 6b), presumably because the neutrophils were rapidly cleared from the lung, as the fibrin was lysed. This finding indicates fibrin contributes to neutrophil sequestration in the lung. Other findings using cultured endothelial monolayers on which fibrin was layered on the cell surface have also shown that fibrin contributes to neutrophil adherence to the normal endothelial monolayer, suggesting fibrin is an important factor in the neutrophil sequestration response.

Neutrophils have been shown to be the effector cells mediating the increase in lung vascular permeability that follows thrombin.[14] The increase in permeability appears to be the result of neutrophil activation and generation of substances from neutrophils subsequent to the thrombin-induced pulmonary microembolism. FIGURE 7 shows the effects of thrombin in an unanesthetized sheep depleted of neutrophils using hydroxyurea. Thrombin challenge in this animal resulted in an increase in pulmonary lymph flow, but the increase in lymph flow was not sustained, as in animals with a normal neutrophil count. The lymph flow (or the net transcapillary filtration rate) is increased, and is associated with a decrease in the lymph-to-plasma protein concentration ratio. The σ_d estimated is identical to that of normal sheep, indicating that the increased lymph flow is due to an increase in the microvascular hydrostatic pressure and not to an increase in the capillary permeability. A similar protection was observed in animals in which neutropenia was induced with antileukocyte serum.[15] Platelet depletion, however, is not protective.[14] Even though platelets may be trapped and activated in the pulmonary microcirculation, they do not appear to mediate the increase in lung vascular permeability induced by thrombin.

The mechanisms of the neutrophil-mediated increase in pulmonary vascular permeability are unclear, but there are some likely possibilities. Substance(s) are released into pulmonary lymph (*i.e.*, the microvascular filtrate) following thrombin challenge, which are capable of altering the neutrophil functions. These substance(s) released into pulmonary lymph following thrombin have been shown to induce chemotaxis of isolated normal neutrophils, to induce neutrophils to aggregate *in vitro*, and also to generate superoxide anion from isolated neutrophils. There is a time-dependent appearance of the neutrophil-activating substance(s) in the pulmonary lymph, peaking at 20-30 minutes after thrombin. Because all samples were collected with hirudin (a

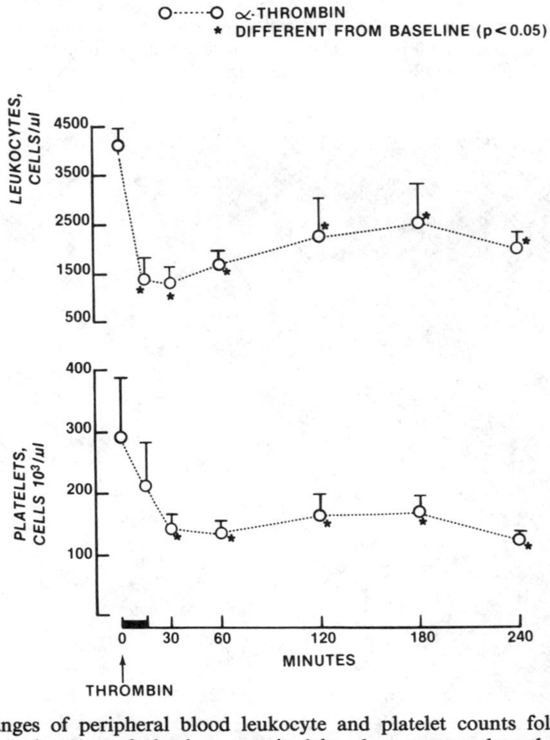

FIGURE 4. Changes of peripheral blood leukocyte and platelet counts following thrombin infusion. Note that the drop of platelet count is delayed as compared to the decrease in the leukocyte count.

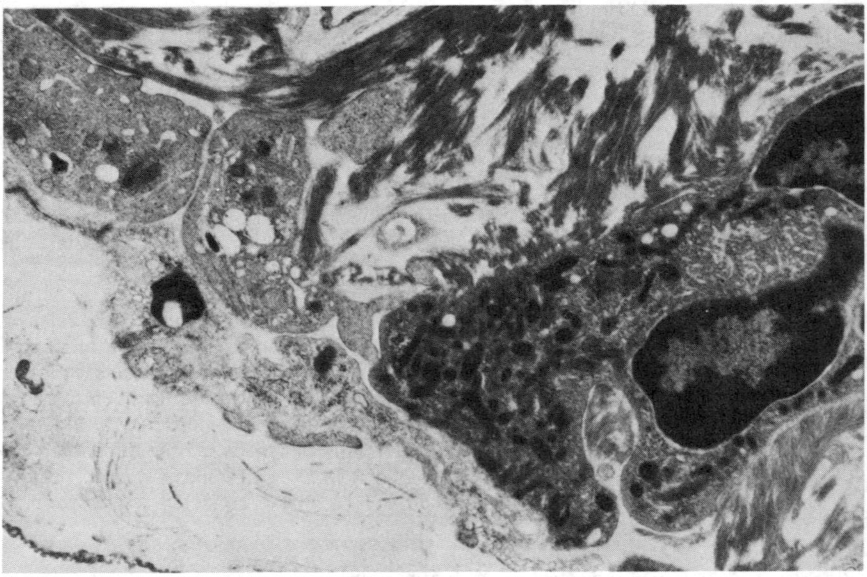

FIGURE 5a. Electron micrograph of a pulmonary vessel in a dog following thrombin infusion; neutrophils and platelets are found associated with fibrin. A neutrophil is observed forming a phagocytic vacuole engulfing fibrin fibrils, indicating active phagocytosis of fibrin by neutrophils.

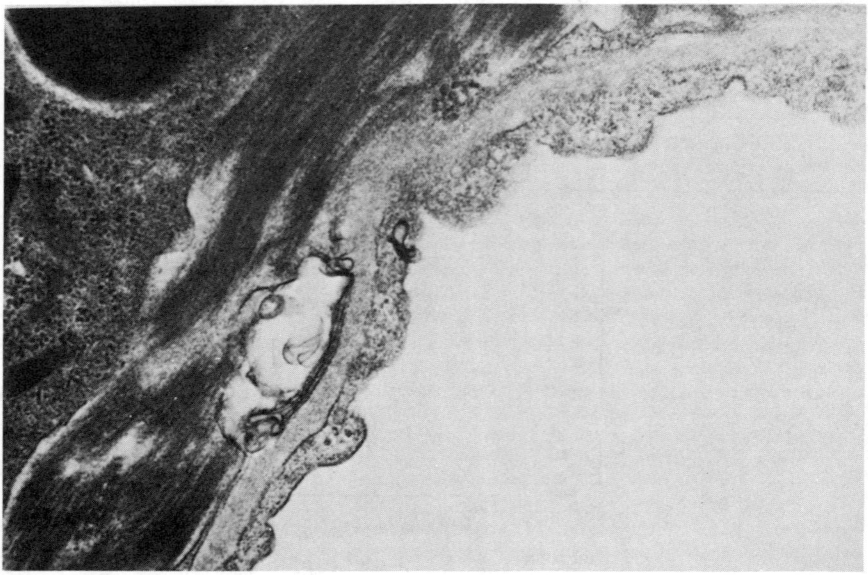

FIGURE 5b. Electron micrograph of a pulmonary vessel in a dog following thrombin infusion. Fibrins are seen in close proximity to endothelial cells, and endothelial injury is noted at the point of contact of fibrin with endothelium.

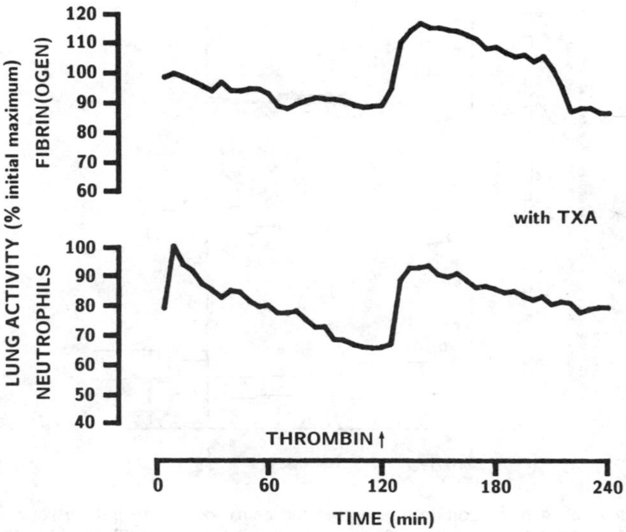

FIGURE 6a. Activity of ^{111}In-labeled sheep neutrophils (PMN) in the sheep lung. Thrombin is infused into sheep at 120 min. The sheep has been pretreated with an antifibrinolytic agent (tranexamic acid, 100 mg). The lung PMN activity is expressed as percentage of maximal lung PMN activity. Thrombin (80 U/kg) caused an immediate and sustained increase of neutrophil activity, indicating a rapid pulmonary neutrophil uptake and a prolonged neutrophil sequestration in the lung.

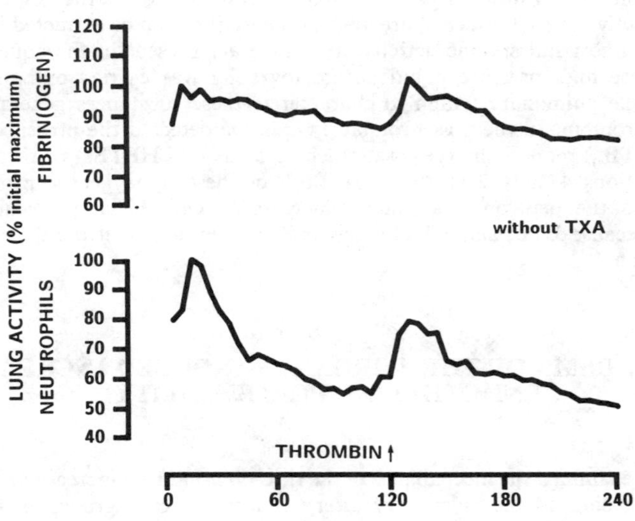

FIGURE 6b. Activity of ^{111}In-labeled sheep neutrophils in the sheep lung. Unlike the fibrinolytically depressed sheep, thrombin infusion in normal sheep only caused a transient increase in pulmonary neutrophil activity.

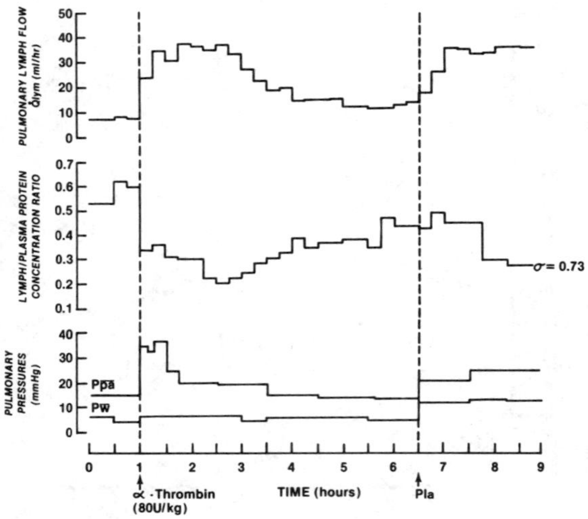

FIGURE 7. Effect of thrombin on an unanesthetized neutropenic sheep. Neutropenia is induced by daily administration of hydroxyurea (200 mg/kg/day) for 4 days. Thrombin infusion caused an immediate increase of pulmonary lymph flow, which was associated with a decrease in the lymph-to-plasma concentration ratio. A sustained increase of pulmonary lymph flow did not occur in the neutropenic sheep. Raising the pulmonary microvascular pressure by inflating the left atrial balloon allows the estimation of the protein reflection coefficient, and this value is comparable to that in normal sheep (0.70-0.73).

thrombin inhibitor), thrombin *per se* cannot be responsible for the response. These neutrophil-activating substance(s) are lipids, because they can be extracted in the ether fraction to almost full specific activity, and none are present in the aqueous phase. Reverse phase high pressure liquid chromatography was carried out on the ether fraction of the pulmonary lymph to characterize these substances generated *in vivo* following thrombin. In the postthrombin lymph, we detected the presence of leukotriene B_4 (LTB$_4$)) monohydroxyeicosatetraenoic acids (*i.e.* HETEs) in the chromatographic fractions 4 and 12 (FIGURE 8). Both of these lipoxygenase products may contribute to the neutrophil-dependent increase in endothelial permeability after thrombin, because LTB$_4$ and HETEs are known to induce neutrophil sequestration and activation.[16-18]

MECHANISMS OF THE THROMBIN-INDUCED INCREASE IN ENDOTHELIAL PERMEABILITY

We have examined the mechanisms of the thrombin-induced increase in endothelial permeability using bovine pulmonary artery endothelial cells grown on nucleopore filters as shown in FIGURE 9. A transmission electron microscopic section of the endothelium grown on a gelatinized nucleopore filter is shown in FIGURE 10a. The endothelial cells form a confluent monolayer on the filter. In addition, there is an

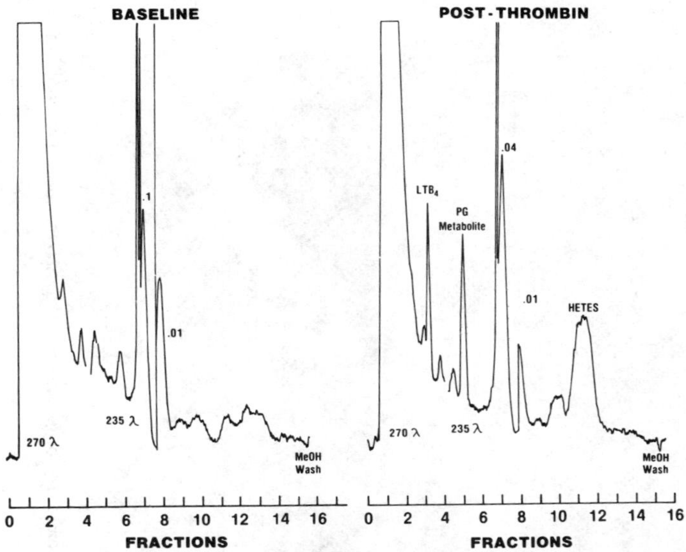

FIGURE 8. Reverse-phase high pressure liquid chromatography (HPLC) of the pulmonary lymph from sheep before and after thrombin challenge. The pulmonary lymph was extracted with ether before assay on HPLC. Note the appearance of three peaks in the postthrombin pulmonary lymph, which correspond to that coeluted with LTB_4, pzostaglandin metabolites, and HETEs.

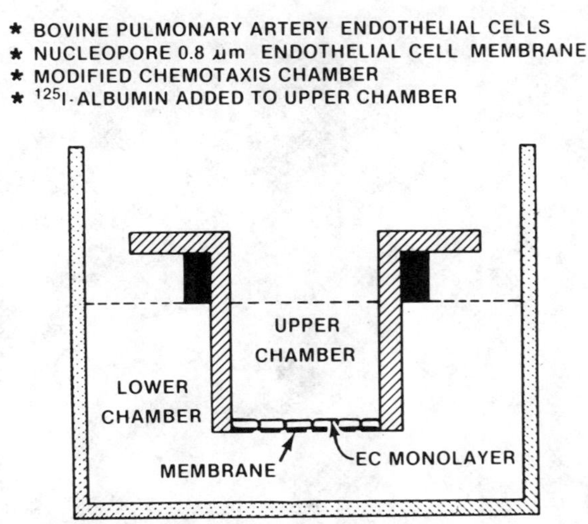

FIGURE 9. Schematic depiction of the endothelial monolayer system.

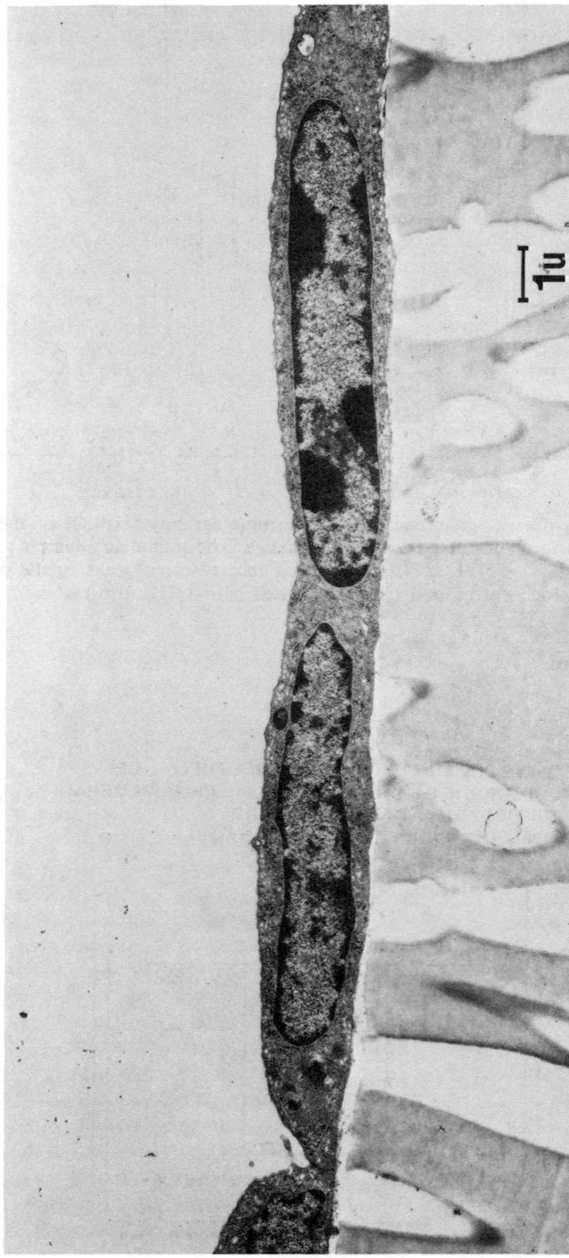

FIGURE 10a. Electron micrograph showing an intact endothelial monolayer grown to confluency on a micropore filter. Note the appearance of the interendothelial junctional complex. These endothelial cells are seeded for four days.

indication of the formation of junctional complexes. The permeability chamber consists of a modified chemotaxis chamber in which the upper (luminal) chamber is floated in the lower (abluminal) chamber so that the fluid levels of the two chambers are identical. Because the fluid levels are the same, the transendothelial albumin flux (from the luminal to the abluminal side) is governed by diffusive factors, that is, a hydrostatic factor does not play a role. [^{125}I]albumin tracer is added on the luminal side of the endothelial monolayer, and the time-dependent appearance of the labeled albumin is measured on the abluminal side. The transendothelial clearance rate of the [^{125}I]albumin is calculated. The surface area of the endothelial monolayer is known, and the permeability coefficient can be determined. Test agents are added to the upper chamber, and it is possible to assess the biological activity of these agents in increasing permeation of albumin across the endothelial monolayer. This system is also useful for studying the role of neutrophil-endothelial interactions in mediating alteration in endothelial permeability.

The gelatinized nucleopore filter is more permeable to albumin than the endothelium (FIGURE 11). The endothelium grown on the gelatinized filter restricts albumin

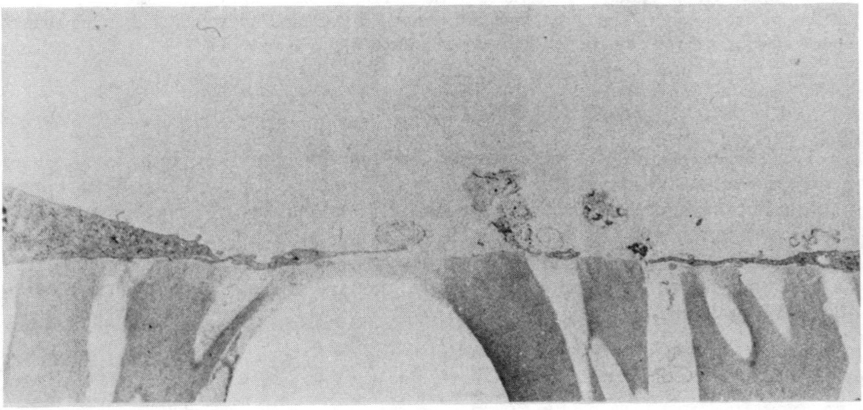

FIGURE 10b. Electron micrograph of the endothelial monolayer following addition of thrombin (10^{-8} M) on the luminal side of the endothelium. Interendothelial "gaps" appear to be due to retraction of endothelial cells.

permeation across the endothelial monolayer by 15-fold as compared to the filter alone. The endothelium monolayer provides restriction to albumin permeability as does the endothelial monolayer *in vivo,* although the albumin permeability of the endothelium *in vitro* [permeability coefficient of 3×10^{-7} cm/sec for the endothelial monolayer] is greater than other values [permeability coefficient of 1.4×10^{-8} cm/sec for lung vessels[8,19,20] and of 18×10^{-8} cm/sec for skeletal muscle vessels[21]] obtained using intact organs.

The addition of postthrombin pulmonary lymph (*i.e.* the 15-30 min lymph samples in which the LTB_4 and HETEs were detected using HPLC) to the luminal side of the endothelial monolayer in the presence of neutrophils resulted in an increase in the endothelial permeability (FIGURE 12). The prethrombin lymph had no significant effect. These results support the hypothesis that neutrophil activating substance(s) generated in pulmonary lymph following thrombin challenge appear to induce an increase in endothelial permeability by a neutrophil-dependent mechanism.

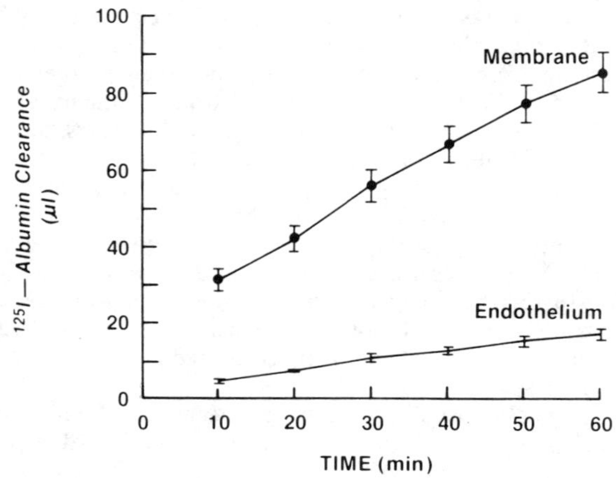

FIGURE 11. The [^{125}I]albumin clearance of the micropore filter and the endothelial monolayer on the micropore filter. The endothelial cell reduces the albumin clearance, indicating that the endothelial cells form a restrictive barrier to albumin flux.

The results of these *in vitro* studies indicate that thrombin induces fibrin and neutrophil sequestrations in the pulmonary microcirculation, and that fibrin appears to be an important determinant of neutrophil sequestration. The lipoxygenase products, leukotriene B_4 and HETEs, are generated following thrombin infusion, and these may contribute to neutrophil aggregation and activation. Neutrophil activation appears to be necessary for the development of the pulmonary microvascular injury following thrombin challenge.

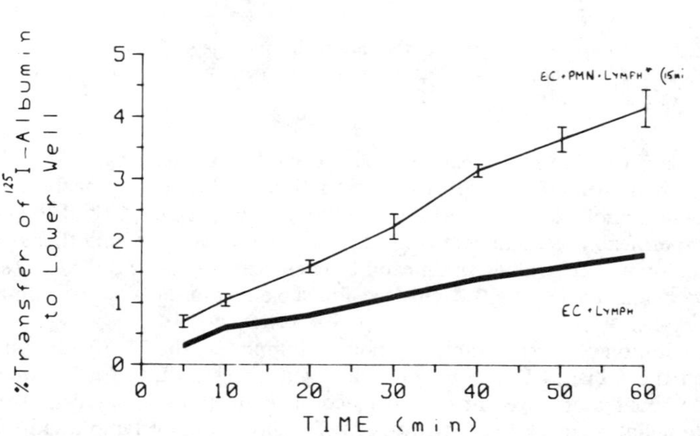

FIGURE 12. Addition of postthrombin lymph to the luminal side of the endothelium in the presence of neutrophils increases the albumin flux across the endothelial monolayer (thin line). Postthrombin lymph does not possess the permeability-increasing effect (thicker line).

DIRECT EFFECTS OF THROMBIN ON ENDOTHELIAL PERMEABILITY

Thrombin may also have direct effects on endothelial permeability independent of its effects on the neutrophil. Thrombin becomes sequestered in the clot during thrombus formation,[1] and therefore thrombin released during clot lysis may attain high concentrations.[1] Addition of thrombin to the endothelial monolayer *in vitro* at high concentration (beginning at 10^{-8} M) resulted in an increase in endothelial permeability (FIGURE 13). This response was the direct result of thrombin on the endothelium because the coincubation with neutrophils did not enhance the response. Moreover, the response was not the result of proteolytic activity of the molecule or its fibrinogen recognition site, for the proteolytically inactivated form of thrombin and gamma thrombin (lacking the fibrinogen recognition site)[22] induced similar increases in the

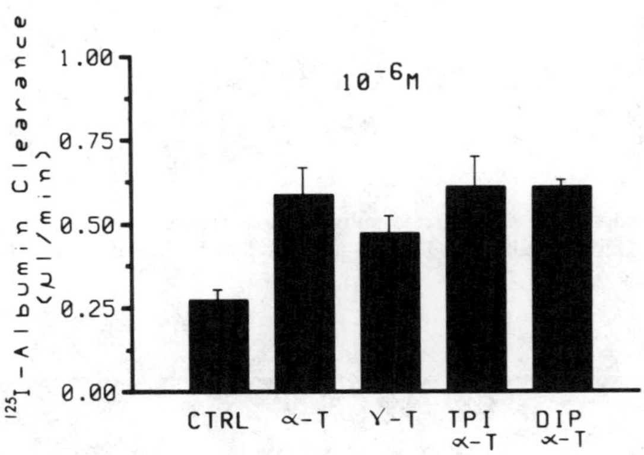

FIGURE 13. Alterations of albumin clearance when the endothelial monolayer is exposed to different forms of thrombin. α-Thrombin molecules lacking the catalytic sites (*i*-Pr_2 P-α-thrombin, DIP, or D-Phe-Pro-Arg-CH_2-α-thrombin, TPI) induce similar increases in albumin clearance. The permeability-increasing effect of α-thrombin is independent of its proteolytic activity. α-Thrombin lacking the fibrinogen recognition site (γ-thrombin) also has a permeability-increasing effect.

permeability of the endothelial monolayer (FIGURE 13). The increase in permeability was associated with the formation of interendothelial gaps (FIGURE 10b), which may result from the "rounding up" of the endothelial cells induced by thrombin.[24,25] Rhodamine staining of actin filaments of the normal endothelium indicated normal-appearing actin microfilaments and cytoskeletal stress fibers (FIGURE 14a). Alterations in these stress fibers were evident after the endothelium was exposed to thrombin (10^{-8} M) (FIGURE 14b), and there was also evidence of change in the cell shape. These findings are consistent with the hypothesis that thrombin causes endothelial cell contraction that leads to formation of interendothelial gaps through which macromolecular "leakage" may occur. This is a reversible phenomenon implying that the response is not the result of endothelial injury and that it may be physiologically important. The thrombin-mediated endothelial shape change may be a receptor-mediated phenomenon,[12,23,24] but it was shown to be independent on the proteolytic and catalytic sites of thrombin.

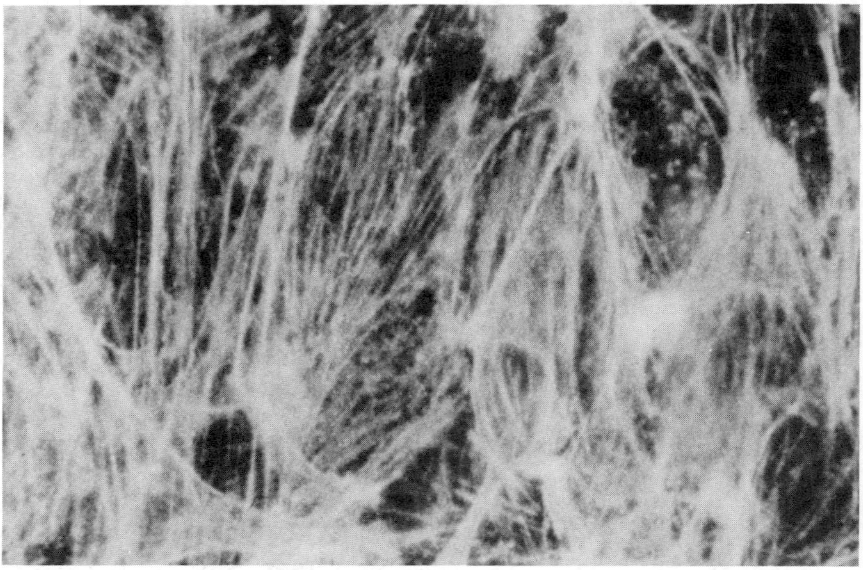

FIGURE 14a. Endothelial cells (bovine pulmonary arterial endothelial cells) after fixation and staining with rhodamine-phalloidin. There is an even distribution of the F-actin in the endothelial cells.

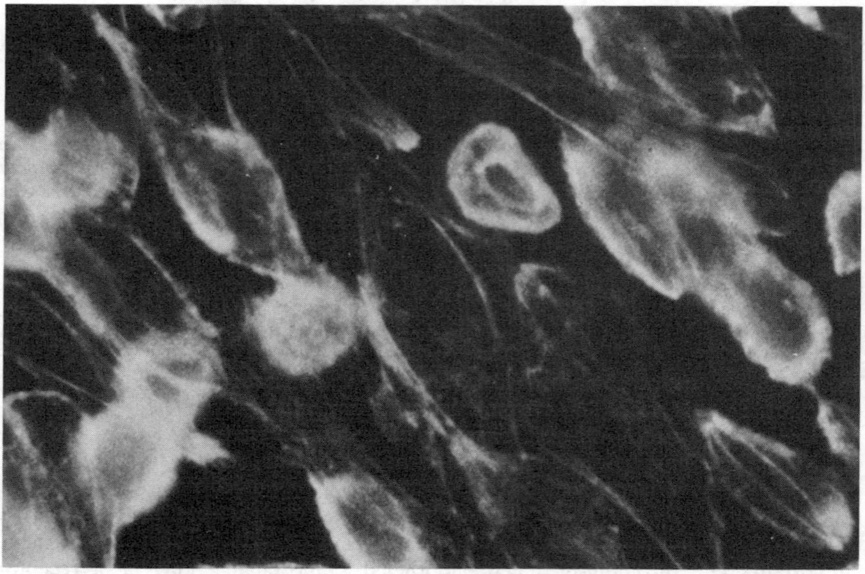

FIGURE 14b. Endothelial cells after exposure to α-thrombin (10^{-8}M). There is less rhodamine staining, indicating loss of F-actin and endothelial cell contracture.

SUMMARY

FIGURE 15 summarizes the current understanding of mechanisms of endothelial permeability alterations induced with thrombin. If thrombin generation exceeds the antiprotease activity, thrombin results in clotting of fibrinogen and intravascular fibrin accumulation. Pulmonary neutrophil sequestration also occurs after fibrin deposition, and this is related to the degree and duration of fibrin sequestration. Neutrophil activation appears to be an essential requirement for the mediation of the pulmonary vascular injury. Thrombin-induced intravascular coagulation results in the generation of lipid mediators (LTB_4 and HETEs), which may be involved in increasing endothelial permeability. The release of thrombin in higher concentrations during lysis of fibrin

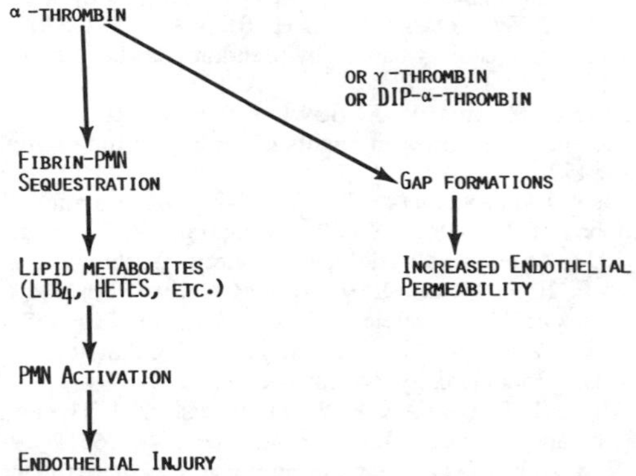

FIGURE 15. Hypothesis showing mechanisms of thrombin-induced increase in endothelial permeability to proteins. Thrombin may have direct effects on endothelial permeability, or thrombin induces fibrinogen clotting, activation of neutrophils, and the release of lipid metabolites that subsequently lead to an increase in endothelial permeability.

clots may induce a direct formation of interendothelial "gaps." Therefore, the vascular injury induced by neutrophil activation and the formation of endothelial "gaps" induced directly by thrombin can both increase the endothelial permeability to proteins.

Thrombin is an important mediator of increased endothelial permeability to macromolecules, and may participate in the inflammatory response. In this regard, thrombin may be similar to other mediators (such as histamine and serotonin) that have been previously documented to increase macromolecule transport across the endothelium. The implications of free thrombin in increasing endothelial permeability may be greater because thrombin not only has a direct effect on endothelial permeability, but also induces clotting of fibrinogen and the subsequent generation of mediators that activate neutrophils and that in turn can induce endothelial injury.

REFERENCES

1. FENTON II, J. W. 1981. Thrombin specificity. Ann. N.Y. Acad. Sci. **370:** 468-495.
2. BAR-SHAVIT, R., A. KAHN, G. D. WILNER & J. W. FENTON II. 1983. Monocyte chemotaxis: stimulation by specific exosite region in thrombin. Science **220:** 728-731.
3. BAR-SHAVIT, R., A. KAHN, M. S. MUDD, G. D. WILNER, K. G. MANN & J. W. FENTON II. 1984. Localization of a chemotactic domain in human thrombin. Biochemistry **23:** 397-400.
4. BIZIOS, R., L. LAI, J. W. FENTON II & A. B. MALIK. 1986. Thrombin-induced chemotaxis and aggregation of neutrophils. J. Cell. Physiol. **128:** 485-490.
5. RENKIN, E. M. 1979. Lymph as a measurement of the composition of interstitial fluid. *In* Pulmonary Edema. A. P. Fishman & E. M. Renkin, Eds.: 145-159. Am. Physiol. Soc. Bethesda, Md.
6. TAYLOR, A. E. 1981. Capillary fluid filtration. Starling forces and lymph flow. Circ. Res. **49:** 557-575.
7. LO, S. K., M. B. PERLMAN, G. D. NIEHAUS & A. B. MALIK. 1985. Thrombin-induced alterations in lung fluid balance in awake sheep. J. Appl. Physiol. **58**(5): 1421-1427.
8. BRIGHAM, K. L., W. C. WOOLVERTON, L. H. BLAKE & N. C. STAUB. 1974. Increased sheep lung vascular permeability caused by pseudomonas bacteremia. J. Clin. Invest. **54:** 792-804.
9. BRIGHAM, K. L., T. R. HARRIS, R. E. BOWERS & R. E. RUSELLI. 1979. Lung vascular permeability inferences from measurements of plasma to lung lymph protein transport. Lymphology **12:** 177-190.
10. LANDIS, E. M. & J. R. PAPPENHEIMER. 1963. Exchange of substances through the capillary walls. *In* Handbook of Physiology, Sect 2, Circulation. W. F. Hamilton & P. Dow. Eds.: II ch. 9: 961-1034. American Physiological Society. Washington, D.C.
11. DAVEY, M. G. & E. F. LUSCHER. 1967. Actions of thrombin and other coagulant and proteolytic enzymes on blood platelets. Nature (London) **216:** 857-858.
12. MARTIN, B. M., R. D. FEINMAN & T. C. DETWILER. 1975. Platelet stimulation by thrombin and other proteases. Biochemistry **14:** 1308-1314.
13. TOLLEFSEN, D. M., J. R. FEAGLER & P. W. MAJERUS. 1974. The binding of thrombin to the surface of human platelets. J. Biol. Chem. **249:** 2646-2651.
14. TAHAMONT, M. V. & A. B. MALIK. 1983. Granulocytes mediate the increase in pulmonary vascular permeability after thrombin embolism. J. Appl. Physiol. **54:** 1489-1495.
15. HEATH, C. A., L. LAI, R. BIZIOS & A. B. MALIK. 1986. Pulmonary hemodynamic effects of anti-leukocyte serum induced leukopenia. J. Leukocyte Biol. **39:** 385-397.
16. GOETZL, E. J., J. M. WOODS & R. R. GORMAN. 1977. Stimulation of human eosinophil and neutrophil polymorphonuclear leukocyte chemotaxis and random migration by 12-L-hydroxy-5,8,10,14-eicosatetraenoic acid (HETE). J. Clin. Invest. **59:** 179-183.
17. GOETZL, E. J., A. R. BRASH, A. I. TAUBER, J. A. OATES & W. C. HUBBARD. 1980. Modulation of human neutrophil function by mono-hydroxy-eicosatetraenoic acids. Immunology **39:** 141.
18. PALMER, R. M. J. & D. A. YEATS. 1981. Leukotriene B_4: a potent chemotactic agent and stimulus for lysosomal enzyme secretion for human neutrophils. Br. J. Pharmacol. **73:** P260-P261.
19. KERN, D. F., D. LEVITT & D. WANGENSTEEN. 1983. Endothelial albumin permeability measured with a new technique in perfused rabbit lung. Am. J. Physiol. **245:** H229-236.
20. RENKIN, E. M. 1977. Multiple pathways of capillary permeability. Circ. Res. **41:** 735-743.
21. SEJRSEN, P., W. P. PAASKE & O. HENRIKSEN. 1985. Capillary permeability of 131-I-albumin in skeletal muscle. Microvasc. Res. **29:** 265-281.
22. GARCIA, J. G., A. SIFLINGER-BIRNBOIM, R. BIZIOS, P. DEL VECCHIO, J. W. FENTON II & A. B. MALIK. 1986. Thrombin-induced increases in albumin transport across cultured endothelial monolayers. J. Cell. Physiol. **128:** 96-104.

23. AWBREY, B. J., J. C. HOAK & W. G. OWEN. 1979. Binding of human thrombin to cultured human endothelial cells. J. Biol. Chem. **254**(10): 4092-4095.
24. GALDAL, K. S., S. A. EVANSON & E. NILSEN. 1983. Thrombin-induced shape changes of cultured endothelial cells: Metabolic and functional observations. Thromb. Res. **32:** 57-66.
25. LAPOSATA, M., D. K. DOVNARSKY & H. S. SHIN. 1983. Thrombin-induced gap formation in confluent endothelial cell monolayers *in vitro.* Blood **82:** 549-556.

Thrombin Effects on Cultured Nerve Cells: Clinical Implications and Evidence for a Novel Mechanism of Neuronal Activation[a]

R. MICHAEL SNIDER[b]

Neuroscience Lab
Mental Health Research Institute
University of Michigan
Ann Arbor, Michigan 48104-1687

Central nervous system tissue *in vivo* is composed of a wide heterogeneity of cell types, such as neurons, glia, and vascular endothelium. One experimental approach that is commonly used to circumvent the inherent problems encountered in studying neuronal phenomena is the use of cloned nerve cells such as have been derived from the C-1300 murine neuroblastoma. One clone, designated N1E-115, has been extensively characterized both biochemically and electrophysiologically, and represents a widely used cell culture system for neurobiological studies.[1] Inasmuch as cloned cells constitute a population of neurons derived from a single cell, specific questions can be addressed to a single aspect of neuronal function.

Neurotransmitter Receptor-Mediated Cyclic GMP Synthesis

Clone N1E-115 cells have been shown to possess functional muscarinic and histamine H_1 receptors that, when activated, cause a rapid and marked increase in the intracellular concentration of cyclic guanosine monophosphate (GMP).[2–4] The molecular hypothesis for receptor-mediated cyclic GMP formation that researchers have held for the past several years involves calcium channel activation as the effector that couples receptor activation to cyclic GMP formation.[5] This hypothesis results primarily from the observations that extracellular calcium ions (Ca^{2+}) are necessary for receptor responses, and that Ca^{2+} ionophores (such as A23187 or X537A) can cause cyclic GMP formation.

In the course of investigating the molecular mechanism of neuronal activation, we gathered direct evidence indicating that a large Ca^{2+} influx did not occur as a result of neurotransmitter agonist stimulation.[6] Instead, results were obtained suggesting that neurotransmitter agonists may be coupled to guanylate cyclase (the enzyme that synthesizes cyclic GMP from guanosine triphosphate (GTP) by involvement of phospholipase A_2 and the release of arachidonic acid metabolites.[6] Phospholipase A_2 is the

[a] This work was supported by USPHS Grant NS 20920.

[b] Present address: T Cell Sciences, Inc., 840 Memorial Dr., Cambridge, MA 02139.

enzyme that catalyzes the release of arachidonic acid from the R_2 position of membrane phospholipids. Thrombin is a serine protease and is the central regulatory enzyme in hemostasis. Among the major biological effects of thrombin in causing coagulation of blood are cleavage of fibrinopeptide A to convert fibrinogen into clotable fibrin and stimulation of platelet degranulation and aggregation. Moreover, thrombin stimulation of platelets is known to result in the activation of phospholipase A_2 and cause the release of arachidonic acid.[11,12]

Thrombin Effects on Neuroblastoma Cells

To explore further the possible involvement of phospholipase A_2 and arachidonic acid release in neurotransmitter action, we tested the ability of thrombin to stimulate cyclic GMP formation in intact N1E-115 cells. Thrombin incubation with intact neuroblastoma cells caused a marked Ca^{2+}-dependent elevation in cyclic GMP levels with a peak around 30-60 seconds.[7] The time course and Ca^{2+} dependency of the thrombin-induced cyclic GMP response was virtually identical with other neurotransmitter agonists, such as carbachol and histamine, which stimulate cyclic GMP formations.[2,4] The EC_{50} (median effective concentration) for the thrombin response ranged from 0.08-0.44 NIH units/ml, which averaged 1.0-1.5 nM, and the cyclic GMP levels increased by 4.1 to 19-fold over basal levels measured in intact cells.[7]

We sought to establish that this effect was specific for thrombin and to determine if receptors for this protease existed on nerve cells. Trypsin, which is another serine protease, but with a broad specificity, was about 100-fold less potent and less effective in stimulating the cyclic GMP response as compared with α-thrombin. Moreover, thrombin treated with diisopropylphosphofluoridate, to inactivate the enzymatic site, was 300- to 500-fold less potent as compared with thrombin.[8] Thus, it is likely that the enzymatic activity of thrombin is involved in the cyclic GMP response of neuroblastoma cells. Thrombin antagonists also were evaluated for effects in this experimental preparation. Hirudin, a specific thrombin antagonist isolated from the leech salivary gland, inhibited cyclic GMP formation in approximately 1:1 stoichiometry, and a competitive inhibitor of thrombin, termed DAPA (dansylarginine-*N*-(3-ethyl-1,5-pentanediyl) amide) produced a shift to the right in the thrombin concentration cyclic GMP response and yielded a K_i value of 17 nM.[7]

Thrombin binding to intact neuroblastoma cells studied using [^{125}I]thrombin in a radioligand binding assay, are characterized as high-affinity receptors with a K_d (equilibrium dissociation constant) of 1.4 nM that number approximately 30 000 per cell.[9] In addition, low-affinity binding with a very high capacity was also found. We believe that the high-affinity binding site (K_d = 1.4 nM) is the functional receptor coupled to the cyclic GMP response (EC_{50} = 1.2 nM). Moreover, [^{125}I]thrombin also binds to human brain and spinal cord homogenates,[10] suggesting that our findings in neuroblastoma cells are not artifactual but, in fact, may represent an aspect of normal or pathological neuronal physiology.

Significance and Clinical Implications

It is unlikely that under normal conditions blood-born clotting factors ever come into direct contact with nerve cells in the brain. The possibility exists, however, that one or more proteases with thrombin-like specificity might be synthesized by neurons, released, and cause activation of other neurons (*i.e.,* a neuromodulatory function). A point of greater interest concerns the function that thrombin interaction may play in the neuropathology subsequent to cerebrovascular accidents, head trauma, or similar events in which the blood comes into direct contact with the brain.

Trauma to the central nervous system such as following cerebrovascular hemorrhage and concussive or projectile head injury clearly results in a compromised blood-brain barrier. Consequently, nerve cells are directly exposed to blood-borne factors. The resultant *in vivo* situation is profoundly complex and, for that reason, it has been difficult to ask questions designed to provide discrete answers concerning the neuronal pathophysiology involved in the injury and healing process.

An extremely exciting possibility concerns whether thrombin may possess mitogenic activity in nerve cells. As stated above, little is known about the neuronal cellular pathophysiology following stroke or traumatic nervous system injury. If thrombin is capable of stimulating differentiated neurons, as we have shown, neurons surviving the initial traumatic event may be induced to restore functional synaptic contacts. These processes may, in part, underlie a regenerative function that occurs with time following a cerebrovascular accident.

A New Hypothesis of Neurotransmitter Receptor-Mediated Cyclic GMP Formation

The Ca^{2+} dependency and time course of thrombin's activation of neuroblastoma cells is similar to that of muscarinic or histaminergic stimulation. Moreover, the receptor-mediated biochemical effects of thrombin in causing platelet activation are well characterized and involve activation of phospholipase A_2 and release of arachidonic acid.[11,12] Interestingly, phospholipase A_2 activity is the rate-limiting step in the generation of free arachidonic acid, and it is known to be a highly Ca^{2+}-dependent enzyme. Released arachidonic acid can undergo oxidative metabolism by way of the cyclooxygenase or lipoxygenase pathways to form the prostaglandins or the hydroxyeicosatetraynoic acids, respectively.

Pharmacologic studies were carried out to evaluate the involvement of phospholipase A_2 and arachidonic acid metabolites in cyclic GMP formation. Inhibition of phospholipase A_2 with quinacrine resulted in a concentration-dependent attenuation of receptor-mediated cyclic GMP formation. Quinacrine was effective in blocking the response elicited by thrombin, carbachol, and histamine with nearly equal potency.[6,8] This observation suggests that all the above agents that cause a receptor-mediated cyclic GMP response do so by the same mechanism. We conducted experiments to examine whether quinacrine inhibited the cyclic GMP response to receptor agonists in a nonspecific manner. Quinacrine did not inhibit the cyclic GMP response caused by sodium nitroprusside (a guanylate cyclase stimulant) at concentrations that totally blocked receptor responses.

Involvement of arachidonic acid metabolites in cyclic GMP formation was also investigated. Indomethacin, a drug that inhibits cyclooxygenase and formation of prostaglandins, did not inhibit the receptor-mediated response.[6,8] In fact, in many experiments, indomethacin actually potentiated by 10-40% the cyclic GMP levels measured in response to agonist stimulation. Inhibition of the lipoxygenase pathway of arachidonate metabolism with nordihydroguaiaretic acid (NDGA) or eicosatetraynoic acid (ETYA) blocked receptor-mediated cyclic GMP synthesis in a concentration-dependent manner. As was observed with quinacrine, the responses evoked by thrombin, carbachol, and histamine were affected similarly by NDGA or ETYA. We believe this observation also supports the hypothesis that neurotransmitter receptors couple to their respective cyclic GMP responses by a similar molecular mechanism.

Based on the observations detailed above, we have proposed a new hypothesis for the molecular mechanism of neurotransmitter receptor-mediated cyclic GMP formation.[6] We believe this scheme of molecular events following receptor activation and leading to cyclic GMP formation is consistent with all of the experimental observations outlined above.

REFERENCES

1. RICHELSON, E. 1979. The use of cultured cells in neurobiological studies. Physiol. Pharmacol. Biochem. **26:** 81-120.
2. MATSUZAWA, H. & M. NIRENBERG. 1975. Receptor-mediated shifts in cGMP and cAMP levels in neuroblastoma cells. Proc. Nat. Acad. Sci. USA **72:** 3472-3476.
3. RICHELSON, E., F. G. PRENDERGAST & S. DIVINETZ-ROMERO. 1978. Muscarinic receptor-mediated cyclic GMP formation by cultured nerve cells—ionic dependence and effects of local anesthetics. Biochem. Pharmacol. **27:** 2039-2048.
4. RICHELSON, E. 1978. Histamine H_1 receptor-mediated guanosine 3′,5′-monophosphate formation by cultured mouse neuroblastoma cells. Science **201:** 69-71.
5. RICHELSON, E. & E. EL-FAKAHANY. 1981. The molecular basis of neurotransmission at the muscarinic receptor. Biochem. Pharmacol. **30:** 2887-2991.
6. SNIDER, R. M., M. MCKINNEY, C. FORRAY & E. RICHELSON. 1984. Neurotransmitter receptors mediate cyclic GMP formation by involvement of arachidonic acid and lipoxygenase. Proc. Nat. Acad. Sci. USA **81:** 3905-3909.
7. SNIDER, R. M. & E. RICHELSON. 1983. Thrombin stimulation of guanosine, 3′,5′-monophosphate formation in murine neuroblastoma cells (clone N1E-115). Science **221:** 566-568.
8. SNIDER, R. M., M. MCKINNEY, J. W. FENTON II & E. RICHELSON. 1984. Activation of cyclic nucleotide formation in murine neuroblastoma N1E-115 cells by modified human thrombins. J. Biol. Chem. **259:** 9078-9081.
9. SNIDER, R. M., M. MCKINNEY & E. RICHELSON. 1986. Thrombin binding and stimulation of cyclic guanosine monophosphate formation in neuroblastoma cells. Semin. Thromb. Hemostasis. **12:** 253-262.
10. MCKINNEY, M., R. M. SNIDER & E. RICHELSON. 1983. Thrombin binding to human brain and spinal cord. Mayo Clin. Proc. **58:** 829-831.
11. LAPETINA, E. G., M. M. BILLAH & P. CUATRECASAS. 1981. The initial action of thrombin on platelets. J. Biol. Chem. **256:** 5037-5040.
12. BILLAH, M. M. & E. G. LAPETINA. 1982. Formation of lysophosphatidylinositol in platelets stimulated with thrombin or ionophore A_{23187}. J. Biol. Chem. **257:** 5196-5200.

Thrombin Interactions with Central Nervous System Tissue and Implications of These Interactions[a]

EUGENE D. MEANS AND DOUGLAS K. ANDERSON

Veterans Administration Medical Center
Cincinnati, Ohio 45220
and
University of Cincinnati College of Medicine
Cincinnati, Ohio 45267

INTRODUCTION

Recent data suggests that thrombin has the potential for causing injury to the central nervous system (CNS). Snider and colleagues observed that neuroblastoma cells[1] and human brain and spinal cord[2] bind thrombin. Our laboratory reported that a monospecific antibody stained neurons in murine spinal cord cultures following incubation with thrombin.[3,4] We also showed that thrombin caused the release of arachidonic acid from murine spinal cord cultures. One could postulate that, with the release of arachidonate from the neuronal membrane by thrombin, a number of potentially injurious prostanoids are formed. In fact, there are a number of CNS afflictions in which blood (thrombin) extravasates into neural parenchyma and could potentially contact neural and glial membranes, causing the release of arachidonate. It seems reasonable, therefore, to suggest that thrombin may play a role in the pathogenesis of CNS injury in instances where blood extravasates into the neural parenchyma.

This paper will describe an immunocytochemical study of thrombin binding to neurons in murine spinal cord cultures. Additionally, the potential for thrombin to be an injury agent in the CNS is discussed.

MATERIAL AND METHODS

Preparation of Antibody

Highly purified human α-thrombin (2.29 mg/ml in NaCl) was combined by sonification with Freund's complete adjuvant and administered to white, female New Zealand rabbits in multiple subcutaneous injections. Rabbits were bled one week after

[a]This work was supported by the Veterans Administration.

injection through the ear using a Belco rabbit bleeding apparatus attached to a millipore vacuum pump. Sera was pooled and stored at -70° C. Antithrombin sera was tested for antibody activity against thrombin using New England Nuclear's enzyme-linked immunosorbent assay (ELISA). Isolation of IgG was accomplished using the technique of Steinbunch & Audran.[5] Immunoglobulin G was further purified against thrombin-conjugated CNB_R-activated sepharose 4B.

Preparation of Cultures

Ventral horn cells are dissociated from 12-14 day mouse embryos by the following procedure. The embryos are removed from timed, pregnant CD-1 mice and placed in sterile HEPES buffered salt solution (D_1SHG:137 mM NaCl, 5.35 mM KC1, 2.2 mM KH_2PO_4). The embryo is placed under a stereomicroscope for ease of dissection. The cord is teased very gently away from the embryo but left connected at the cephalad end. The meninges are eased apart along the central canal and then stripped away. This procedure also removes all dorsal root ganglia. The cords are then transferred to a fresh dish of HEPES coated with Sylgard resin. The cords are pinned dorsal side up on the resin using minuten pins (4 mm in length, 000), and the dorsal horns are cut away using a #15 scalpel blade. The dorsal horns are discarded and the ventral horns (10 cords/dish) are placed in free HEPES, minced, and trypsinized in 2 ml of 0.25% trypsin for 30 minutes in a 35°C incubator with 10% CO_2. After trypsinization, the tissue is transferred to 3 ml bicarbonate-buffered minimum essential media (MEM) with Earle's salts containing 10% horse serum, 10% calf serum, 1% L-glutamine and 1% deoxyribonuclease (10/10 MEM) and allowed to settle. The settled tissue is then transferred to 2.0 ml of 10/10 MEM and triturated with a sterile plugged Pasteur pipette to dissociate the cells. Subsequently, the tissue is allowed to settle again, and the supernatant of dispersed cells is transferred to a sterile glass bottle. The process of trituration and settling out is repeated three times; each time the pellet is resuspended with 2.0 ml of 10/10 MEM. The pooled cell suspension is further diluted with 10/10 MEM, and cell density is determined using a hemocytometer.

The cells are plated at approximately 5×10^5 cells/ml on a collagen-coated Aclar coverslips in 35 mm culture dishes (2 ml/dish) and kept at 35°C in 10% CO_2. At 72 hrs, the media is changed to 1.5 ml MEM containing 5% horse serum, 1% L-glutamine and 1% nutrient mixture (N_3: 20 mg/ml transferrin, 20 mM putrescine, 6 μM sodium selenite, 20 μg/ml triiodothyronine, 1 mg/ml insulin, 4 μM progesterone, 4 μg/ml corticosterone, and 0.1% BSA) (5HS/N_3/MEM). Cultures are left undisturbed for five days, at which time they are changed to 0.5 ml MEM containing 5% horse serum, 20 μ/ml FUDR, and 50 μg/ml uridine to inhibit the growth of dividing background cells. After 48 hrs, the media is changed to 5HS/N_3/MEM. Cultures are used at 3 weeks after plating.

Immunocytochemistry

Cultures on Aklar cover slips are rinsed in HEPES buffer for 5 min and then fixed for 30 min in 4% paraformaldehyde-0.25% glutaraldehyde in 0.1 M phosphate buffer, pH 7.4 at room temperature. The slides are rinsed twice for 5 min in phosphate buffered saline (PBS) followed by a reaction with 0.05% sodium borohydride in PBS for 5 minutes. The slides are incubated for 30 min in 1-10 nM α-thrombin for 30 min and then rinsed four times for 5 min in PBS followed by incubation in 5% goat serum in PBS for 30 minutes. The slides are incubated overnight at 4° C in an affinity-purified monospecific antibody to α-thrombin using serial dilutions. These are brought to room temperature and incubated in biotinylated goat antirabbit IgG 1:2000 for 30 min and rinsed four times for 5 min in PBS. The slides are incubated in avidin/peroxidase 1:100 for 60 min (made 30 min before use), rinsed four times for 5 min in PBS, and treated with 5 mg diaminobenzadine in 0.1 M Tris/HC1, pH 7.6 plus 5 ml of 0.02% H_2O_2 for 10 minutes. These are rinsed twice for 5 min and mounted on glass slides in glycerogel.

RESULTS

Cultures incubated with 1-10 nM α-thrombin followed by a monospecific antibody to α-thrombin prominently stained neurons (FIGURE 1) using the avidin-biotin-peroxidase (ABC) technique. Astrocytes failed to stain, although a small round cell believed to be a macrophage showed heavy staining. No staining was observed if the primary or linking antibodies were eliminated. Absorption of the antithrombin antibody with α-thrombin abolished neuronal staining. Similar results were obtained with a rabbit Pro-Blot Test (Cappel) (FIGURE 2). Treatment of the cultures with equimolar or excess concentrations of hirudin prior to incubation with α-thrombin or reaction of α-thrombin with hirudin either eliminated staining or caused the reaction product to clump on the neuronal surface. Incubation of the cultures with the primary antibody, but eliminating thrombin incubation, produced staining, although reduced. This suggests either a contaminant or the presence of an endogenous protease associated with the neurons.

DISCUSSION

The role of thrombin in the pathogenesis of central nervous system (CNS) injury is, to date, theoretical. The potential for thrombin to produce an adverse effect on the CNS is, however, well-established. We[3,4] as well as McKinney and colleagues[2] have proposed that thrombin may lead to neuronal injury in hemorrhagic afflictions of the CNS such as cerebral hemorrhage or trauma. In these circumstances, blood may escape through the ruptured vessel into the neural parenchyma and lie adjacent to neuronal or glial membranes. The effect of thrombin on endothelial cells of the blood vessel, *per se,* has been well described. Lough and Moore showed extensive subendothelial vesiculation with focal ulceration of the endothelium of rabbit aorta exposed to thrombin.[6] Endothelial cell injury in the cerebral vasculature, secondary to the effect of thrombin, may lead to a compromise of the blood-brain barrier. Blood products could reach the abluminal surface through widened interendothelial junctions

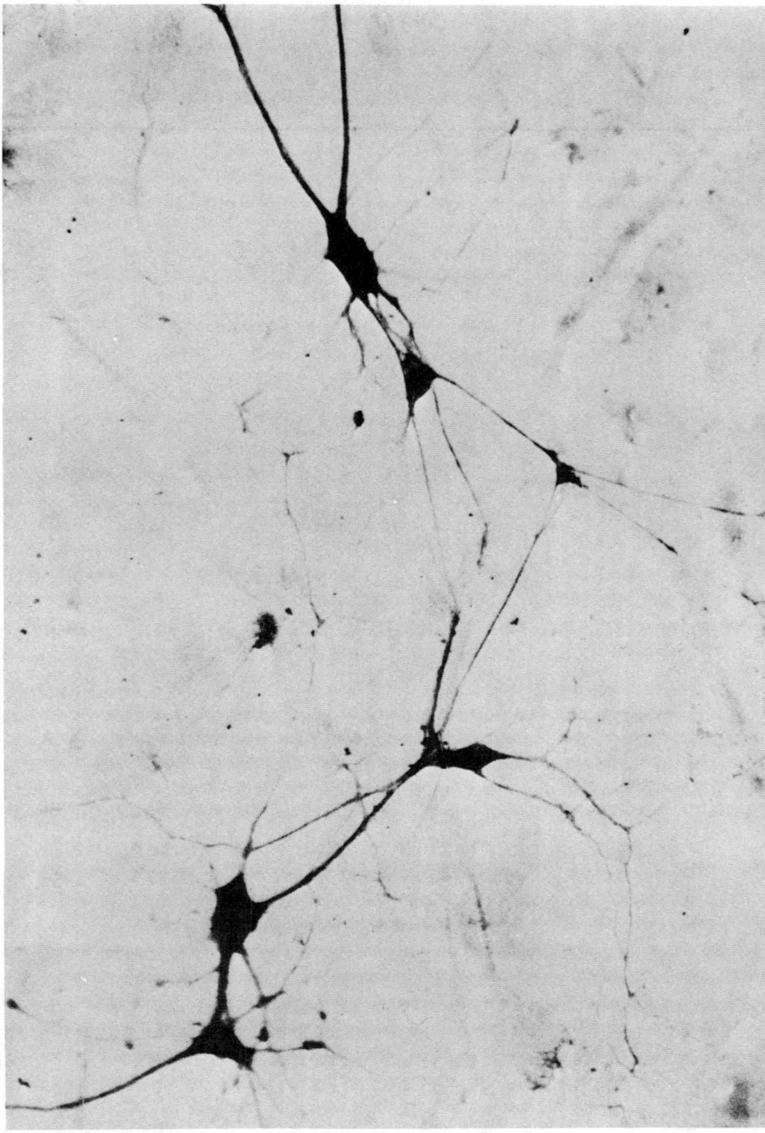

FIGURE 1. Several multipolar neurons including the cell soma and processes are stained following incubation with α-thrombin, a monospecific antibody to thrombin, a biotinylated linked antibody, and avidin-peroxidase (ABC technique). The cells were fixed with paraformaldehyde-gluteraldehyde prior to staining. Murine spinal cord culture, $\times$ 1000.

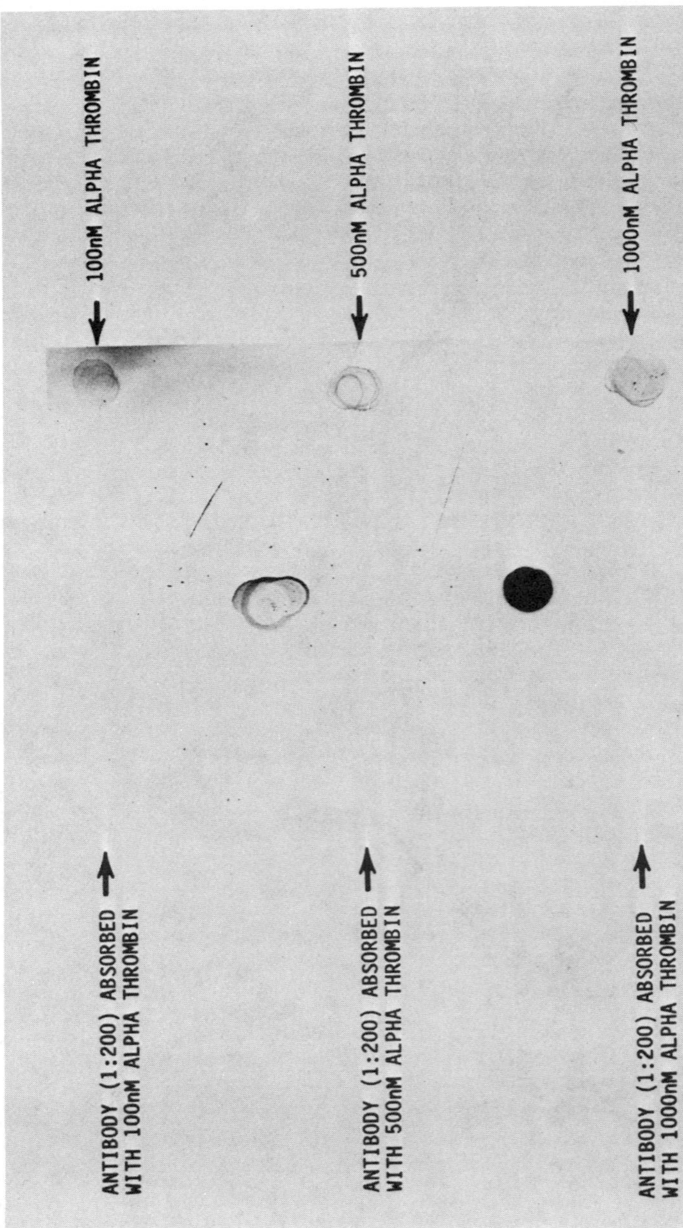

FIGURE 2. Rabbit Pro-Blot (Cappel) showing absorption of antithrombin antibody (1:200) with 100, 500, and 1000 nM α-thrombin. Undiluted α-thrombin is seen at upper center. Pro-Blot control is noted at lower center.

or by vesicular transport directly across the endothelial cell. By whatever mechanism, (direct rupture of the vessel or the effect of thrombin on the endothelial cell), once in contact with the cell, thrombin could have a deleterious effect on the neuronal or glial membrane, leading to increased cell permeability to divalent cations such as Ca^{+} (*vide infra*). A theoretical scheme of cellular injury and tissue necroses in experimental spinal cord injury is displayed in FIGURE 3. The potential role of thrombin and other proteases in this injury process is shown.

Snider and colleagues were the first to show that α-thrombin binds to a clone of neuroblastoma cells[1] or to human brain and spinal cord.[2] Based on the later study,[2] we were curious to know which of the cellular elements in the CNS bind thrombin. The current study showed that only neurons as opposed to astrocytes bind thrombin. This observation suggests that any deleterious effect of thrombin on the CNS is probably due to neuronal, as opposed to glial injury. A small round cell, probably a macrophage, also bound thrombin, but the significance of this observation is unknown.

The mechanism by which thrombin might lead to membrane damage is speculative. We showed in preliminary experiments that a 4- to 10-fold increase in arachidonic acid occurred in spinal cord cultures when incubated with 20 nM α-thrombin. Snider and colleagues also described arachidonate release from neuroblastoma cells exposed to thrombin.[16] This was a mepacrine-sensitive mechanism suggesting thrombin activation of phospholipase A_2. The mechanism of thrombin release of arachidonic acid from the neuronal membrane is, therefore, most likely secondary to the activation of membrane lipases similar to the well-established effect of thrombin on the platelet membrane.[8] Both platelets and neurons contain high concentrations of arachidonic acid and the enzymes phospholipases A_2 and C[9–12] and diglyceride lipase[13,14] to liberate this fatty acid. It, therefore, is reasonable to postulate a similar mechanism for arachidonic acid release in both platelets and neurons. Arachidonate then serves as a substrate for cyclooxygenase and 5-lipoxygenase enzymes, the initial enzymes in the prostaglandin and leukotriene pathways, respectively. Prostanoids have a number of deleterious effects on CNS tissue.[15]

Snider and coworkers described a Ca^{++}-dependent increase in cyclic guanosine monophosphate (GMP) formation to thrombin stimulation in a clone of neuroblastoma cells.[1,7,16] The receptor-mediated increase in Ca^{++} was thought to act by way of inositol phospholipid metabolism. To our knowledge, these are the only studies in neuronal cells showing a receptor-mediated response to thrombin. Modified thrombin was less active in producing this response. We have not yet characterized the receptor-mediated metabolic response to thrombin in our cultures. The fact that hirudin blocked thrombin binding to neuronal cells in our cultures and arachindonate release occurred in response to thrombin stimulation suggests that a mechanism similar to that described by Snider[1,7,16] may be operative in these cells. The role of thrombin receptors on neuronal cells is unclear, but these receptors may play several roles. For example, thrombin has been shown to be a mitogen in some cell types[8] and might participate in the growth or repair of nerve cells. Thrombin might also function in neurotransmission or neuromodulation.[2] It is intriguing to speculate as to why thrombin or thrombin-like protease receptors exist in tissues not normally exposed to thrombin. There could be a limited number of receptor types common to all tissues, which respond to different agonists unique to a specific tissue, for example, a thrombin-like protease in the CNS.[17]

In summary, we have shown thrombin labeling of neurons, but not astrocytes, in murine spinal cord cultures. The possible role of thrombin in central nervous system injury is discussed. It is proposed that thrombin may act to release arachidonic acid from the neuronal membrane leading to membrane damage and, moreover, prostanoids are released that may have other deleterious effects on cellular elements and blood vessels.

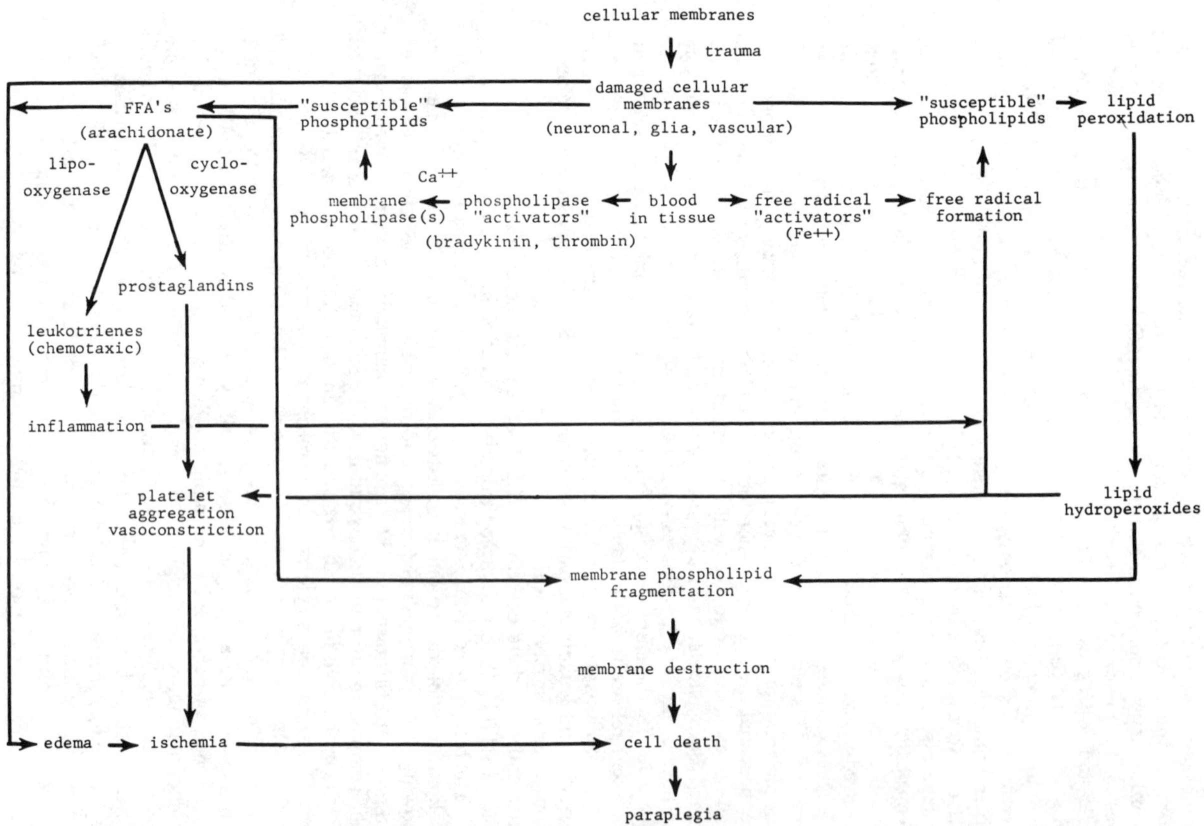

FIGURE 3. Diagram of proposed mechanisms leading to damage of cellular membranes following trauma to the spinal cord. Secondary pathophysiological events occur (autodestructive) such as edema, ischemia, and inflammation that lead to tissue necrosis and paraplegia.

SUMMARY

A monospecific antibody was developed to human α-thrombin. This antibody stained neurons but not astrocytes in murine spinal cord cultures incubated with 1-10 nM α-thrombin using the avidin-biotin-peroxidase technique. Staining did not occur when the primary or linking antibodies were eliminated, and staining was blocked with hirudin. Preliminary studies showed release of arachidonic acid from the cultures when exposed to thrombin. It was proposed that arachidonate release from the membranes of neurons upon exposure to thrombin was similar to that observed in platelets, for example, by activation of phospholipases. Moreover, prostanoids were formed that could have a deleterious effect on cellular elements in the central nervous system. The potential role of thrombin receptors on neurons was discussed.

ACKNOWLEDGMENT

The authors wish to thank Dr. John Fenton for supplying the thrombin and Ms. Maureen Fitzgerald and Ms. Sheryl Helsinger for their technical support.

REFERENCES

1. Snider, R. M. & E. Richelson. 1983. Thrombin stimulation of guanosine 3',5'-monophosphate formation in murine neuroblastoma cells (Clone N1E-115). Science **221:** 566-568.
2. McKinney, M., R. M. Snider & E. Richelson. 1983. Thrombin binding to human brain and spinal cord. Mayo Clin. Proc. **58:** 829-831.
3. Means, E. D., D. K. Anderson & M. Fitzgerald. 1983. Thrombin binding to cells in murine spinal cord cultures. Soc. Neurosci. (Absts.) **9:** 348
4. Means, E. D., D. K. Anderson & M. Fitzgerald. 1985. Thrombin may be an injury agent in stroke and trauma. Neurology **35** (Suppl. 1): 141.
5. Steinbuch, M. & R. Audran. 1969. The isolation of IgG from mammalian sera with the aid of caprylic acid. Arch. Biochem. Biophys. **134:** 279-284.
6. Lough, J. & S. Moore. 1975. Endothelial injury induced by thrombin or thrombi. Lab. Invest. **33:** 130-140.
7. Snider, R. M., M. McKinney, J. W. Fenton II & E. Richelson. 1984. Activation of cyclic nucleotide formation in murine neuroblastoma N1E-115 cells by modified human thrombins. J. Biol. Chem. **259:** 9078-9081.
8. Fenton II, J. W. 1981. Thrombin specificity. Ann. N.Y. Acad. Sci. **370:** 468-495.
9. Kunze, H. & W. Vogat. 1971. Significance of phospholipase A_2 for prostaglandin formation. Ann. N.Y. Acad. Sci. **180:** 123-125.
10. Moskowitz, N., W. Schook & S. Puszkin. 1982. Interaction of brain synaptic vesicles induced by endogenous Ca^{2+}-dependent phospholipase A_2. Science **216:** 305-307.
11. Rittenhouse-Simmons, S. 1979. Production of diglyceride from phosphatidylinositol in activated human platelets. J. Clin. Invest. **63:** 580-587.
12. Edgar, A. D. & L. Freysz. 1982. Phospholipase activities of rat brain. Cytosol occurrence of phospholipase C activity with phosphatidycholine. Biochim. Biophys. Acta **711:** 224-228.

13. BELL, R. L., D. A. KENNERLY, N. STANFORD & P. MAJERUS. 1979. Diglyceride lipase: A pathway for arachidonic acid from human platelets. Proc. Nat. Acad. Sci. USA **76:** 3238.
14. SUN, G. Y., K. L. SU, O. M. DER & W. TANG. 1979. Enzymic regulation of arachidonate metabolism in brain membrane phospholipids. Lipids **14:** 229-235.
15. WOLFE, L. 1982. Eicosanoids: prostaglandins, thromboxanes, leucotrienes and other unsaturated fatty acids. J. Neurochem. **38:** 1-14.
16. SNIDER, R. M., M. MCKINNEY, C. FORRAY & E. RICHELSON. 1984. Neurotransmitter receptors mediate cyclic GMP formation by involvement of arachidonic acid and lipoxygenase. Proc. Natl. Acad. Sci. USA **91:** 3905-3909.
17. SIMMER, R. L., J. B. BAKER & D. D. CUNNINGHAM. 1979. Direct linkage of thrombin to its cell surface receptors in different cell types. J. Supramol. Struct. **12:** 245-257.

Responses of Aortic Smooth Muscle to Thrombin and Thrombin Analogues[a]

DANIEL A. WALZ,[b] GORDON F. ANDERSON,[b]
AND JOHN W. FENTON II[c]

[b]*Departments of Physiology and Pharmacology*
Wayne State University School of Medicine
Detroit, Michigan 48201
and
[c]*Wadsworth Center for Laboratories and Research*
New York State Department of Health
Albany, New York 12201

Thrombin is the serine proteinase generated from the carboxy-terminal portion of its circulating zymogen prothrombin.[1,2] The generation of procoagulant α-thrombin is controlled by the hepatic synthesis of prothrombin, the presence of the vitamin K-dependent gamma-carboxyglutamic acid residues within the amino-terminal fragment of prothrombin, and the assembly of the prothrombinase activation complex.[3–5] Prothrombin activation, unlike the activation of the other coagulation zymogens, generates an enzyme that is not linked to surface-binding fragments of the zymogen. Thrombin is generated in concentrations that exceed that of the preceding activation pathway enzymes.[6–9] Human plasma contains a sufficient amount of prothrombin to generate approximately 150 clotting units/ml,[10,11] corresponding to 1.37 μM.[12] During the spontaneous clotting of whole blood or plasma, however, measurable clotting activities do not exceed 15 units/ml[11] despite the fact that >90% of the prothrombin is consumed during the clotting process, as measured by the formation of prothrombin fragments 1 and 2.[13] This prothrombin consumptive process is directly correlated with fibrin formation from fibrinogen.[13]

The procoagulant α-thrombin has several functions in hemostasis, including the conversion of fibrinogen to fibrin, the activation of other plasma coagulation proteins (factors V, VIII, XIII and protein C), and the activation of platelets.[6] Thrombin has also been shown to interact with virtually all mammalian tissue or cell types including endothelial cells,[14] nerve cells,[15,16] smooth muscle,[14,17,18] leukocytes,[19,20] and fibroblasts.[21–24]

[a]This work was supported by NIH Grants HL 27073, AG 03539, and HL 13160 and a Grant-in-Aid from the American Heart Association of Michigan.

INTERACTIONS OF BLOOD CONSTITUENTS WITH VASCULAR TISSUE

The direct effects of whole blood or its components on the endothelium are summarized in TABLE 1. Lough and Moore[25] injected a variety of blood constituents into isolated rabbit aorta segments in order to evaluate their effects on early endothelial injury. They noted that the perfusion of vessel segments with platelet-rich plasma or platelet-poor plasma had little effect on the subendothelium, whereas thrombin alone, or thrombin in concert with platelet-rich plasma, resulted in extensive subendothelial vesiculation, focal alterations, and the adherence of a thrombus to the endothelium. Hagen *et al.*[26] observed that blood substances including thrombin, when injected into the cerebrospinal fluid, caused cerebral vasospasm and suggested that this might be due to the marked elevation of prostaglandin levels specifically caused by thrombin. Linder and Alksne[27] used isolated canine carotid artery preparations to measure arterial constriction and demonstrated the importance of platelet function in maintaining cerebral smooth muscle contraction after whole blood injections into these preparations. Whole blood from rabbits or monkeys produced a persistent arterial contraction, whereas whole blood from these animals pretreated with aspirin or phthalazinol failed to generate any significant contraction. Thrombin was capable of mimicking these same effects. Weksler *et al.*[28], using monolayers of cultured human endothelial cells, showed that thrombin stimulated the production of prostacyclin, and this increased production was dependent upon the use of an active thrombin. Awbrey *et al.*[29] demonstrated that thrombin bound specifically to cultured endothelial cells with high affinity and achieved binding equilibrium within 1 minute. This specific binding was

TABLE 1. Interactions of Thrombin with Vascular Tissue

Investigators	Observations	Reference
Lough and Moore	Suggested that blood components, especially thrombin, could directly damage endothelial cells.	25
Hagen *et al.*	Intracisternal injection of thrombin resulted in elevated $PGF_{2\alpha}$ and PGE_2 levels in dog cerebrospinal fluid.	26
Linder and Alksne	Platelets liberated by-products that produced cerebral vessel contraction; action mimicked by thrombin.	27
Weksler *et al.*	Increased synthesis in cultured endothelial cell production of prostacyclin in presence of thrombin.	28
Awbrey *et al.*	Thrombin and diisopropyl fluorophosphate-thrombin bind to umbilical vein endothelial cells with high (0.1 nM) and low (10 nM) K_d.	29
Esmon *et al.*	Thrombomodulin binding site on endothelium.	31
Groves *et al.*	Thrombin is generated after aortic endothelium is damaged in rabbits.	33
Bauer *et al.*	Thrombin bound to endothelial cells with a K_d of 30 nM and achieves equilibrium within 1 minute.	32

TABLE 2. Contractile Responses of Blood Vessels to Thrombin

Investigators	Observations	References
White *et al.*	Thrombin causes sustained contraction in dog cerebral basilar artery.	34,35
DeMay *et al.*	Thrombin causes partial relaxation of norepinephrine-contracted dog femoral arteries; endothelium dependent.	36
Rapoport *et al.*	Thrombin caused a relaxation of precontracted rat aortic tissue by an endothelium-dependent mechanism.	37
Haver and Namm	Thrombin-promoted contraction of dog and rabbit aorta is not antagonized by cyclooxygenase inhibitors.	18,39
White *et al.*	Thrombin produces initial relaxation then contraction of dog coronary and cerebral, but not mesenteric, arteries.	40
Walz *et al.*	Thrombin at pM concentrations causes relaxation and at nM concentrations causes contraction of rabbit aorta. Dependent upon functional enzyme site in thrombin.	12

similar for active and inactivated thrombin analogues and was 100 times greater for endothelium than it was for either smooth muscle cells or fibroblasts. Swedenborg *et al.*[30] used washed porcine aorta preparations to show that the specific binding of thrombin to this tissue resulted in a loss of thrombin amidolytic activity, which correlated well with the previous observations of Esmon *et al.*[31] on the role of the endothelial cell protein thrombomodulin, which binds thrombin and results in the concomitant loss of fibrinogen clotting activity. Bauer *et al.*[32] used isolated minipig aortic endothelial cell cultures to study the relationship between heparin-binding sites within thrombin and the endothelial interactive sites of thrombin. These investigators found that both classes of binding sites were dependent on the intact lysine residues within the thrombin molecule; they also reported that endothelium-bound thrombin could be released by the addition of antithrombin to the medium.

CONTRACTILE RESPONSES OF BLOOD VESSELS TO THROMBIN

White *et al.*[34,35] first observed the ability of a number of blood components to produce vasospasm and noted that, of all the vasoactive blood components examined, thrombin produced spasms that were more delayed in onset, whereas serotonin and selected prostaglandins induced spasms more nearly resembling those observed when whole blood was used (TABLE 2). When thrombin was added directly to isolated canine basilar arteries,[35] its effect was slower in onset but more prominent than either serotonin or prostaglandins for inducing sustained contracture. These thrombin-induced contractions could not be terminated by prolonged and repeated tissue washing.

On the other hand, DeMey *et al.*[36] and Rapoport *et al.*[37] have reported on the ability of thrombin to relax arterial preparations that had been previously contracted by norepinephrine. This relaxation was dependent upon the presence of an intact endothelium, because in scraped preparations, the relaxation was absent. The relaxation was possibly mediated by an arachidonate metabolite, inasmuch as eicosatetraenoic acid, a lipoxygenase and cyclooxygenase inhibitor, inhibited thrombin-induced relaxation. Goldsmith and Kisker[38] have shown that the interaction of thrombin with endothelial cells was critically dependent upon the vessel of origin; using prostacyclin release as the indicator, thrombin markedly increased the synthesis of prostacyclin in perfused sheep umbilical veins, but was without effect on the same animal's aorta. Haver and Namm[18,39] quite convincingly demonstrated that a potent vasoactive substance was generated during the clotting of plasma that was inhibited by either heparin or hirudin, suggesting that this vasoactive substance was thrombin. They subsequently reported[18] that dog coronary arteries treated with thrombin contracted slowly and were refractory to a second thrombin exposure after washing. They also showed that thrombin-induced contractions were dependent upon active thrombin, for *N*α-*p*-tosyl-L-lysine chloromethyl ketone (TLCK)-modified thrombin was without contractile effects in their preparations. White *et al.*[40] demonstrated that thrombin had no effect on canine mesenteric arteries, which was inconsistent with its relaxation effect on canine renal arteries and the contractile effect on coronary and basilar arteries. We have elaborated on these studies,[12] using well-characterized preparations of human thrombin (TABLE 3) in order to focus on the structural requirements of thrombin necessary to induce contraction, as well as to correlate the contractile and relaxation responses of rabbit aortic tissue preparations to human thrombins.

SAMPLE PREPARATIONS

Rabbit thoracic aorta samples were excised from freshly sacrificed New Zealand White male rabbits and immersed in chilled balanced salt solution as previously described.[12] The artery was carefully dissected clean of connective tissue, cut into 45° spiral helical segments and then longitudinally divided into 2.5 mm wide strips. Unstretched 15 mm segments were mounted in isolated organ baths containing balanced salt solution aerated with 95-5% O_2-CO_2 pH 7.4 and maintained at 37°C for 60 minutes prior to passive tension loading on each muscle strip. Norepinephrine at a final bath concentration of 1.0 μM was used to standardize all contractile responses. All thrombin samples and pharmacological agents were dissolved in balanced salt solution and their contractile activity expressed relative to the 100% norepinephrine response.

AORTIC TISSUE RESPONSES TO THROMBIN

The response of vessel preparations, from different species and using a variety of vascular smooth muscle preparations, can be divided into two fundamental responses: aortic relaxation, which appears to be dependent upon an intact endothelium, and aortic contractile responses, which are endothelium-independent.

Relaxation

Thrombin has been reported by a number of investigators[12,36,37,40] to relax vascular smooth muscles that have been contracted prior to their exposure to thrombin. DeMey and coworkers,[36] for example, used canine femoral artery ring preparations in which contraction was induced with 0.5 μM norepinephrine. Bovine thrombin caused a dose-dependent relaxation of these precontracted vessels, with approximately 50% relaxation occurring with only 1 unit/ml thrombin. This relaxation response was not seen

TABLE 3. Characteristics of Thrombin and Thrombin Analogues Tested for Contractile Activity[12]

Preparations and characterization	Modification and description
α-Thrombin (94.4% α : 2.8 β : 2.9% γ) 91.7% NPGB[a] active 3,400 clotting units/mg	Native enzyme form with high fibrinogen clotting and all other thrombin-ascribed activities.
γ-Thrombin (0.01% α : 15.7% β : 87.3% γ) 80.0% NPGB active 1.74 clotting units/mg	Thrombin B chain proteolytically cleaved into three noncovalently associated fragments. This enzymically active form has essentially no clotting activity.
NO_2-α-Thrombin (99.6% α : 0.2% β : 0.2% γ) 57.3% NPGB active 34.3 clotting units/mg	Nitration of 4 out of 10 tyrosines in α-thrombin with tetranitromethane causes differential loss of clotting versus catalytic activity.
iPr$_2$P-α-Thrombin (96.5% α : 2.8% β : 0.7% γ) 0.1% NPGB active 0.5 clotting units/mg	Covalent conjugation of active-site serine (Ser_{195} in chymotrypsin) with iPr$_2$P-F causes enzymic inactivation with a large obstructive conjugated group at the catalytic site.
$MeSO_2$-α-Thrombin (97.6% α : 0.8% β : 1.6% γ) 0.2% NPGB active 0.3 clotting units/mg	Covalent conjugation of the active-site serine with $MeSO_2F$ causes enzymic inactivation with a small conjugated group at the catalytic site.
D-Phe-Pro-Arg-CH_2-α-Thrombin (95.7% α : 2.8% β : 1.5 γ) 9% NPGB active 0.1 clotting units/mg	Fibrinopeptide groove obstructed by affinity labeling with D-Phe-Pro-Arg-CH_2-Cl at or near the catalytic site, such that the ligand cannot be displaced, causing essentially complete enzymic inactivation.

[a] NPGB = *p*-nitrophenyl *p*′-guanidinobenzoate

in artery preparations in which the endothelium had been removed.[36] Thrombin also relaxed vascular muscle previously contracted with 1 mM $BaCl_2$ in the presence of 3 μM phentolamine, showing that alpha adrenergic receptors were not involved in the relaxation. Repeated exposure to thrombin (1 unit/ml) resulted in a progressive loss of the observed thrombin-induced relaxation,[36] suggesting a consumptive process of the mediator. Thrombin-induced relaxation was prevented by preincubation of thrombin with heparin, but thrombin-induced relaxations were unaffected by pre-exposure of the tissue to atropine, indomethacin, or mipacrine,[36] therefore suggesting that the thrombin-released endothelial factor promoting relaxation was not mediated by prostaglandins, leukotrienes, or a cholinergic mechanism. Rapoport and coworkers[37] studied bovine thrombin-induced relaxation using rat thoracic aorta preparations. In tissues that were precontracted with 0.1 μM norepinephrine, thrombin (3 units/ml) caused a 29.5% relaxation, an effect that could be abolished by removal of endothelium. Thrombin-induced relaxation was also prevented by preincubation of thrombin with either antithrombin or hirudin prior to placing thrombin in the bath, further supporting the need of an active enzymatic site on thrombin to mediate the release of the endothelial factor.[37] The thrombin-induced relaxation demonstrated in these studies was transient in nature and reached a maximum within 30 seconds. These same tissues did not relax upon a second exposure to thrombin, yet were frequently more responsive to further norepinephrine contractions. Relaxation caused by thrombin has been shown to be associated with increased levels of cyclic guanosine monophosphate (cGMP), whereas cyclic adenosine monophosphate (cAMP) levels were unaltered, and removal of the endothelium abolished the changes in cGMP levels.[37] Neither of these studies examined the effects of chemically modified thrombins, although the observations made using heparin, antithrombin, and hirudin-inhibited thrombins suggests that, in the case of vascular relaxation, thrombin is having a direct, active-site dependent pharmacologic effect on the vascular endothelium.

White *et al.,*[40] using human α-thrombin, observed a biphasic response in basilar and coronary arteries; additions of increasing concentrations of thrombin (from 0.1 to 10 units/ml) resulted in an initial relaxation, followed by contraction, as the concentration of thrombin was increased in tissues untreated with norepinephrine. Removal of the endothelium resulted in the specific loss of the relaxation response only; contractile amplitude and duration was the same in each type of tissue preparation.[40] In four different types of artery preparations, α-thrombin (100 units/ml) induced maximal relaxation of vascular tissue precontracted with $PGF_{2\alpha}$. In basilar arteries, heparin, hirudin, heated thrombin, and D-phenylalanyl-L-propyl-L-arginine chloromethyl ketone (PPACK)-inhibited thrombin[41] were all significantly blocked with respect to relaxation of precontracted tissue.[40]

In our experience,[12] extremely low concentrations of thrombin (7.5-75 pM; 0.0008-0.008 units/ml) caused a noticeable and persistent relaxation of rabbit aorta tissue when the endothelium was intact; denuded tissue did not relax in the presence of these picomolar concentrations of human α-thrombin. Relaxation of unstimulated aorta could also be induced by γ-thrombin and NO_2-α-thrombin but not by $i\mathrm{Pr}_2\mathrm{P}$-α-thrombin; these thrombins did not cause relaxation of aortic tissue that had the endothelium removed. This supports the concept that thrombin relaxation is a secondary response to some enzymatically generated factor that is an endothelium-dependent product of the vessel wall.

Contraction

Thrombin-induced contraction of rabbit aortic muscle preparations was, typically, a slowly developing sustained contracture, achieving maximal contractile tension between 17 and 18 minutes[12] after the thrombin addition (FIGURE 1). Purified human α-thrombin at 75 nM (8 units/ml) resulted in a response approximately equal to 50% that generated by 1.0 μM norepinephrine. All of the aortic smooth muscle preparations tested proved refractory to a second α-thrombin exposure following repeated bath washings. Using rabbit aorta and human α-thrombin at 10 units/ml, Haver and

Namm showed[18] that their aortic preparations were severely attenuated, yet gave approximately one-third the original contractile response upon re-exposure to thrombin. Part of this difference may lie in the observed dose-responses for α-thrombin; whereas our maximal contraction occurred at 8 units/ml α-thrombin (75 nM; 49.6% maximal tension),[12] Haver and Namm[18] obtained approximately 55% maximal tension at thrombin concentrations greater than 100 units/ml. They did report[18] that the dog coronary artery exhibited a greater sensitivity to thrombin, with 54.9% maximal tension developed in response to 10 units/ml thrombin. White *et al.*[35,40] have reported that thrombin added to canine basilar arteries generated a relative tension of nearly 100% at 13 units/bath (5-hydroxytryptamine defined as 100%) and approximately 55% at 1 unit/ml ($PGF_{2\alpha}$ defined as 100%). In their experiments, dog coronary arteries were less responsive than were basilar arteries both in terms of maximal tension generated and the thrombin concentrations required for optimal response.[40] We have reported[12] that concentrations of human α-thrombin that would mimic the highest measurable quantities of free thrombin during whole blood clotting,[11,13] 22 units/ml (180 nM), were not reversible in rabbit aorta smooth muscle as determined by the inability of these tissues to return to initial resting tension levels within 120 minutes following repeated muscle bath rinsings after the initial thrombin addition.

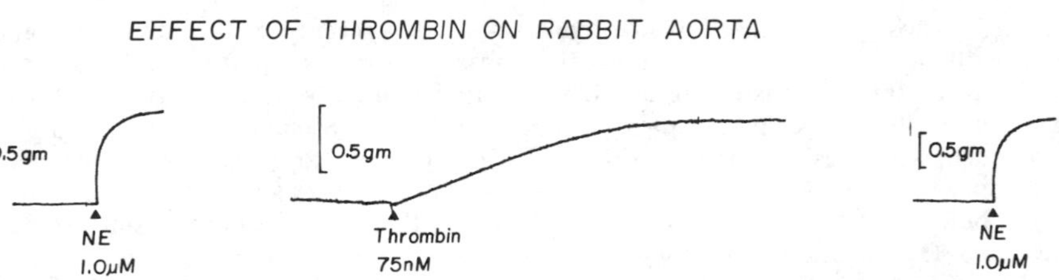

FIGURE 1. Contractile response of rabbit thoracic aorta to norepinephrine (NE) followed by a single dose of human α-thrombin. The thrombin response was maximal at 17 minutes and was approximately 43% that of the NE response.

The contractile response of aortic tissue preparations is not dependent upon an intact endothelium[12] (FIGURE 2); this is precisely the opposite observation made for the relaxation of precontracted arterial preparations. All tissue preparations, with or without endothelium, contracted in response to 75 nM α-thrombin. The time interval necessary to achieve the maximal thrombin response did not differ significantly between these two types of preparations nor did the percentage maximal tension generation differ significantly.

Thrombin analogues were examined for their respective contractile-eliciting potencies in order to determine whether the contraction required a catalytically active enzyme or was restricted to α-thrombin as is the case for thrombin-fibrinogen interaction or involved occupancy of high- or low-affinity binding sites. Of the thrombin analogues examined (see TABLE 3), γ-thrombin and nitro-thrombin were each as potent as α-thrombin in eliciting contractile activity[12] (FIGURE 3). Catalytically inactive thrombin analogues, on the other hand, were essentially without effect in this assay (FIGURE 3). Thus, enzymic activity, but not that activity restricted to fibrinogen,[3,6-8] is required for contractile activity. This is unlike the observations reported for other proteins, where γ-thrombin has no proteolytic effect on thrombospondin[42] and restricted activity towards protein C in the absence of thrombomodulin[43] In our expe-

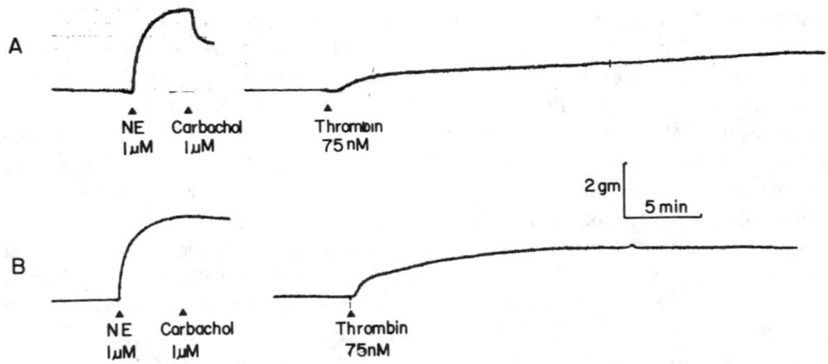

FIGURE 2. Response of rabbit aortic muscle strips to α-thrombin. (A) The endothelium was intact as evidenced by the relaxation induced when carbachol was added to norepinephrine-contracted tissue. (B) Carbachol was without effect in scrapped aortic strips. The effect of α-thrombin in both types of preparation was identical. (Walz *et al.*[12]. With permission from the *Proceedings of the Society for Experimental Biology and Medicine.*)

riences,[12] those tissues that failed to contract in the presence of thrombin analogues were still capable of initiating a normal contractile response upon the addition of 75 nM α-thrombin, demonstrating that the thrombin analogues were not competing with α-thrombin for a specific-receptor binding site. These observations are in complete agreement with those of Haver and Namm[18] who reported that they found no significant difference between native thrombin contraction of rabbit aorta and that of the autolytic thrombin form (termed β-thrombin) or thrombin that had specific tyrosine residues modified. On the other hand, they also observed[18] the absence of contractile responses in catalytically inactivated thrombin as well as thrombin in the presence of hirudin

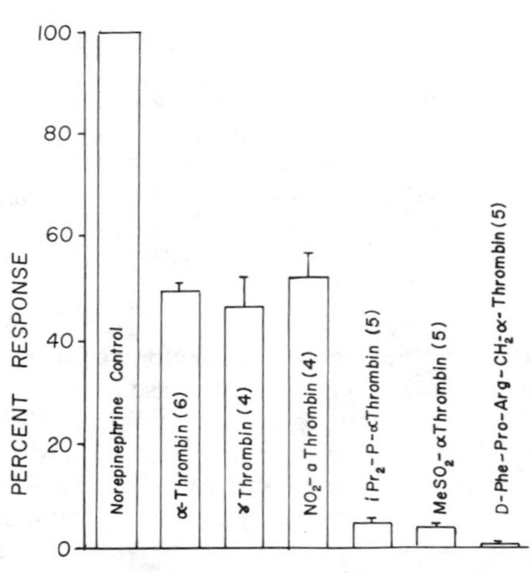

FIGURE 3. The contractile response of aortic strips to α-thrombin and thrombin analogues. See TABLE 3 for description of thrombin analogues. Numbers in parentheses are the number of different tissue preparations examined with each thrombin.

TABLE 4. Antagonism of Aortic Smooth Muscle Contractures by Selected Pharmacologic Inhibitors[12]

Antagonist	Incubation Conc[a] μM	Incubation time[b] min	Mechanism of action
Atropine	10	5	Muscarinic inhibitor
Indomethacin	10	5 to 15	Arachidonate cyclooxygenase inhibitor
Phentolamine	10	5	α-Adrenergic receptor inhibitor
D-600	10	5	Ca^{2+} channel blocker

[a] Final bath concentration.
[b] Amount of preincubation time prior to addition of α-thrombin.

and heparin/antithrombin III. White *et al.*[40] reported similar findings in canine basilar arteries, although they found the retention of contractile activity following heat inactivation of thrombin. This latter observation is inconsistent with that of active-site inhibition of thrombin being inactive in the contractile tissue assays.

High concentrations of specific pharmacologic antagonists (TABLE 4) were used to attempt to determine the mechanism underlying the thrombin-induced contractile response.[12,18,35] Of the agents tested,[12] only the Ca^{++}-channel blocker D-600 significantly blocked the thrombin-induced contraction (FIGURE 4). These observations are consistent with others,[18] which have also reported that prostaglandin inhibitors had essentially no inhibitory effects in thrombin-elicited contractions, whereas Ca^{++}-free bathing media, produced in the presence of EGTA, gave an attenuated thrombin response. In a series of experiments using canine basilar arteries, White *et al.*[35] added pharmacological inhibitors to thrombin-contracted arteries and suggested that thrombin-induced contractions were inhibited by prostacyclin and to a lesser extent by phenoxybenzamine, meclofenamate and glycerol. In a single series of experiments in our hands, the pharmacologic antagonist effects observed on α-thrombin-induced contractures were similar when tested with γ-thrombin, at the same concentrations of enzymes.

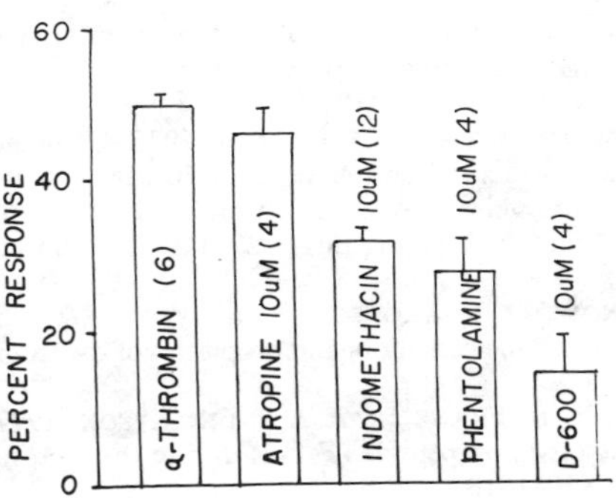

FIGURE 4. The α-thrombin response of aortic tissue in the presence of different pharmacologic antagonists. See TABLE 4 for sample description. Parenthetic numbers indicate the number of trials per sample.

CONCLUSIONS

Based upon our observations,[12] and those of others,[18,34,35,39,40] a number of conclusions regarding the action of thrombin on vessel wall tone can be summarized as follows: (1) Thrombin-elicited aortic contractions are dependent upon a catalytically active enzyme, and are evoked by physiologically relevant concentrations of thrombin. (2) Thrombin-induced aortic relaxation of precontracted tissue is dependent upon an intact endothelium. (3) Aortic contraction is not dependent upon an intact endothelium, suggesting a direct action on the underlying smooth muscle cells. (4) Contraction does not appear to be mediated by an arachidonate metabolite or α-adrenergic receptor, but probably is dependent upon calcium ion mobilization. (5) Catalytically inactivated thrombins and thrombin analogues neither diminish nor enhance subsequent tissue contraction, implying that occupancy of low-affinity receptors is not of limiting importance. (6) The observation that γ-thrombin was as active as (or more active than) α-thrombin favors a high-affinity model, where a catalytically active enzyme carries out a proteolytic function that generates a stimulatory signal, resulting in muscle contraction.

REFERENCES

1. SEEGERS, W. H. 1981. A personal perspective on hemostasis and thrombosis (1937-1981). Semin. Thromb. Hemostasis **7:** 178-307.
2. SEEGERS, W. H., H. I. HASSOUNA, D. HEWETT-EMMETT, D. A. WALZ & T. J. ANDARY. 1975. Prothrombin and thrombin. Selected aspects of thrombin formation, properties, inhibition, and immunology. Semin. Thromb. Hemostasis **1:** 211-283.
3. FENTON, J. W. & B. H. LANDIS. 1981. Prothrombin and thrombin transformations: bioregulations and function. *In* Perspectives in Hemostasis. J. Fareed, H. L. Messmore, J. W. Fenton & K. M. Brinkhous, Eds.: 31-52. Pergamon Press. New York.
4. MANN, K. G., M. E. NESHEIM, L. S. HIBBARD & P. B. TRACEY. 1981. The role of factor V in the assembly of the prothrombin complex. Ann. N.Y. Acad. Sci. **370:** 378-388.
5. SUTTIE, J. W. & C. M. JACKSON. 1977. Prothrombin structure, activation, and biosynthesis. Physiol. Rev. **57:** 1-70.
6. FENTON, J. W. 1981. Thrombin specificity. Ann. N.Y. Acad. Sci. **370:** 468-495.
7. FENTON, J. W., B. H. LANDIS, D. A. WALZ, D. H. BING, R. D. FEINMAN, M. P. ZABINSKI, S. A. SONDER, L. J. BERLINER & J. S. FINLAYSON. 1979. Human thrombin: preparative evaluation, structural properties, and enzymic specificity. *In* The Chemistry and Physiology of Human Plasma Proteins. D. H. Bing, Ed.: 151-183. Pergamon Press. New York.
8. FENTON, J. W., B. H. LANDIS, D. A. WALZ & J. S. FINLAYSON. 1977. Human thrombins. *In* Chemistry and Biology of Thrombin. R. L. Lundblad, J. W. Fenton & K. G. Mann, Eds.: 43-70. Ann Arbor Science Publishers. Ann Arbor, MI.
9. MAGNUSSON, S., T. E. PETERSEN, L. SOTTRUP-JENSEN & H. CLAEYS. 1975. Complete primary structure of prothrombin: isolation, structure, and reaction of 10 carboxylated glutamic acid residues and regulation of prothrombin activation by thrombin. *In* Proteases and Biological Control. E. Reich, D. B. Rifkin & E. Shaw, Eds.: 123-149. Cold Spring Harbor Laboratory. Cold Spring Harbor, NY.
10. FENTON, J. W., M. J. FASCO, A. B. STACKOW, D. L. ARONSON, A. M. YOUNG & J. S. FINLAYSON. 1977. Human thrombins: production, evaluation, and properties of α-thrombin. J. Biol. Chem. **252:** 3587-3598.
11. ARONSON, D. L., L. STEVAN, A. P. BALL, B. B. FRANZ JR. & J. S. FINLAYSON. 1977. Generation of the combined prothrombin activation peptide (F 1·2) during the clotting of blood and plasma. J. Clin. Invest. **60:** 1410-1418.

12. WALZ, D. A., G. F. ANDERSON, R. E. CIAGLOWSKI, M. AIKEN & J. W. FENTON. 1985. Thrombin-elicited contractile responses of aortic smooth muscle. Proc. Soc. Exp. Biol. Med. **180:** 518-526.
13. WALZ, D. A., J. N. LOVE, W. H. SEEGERS & T. R. BROWN. 1981. Radioimmunoassays for human prothrombin fragments: development and implementation. Ann. N.Y. Acad. Sci. **370:** 398-413.
14. LEVIN, E. G., V. MARZEC, J. ANDERSON & L. A. HARKER. 1984. Thrombin stimulates tissue plasminogen activator release from cultured human endothelial cells. J. Clin. Invest. **74:** 1988-1995.
15. SNIDER, R. M., M. MCKINNEY, J. W. FENTON & E. RICHELSON. 1984. Activation of cyclic nucleotide formation in murine neuroblastoma NIE-115 cells by modified human thrombins. J. Biol. Chem. **259:** 9078-9081.
16. SNIDER, R. M., M. MCKINNEY, C. FORRAY & E. RICHELSON. 1984. Neurotransmitter receptors mediate cyclic GMP formation by involvement of arachidonic acid and lipoxygenase. Proc. Natl. Acad. Sci. USA **81:** 3905-3909.
17. FAREED, J., H. L. MESSMORE, G. KINDEL, A. G. KARCZMAN & J. W. FENTON. 1981. Thrombin induced contraction of isolated smooth muscles. Thromb. Haemostasis **46:** 201.
18. HAVER, V. M. & D. H. NAMM. 1984. Characterization of thrombin-induced contraction of vascular smooth muscle. Blood Vessels **21:** 53-63.
19. BAR-SHAVIT, R., A. KAHN, G. D. WILNER & J. W. FENTON. 1983. Monocyte chemotaxis: stimulation by specific exosite region in thrombin. Science **220:** 728-731.
20. BIZIOS, R., L. LAI, J. W. FENTON, S. A. SONDER & A. B. MALIK. 1985. Thrombin-induced aggregation of lymphocytes: nonenzymatic induction by a hirudin-blocked thrombin exosite. Thromb. Res. **38:** 425-431.
21. CARNEY, D. H., K. C. GLENN & D. D. CUNNINGHAM. 1978. Conditions which affect initiation of animal cell division by trypsin and thrombin. J. Cell. Physiol. **95:** 13-33.
22. CARNEY, D. H., J. STIERNBERG & J. W. FENTON. 1984. Initiation of proliferative events by α-thrombin requires both receptor binding and enzymic activity. J. Cell. Biochem. **26:** 181-195.
23. CHEN, L. B. & J. M. BUCHANAN. 1975. Mitogenic activity of blood components. I. Thrombin and prothrombin. Proc. Natl. Acad. Sci. USA **72:** 131-135.
24. PERDUE, J. F., W. LUBENSKYI, E. KIVITY & J. W. FENTON. 1981. Characterization of human α-thrombin binding on cultured avian and mammalian cells. *In* Plasma and Cellular Modulatory Proteins. D. H. Bing & R. A. Rosenbaum, Eds.: 109-123. Center for Blood Research. Boston, MA.
25. LOUGH, J. & S. MOORE. 1975. Endothelial injury induced by thrombin and thrombi. Lab. Invest. **33:** 133-135.
26. HAGEN, A. A., J. N. GERBER, C. C. SWEELEY, R. P. WHITE & J. T. ROBERTSON. 1977. Pleocytosis and elevation of prostaglandins $F_{2\alpha}$ and E_2 in cerebrospinal fluid following intracisternal injection of thrombin. Stroke **8:** 236-238.
27. LINDER, M. & J. F. ALKSNE. 1978. Prevention of persistent cerebral smooth muscle contraction in response to whole blood. Stroke **9:** 472-477.
28. WEKSLER, B. B., C. W. LEY & E. A. JAFFE. 1978. Stimulation of endothelial cell prostacyclin production by thrombin, trypsin, and the ionophore A23187. J. Clin. Invest. **62:** 923-930.
29. AWBREY, B. J., J. C. HOAK & W. G. OWEN. 1979. Binding of human thrombin to cultured human endothelial cells. J. Biol. Chem. **254:** 4092-4095.
30. SWEDENBORG, J., M. DRYJSKI & P. OLSSON. 1983. Inactivation of thrombin by the aortic endothelium. Thromb. Haemostasis **50:** 635-638.
31. ESMON, C. T., N. L. ESMON & K. W. HARRIS. 1982. Complex formation between thrombin and thrombomodulin inhibits both thrombin-catalyzed fibrin formation and factor V activation. J. Biol. Chem. **257:** 7944-7947.
32. BAUER, P. I., R. MACHOVICH, P. ARANYI, K. G. BUKI, E. CSONKA & I. HORVATH. 1983. Mechanism of thrombin binding to endothelial cells. Blood **61:** 368-372.
33. GROVES, H. M., R. L. KINLOUGH-RATHBONE, M. RICHARDSON, L. JORGENSEN, S. MOORE & J. F. MUSTARD. 1982. Thrombin generation and fibrin formation following injury to rabbit neointima. Lab. Invest. **46:** 605-612.

34. WHITE, R. P., A. A. HAGEN, H. MORGAN, W. N. DAWSON & J. T. ROBERTSON. 1975. Experimental study on the genesis of cerebral vasospasm. Stroke **6:** 52-57.
35. WHITE, R. P., C. E. CHAPLEAU, M. DUGDALE & J. T. ROBERTSON. 1980. Cerebral arterial contractions induced by human and bovine thrombin. Stroke **11:** 363-368.
36. DEMEY, J. G., M. CLAEYS & P. M. VANHOUTTE. 1982. Endothelium-dependent inhibitory effects of acetylcholine, adenosine triphosphate, thrombin and arachidonic acid in canine femoral artery. J. Pharmacol. Exp. Ther. **222:** 166-173.
37. RAPOPORT, R. M., M. B. DRAZNIN & F. MURAD. 1984. Mechanisms of adenosine triphosphate-, thrombin-, and trypsin-induced relaxation of rat thoracic aorta. Circ. Res. **55:** 468-479.
38. GOLDSMITH, J. C. & C. T. KISKER. 1982. Thrombin-endothelial cell interactions: critical importance of endothelial cell vessel of origin. Thromb. Res. **25:** 131-136.
39. HAVER, V. M. & D. H. NAMM. 1983. Generation of a vasoactive substance in human plasma during coagulation. Blood Vessels **20:** 92-98.
40. WHITE, R. P., Y. SHIRASAWA & J. T. ROBERTSON. 1984. Comparison of responses elicited by alpha-thrombin in isolated canine basilar, coronary, mesenteric, and renal arteries. Blood Vessels **21:** 12-22.
41. COLLEN, D., O. MATSUO, J. M. STASSEN, C. KETTNER & E. SHAW. 1982. *In vivo* studies of a synthetic inhibitor of thrombin. J. Lab. Clin. Med. **99:** 76-83.
42. TAKAHASHI, K., M. AIKEN, J. W. FENTON & D. A. WALZ. 1984. Thrombospondin fragmentation by α-thrombin and resistance to γ-thrombin. Biochem. J. **224:** 673-676.
43. BEZEAUD, A., M. H. DENNINGER & M. C. GUILLIN. 1985. Interaction of human α-thrombin and γ-thrombin with antithrombin III, protein C and thrombomodulin. Eur. J. Biochem. **153:** 491-496.

Hormone-Like Activity of Human Thrombin[a]

RACHEL BAR-SHAVIT,[b,e] KEITH A. HRUSKA,[c]
ARNOLD J. KAHN,[d] AND GEORGE D. WILNER[b,c]

Departments of [b]Pathology and [c]Medicine
Washington University School of Medicine
St. Louis, Missouri 63110
and
[d]Pediatric Research Institute
St. Louis University School of Medicine
St. Louis, Missouri 63110

INTRODUCTION

Thrombin, the major procoagulant serine esterase elaborated by activation of the clotting cascade, is also a potent activator/regulator of a variety of cellular mediated events.[1-4] For the induction of the majority of these effects, the proteolytic activity of this enzyme is a strict requirement. By contrast, we have observed that esterolytically inactivated or proteolytically degraded thrombin forms have potent stimulatory and growth-promoting effects specifically on cells of monocyte/macrophage lineage.[1,5,6] What emerges from our studies of the past several years using protein chemistry and computer modeling techniques is the definition and structural delineation of unique cell interaction exosite within the thrombin molecule which, on a molar basis, is equivalent to its parent protein in mediating these biological functions.[5,6] Although the presence of structurally distinct cell-interactive domains within protein molecules is not unusual (*e.g.*, fibronectin and immunoglobulins), this is the first instance of description of such a region in a major enzyme in the blood coagulation pathway. This finding has important physiological implications insofar as it directly links activation of the procoagulant cascade with the cellular events of inflammation and wound healing.

In the present communication, we will provide an updated overview of two important areas regarding the biological functioning of this cell-interactive exosite in thrombin. Our previous studies have suggested that this region in thrombin, which is contained within residues 338-400 of the human prothrombin sequence, is a selective

[a]This investigation was supported by SCOR Grant HL-14147, HL-34282, and HL-34575 from the NHLBI, NIH; Grant DE-04629 from the NIDR, NIH; and the Monsanto-Washington University Agreement Grant. Dr. Bar-Shavit is recipient of a Postdoctoral Fellowship Award from the American Heart Association.

[e]Address for correspondence: Rachel Bar-Shavit, Ph.D., Department of Pathology, The Jewish Hospital, 216 South Kingshighway, St. Louis, MO 63110.

stimulator of directed movement for cells of monocyte/macrophage origin, but not for granulocytes.[1,7,8] Thrombin's ability to function as a chemotaxin specifically for these cell types is worthy of further exploration because this behavior is unlike that of most well-characterized chemotactic agents (*e.g.,* FMLP, C5 fragments, and LTB4) that are chemotactic for both granulocytes and monocytes.[9] Toward this end, we have studied the human promyelocytic leukemia cell line HL-60 as a model system. This cell line is capable of differentiating upon treatment with phorbolmyristate acetate (TPA)[10] or 1,25$(OH)_2D_3$[11] along a monocytic pathway, or along a granulocytic lineage upon treatment with dimethyl sulfoxide (DMSO)[12] or retinoic acid.[13] Therefore, HL-60 cells are a convenient tool for assessing, within the context of cell lineage and differentiation, the early events associated with development of chemotactic responsiveness to thrombin.

In addition to thrombin's chemotactic activity on monocytes/macrophages, we will provide data demonstrating that it is also a potent growth factor for these cells. As with chemotaxis, these growth-promoting effects are completely independent of thrombin's esterolytic function and are mediated by the same cell-interactive region in thrombin. Whereas the sequences required for chemotaxis and mitogenicity overlap, however, they are separable. In the present communication, we will show that although most, if not all, of the surface-expressed portions of the thrombin cell-interactive exosite are required for mediation of directed cell movement, a small portion of this region containing the loop B insertion sequence[14] is itself sufficient to promote DNA synthesis and cell proliferation in growth-arrested macrophages.

MATERIAL AND METHODS

Reagents

All chemicals were of reagent grade or better. The following were obtained from the sources listed: bovine serum albumin (BSA) (fraction V) from Miles, Naperville, IL; Iscore modified Dulbecco's medium (IMDM) from KC Biologicals, Kansas City, MO; fetal calf serum (FCS) from Hyclone, Logan, UT; Triton X-100, imidazole, f-Met-Leu-Phe-OH, actin, transferrin, glutamine, acrylamide, sodium dodecyl sulfate (SDS), and reagents for gel electrophoresis from Sigma Chemical Co., St. Louis, MO; quin-2 from Amersham, Arlington, IL; 1,25$(OH)_2D_3$(vitamin D_3), a gift from Dr. Milan Uskovic, Hoffmann-LaRoche, Nutley, NJ; methyl-^{3}[H]-TdR (specific activity, 6.7 Ci/mmol) from New England Nuclear, Boston, MA.

Cell Lines

HL-60 cells were maintained in IMDM containing BSA (5 mg/ml), transferrin (5 μg/ml), and glutamine (2 mM).[15] Cultures were maintained at 37°C in a humidified 5% CO_2 atmosphere. The cells were differentiated toward monocytes (HL-60/mono) by addition of 1.25 $(OH)_2D_3$ to the medium in ethanol at a final concentration of 50 nM. The ethanol concentration did not exceed 0.1 percent. Alternatively, the cells were differentiated along a granulocytic pathway (HL-60/gran) by addition of DMSO (final concentration, 1.25%) to the medium. Differentiation of HL-60 to either HL-60/mono or HL-60/gran occurred in > 90% of the resting cell population following incubation with the appropriate differentiating agent for a period of 3-6 days. The criteria used to establish either HL-60/mono or HL-60/gran differentiation were as previously described.[11-13] J-774 murine macrophage-like cells were a gift from Dr. Jay Unkeles, Rockefeller University, New York, NY. Murine macrophage-like cell lines P-388D, RAW, and PU5 were obtained from the American-Type Culture Collection (ATCC), Rockville, MD.

Human Thrombin Preparations

Preparations of active human α-thrombin and esterolytically inactive human di-isopropyl phosphorofluoridate (iPR_2P)-α-thrombin were generously provided by Dr. John Fenton, New York State Department of Health, Albany, NY. Their preparation and characterization have been described in detail.[16]

Thrombin Fragments

The isolation and purification of peptide CB67-129 from human prothrombin 1, and the preparation of limited tryptic digests of this peptide following citraconylation and subsequent removal of the reversible blocking groups were carried out as described.[6,17,18] Fractionation and isolation of peptides from this digest were performed by semipreparative reverse-phase high performance liquid chromatography (HPLC)[19] using a 250 × 10 mm Hi-Pore RP-318 column (Bio-Rad, Richmond, CA).

Chemotaxis Assays

Chemotaxis was determined using a double filter technique in modified Boyden chambers (Ahlco Manufacturing Co., Southington, CT) as previously described.[7]

Cytoskeletal-Associated Actin Assay

Cytoskeletal proteins were isolated as described by White *et al.*[20] Briefly, cells (10^7) suspended in 500 μl of medium in microcentrifuge tubes were incubated with the appropriate test agent at 37°C for the times indicated. The cytoskeletal fraction was then isolated by addition of 500 μl of an ice cold buffer solution (40 mM imidazole and 160 mM HCl, final pH 7.0) containing 2% Triton X-100, 20 mM EGTA, and 8 mM sodium azide. The tubes were incubated at 0°C for 10 minutes, then centrifuged (g × 8000) for 3 minutes in a high-speed microcentrifuge (Fisher Scientific Co., Springfield, NJ). The pellet was dissolved by boiling (with vigorous stirring) for 5 minutes in 50 μl of a solution containing 10% SDS, 13 mM 2-mercaptoethanol and

20% glycerol, in 86 mM Tris-HCl buffer, pH 7.6, and resolved by gradient polyacrylamide gel electrophoresis SDS (PAGE), using a 5-20% gradient. The 42 000 mol wt actin band was identified in the Coomassie-stained gel, and quantitated by absorption at 590 nm using an LKB laser densitometer (LKB Instruments, Houston, TX).

Fluorometric Measurement of Free Cytosolic Ca^{2+}

Cells (2.5×10^7) were preloaded with the acetoxymethyl ester of quin-2 (25 μM) by incubation in 0.5 ml volume Hanks'-HEPES buffer at 37°C with vigorous shaking. After 20 minutes, an additional 4.5 ml of Hanks'-HEPES buffer was added, and the incubation continued for an additional 60 minutes. The cells were then washed and resuspended in 2 ml Krebs-Henslit buffer in 1 cm quartz cuvettes. Intracellular quin-2 fluorescence changes were measured at 37°C in 2 ml samples of continuously stirred cell suspensions using an SLM 4880 spectrofluorometer (SLM Instruments, Urbana, IL). The assay was carried out as described by Tsein *et al.*[21] and modified by Hruska *et al.*[22]

Tritiated Thymidine ([^{3}H]TdR) Incorporation

Cells were plated in Dulbecco's modified Eagle's medium (DMEM) containing 10% FCS in 95% CO_2-humidified atmosphere at 37°C at an initial density of 5×10^5 per well in 24-well disposable plastic plates (Falcon, Oxnard, CA). Arrest of DNA synthesis (*i.e.*, G_0/G_1) was achieved by incubating cells for 48 hours in serum-free DMEM containing 0.1% BSA. The cells were then exposed to various thrombin forms, peptide, or FCS for 48 hours. Enhanced thymidine incorporation was assessed following a 2-hour pulse of *N*-methyl-[^{3}H]TdR (1 μCi/ml). The cells were washed three times in phosphate-buffered saline (PBS) at 4°C, precipitated with 10% trichloroacetic acid (TCA) (30 minutes at 4°C), and the insoluble material extracted twice with ETOH:ET_2O (3:1 v/v). The precipitate was solubilized in 1 N NaOH and aliquots withdrawn for protein determinations using a dye-binding assay (Bio-Rad, Richmond, CA) and liquid scintillation spectrometry.

Peptide Synthesis

Peptide H-Tyr-Pro-Pro-Trp-Asn-Lys-Asn-Phe-Thr-Glu-Asn-Asp-Leu-Leu-OH, representing residues 367-380[f] of the human thrombin B chain, and containing the loop B insertion sequence, was synthesized by a modification of the method of Merrifield, as previously described.[23,24] The fully protected peptide was simultaneously deprotected and cleaved from its resin support by the two-step hydrofluoric acid (HF)-catalyzed S_N2 procedure described by Tam.[25] The crude peptide was definitively purified by ion exchange chromatography on a DEAE Sephacel column as previously

[f] Prothrombin nomenclature.[26] The sequence used for synthesis is according to the protein sequence data of Butkowski *et al.*[17]

described.[24] Peptide purity was ascertained by reverse-phase (C_{16}) HPLC,[19] where it chromatographed as a single peak. The peptide was also found to be homogeneous by thin-layer chromatography (TLC), migrating as a single spot using two different solvent systems.[23,24] Amino acid analysis yielded the expected molar ratios.

RESULTS

Specificity of Thrombin Chemotactic Effects on Cells of Monocyte/Macrophage Lineage

Chemotactic Responses of Differentiated HL-60 Cells

HL-60, a human promyelocytic tumor cell line capable of bidirectional differentiation, was induced to differentiate toward monocytes (HL-60/mono) by treating the cells for 3-4 days with $1,25(OH)_2D_3$[11] or toward granulocytes (HL-60/gran) by exposure to DMSO for 5-6 days.[12] Alpha-thrombin as well as the esterolytically inactive iPR_2P-α-thrombin stimulate directed cell migration in HL-60/mono but not in undifferentiated HL-60 cells (FIGURE 1A, 1B). The response occurs over a broad range of thrombin concentration (10^{-10} M to 10^{-6} M) with an optimal response occurring at 10^{-6} M. By contrast, HL-60/gran show insignificant movement toward thrombin (FIGURE 1A, 1B). Both HL-60/mono and HL-60/gran respond chemotactically to f-Met-Leu-Phe-OH (FMLP) in contrast to nontreated HL-60 cells (FIGURE 1d). These results are consistent with FMLP being an active chemoattractant for both macrophages and neutrophils, and with our previous observations on thrombin being a specific chemoattractant for monocytes and certain macrophage-like cell lines but not for granulocytes.[7,8]

Our earlier studies have indicated that the thrombin cell-interactive exosite (which is responsible for thrombin's chemotactic effects) is contained within a cyanogen bromide-derived cleavage fragment of the thrombin B chain. This fragment, known as peptide CB 67-129, represents residues 367-380 of the human prothrombin sequence[26] (FIGURE 2). As shown in FIGURE 1C, this peptide is chemotactic for HL-60/mono at the same concentration range as intact thrombin (FIGURE 1C). These data imply that the characteristics of HL-60/mono chemotactic responses to FMLP and thrombin are similar to those we have observed with peripheral blood monocytes and murine macrophage-like cell lines such as J-774, providing further evidence for the unique selectivity of thrombin as a chemotaxin.

Early Events Associated with Thrombin-Mediated Chemotaxis in HL-60/Mono

Thrombin Effects on the Cytoskeleton

Because chemotaxis involves cell mobility and changes in cell shape, it is dependent on the ability of cytoskeletal actin to polymerize into filaments capable of bearing tension (F-actin). Association of actin with the cytoskeleton was assessed by SDS-

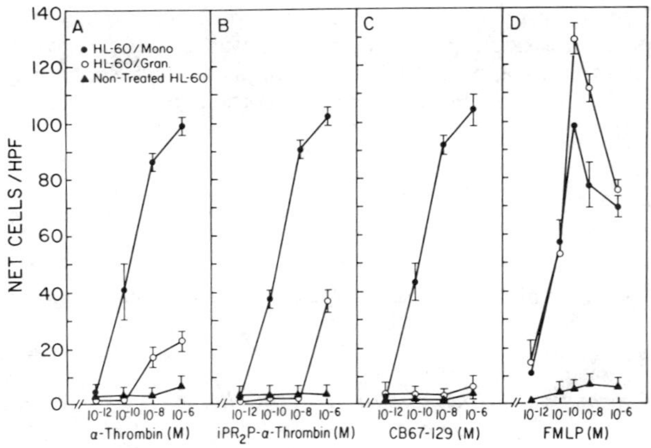

FIGURE 1. Chemotaxis of HL-60/mono (●—●), HL-60/gram (○—○) and non-treated HL-60 (▲—▲) toward **(a)** α-thrombin, **(b)** iPR$_2$P-α-thrombin, **(c)** the cyanogen bromide-derived peptide CB67-129, and **(d)** FMLP.

PAGE analysis of the insoluble fraction of Triton X-100 buffer of cells. Exposure of HL-60/mono to thrombin for 30 seconds induces an increase in cytoskeletal-associated actin. Densitometric quantitation of the 42 K actin band on gradient gels indicates that the highest response to thrombin is obtained at 10^{-6} M (75% increase over control, FIGURE 3); the same concentration elicits optimal HL-60/mono chemotactic response (FIGURE 1b). No significant effect was produced by these agents on undifferentiated HL-60 cells (data not shown).

Thrombin effect on actin polymerization occurs very rapidly and in a transient fashion. As shown in TABLE 1, the effect occurs in the range of 15-150 seconds with a maximum occurring at 60 seconds. Subsequently, after 5 minutes it declines back to control values.

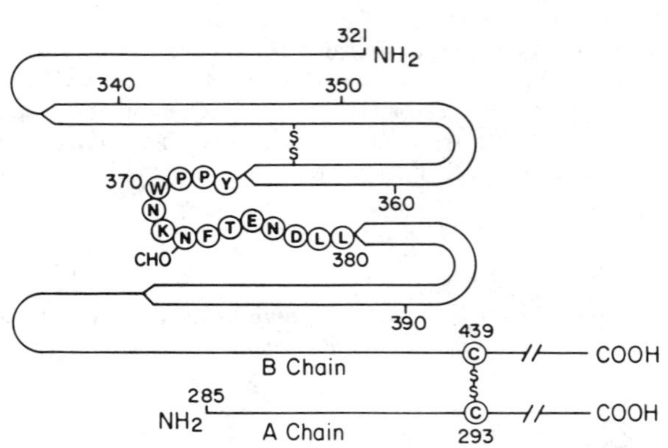

FIGURE 2. Model of α-thrombin, based on the protein sequence data of Butkowski *et al.*[17] The sequence nomenclature is that of prothrombin.[26] The location of peptide CB67-129 is shown by the double solid lines. The sequence of the loop B synthetic homologue residues (367-380) is indicated by beads.

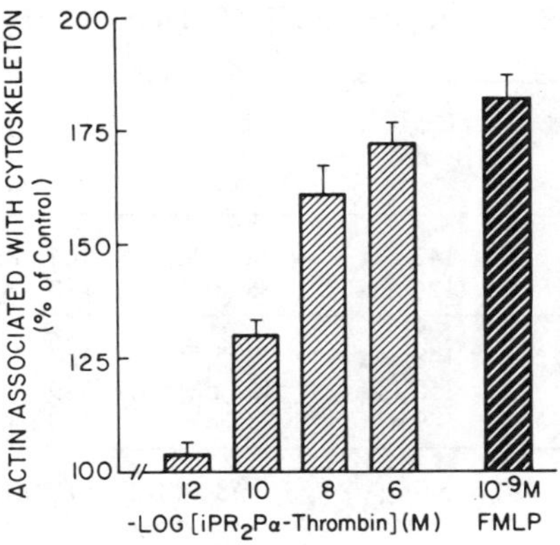

FIGURE 3. Actin association to the Triton-insoluble cytoskeletal fraction of HL-60/mono following 30 seconds stimulation with iPR_2P-α-thrombin or FMLP. Each point was determined by densitometric quantitation of the actin band, separated on gradient SDS-PAGE. Results are expressed as a mean of triplicate determinations ± SEM.

Thrombin Effects on Cytosolic Ca^{2+}

Exposure of HL-60/mono to thrombin elicits an increase in cytosolic Ca^{2+} levels, reaching a maximum within 20-30 seconds, then declining back to control levels by 5 minutes (TABLE 2). The elevation of free cytosolic Ca^{2+} occurs in a dose-dependent manner as a function of thrombin concentration (data not shown), and reaches maximum at 10^{-6} M (similarly to thrombin-induced chemotaxis in HL-60/mono). As indicated in TABLE 2, 10^{-6} M iPR_2P-α-thrombin elevates free intracellular Ca^{2+} levels from 142 nM to 281 nM in 20 seconds of stimulation, then declines back to basal levels. A similar effect is obtained by 10^{-9} M FMLP (from 124 nM to 264 nM). We have previously shown that chemotaxis by thrombin or FMLP is mediated through different receptors. Exposure of HL-60/mono cells to a micromolar concentration of thrombin or a nanomolar concentration of FMLP (optimal concentration for both agents) induces a rapid burst in free cytosolic Ca^{2+} (TABLE 2). A second stimulation of the cells with thrombin causes only a slight elevation in free cytosolic Ca^{2+} concentration. When a different chemotaxin (FMLP) is used for the second stimulation, however, a rapid large burst of free cytosolic Ca^{2+} is observed (from 145 nM to 258

TABLE 1. Kinetics of Actin Association[a]

Time (seconds)	Amount of Actin Associated with Cytoskeleton (relative to control)
0	1.0
15	1.75 ± 0.3
30	2.0 ± 0.25
60	1.80 ± 0.1
150	1.5 ± 0.18
300	1.25 ± 0.32
500	1.1 ± 0.09

[a] Kinetics of actin association with the triton-insoluble cytoskeletal fraction of HL-60/mono, following exposure of 10^{-6} M iPR_2P-α-thrombin. Assay conditions are similar to those of FIGURE 2.

TABLE 2. Effects of iPR_2P-α-Thrombin and FMLP-Stimulated HL-60/mono on Free Cytosolic Ca^{2}[a]

Chemotaxin	Time:	$[Ca^{2+}]i$ nM 0	$[Ca^{2+}]i$ nM 20 sec	$[Ca^{2+}]i$ nM 5 min
iPR_2P-α-thrombin, (10^{-6} M)		142 nM	281 nM	144 nM
FMLP, (10^{-9} M)		124 nM	364 nM	240 nM
iPR_2P-α-thrombin, 1st pulse (10^{-6} M)		148 nM	220 nM	150 nM
iPR_2P-α-thrombin, 2nd pulse (10^{-6} M)		150 nM	152 nM	149 nM
FMLP, 3rd pulse (10^{-9} M)		149 nM	258 nM	190 nM

[a] Stimulated free cytosolic Ca^{2+} levels by iPR_2P-α-thrombin (10^{-6} M) and FMLP (10^{-9} M) on HL-60/mono. Cells were preloaded with quin-2 and their relative fluorescence analyzed as described in METHODS. The effect of consecutive pulse stimulation of HL-60/mono cells with iPR_2P-α-thrombin followed by FMLP is indicated. In this experiment, the repeated pulses of chemotactic agents were given following return of the Ca^{2+} levels to basal. Representative experiments are shown.

nM). A possible explanation for these results is that whereas thrombin receptors are desensitized at the second pulse and incapable of inducing the receptor-mediated elevation of Ca^{2+}, FMLP receptors would remain free and available for response.

Thus, thrombin appears to be a selective and specific chemotaxin for cells of macrophage/monocyte lineage. The specificity of this effect is clearly indicated by absence of significant stimulation of mobility by thrombin of either peripheral blood neutrophils, or of granulocytic differentiated HL-60 cells. Concomitant early events known to parallel chemotaxis, including cytoskeletal actin association and free Ca^{2+} mobilization, are likewise observable following thrombin stimulation of monocytic differentiated HL-60 cells.

Thrombin Mitogenic Activity on Macrophages

Addition of esterolytically inactive iPR_2P-α-thrombin to macrophage-like cells stimulates DNA synthesis.[6] This stands in contrast to fibroblasts where the enzymatic activity is essential for cell proliferation.[2] The observation that thrombin promotes cell division in J-774 cells (and other macrophage-like cell lines, including P-388D, RAW and PU-5) independent of its esterolytic function, suggests that the region in thrombin responsible for these effects may either coincide or overlap with thrombin chemotactic exosite.[5] Therefore, the thrombin-derived chemotactic fragment peptide CB67-129 (corresponds to residues 338-400 of human prothrombin, see FIGURE 2) was assessed for its mitogenic activity. Indeed, as shown in FIGURE 4 (insert), the peptide at 10^{-8} M is capable of inducing [^{3}H]TdR incorporation 128% over arrested cells. The response was observed over a concentration range of 10^{-11} M to 10^{-6} M (data not shown) with optimum at 10^{-8} M. Next, we assessed whether this mitogenic activity required the entire CB67-129 fragment, or whether it could be expressed in a smaller peptide derived from this cyanogen bromide-derived polypeptide. CB67-129 peptide was therefore further digested with trypsin (under reversible blockage by citraconylation of lysine groups, which will permit cleavage only at arginyl bonds).[18] This digest (upon removal of the lysine side-chain blocking group), when tested for mitogenic activity, showed stimulation of [^{3}H]TdR incorporation equivalent to the parent molecule (FIGURE 4, insert). The mitogenic digest was not chemotactic (TABLE 3), demonstrating that separate but overlapping regions in the cell-interaction exosite are required for mediating these chemotactic and mitogenic effects. Fractionation of the digest by reverse-phase HPLC showed that the mitogenic activity was present in fractions containing residues 356-382 (FIGURE 2) of thrombin B chain (data not shown). This region of thrombin chain differs from homologous regions in two closely related (but chemotactically and mitogenically inactive) serine esterases, chymotrypsin and trypsin, principally by the presence of a unique 9-10 residue insertion sequence termed loop B[14,27] (FIGURE 2). This suggested to us that the loop B sequence may play a critical role in the biological functioning of the cell-interactive exosite.

In order to establish whether the loop B sequence itself might account for the biological activity of thrombin, a loop-B-containing homologue representing residues 367-380 of human prothrombin sequence (FIGURE 2) was prepared synthetically. This peptide proves capable of stimulating [^{3}H]TdR incorporation in G_0/G_1-arrested J-774 cells (FIGURE 4) with a comparable dose-response effect to that observed with intact iPR$_2$P-α-thrombin. Additionally, a dose-dependent increase in cell number is also observed. In a representative experiment, 24 hours following exposure to the peptide at 10^{-8} M, the cell number was increased from 1.2×10^5 M to 2×10^5 cells/well.

From these experiments, it is apparent that thrombin, or more specifically, the loop B sequence within the cell-interactive exosite region of the thrombin B chain

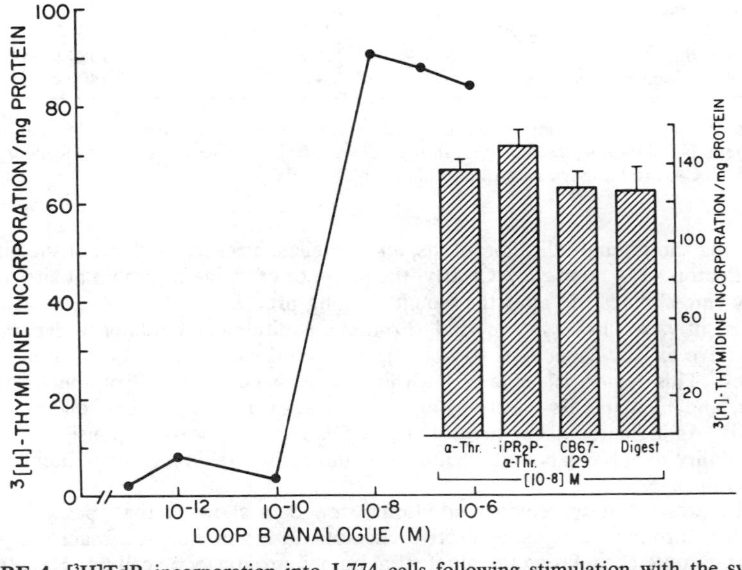

FIGURE 4. [^{3}H]TdR incorporation into J-774 cells following stimulation with the synthetic homologue of thrombin loop B insertion sequence. Insert: [^{3}H]TdR incorporation to J-774 stimulated by the optimal concentration (10^{-8} M) of α-thrombin, iPR$_2$P-α-thrombin, CB67-129, and the tryptic digest of peptide CB67-129.

appears to be a specific growth promoter for cells of macrophage lineage. It is worth noting that in contrast to thrombin, other well-characterized growth factors, including EGF, FGF, NGF, and PDGF fail to stimulate G_0/G_1-arrested J-774 cells (data not shown).

DISCUSSION

Given thrombin's role as the major procoagulant enzyme of the clotting cascade coupled with its ubiquity at sites of inflammation and tissue repair, it is, therefore, important to explore thrombin's alternate role in modulating or regulating these latter processes. That enzymatically active α-thrombin is a potent mitogen for a variety of fibroblasts, and elicits a variety of important biological responses in other cell types,

TABLE 3. Thrombin-Directed Cell Migration and Mitogenesis on Monocytes/Macrophages[a]

	Migration (cells/hpf)	[^{3}H]TdR Incorporation by J-774 Cells (percent increase)
α-thrombin	120 ± 10	142 ± 9
iPR$_2$P-α-thrombin	135 ± 9	170 ± 8
Hirudin-α-thrombin complex	9 ± 3	12 ± 2
Prothrombin	10 ± 2	12 ± 3
AT3-α-thrombin complex	4 ± 0.5	10 ± 3
CB67-129	110 ± 6	138 ± 7
CB67-129 digest	2 ± 0.5	139 ± 11
Synthetic B-loop peptide	3 ± 0.4	140 ± 9

[a] Chemotaxis was determined as described[7] using modified Boyden chambers and human peripheral blood monocytes. Mitogenesis was established by the degree of [^{3}H]TdR incorporation into the TCA-insoluble fraction of stimulated J-774 cells.

including endothelial cells, fibroblasts, and platelets, has been well established by other investigators (2-4 *inter alia*). Clearly, the presence of active thrombin at sites of tissue injury can significantly alter the wound healing process.

Recently, we have shown that thrombin additionally contains a separate cell-interactive exosite capable of stimulating biological effects in monocytes and macrophages.[5] This region is contained within the sequence 338-400 of the thrombin B chain, and mediates its effects as an isolated segment independent of any enzymic activity. As indicated in the present study, this region appears responsible for thrombin's ability to act as a potent chemotaxin, and additionally, a growth factor, for cells of this lineage.

The present study provides additional new data showing that, despite common ancestry, thrombin acts as a selective chemotaxin for monocytes/macrophages, but not for granulocytes. Using the bipotential human promyeloctic cell line HL-60, which can be induced to differentiate either toward monocytes or toward granulocytes by treating the cells with an appropriate chemical inducer, we have shown that only monocyte-differentiated HL-60 cells (HL-60/mono), but not undifferentiated or granulocyte-differentiated cells, respond chemotactically to either intact thrombin or an isolated cell-interactive cyanogen bromide fragment. Moreover, concomitant events that are associated with directed cell movement, such as association of cytoplasmic actin with monomeric actin (G-actin) into cytoskeletal filamentous actin,[20] and mobilization of free cytosolic Ca^{2+},[28,29] are likewise seen in HL-60/mono cells exposed to esterolytically inactivated thrombin. The reason for the selective chemotactic response of HL-60/mono as compared to granulocyte-differentiated or undifferentiated HL-60 is unclear at this time. Preliminary radioligand binding studies comparing monocyte-differentiated, granulocyte-differentiated, and undifferentiated HL-60 cells using $[^{125}I]\alpha$-thrombin suggest that differences exist in the expression of specific thrombin binding sites on the cell surfaces. Presumably, differences in receptor number might account for variations in biological activity, but these findings will have to be confirmed.

We also present evidence that thrombin, or more specifically, the cell-interactive exosite (residues 338-400, see FIGURE 2), located in the thrombin B chain, is a mitogen for macrophage-like cell lines. This effect stands in sharp contrast to what has been observed with fibroblasts, where thrombin's mitogenic activity is totally dependent on retention of its enzymic activity.[2] It is also clear that chemotactic and mitogenic activities are expressed by distinct but overlapping segments of this exosite region. As was shown in detail in earlier studies,[5,30] eliciting chemotactic movement in monocytes/macrophages requires the availability of most of sequence 338-400, including the loop B insertion sequence (FIGURE 2). As indicated in the present study, in contrast to observations regarding stimulation of directed cell movement, the loop B insertion sequence alone appears to be sufficient to stimulate DNA synthesis and proliferation in growth-arrested macrophages. This assumption is supported by the following findings: Native α-thrombin, esterolytically inactive iPR_2P-α-thrombin, and fragment CB67-129 (consisting of the entire sequence 338-400) are approximately equivalent in their abilities to stimulate proliferation of G_0/G_1, and limited tryptic digests of fragment CB67-129, which retain intact the loop B insertion sequence, are also mitogenic for these cells. These effects can be reproduced in a synthetic tetradecapeptide homologue of this thrombin B chain sequence.

Delineation of the thrombin B chain cell-interactive exosite has important physiologic implications. This sequence is expressed in noncoagulant, proteolytically degraded thrombins,[1] and possibly in other thrombin degradation products as well.[3] Possessing biological activity, these fragments will escape inhibition by the traditional thrombin inhibitors, such as protease nexin,[32] AT3,[33] or heparin cofactor II.[34] From these considerations, it is likely that thrombin and its derivatives can function effectively as a stimulator/regulator of monocytes/macrophages at injury sites.

SUMMARY

Recently, we have shown that thrombin is a chemotaxin and growth-promoting agent for cells of the mononuclear phagocytic lineage. These activities are independent of thrombin's enzymatic activity. Unlike other chemotactic factors, thrombin is specific for monocytes and does not attract granulocytes. To further explore the cellular specificity we have used a human leukemia cell line HL-60 that is capable of *in vitro* differentiation toward either monocytes (HL-60/mono) following incubation with $1,25(OH)_2D_3$, or granulocytes (HL-60/gran) following incubation with DMSO. In contrast to undifferentiated HL-60 cells or HL-60/gran, we find that HL-60/mono respond chemotactically to intact human α-thrombin, esterolytically inactive iPR_2P-α-thrombin, and the thrombin-derived peptide CB67-129, previously shown to contain the thrombin chemotactic exosite. In addition, thrombin induces in HL-60/mono association of actin with the cytoskeleton and causes an increase in levels of free cytosolic Ca^{2+}. These phenomena are well characterized as early events occurring concomitant with directed cell movement associated with exposure to chemotactic agents such as FMLP.

Furthermore, in contrast to fibroblasts, both iPR_2P-α-thrombin and the thrombin chemotactic peptide CB67-129 evoke dose-dependent [^{3}H]TdR incorporation, protein synthesis, and cell replication in growth-arrested J-744 cells, a murine macrophage-like cell line. Limited tryptic digests of CB67-129 lose chemotactic activity but retain full mitogenic activity, demonstrating that as with PDGF, the sites on CB67-129 required for chemotaxis and mitogenesis are clearly dissociable. The mitogenic effects of the CB67-129 digest can be mimicked by a synthetic tetradecapeptide analogue of CB67-129 (residues 367-380) that includes the loop B insertion sequence, previously shown to be critical for thrombin's chemotactic effects. From these data, it is apparent that the loop B insertion is critical for thrombin's nonenzymic biological effects on cells, but additional sites are required for stimulation of cell movement.

ACKNOWLEDGMENTS

The technical assistance of Ms. M. S. Mudd and Ms. A. Jernigan, and the secretarial assistance of Ms. M. Hammer is gratefully acknowledged.

REFERENCES

1. Bar-Shavit, R., A. Kahn, G. D. Wilner & J. W. Fenton II. 1983. Monocyte chemotaxis: stimulation by specific exosite region in thrombin. Science **220:** 728-731.
2. Perdue, J. F., W. Lubensky, E. Kivity, S. A. Sonder & J. W. Fenton. 1981. Protease mitogenic response of chick embryo fibroblasts and receptor binding/processing of human α-thrombin. J. Biol. Chem. **256:** 2767-2776.
3. Weksler, B. B., C. W. Ley & E. A. Jaffe. 1978. Stimulation of endothelial cell prostacycline production by thrombin, trypsin, and ionophore A23187. J. Clin. Invest. **62:** 923-930.
4. Martin, B. M., R. D. Feinman & T. C. Detwiler. 1975. Platelet stimulation by thrombin and other proteases. Biochemistry **14:** 1308-1314.
5. Bar-Shavit, R., A. Kahn, G. D. Wilner, K. G. Mann & J. W. Fenton II. 1984. Thrombin chemotactic domain is localized within a B chain CNBr fragment. Biochemistry **23:** 397-400.
6. Bar-Shavit, R., A. J. Kahn, K. G. Mann & G. D. Wilner. 1986. Identification of a thrombin sequence with growth factor activity on macrophages. Proc. Natl. Acad. Sci. USA **83:** 976-980.
7. Bar-Shavit, R., A. J. Kahn, J. W. Fenton II & G. D. Wilner. 1983. Chemotactic responses of monocytes to thrombin. J. Cell Biol. **96:** 282-285.
8. Bar-Shavit, R., A. J. Kahn, J. W. Fenton II & G. D. Wilner. 1983. Receptor-mediated chemotactic response of a macrophage cell line (J-774) to thrombin. Lab. Invest. **49:** 702-707.

9. Becker, E. L. & T. P. Stossel. 1980. Chemotaxis. Fed. Proc. Fed. Am. Soc. Exp. Biol. **39:** 2949-2952.
10. Lotem, J. & L. Sachs. 1979. Regulation of normal differentiation in mouse and human myeloid leukemia cells by phorbol esters and the mechanism of tumor promotion. Proc. Natl. Acad. Sci USA **76:** 5158-5162.
11. Bar-Shavit, Z., S. L. Teitelbaum, P. Reitsma, A. Hall, L. E. Pegg, J. A. Trial & A. J. Kahn. 1983. Induction of monocyte differentiation and bone resorption by 1,25-dihydroxyvitamin D3. Proc. Natl. Acad. Sci. USA **80:** 5907-5911.
12. Collins, S. J., F. W. Ruscetti, R. E. Gallagher & R. C. Gallo. 1978. Terminal differentiation of human promyelocytic leukemia cells induced by dimethyl sulfoxide and other polar compounds. Proc. Natl. Acad. Sci. USA **75:** 2458-2462.
13. Honma, Y., K. Takenaga, T. Kasukabe & M. Hozumi. 1980. Induction of differentiation of cultured human promyelocytic leukemia cells by retinoids. Biochem. Biophysics Res. Commun. **95:** 507-512.
14. Elion, J., M. R. Downing, R. J. Butkowski & K. G. Mann. 1977. *In* Chemistry and Biology of Thrombin. R. L. Lundblad, J. W. Fenton II & K. G. Mann, Eds.: 97-111. Ann Arbor Science Publishers. Ann Arbor, Michigan.
15. Bar-Shavit, Z., S. L. Teitelbaum, G. P. Stricklin, A. Z. Eisen, A. J. Kahn & H. G. Welgus. 1985. Differentiation of a human leukemia cell line and expression of collagenase inhibitor. Proc. Natl. Acad. Sci. USA **82:** 5380-5384.
16. Fenton II, J. W., M. J. Fasco, A. B. Stackrow, D. L. Aronson, A. M. Young & J. S. Finlayson. 1977. Human thrombins: production, evaluation and properties of α-thrombin. J. Biol. Chem. **252:** 3587-3598.
17. Butkowski, R. J., J. Elion, M. R. Downing & K. G. Mann. 1977. The primary structure of human prethrombin 2 and α-thrombin. J. Biol. Chem. **252:** 4942-4957.
18. Gibbons, I. & R. N. Perham. 1970. The reaction of aldolase with 2-methylmaleic acid. Biochem. J. **116:** 843-849.
19. Fulmer, C. S. & R. H. Wasserman. 1979. Analytical peptide mapping by high performance liquid chromatography: application to intestinal Ca-binding proteins. J. Biol. Chem. **254:** 7208-7212.
20. White, J. R., P. H. Naccache & R. I. Sha'afi. 1983. Stimulation by chemotactic factor of actin association with the cytoskeleton in rabbit neutrophils. J. Biol. Chem. **258:** 14041-14047.
21. Tsien, R. Y., T. Pozzan & T. J. Rink. 1982. Calcium homeostasis in intact lymphocytes: cytoplasmic free calcium monitored with a new intracellulary fluorescent indicator. J. Cell Biol. **94:** 325-334.
22. Hruska, K. A., M. Goligorskij, J. Scoble, D. Moskowitz, S. Westbrook & S. Mills. The effects of parathyroid hormone on cytosolic calcium in renal proximal tubular primary cultures. Manuscript submitted.
23. Wilner, G. D., H. L. Nossel, R. E. Canfield & V. P. Butler Jr. 1976. Immunochemical studies of human fibrinopeptide A using synthetic peptide homologues. Biochemistry **15:** 1209-1213.
24. Wilner, G. D., D. W. Thomas, H. L. Nossel, P. F. Robbins & M. S. Mudd. 1979. Immunochemical analysis of rabbit antihuman fibrinopeptide B antibodies. Biochemistry **18:** 5078-5082.
25. Tam, J. P., W. F. Heath & R. B. Merrifield. 1983. S_N2 deprotection of synthetic peptides with a low concentration of HF in dimethyl sulfide: evidence and application in peptide synthesis. J. Am. Chem. Soc. **105:** 6442-6454.
26. Degen, S. J. F., R. T. A. MacGillivray & E. W. Davie. 1983. Characterization of the complementary deoxyribonucleic acid and gene coding for human prothrombin. Biochemistry **22:** 2087-2097.
27. Furie, B., D. H. Bing, R. J. Feldmann, D. J. Robison, J. P. Burnier & B. C. Furie. 1982. Computer-generated models of blood coagulation factor Xa, factor IXa, and thrombin, based upon structural homology to other serine proteases. J. Biol. Chem. **257:** 3875-3882.
28. Naccache, P. H., T. F. P. Molski, P. Borget & R. I. Sha'afi. 1985. Intracellular calcium redistribution and its relationship to fMet-Leu-Phe, leukotriene B4, and phorbol ester-induced rabbit neutrophil degranulation. J. Cell. Physiol. **122:** 273-280.

29. SHA'AFI, R. I. & P. H. NACCACHE. 1981. Ionic events in neutrophil chemotaxis and secretion. Adv. Inflamm. Res. **2:** 115-148.
30. BAR-SHAVIT, R., D. H. BING, A. J. KAHN & G. D. WILNER. 1985. Thrombin-mediated chemotaxis. Relationship of ligand structure to biological activity. *In* Membrane Receptors and Cellular Regulation. M. P. Czech & C. R. Kahn, Eds.: **23:** 329-338. Alan R. Liss. New York.
31. MARUYAMA, I. & P. W. MAJERUS. 1985. The turnover of thrombin:thrombomodulin complex in cultured human umbilical cells and A549 lung cancer cells: endocytosis and degradation of thrombin. J. Biol. Chem. **260:** 15432-15438.
32. BAKER, J. B., D. A. LOW, R. L. SIMMER & D. D. CUNNINGHAM. 1980. Protease nexin: a cellular component that links thrombin and plasminogen activator and mediates their binding to cells. Cell **21:** 37-45.
33. BJORK, I., C. M. JACKSON, H. JORNVALL, K. K. LAVINE, K. NORDLING & W. J. SALSGIVER. 1982. The active site of antithrombin: release of the same proteolytically cleaved form of the inhibitor from complexes with factor IXa, Xa, and thrombin. J. Biol. Chem. **257:** 2406-2411.
34. TOLLEFSEN, D. M., P. W. MAJERUS & M. K. BLANK. 1982. Heparin cofactor II. J. Biol. Chem. **257:** 2162-2169.

Thrombin Stimulates Neutrophil Adherence by an Endothelial Cell-Dependent Mechanism: Characterization of the Response and Relationship to Platelet-Activating Factor Synthesis[a]

GUY A. ZIMMERMAN, THOMAS M. McINTYRE, AND STEPHEN M. PRESCOTT

Nora Eccles Harrison Cardiovascular Research and Training Institute
Department of Internal Medicine
University of Utah School of Medicine
Salt Lake City, Utah 84112

INTRODUCTION

Thrombin, the terminal protease generated in the coagulation cascade,[1] interacts directly with human endothelial cells (EC), stimulating biochemical events and functional alterations.[2] Thrombin binds rapidly to cultured human EC.[3,4] Approximately 50-60% of the binding sites on umbilical vein EC in primary culture are thrombomodulin, although the number and identity of each of the distinct receptor molecules for thrombin on human endothelium are not yet clear.[5] Thrombin causes the release of arachidonate and its synthesis to prostacyclin (PGI_2) and other prostaglandins in primary and passed umbilical vein and adult systemic macrovascular EC,[6-10] although passed human EC from some other sources are reported to be unresponsive.[11,12] Thrombin also stimulates the release of tissue plasminogen activator from human endothelium,[13] but inhibits the release of a lipoxygenase chemorepellent factor.[14] Under some conditions thrombin stimulates human EC to contract[15,16] and is reported to cause EC injury,[17] whereas under other conditions, it is mitogenic for human endothelium.[18] Thrombin causes a variety of alterations in endothelium from other spe-

[a]This work was supported by awards from the Nora Eccles Treadwell Foundation and the Richard A. and Nora Eccles Harrison Fund for Cardiovascular Research, a Grant-in-Aid (#84 975) from the American Heart Association (AHA) with funds contributed in part by the Utah Heart Association, and a Public Health Service Clinical Investigator Award (#HL00696) from the National Heart, Lung, and Blood Institute. Part of this work was done during the tenure of an Established Investigatorship of the American Heart Association (G. A. Zimmerman).

cies,[2,19–23] although certain responses differ when animal and human EC are compared.[18,24,25]

We have found that thrombin stimulates the adherence of neutrophils (polymorphonuclear leukocytes, PMNs) to human endothelial cells,[26,27] a previously unrecognized biologic activity. In this paper we describe experiments that extend our original observations and discuss the relationships of thrombin-stimulated PMN adherence to another novel response of human endothelium to thrombin: the production of platelet-activating factor.[26,28,29] These observations demonstrate newly identified bioregulatory functions of thrombin and suggest that the endothelial responses may be important mechanisms that link the coagulation cascade and the acute inflammatory response.

METHODS

Materials

Purified human thrombin was generously provided by Dr. George J. Broze, Washington University, St. Louis, Missouri. The stock solution of thrombin, preserved at −70°C, contained 1050 U/ml with a specific activity of 2920 U/mg. It was diluted in Hank's balanced salt solution (HBSS) and used immediately or stored in aliquots at −20°C for use in the experiments to be described. Leukotriene B_4 (LTB_4) and leukotriene C_4 (LTC_4) were the kind gifts of Dr. Joshua Rokach (Merck-Frosst Canada, Inc., Quebec, Canada). Platelet-activating factor (PAF) was from Avanti Polar Lipids, Inc., (Birmingham, AL.). *N*-formylmethionyl-leucyl-phenylalanine (fMLP) was purchased from Sigma Chemical Co., (St. Louis, MO). Human albumin was purchased as a 25% stock solution (Albuminar 25) from Armour Pharmaceuticals (Kankakee, IL). Medium 199, L-glutamine, antibiotic solutions, and HBSS were from MA Bioproducts (Walkersville, MD) or Gibco Laboratories (Chagrin Falls, OH). All reagents were the purest grade available.

Human Endothelial Cell Culture

Human umbilical vein endothelial cells were isolated and cultured as described.[26–29] Only primary cultures were used for these experiments.

Isolation and Indium Labeling of Human Neutrophils

Suspensions of ^{111}Indium-labeled PMNs were prepared as described.[27] Briefly, leukocyte suspensions that contained 95-100% PMNs were prepared by dextran sedimentation, hypotonic lysis, and Hypaque-Ficoll centrifugation. The neutrophils were radiolabeled by incubating them with [^{111}In]oxine or [^{111}In]tropolonate (0.2-0.5 μCi/10^6 PMNs) for 5-15 minutes at 37°C, centrifuged, washed, and resuspended in

HBSS/A (HBSS with 0.5% human albumin) at a concentration of 5.5×10^6 PMNs/ml. Neutrophils isolated and labeled by this method behaved as did unlabeled PMNs in several functional assays and released 6% or less of the incorporated indium when stimulated.[27] When PMN suspensions prepared in this way were treated with 10 μM ionophore A23187 and the extracted lipids analyzed by HPLC,[30] no 12-hydroxyeicosatetraenoic acid (HETE) was detected, whereas the PMNs produced 5-HETE and LTB_4 as expected.[31] Also, neutrophil suspensions did not aggregate[27] or synthesize 12-HETE when treated with thrombin.[32] These results indicate that the suspensions did not contain functionally significant numbers of platelets.

Adherence of Labeled Neutrophils to EC Monolayers

The adherence of ^{111}In-labeled PMNs to endothelial cells was measured as described.[27] In brief, EC monolayers were washed with HBSS and overlayed with neutrophil suspensions. Control buffer, thrombin, or another agonist solution was added to start the reaction, and the incubation was continued for 5 minutes, or various times as indicated (FIGURES 1,8). In a second experimental protocol, washed EC monolayers were incubated with control buffer, thrombin, or another agonist for 5-60 minutes; the solutions were then removed, the monolayers were washed 1-3 times with HBSS, ^{111}In-labeled PMNs were added, and adherence was determined after an additional incubation period, usually 5 minutes (FIGURES 3,6,7). EC monolayers were inspected by phase contrast microscopy in each experiment to document that PMNs adhered to the EC and to correlate the neutrophil adherence by inspection with the values derived by measuring the radioactivity associated with the monolayer. The monolayers remained intact during both protocols.

Quantitation of ^{111}In-labeled neutrophil adherence[27] was done in the same way with both experimental protocols. The nonadherent PMNs were aspirated from the monolayers at the end of the incubation and saved. The monolayers were washed twice with HBSS, and the washings were collected and pooled. The EC and remaining adherent PMNs were dissolved by incubation with 1M NH_4OH for 30-60 minutes. The plates were scraped and washed again with NH_4OH. The amount of radioactivity in the nonadherent PMN suspension, the wash fractions, and the pooled NH_4OH washings and scrapings were individually measured. The fraction of adherent PMNs was calculated as the radioactivity (cpm) associated with the EC monolayer (NH_4OH washings and scrapings) divided by the total radioactivity. Three percent or fewer of the PMNs remained associated with the monolayers when neutrophil suspensions were added to EC and removed as rapidly as possible (FIGURES 7,8), indicating that there was little nonspecific trapping.

In some experiments nonadherent neutrophils were removed after the incubation, NH_4OH was added without washing the monolayers, and the remainder of the quantitation procedure was done as described. This allowed the measurement of the fraction of loosely adherent PMNs[33] and comparison of this value to experiments in which the fraction of tightly adherent PMNs was measured (*i.e.,* neutrophils that remained adherent after two washes of the monolayer).

In experiments examining the time course of thrombin-stimulated PMN adherence to EC, the experiments were varied in three ways: a) EC monolayers were preincubated with thrombin for variable times and washed; labeled PMNs were added for a fixed time (5 minutes). b) EC monolayers were preincubated with thrombin for a fixed time and washed; ^{111}In-labeled PMNs were added and incubated for variable times.

c) Thrombin was added to PMN suspensions over EC monolayers and was continuously present while the two cell types were incubated together. These variations allowed us to examine important aspects of the kinetics of the thrombin-mediated interaction between EC and PMNs, such as the rapidity of the response of each cell type and reversibility.

Adherence of Labeled Neutrophils to Umbilical Vein Smooth Muscle Cells

Primary cultures of umbilical vein smooth muscle cells were grown by a minor modification of the method described by Jaffe *et al.*[34] Adherence of ^{111}In-labeled PMNs was measured as in assays with EC.

Adherence of Neutrophils to Subendothelial Matrices

Subendothelial matrices deposited by primary confluent monolayers of human umbilical vein EC were prepared by a modification of the method described by Vlodavsky *et al.*[35] The culture media was removed from EC monolayers, they were washed once with HBSS, and 0.5% triton X-100 was added to each. After a 30-minute incubation at room temperature on a rocking platform, the triton X solution was removed and the matrices were washed twice with HBSS. Residual cellular debris was removed by treating them with 0.025 M NH_4OH for 2 minutes followed by washing 3 times with HBSS. The matrices were covered with HBSS and kept at 4°C until used.[36] Matrices prepared in this manner supported the growth of human respiratory epithelium[36] (R. B. Turner, personal communication). The quantitation of adherent ^{111}In-labeled PMNs to these surfaces was measured as in experiments with EC monolayers.

Adherence of Labeled Neutrophils to Nonbiologic Surfaces

Thirty-five mm polystyrene petri dishes (Corning Glassworks, Corning, NY) were preincubated with 1.5 ml HBSS/A for 60-120 minutes at 37°C. The HBSS/A was removed, the dishes were washed once with 1.0 ml HBSS, and 0.9 ml of ^{111}In-labeled PMNs was added followed by 0.1 ml of control buffer or agonist solution (thrombin or fMLP). After a 5-minute incubation the nonadherent PMNs were removed, the dishes were washed twice with 1.0 ml volumes of HBSS, and the adherent PMNs were dissolved with 1.0 N NH_4OH and scraped from the dish as previously described. The radioactivity in the nonadherent PMN fraction, the washes, and the adherent PMN fraction was determined, and the total radioactivity was calculated. The fraction of adherent neutrophils was quantitated by dividing the radioactivity recovered in the NH_4OH washings and scrapings by the total radioactivity. In each experiment the plates were examined by phase contrast microscopy before the addition of NH_4OH. The number of adherent PMNs observed by microscopy correlated closely with the calculated values for PMN adherence.

RESULTS

Thrombin Stimulates PMN Adherence to Cultured Human Endothelial Cells

The addition of thrombin to suspensions of Indium-labeled neutrophils overlying endothelial monolayers resulted in enhanced adherence of PMNs to the endothelial cells. In 18 experiments, the adherence after a 5-minute incubation with thrombin (2 U/ml) was 33 ± 14% compared to 8 ± 3% in response to control buffer ($p <$

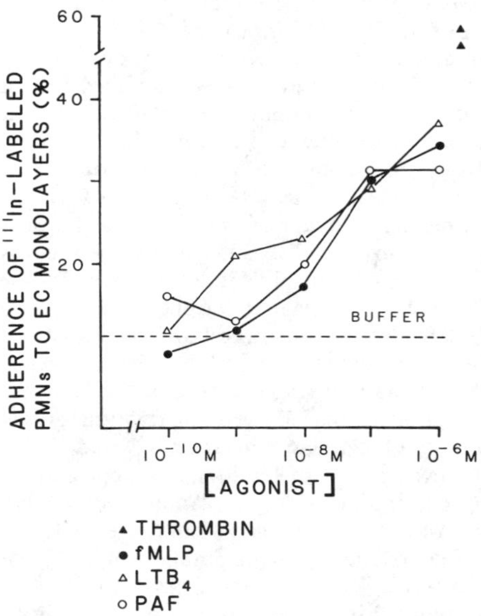

FIGURE 1. Thrombin is a potent agonist for the adherence of neutrophils to endothelial cells. Replicate EC monolayers in 35 mm petri dishes were washed with HBSS, 1 ml aliquots of ^{111}In-labeled PMNs were layered over them, and control buffer, thrombin (2 U/ml;18.5 nM), or other agonist solutions were added in 0.1 ml volumes. The concentrations shown on the horizontal axis were the final concentrations of fMLP, LTB_4 and PAF in the incubation mixture. After a 5-minute incubation at 37° in 5% CO_2, 95% air, the nonadherent PMNs were aspirated from the monolayer, loosely adherent PMNs were removed with two 1.0 ml washes of HBSS, and the binding of tightly adherent neutrophils was measured as described (METHODS and reference 27). The duplicate values for thrombin-stimulated adherence were 56 and 58 percent.

0.01). In only one of the experiments was the neutrophil adherence in response to thrombin less than twice the adherence in dishes treated with control buffer. The response to thrombin was similar in replicate dishes from the same endothelial culture, and was frequently equivalent to, or greater than, the adherence stimulated by agonists that directly stimulate neutrophil adhesiveness such as PAF, fMLP, and LTB_4 (FIGURE 1).

In an experiment to determine if thrombin stimulated both loosely- and tightly-bound PMNs,[33] we measured neutrophil adherence after simply removing the neutrophil suspension following a 5-minute incubation with thrombin, rather than after removing the PMN suspension and washing the monolayers with buffer (METHODS). Under this condition, 61% of the neutrophils were adherent in response to thrombin (2 U/ml) compared to 25% in response to control buffer. In dishes that were washed twice after removing the PMN suspension, the adherence in response to thrombin was 34%, and was 5% in response to buffer. Thus, thrombin enhanced both weak and avid adherence of the leukocytes.

Thrombin also caused stimulated adherence when the number of neutrophils added to the monolayer was reduced (1×10^6 or 5.5×10^5 PMNs/ml, rather than the usual 5.5×10^6 PMNs/ml). In this experiment, the fraction of the neutrophils that adhered in response to thrombin (2 U/ml) increased as the number of neutrophils in suspension was decreased, whereas the fraction of adherent neutrophils remained constant in response to fMLP 10^{-6}M (not shown).

The thrombin-stimulated adherence was clearly demonstrable by phase contrast microscopy and correlated closely with values calculated for the number of Indium-labeled PMNs associated with the monolayers.[27] The adherence of unlabeled as well as radiolabeled neutrophils was enhanced by thrombin (reference 27 and FIGURE 2). Using scanning electron microscopy, we found that adherent neutrophils were intimately associated with the plasma membranes of the EC.[27] As shown in FIGURE 2, the morphology of adherent neutrophils was variable. Approximately 75% of the adherent PMNs in thrombin-treated dishes had a globular, ruffled appearance[27] similar to the morphology of adherent neutrophils in buffer-treated dishes (FIGURE 2A). This appearance is characteristic of unactivated peripheral blood neutrophils.[37] Twenty-five percent of the adherent neutrophils in thrombin-treated dishes, however, had undergone dramatic membrane reorganization with the development of lamillopodia (FIGURE 2B) or both lamillopodia and uropods (FIGURE 2C and 2D). This morphology was not observed in buffer-treated dishes. Polarization of neutrophils is an early morphologic concomitant of cellular activation,[37,38] and is important for effective chemotaxis.[37,39,40] The development of lamillopodia appeared to precede uropod formation, because many neutrophils with only lamillopodia or lamillopodia with small uropods were seen (FIGURE 2B), whereas all leukocytes with well-developed uropods also had large areas of coarse, anterior membrane ruffling (FIGURES 2C and 2D). A similar temporal sequence has been reported from sequential or continuous observations of neutrophils stimulated in suspension[38,40,41] or during adherence to nonbiologic surfaces.[37,39] A few adherent neutrophils had developed extensive membrane spreading in all quadrants (not shown) without the polarization shown in FIGURES 2C-D.

FIGURE 2A-D. Unlabeled neutrophils adhere to thrombin-stimulated EC. Thrombin (2 U/ml) or control buffer (HBSS) was added to suspensions of neutrophils overlying EC monolayers. The neutrophils were not labeled with Indium, but were otherwise similar to those used in experiments with ^{111}In-labeled leukocytes. After a 5-minute incubation, the nonadherent neutrophils were removed and the monolayers were washed twice with buffer. They were inspected and photographed by phase contrast microscopy, which demonstrated that the PMN adherence in thrombin-treated dishes was markedly increased compared to the adherence in buffer-treated dishes. The monolayers were then fixed with Karnovsky's fixative and photographed using a JEOL-JSM35 scanning electron microscope.[27] **A:** PMNs adherent to EC in dishes treated with control buffer. **B,C,** and **D:** Adherent PMNs in thrombin-treated dishes. The neutrophil shown in **C** has a large area of coarse membrane ruffling on its superior, anterior surface that was more easily visible on tangential view (not shown). Tangential views also demonstrated that there were multiple plasma membrane projections from the neutrophil in **D** that were in intimate contact with the surface of the EC (see reference 27).

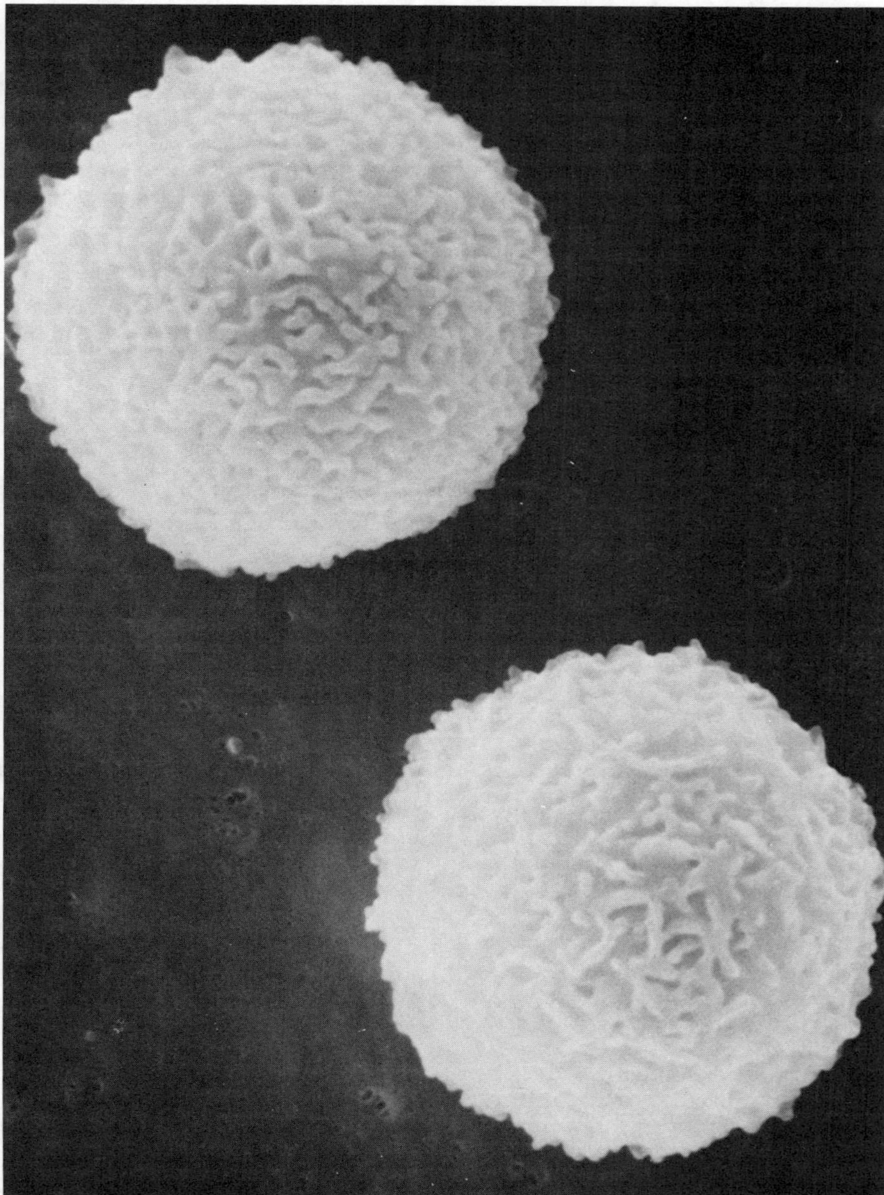

FIGURE 2A. See legend on page 354.

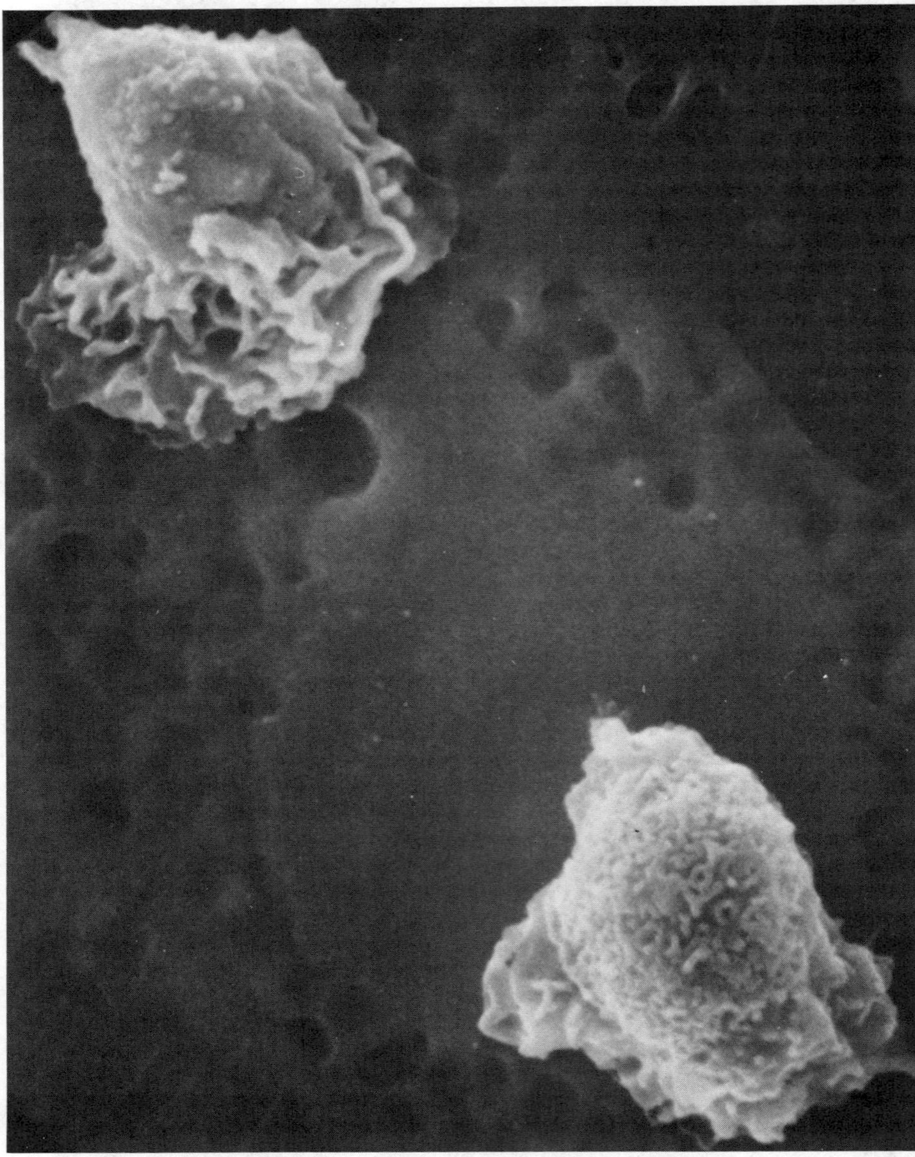

FIGURE 2B. See legend on page 354.

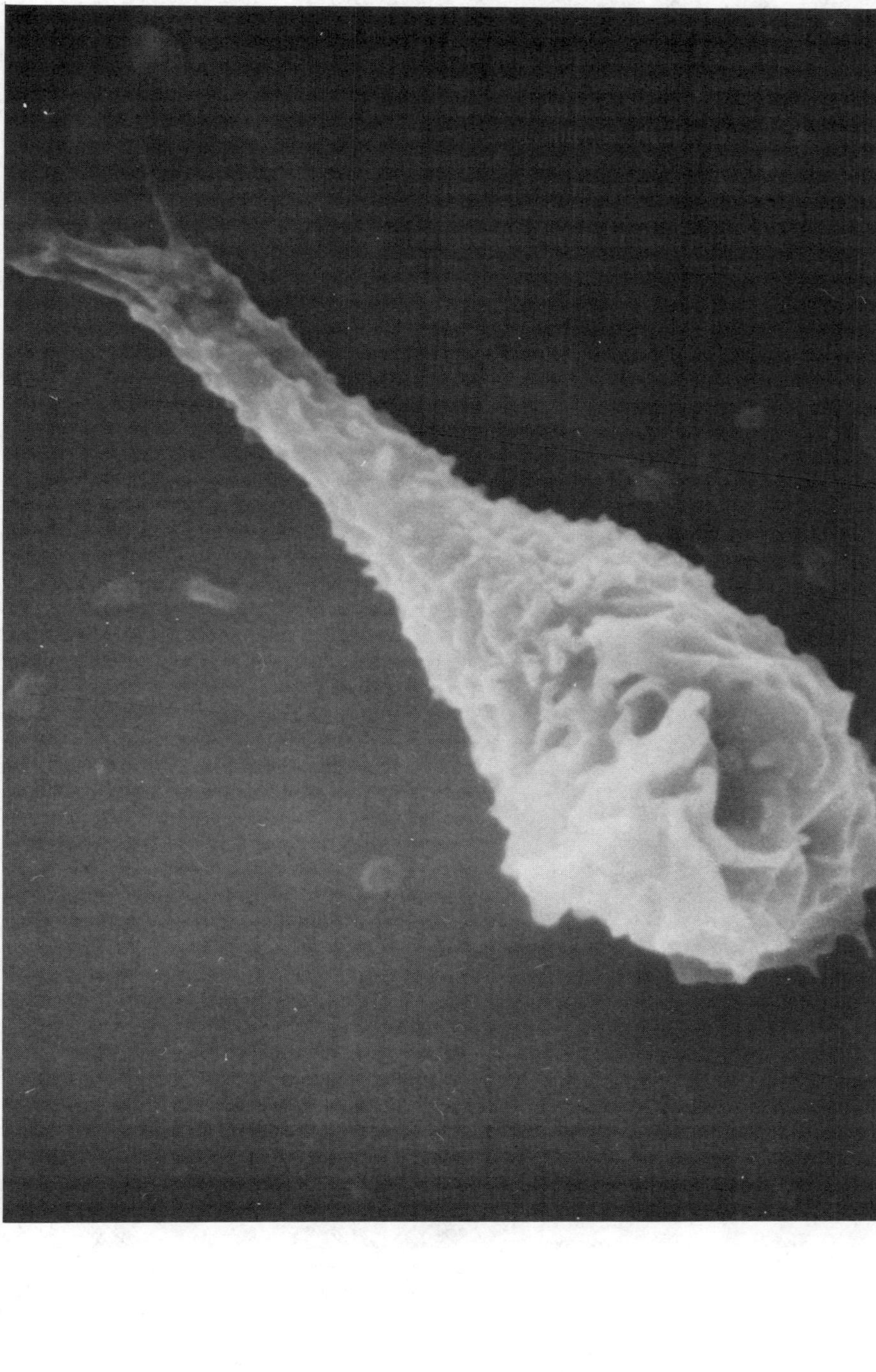

FIGURE 2C. See legend on page 354.

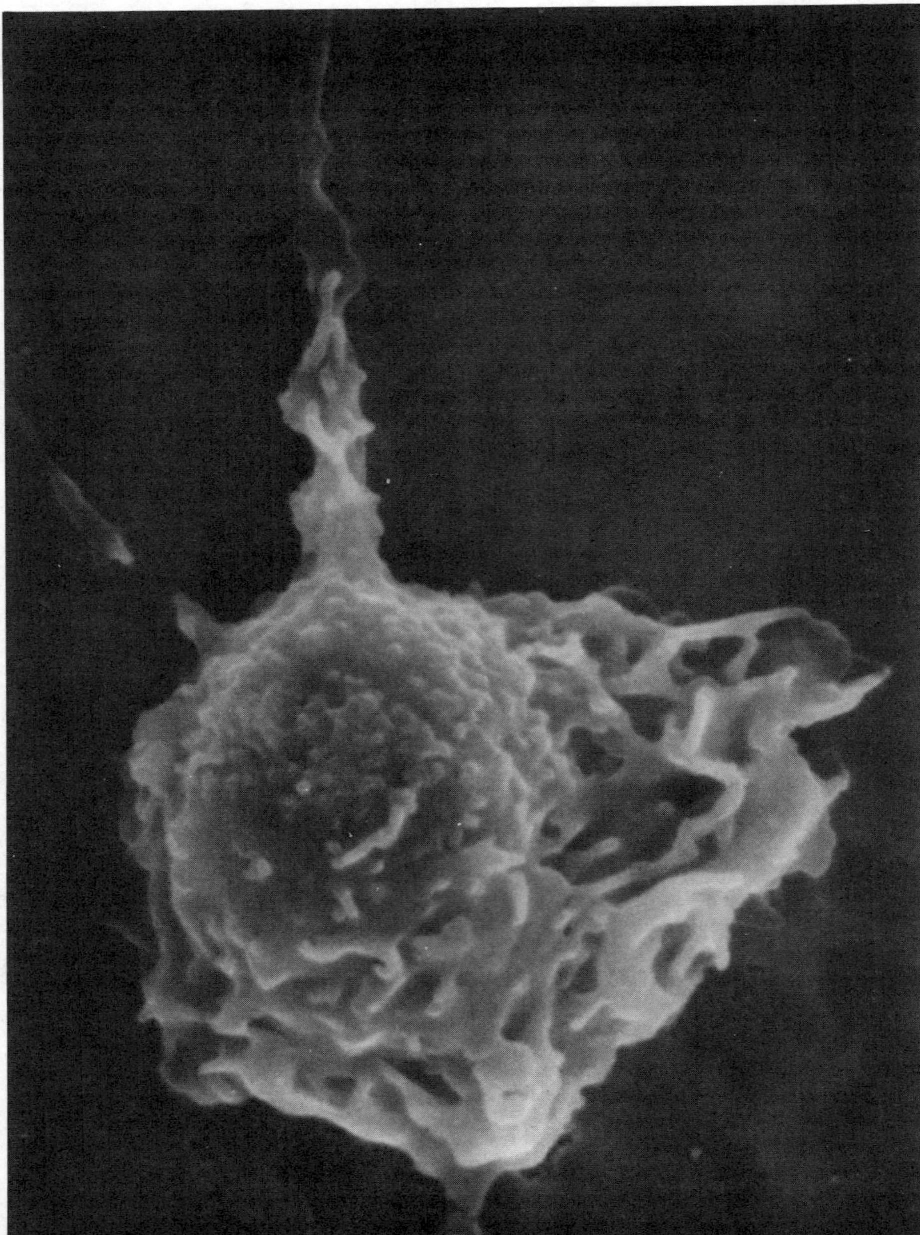

FIGURE 2D. See legend on page 354.

Thrombin-Stimulated Neutrophil Adherence Is Dependent on the Endothelial Cells and Does Not Result from Direct Activation of the Leukocytes by Thrombin

Treatment of the endothelial cells with thrombin, followed by washing the monolayers prior to adding ^{111}In-labeled PMNs, reproducibly resulted in enhanced neutrophil adherence (FIGURE 3) that was comparable in magnitude to stimulated adherence caused by adding thrombin to neutrophil suspensions in the presence of endothelial cells (FIGURE 1). Thrombin also stimulated the adherence of unlabeled neutrophils under conditions similar to those in FIGURE 3, using an assay technique that involved counting the number of PMNs remaining in suspension after incubation with thrombin-treated and control monolayers.[26] In contrast to incubations with EC monolayers,

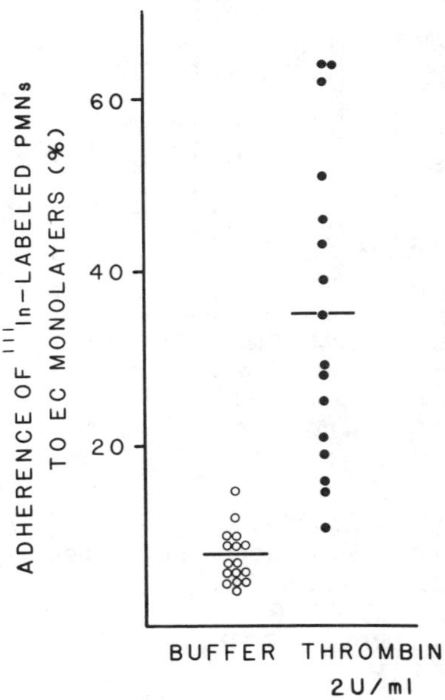

FIGURE 3. Pretreatment of endothelial monolayers with thrombin results in the enhanced adherence of ^{111}In-labeled neutrophils. EC monolayers were washed with HBSS, and a 1 ml aliquot of HBSS/A containing 2 U/ml thrombin or control buffer was added. After a 5-minute incubation at 37° in 5% CO_2 and 95% air, the solutions were aspirated and the monolayers were washed again 1-3 times with 1 ml volumes of HBSS. 1 ml volumes of ^{111}In-labeled PMNs were added, and the incubation was continued for an additional 5 minutes. The PMN suspensions were removed, loosely adherent PMNs were removed with two 1 ml washes of HBSS, and the adherence of the remaining PMNs was quantitated as described (METHODS).

thrombin did not significantly stimulate the adherence of neutrophils to plastic petri dishes that did not contain EC (FIGURE 4A) or to subendothelial matrices (FIGURE 4B). Pretreatment of EC matrices with control buffer or thrombin (2 U/ml) for 5 minutes prior to addition of PMNs to the matrices resulted in adherence similar to that shown in FIGURE 4B. In an additional experiment, primary cultures of umbilical vein smooth muscle cells (SMC) were treated with buffer or thrombin (2 U/ml) for 5 minutes, washed, and incubated with ^{111}In-labeled PMNs for 5 minutes as in FIGURE 3. The neutrophil adherence to buffer-treated SMC was 12% and to thrombin-treated SMC was 13.5 percent. These observations demonstrate that thrombin-stimulated PMN adherence is dependent on the presence of endothelial cells under the conditions of these experiments.

We also found that thrombin did not cause PMNs to produce LTB_4, a major metabolite of arachidonic acid in stimulated neutrophils[31,42] that can enhance leukocyte

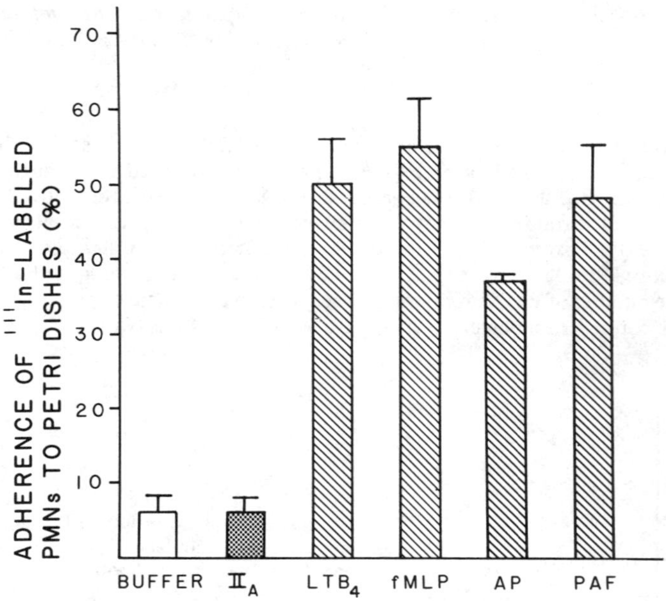

FIGURE 4A. Thrombin does not enhance neutrophil adherence in the absence of endothelial cells. PMN suspensions were treated with control buffer, thrombin, or another agonist in 35 mm plastic petri dishes pretreated with HBSS/A as described in METHODS. The bars indicate the mean results from four experiments using PMNs isolated from different donors. Zymosan-activated plasma (AP), used as a source of C5a desarg, was prepared as described.[27] The concentration of other agonists: thrombin (IIa)-2 U/ml; LTB_4, fMLP, and PAF, 1 μM each.

adhesion.[43,44] Neutrophils were incubated with thrombin (2 U/ml), ionophore A23187 (10 μM), or buffer for 5 minutes, and the oxygenated metabolites of arachidonic acid were extracted and separated by high performance liquid chromatography (HPLC). Thrombin-stimulated PMN suspensions did not produce LTB_4, whereas ionophore-stimulated neutrophils synthesized approximately 160 ng of $LTB_4/10^7$ PMNs (the sensitivity of the assay was as little as 4 ng of LTB_4 per 10^7 PMNs). These data indicate that thrombin did not directly activate the neutrophils or promote adhesion by causing endogenous generation of LTB_4.

Thrombin-Stimulated Neutrophil Adherence to Human Endothelial Cells Is Concentration-Dependent

The enhanced neutrophil adherence was dependent on the concentration of thrombin (FIGURE 5) with a half-maximal effect at 0.2-0.25 U/ml and maximal stimulation at 2 U/ml. The shape of the concentration-response curve was similar when the incubations were done by directly adding thrombin to neutrophil suspensions overlying EC monolayers (*i.e.,* as in FIGURE 1) or when the EC were pretreated with thrombin (*i.e.,* as in FIGURE 3).

The Thrombin-Stimulated Adhesiveness of Endothelial Cells Is a Time-Dependent Response

The enhanced adhesiveness of thrombin-stimulated EC increased rapidly when monolayers were treated with thrombin for various periods, with a peak at 5 minutes and a decline thereafter (FIGURE 6). Pretreatment of the EC for a fixed two-minute period, followed by washing of the monolayers and incubation with neutrophils for various periods, demonstrated that increased binding of the neutrophils could be measured as early as one minute after adding the PMNs. Furthermore, neutrophil adherence was reversible under these conditions (FIGURE 7). A similar result was consistently found when thrombin was continuously present in solution in the incubation (FIGURE 8). Under this condition we found the same general time relationship for thrombin-stimulated PMN adherence as was seen in experiments in which the EC were pretreated with thrombin for various times prior to addition of neutrophils (FIGURE 6).

The gradual decline in neutrophil adherence to thrombin-stimulated EC that occurred after the first 5-10 minutes of incubation (FIGURES 6-8) was not due to injury or impaired responsiveness of the leukocytes resulting from the experimental procedures. This was documented by experiments in which basal, unstimulated adherence,

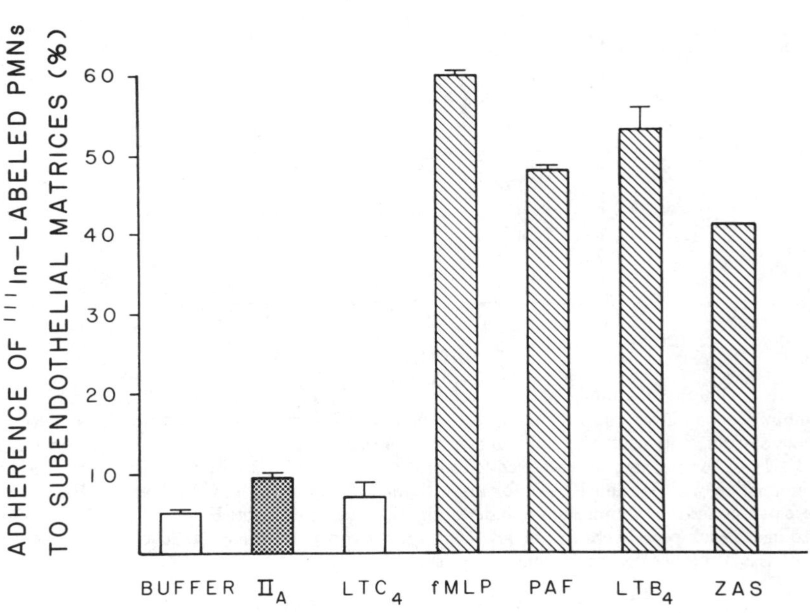

FIGURE 4B. In two experiments, neutrophil suspensions were layered over subendothelial matrices and incubated with buffer, thrombin (2 U/ml), or an agonist for 5 minutes at 37°C, after which neutrophil adherence was determined. The concentration of fMLP, PAF, LTB_4, and LTC_4 was 1 μM in each. Zymosan-activated serum (ZAS) was prepared as in FIGURE 4A, using serum rather than plasma (N = 1). An aliquot of the same thrombin solution used in these experiments caused 64% of the neutrophils to adhere to an EC monolayer, compared to 5% adherence to EC in response to buffer.

and adherence stimulated by the sulfidopeptide leukotriene LTC_4, increased or remained stable during the interval in which thrombin-stimulated neutrophil adherence decreased (FIGURE 8). We have shown that LTC_4 also induces the endothelial cell-dependent adherence of PMNs.[45]

DISCUSSION

In this and earlier reports[26,27] we have shown that thrombin stimulates the adherence of neutrophils to cultured human endothelial cells. The thrombin-stimulated

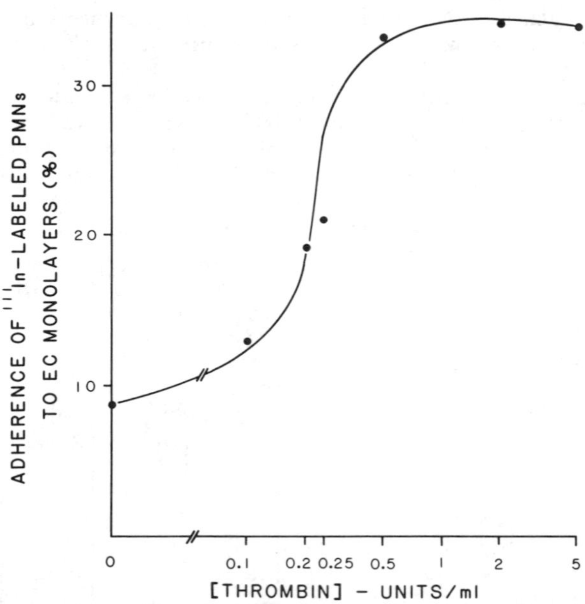

FIGURE 5. Thrombin-stimulated PMN adherence to EC is dependent on the concentration of thrombin. Thrombin or control buffer was added to ^{111}In-labeled PMN suspensions overlying EC monolayers, and neutrophil adherence was measured after a 5-minute incubation (as in FIGURE 1), or the test solutions were added to EC monolayers for 5 minutes followed by washing and incubation with labeled PMNs for an additional 5 minutes (as in FIGURE 3). Each point represents the mean of a minimum of 3 determinations using different EC cultures. The standard deviations at each point were 5% or less at thrombin concentrations of 0.25 U/ml or less, and 16% or less at higher concentrations.

adherence can be demonstrated by assays that measure the recovery of unlabeled PMNs after incubation with thrombin-treated EC,[26] the binding of Indium-labeled neutrophils to the monolayers (reference 27; FIGURES 1,3,5-8), and by direct observation of the adherence of unlabeled and ^{111}In-labeled PMNs to endothelial cells (FIGURE 2; reference 27). Prothrombin, the zymogen precursor of thrombin, factor X_a, fibrinogen, and thrombin that was inactivated with antithrombin III or phenyl-

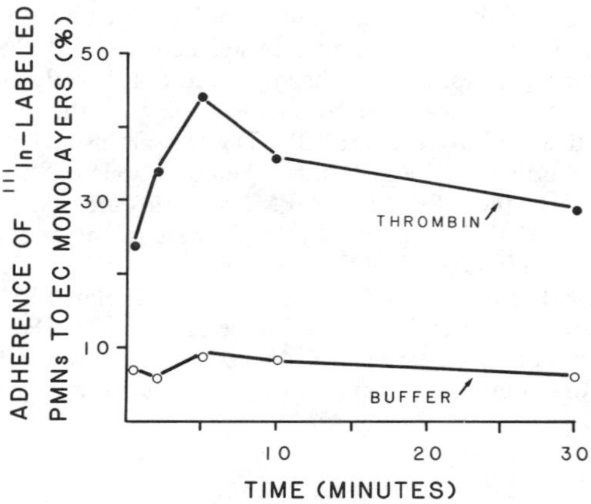

FIGURE 6. Thrombin-stimulated neutrophil adherence is time-dependent. EC monolayers were pretreated with thrombin (1 or 2 U/ml) or buffer for the indicated times, washed, and incubated with ^{111}In-labeled PMNs followed by measurement of the adherent PMNs (METHODS and FIGURE 3). The figure represents the mean results of four experiments. The standard deviation was 16% or less at each point in the thrombin curve and was 4% or less in the buffer curve.

methanesulfonylfluoride did not stimulate adherence, indicating specificity and a requirement for active thrombin. Thrombin stimulated loose binding[33] as well as tight adherence of PMNs (RESULTS) in a time-dependent fashion (FIGURES 6-8). Variations in the experimental procedure demonstrated that enhanced PMN adherence could be detected within 1-3 minutes of the addition of thrombin (FIGURES 7,8). The increased adherence was primarily due to an effect of thrombin on the EC, demonstrated by experiments in which thrombin did not significantly stimulate the adherence

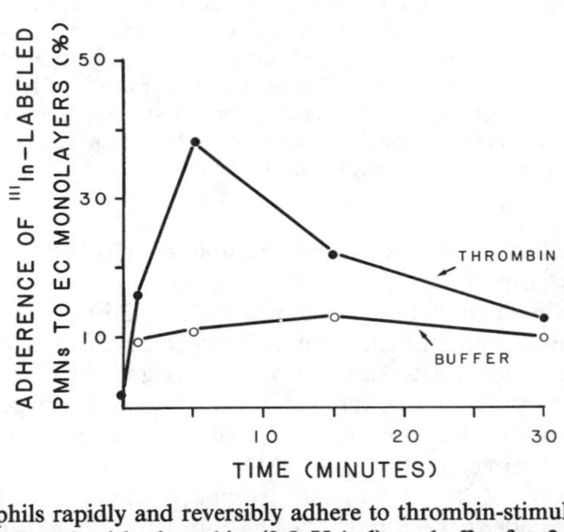

FIGURE 7. Neutrophils rapidly and reversibly adhere to thrombin-stimulated EC. Endothelial monolayers were incubated with thrombin (0.5 U/ml) or buffer for 2 minutes at 37°. The solutions were then removed, the monolayers washed, and ^{111}In-labeled PMNs were added and incubated for the indicated times. The adherence of radiolabeled neutrophils was determined as described (METHODS and FIGURE 3).

of PMNs to plastic petri dishes in the absence of EC (FIGURE 4A), to subendothelial matrices (FIGURE 4B), to human smooth muscle cells (RESULTS), or to nylon fiber columns.[27] In addition, we found that thrombin did not directly activate PMNs when functional activation was measured by aggregation[27] or the synthesis of LTB_4 by thrombin-treated neutrophils (RESULTS).[b] The thrombin-mediated alteration of the EC was not due to injury of the EC under the conditions of these experiments.[29]

The time course of the adherence of PMNs to thrombin-stimulated, washed EC monolayers indicates that the enhanced adhesiveness of the endothelium is transient and that the thrombin-induced PMN adherence is reversible (FIGURES 6-8). In an additional experiment, the adhesiveness of thrombin-stimulated EC returned to control values at 60 minutes.[27] In additional studies we found that HBSS/A removed from thrombin-treated EC did not aggregate PMNs or cause them to adhere to nonbiologic surfaces,[27] suggesting that the enhanced PMN adhesion was due to a proadhesive

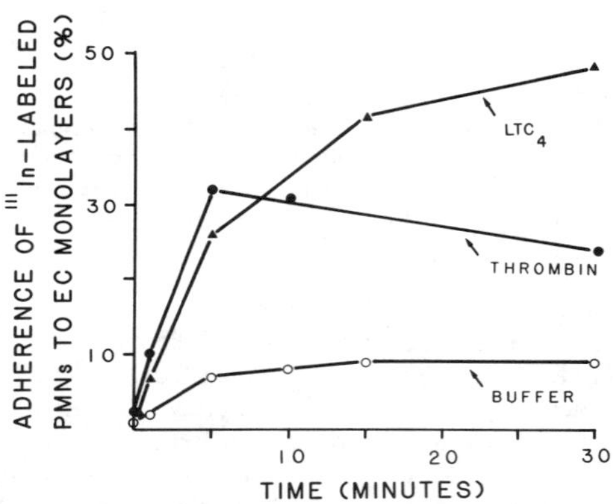

FIGURE 8. The time course of thrombin-stimulated PMN adherence differs from unstimulated adherence and adherence stimulated by leukotriene C_4. Volumes of ^{111}In-labeled PMNs (0.9 ml) were added to washed EC monolayers, 0.1 ml of control buffer or agonist solution was added, and the incubation was continued for the indicated intervals. Neutrophil adherence was determined as in FIGURE 1 and METHODS. The final concentrations of thrombin and LTC_4 were 2 U/ml and 0.1 μM respectively. The mean data from four experiments with each agonist are shown. The standard deviations were 3% or less for each point in the buffer curve, 16% or less in the thrombin curve, and 18% or less in the LTC_4 curve.

factor that remained associated with the endothelial cells rather than being released. Taken together, the experiments indicate that thrombin causes a rapid and gradually reversible increase in the adhesiveness of the endothelial cell surface for neutrophils.

Endothelial cell-dependent neutrophil adherence resulting from the action of fluid phase mediators has been postulated for over 80 years,[46] but has been unequivocally observed only recently. Our experiments with thrombin clearly demonstrate this phenomenon, indicating that EC can provide a transduction mechanism for biochemical signals that do not directly stimulate PMN adhesiveness under some conditions. Bevilacqua *et al.* have observed that interleukin 1 stimulates PMN adherence by an endothelial cell-dependent mechanism.[47] The interleukin 1 effect, however, requires

[b]Thrombin also does not cause human PMNs to synthesize PAF (J. H. Sisson, T. M. McIntyre, S. M. Prescott & G. A. Zimmerman, submitted for publication).

de novo protein synthesis and 2-4 hours to develop, suggesting that the mechanism is different from that of thrombin-stimulated adherence (FIGURES 7 and 8). Although Hoover *et al.* reported that LTB_4-stimulated neutrophil adherence (FIGURE 1) is dependent on endothelial cells,[48] FIGURES 4A and 4B demonstrate that it can directly enhance PMN adhesiveness to surfaces in the absence of endothelium. LTB_4, like C5a fragments and fMLP,[27,33] may have effects on both neutrophils and EC. Tumor necrosis factor enhances the adhesiveness of both cell types.[49]

In addition to stimulating EC-dependent neutrophil adherence, thrombin causes cultured human endothelial cells to produce platelet-activating factor (PAF; 1-O-alkyl-2-acetyl-*sn*-glycero-3-phosphocholine), a phospholipid with a variety of biologic effects.[26,29] PAF synthesis by thrombin-stimulated EC is a time- and concentration-dependent response that requires active thrombin.[26] PAF produced by EC in response to thrombin remains largely cell-associated.[26,28] This feature, and others,[28] differentiate thrombin-stimulated PAF production from thrombin-stimulated PGI_2 production by EC. An unusual characteristic of PAF is the ability to directly activate, and stimulate the adhesiveness of, neutrophils as well as platelets.[29] PAF produced by thrombin-stimulated EC maintains this activity, as measured by its ability to aggregate platelets and neutrophils.[26,29] Thus it is possible that PAF that is produced endogenously by EC participates in the enhanced neutrophil and platelet adherence that occurs in the presence of thrombin (RESULTS and reference 50). Our experiments demonstrate that the concentration-response and time-dependence relationships for thrombin-stimulated PMN adherence and thrombin-stimulated PAF accumulation are tightly coupled (RESULTS and reference 26,27), providing evidence that these two events are related. Exogenous PAF stimulates neutrophil adherence to EC[27,51] with a time course that is consistent with thrombin-stimulated neutrophil adhesion.[27] Furthermore, pretreatment of neutrophils with submaximal concentrations of PAF selectively diminished their subsequent adherence to thrombin-treated EC and adherence stimulated by exogenous PAF, but not adherence stimulated by C5a desarg or fMLP.[27] These experiments are consistent with specific-desensitization of thrombin-stimulated adherence by prior exposure of neutrophils to PAF,[27] and suggest that PAF produced by the EC in response to thrombin and expressed at the cell surface directly participates in the intercellular interaction between neutrophils and the EC. The limitations of this hypothesis, and features suggesting that mechanisms in addition to PAF synthesis are involved in thrombin-stimulated neutrophil adherence, have been reviewed.[27] It is also likely that PAF produced by thrombin-stimulated EC may have important intracellular functions because it remains largely cell-associated.[26,28]

The studies that we have described indicate two novel biologic responses stimulated by thrombin, the endothelial cell-dependent adherence of neutrophils and the production of PAF by the endothelium. In addition to the fact that they may be related at the cellular level, both have potential proinflammatory consequences. The localized, reversible adherence of PMNs to EC (FIGURES 6-8) and the development of polarized morphology (FIGURE 2) are early and requisite steps in the chemotaxis of PMNs to sites of extravascular inflammation, a process required for host defense.[39,40,46] Furthermore, PAF has a variety of proinflammatory effects.[29] Thus, the two EC responses represent new mechanisms by which thrombin generation may be linked to the acute inflammatory process, and suggest that thrombin is a humoral mediator of inflammation in some conditions. Other activities of thrombin that may enhance or modulate the acute inflammatory response include the generation of proinflammatory fibrin degradation products[52] and complement fragments,[53] direct stimulation of mononuclear cell chemotaxis,[54] and stimulation of eicosanoid production by EC.[6–10] It is likely that the recruitment of inflammatory cells to areas of vascular injury is important in the control of thrombus growth and in resolution of thrombi and wound repair.[55] Thus, thrombin-induced neutrophil adherence to EC and PAF production by EC, as well as other mechanisms that link the coagulation and inflammatory system in a controlled fashion, may have homeostatic importance. Neutrophils and other inflammatory cells that are recruited to the endothelial surface, however, may also participate in pathologic thrombosis and inflammatory vascular injury.[27,46,56] For this reason additional knowledge of the regulation of thrombin-stimulated responses of EC[57] may yield insights that are useful in understanding human vascular diseases, as well as biologic events at the cellular level.

SUMMARY

Thrombin, a serine coagulation protease that is generated at sites of tissue injury and inflammation, stimulates the adherence of PMNs and neutrophils to EC. We found that thrombin enhanced the adhesion of neutrophils to primary monolayers of human umbilical vein EC when assayed by the binding of ^{111}Indium-labeled PMNs to the EC, the recovery of unlabeled PMNs after incubation with thrombin-treated EC, and by phase contrast and scanning electron microscopy (SEM). SEM demonstrated that thrombin caused PMNs to intimately adhere to the EC plasma membrane and under some conditions to become polarized. The thrombin-stimulated adherence was a rapid, time-dependent response with an onset within 1 minute of addition of thrombin, a peak at 5-10 minutes, and a decline thereafter. The response was concentration-dependent over the range 0.01-2 U/ml thrombin, and required active thrombin. Prothrombin, factor X_a, and fibrinogen were not effective. Thrombin-stimulated PMN adherence was dependent on the EC, because thrombin did not significantly stimulate neutrophils to adhere to albumin-coated petri dishes, subendothelial matrices, or primary cultures of smooth muscle cells. Human EC, when treated with thrombin, also produce platelet-activating factor (PAF; 1-alkyl-2-acetyl-*sn*-glycero-3-phosphocholine). The concentration-response relationships and time courses for thrombin-stimulated PMN adherence and PAF production were tightly correlated. Furthermore, PAF itself stimulated the adherence of PMNs to EC, and pretreatment of PMNs with PAF selectively inhibited their adherence response to thrombin. These findings demonstrate two novel biologic activities of thrombin, the stimulation of EC-dependent adherence of PMNs and the production of PAF by EC, and suggest that they are functionally related. In addition, they suggest that thrombin may act as a plasma-derived humoral mediator of inflammation under some conditions.

ACKNOWLEDGMENTS

The authors thank Donelle Benson and Tony Seeger for technical assistance, the nurses and staff of the Labor and Delivery Unit, LDS Hospital, for their invaluable collection of umbilical samples, Jeanette Taylor and Dr. Elizabeth Hammond for electron microscopy, Carol Evans for preparation of the figures, and Leona Archuleta for preparation of the manuscript.

REFERENCES

1. JACKSON, C. M. & Y. NEMERSON. 1980. Ann. Rev. Biochem. **49:** 765-811.
2. OWEN, W. G. 1984. Interactions of thrombin, antithrombin III, and protein C with endothelium. *In* Biology of Endothelial Cells. E. A. Jaffe, Ed.: 259-267. Martinus Nijhoff Publishers. Boston, MA.
3. AWBREY, B. J., J. C. HOAK & W. G. OWEN. 1979. J. Biol. Chem. **254:** 4092-4095.
4. LOLLAR, P., J. C. HOAK & W. G. OWEN. 1980. J. Biol. Chem. **255:** 10279-10283.
5. MARUYAMA, I. & P. W. MAJERUS. 1985. J. Biol. Chem. **260:** 15432-15438.
6. WEKSLER, B. B., C. W. LEY & E. A. JAFFE. 1978. J. Clin. Invest. **62:** 923-930.
7. CZERVIONKE, R. L., J. B. SMITH, J. C. HOAK, G. L. FRY & D. L. HAYCRAFT. 1979. Thromb. Res. **14:** 781-786.
8. LOLLAR, P. & W. G. OWEN. 1980. J. Biol. Chem. **255:** 8031-8034.
9. GLASSBERG, M. K., M. M. BERN, S. R. COUGHLIN, C. C. HAUDENSCHILD, L. W. HOYER, H. N. ANTONIADES & B. R. ZETTER. 1982. In Vitro **18:** 859-866.
10. FRY, G., T. PARSONS, J. HOAK, H. SAGE, R. D. GINGRICH, L. ERCOLANI, D. NGHIEM & R. CZERVIONKE. 1984. Arteriosclerosis **4:** 4-13.
11. JOHNSON, A. R., K. S. CALLAHAN, S. C. TSAI & W. B. CAMPBELL. 1981. Bull. Eur. Physiopath. Resp. **17:** 531-551.
12. CHARO, I. F., S. SHAK, M. A. KARASEK, P. M. DAVISON & I. M. GOLDSTEIN. 1984. J. Clin. Invest. **74:** 914-919.
13. LEVIN, E. G., U. MARZEC, J. ANDERSON & L. A. HARKER. 1984. J. Clin. Invest. **74:** 1988-1995.
14. BUCHANAN, M. R., T. A. HAAS, M. LAGARDE & M. GUICHARDANT. 1985. J. Biol. Chem. **260:** 16056-16059.
15. EVENSEN, S. A. 1979. Haemostasis **8:** 203-210.
16. LAPOSATA, M., D. K. DOVNARSKY & H. S. SHIN. 1983. Blood **62:** 549-556.
17. GALDAL, K. S. & S. A. EVENSEN. 1981. Thromb. Res. **21:** 273-284.
18. GOSPODAROWICZ, D., K. D. BROWN, C. R. BIRDWELL & B. R. ZETTER. 1978. J. Cell. Biol. **77:** 774-788.
19. PEARSON, J. D. & J. L. GORDON. 1979. Nature (London) **281:** 384-386.
20. LOSKUTOFF, D. J. 1979. J. Clin. Invest. **64:** 329-332.
21. ISAACS, J., N. SAVION, D. GOSPODAROWICZ & M. A. SHUMAN. 1981. J. Cell. Biol. **90:** 670-674.
22. LOLLAR, P. & W. G. OWEN. 1980. J. Clin. Invest. **66:** 1222-1230.
23. SHIMADA, K. & T. OZAWA. 1985. J. Clin. Invest. **75:** 1308-1316.
24. HONG, S. L. 1980. Thromb. Res. **18:** 787-795.
25. GOLDSMITH, C., C. T. JAFVERT, P. LOLLAR, W. G. OWEN & J. C. HOAK. 1981. Lab. Invest. **45:** 191-197.
26. PRESCOTT, S. M., G. A. ZIMMERMAN & T. M. MCINTYRE. 1984. Proc. Nat. Acad. Sci. USA **81:** 3534-3538.
27. ZIMMERMAN, G. A., T. M. MCINTYRE & S. M. PRESCOTT. 1985. J. Clin. Invest. **76:** 2235-2246.
28. MCINTYRE, T. M., G. A. ZIMMERMAN, K. SATOH & S. M. PRESCOTT. 1985. J. Clin. Invest. **76:** 271-280.
29. ZIMMERMAN, G. A., T. M. MCINTYRE & S. M. PRESCOTT. 1985. Circulation **72:** 718-727.
30. PORTER, N. A., J. LOGAN & V. KONTOYIANNIDOU. 1979. J. Org. Chem. **44:** 3177-3181.
31. PRESCOTT, S. M., G. A. ZIMMERMAN & A. R. SEEGER. 1984. Biochem. Biophysics Res. Commun. **122:** 535-541.
32. ZIMMERMAN, G. A., G. A. WISEMAN & H. R. HILL. 1985. J. Immunol. **134:** 1866-1874.
33. TONNESEN, M. G., L. A. SMEDLY & P. M. HENSON. 1984. J. Clin. Invest. **74:** 1581-1592.
34. JAFFE, E. A., R. L. NACHMAN, C. G. BECKER & C. R. MINICK. 1973. J. Clin. Invest. **52:** 2745-2756.
35. VLODAVSKY, I., G. M. LUI & D. GOSPODAROWICZ. 1980. Cell **19:** 607-616.
36. WIESEL, J. M., H. GAMIEL, I. VLODAVSKY, I. GAY & H. BEN-BASSAT. 1983. Eur. J. Clin. Invest. **13:** 57-63.
37. ZIGMOND, S. H. 1978. J. Cell. Biol. **77:** 269-287.

38. HOFFSTEIN, S. T., R. S. FRIEDMAN & G. WEISSMANN. 1982. J. Cell. Biol. **95:** 234-241.
39. ZIGMOND, S. H., H. I. LEVITSKY & B. J. KREEL. 1981. J. Cell. Biol. **89:** 585-592.
40. SNYDERMAN, R. & E. J. GOETZL. 1981. Science **213:** 830-837.
41. SMITH, C. W., J. C. HOLLERS, R. A. PATRICK & C. HASSETT. J. Clin. Invest. **63:** 221-229.
42. BORGEAT, P. & B. SAMUELSSON. 1979. Proc. Nat. Acad. Sci. USA **76:** 2148-2152.
43. PALMBLAD, J., C. L. MALMSTEN, A. UDÉN, O. RADMARK, L. ENGSTEDT & B. SAMUELSSON. 1981. Blood **58:** 658-661.
44. GIMBRONE, M. A., A. F. BROCK & A. I. SCHAFER. 1984. J. Clin. Invest. **74:** 1552-1555.
45. MCINTYRE, T. M., G. A. ZIMMERMAN & S. M. PRESCOTT. 1986. Proc. Nat. Acad. Sci. USA **83:** 2204-2208.
46. HARLAN, J. M. 1985. Blood **65:** 513-525.
47. BEVILACQUA, M. P., J. S. POBER, M. E. WHEELER, R. S. COTRAN & M. A. GIMBRONE. 1985. J. Clin. Invest. **76:** 2003-2011.
48. HOOVER, R. L., M. J. KARNOVSKY, K. F. AUSTEN, E. J. COREY & R. A. LEWIS. 1984. Proc. Nat. Acad. Sci. USA **81:** 2191-2193.
49. GAMBLE, J. R., J. M. HARLAN, S. J. KLEBANOFF & M. A. VADAS. 1985. Proc. Nat. Acad. Sci. USA **82:** 8667-8671.
50. CZERVIONKE, R. L., J. C. HOAK & G. L. FRY. 1978. J. Clin. Invest. **62:** 847-856.
51. INGRAHAM, L. M., T. D. COATES, J. M. ALLEN, C. P. HIGGINS, R. L. BAEHNER & L. A. BOXER. 1982. Blood **59:** 1259-1266.
52. KAY, A. B., D. S. PEPPER & M. R. EWART. 1973. Nature (London) New Biol. **243:** 56-57.
53. HUGLI, T. E. 1977. Complement factors and inflammation: effects of α-thrombin on components C_3 and C_5. *In* Chemistry and Biology of Thrombin. R. L. Lundblad, J. W. Fenton & K. G. Mann, Eds.: 345-360. Ann Arbor Science Publishers Inc. Ann Arbor, MI.
54. BAR-SHAVIT, R., A. KHAN, J. W. FENTON II & G. D. WILNER. 1983. J. Cell. Biol. **96:** 282-285.
55. DEUEL, T. F. & J. SAN HUANG. 1984. J. Clin. Invest. **74:** 669-676.
56. SCHAUB, R. G., C. A. SIMMONS, M. H. KOETS, P. J. ROMANO & G. J. STEWART. 1984. Lab. Invest. **51:** 218-224.
57. PRESCOTT, S. M., G. A. ZIMMERMAN & T. M. MCINTYRE. 1986. The production of platelet-activating factor by cultured human endothelial cells: Regulation and function. *In* Platelet-Activating Factor. F. L. Snyder, Ed. Plenum Publishing Co. In press.

The Role of Thrombin in Transcellular Metabolism of Eicosanoids[a]

AARON J. MARCUS

Divisions of Hematology-Oncology
Department of Medicine
New York Veterans Administration Medical Center
Cornell University Medical College
New York, New York 10010

INTRODUCTION

Thrombi that form in arterioles morphologically resemble hemostatic platelet plugs and may represent an exaggerated form of a normal process.[1] A thrombotic lesion is initiated by focal vascular damage, which is followed by platelet activation and finally fibrin deposition as catalyzed by thrombin action on fibrinogen. Thus, arterial thrombi consist of platelets that have initially adhered to the subendothelium and then to each other by way of a recruitment process that is a consequence of the platelet release reaction.[2]

Contact and adhesion of platelets to exposed collagen in the subendothelium is a direct stimulus for release of adenosine diphosphate (ADP), formation of the eicosanoid, thromboxane A_2 and 12-hydroxyeicosatetraenoic acid (12-HETE), and release of the biogenic amine, 5-hydroxytryptamine (5-HT). ADP is the final common recruitment pathway for platelet aggregation, because no known platelet agonists will induce a full response if ADP is biochemically removed from an *in vitro* test system. Thromboxane A_2 induces vasoconstriction and is a mild stimulus for platelet aggregation. 5-HT does not aggregate platelets in humans, but does function as a vasoconstrictor. The presence of 5-HT is not mandatory for hemostasis, inasmuch as the bleeding time is normal in its absence. Although thromboxane A_2 only induces about 28% 5-HT release (as compared to 65% for thrombin and collagen), it does contribute to hemostasis for there is a slight prolongation of the bleeding time in its absence, as observed following aspirin ingestion.[1]

As platelet plug or thrombus formation is initiated, the coagulation process is set into motion, eventually leading to thrombin formation at the site of vascular damage. Fibrin strands begin to form, and can be seen interlacing in the interstices of the platelet mass.[2] Fibrin deposition results in consolidation of the platelet plug and renders

[a]Supported by Grants from the Veterans Administration, the National Institutes of Health (HL 18828-10 SCOR), the Edward Gruenstein Fund, and the Sallie Wichman Fund.

it impermeable. At this point, formation of the plug or thrombus is essentially irreversible. Although it had been recognized that neutrophils, mononuclear cells, and erythrocytes are concomitantly present in thrombi and platelet plugs, only recently has it been appreciated that this presence may have functional implications.[3–5]

With regard to the eicosanoid pathway, it can be shown that platelets, neutrophils, endothelial and mononuclear cells can interact biochemically by sharing precursors and intermediates. These cell types are capable of metabolizing molecules in such a way that they can synthesize more of a product that they ordinarily produce when stimulated. In addition, two cells can interact biochemically for synthesis of a product that neither cell can produce alone.[6]

Many of the reactions cited above have been elucidated with the use of thrombin as the agonist.[7] This is due to the specificity of human thrombin, because it will initiate eicosanoid metabolism in platelets and endothelial cells, but not in neutrophils, mononuclear cells, or lymphocytes.[7] Therefore, as will be further discussed, if a platelet is radiolabeled and stimulated with thrombin in the presence of a neutrophil, any radiolabeled product that is synthesized by the neutrophil must have originated from a precursor released by the thrombin-stimulated platelet such as 12-HETE.[6,7]

EICOSANOIDS

Eicosanoids are ubiquitous biological substances that are only produced in stimulated cells and tissues. Their effects in the microenvironment are exerted in nanomolar quantities. Defined biochemically, eicosanoids are oxygenated derivatives of arachidonic acid or other 20-carbon polyunsaturated fatty acids. Arachidonic, and its precursor linoleic acid are classified as essential fatty acids because they cannot be synthesized by humans and must be obtained from the diet.[8] Because they contain a double bond 6 carbons from the methyl group, arachidonic and linoleic acids are also classified as omega-6 fatty acids. Thus, arachidonate contains 20 carbon atoms and 4 double bonds.

Eicosanoids (the term *eicosa* is derived from the Greek word denoting twenty) may be classified as autacoids, inasmuch as their biological activities and metabolism resemble that associated with this group of substances.[9] Autacoids are evanescent biological products, formed locally in a perturbed tissue, and exert their effects in the immediate microenvironment of their site of synthesis. Autacoids differ from hormones, which usually are proteins or polypeptides synthesized and secreted by an endocrine-type gland and subsequently transported in blood to a distal organ or cell, upon which a stimulatory or inhibitory effect is exerted.[6]

BIOSYNTHESIS OF EICOSANOIDS

In contrast to other autacoids such as 5-HT and histamine, eicosanoids are not preformed or stored in cells. Their precursor, arachidonate (or eicosapentaenoate) is almost never found free in the cell. Rather, the arachidonic acid is esterified, mainly in the phospholipid compartment, and is hydrolyzed by an activated phospholipase(s) when the cell is stimulated by way of a receptor mechanism or by chemical or physical perturbation.[10] Upon hydrolysis, the free arachidonate is processed in several ways, all of which eventually result in its removal as a free entity. Thus, it may passively leave the cell intact and become bound by plasma albumin. The arachidonate may also be reesterified by the cell or, in the case of eicosanoid formation, its oxygenation may be catalyzed by two enzymes in the cell (FIGURE 1). One enzyme, known as

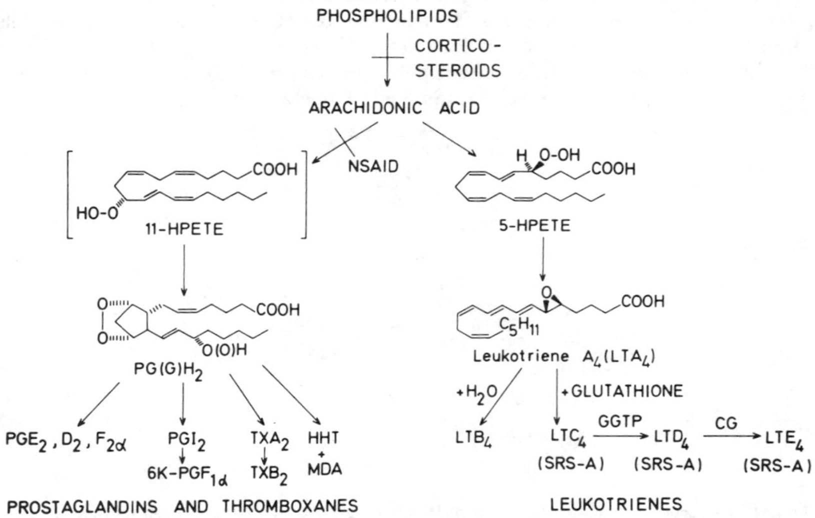

FIGURE 1. Flow sheet depicting biochemical reactions involved in formation of prostaglandins, thromboxanes, hydroxy acids, and leukotrienes from free arachidonic acid. Also shown are the transient intermediate compounds, the endoperoxides ($PG(G)H_2$), and leukotriene A_4 (LTA_4). These intermediates have a short half-life and are processed to end products according to the enzyme(s) present in the tissue under study. The first rate-limiting step in the eicosanoid pathway is hydrolysis of esterified arachidonic acid from cell phospholipids. This step, catalyzed by a phospholipase(s) can be inhibited by corticosteroids. The cyclooxygenation step (blocked by aspirin) shown on the left results in conversion of the endoperoxides into other metabolites and is, as mentioned above, tissue-specific. Formation of PGF_{2alpha} may be nonenzymatic, and PGD_2 may be produced from endoperoxides in the presence of serum albumin. Thromboxane A_2 and prostacyclin are formed enzymatically and measured in the laboratory as their end products thromboxane B_2 and 6-keto-PGF_{1alpha}, respectively. The 5-lipoxygenase pathway, shown on the right is present mainly in cells involved in the inflammatory response and host defense mechanisms. Thrombin does not stimulate leukocytes and therefore is not involved in leukotriene formation. By contrast, thrombin can initiate lipoxygenation of arachidonic acid in platelets, which results in formation of 12-HETE. (Courtesy of Dr. Bengt Samuelsson.)

cyclooxygenase, is particulate and catalyzes transformation of arachidonate to prostaglandins, thromboxane, and prostacyclin. Importantly, the cyclooxygenase is irreversibly inactivated by aspirin by way of an acetylation reaction. The lipoxygenase is cytoplasmic and catalyzes oxygenation of arachidonate to hydroxy fatty acids and leukotrienes. In any given tissue, the nature of the end product formed depends upon converting enzymes indigenous to that tissue.[10]

EFFECTS OF THROMBIN OR IONOPHORE ON PLATELETS AND PLATELET-NEUTROPHIL MIXTURES

If a platelet suspension is radiolabeled with arachidonate and exposed to thrombin (5 units/ml) or ionophore A23187 (1-2 micromolar), free arachidonic acid is released and several eicosanoids are formed. This includes thromboxane, 12-hydroxy-5,8,10-heptadecatrienoic (HHT), malonaldehyde (MDA), and 12-HETE. When a suspension containing 3×10^8 radiolabeled, aspirin-treated platelets and 3×10^7 neutrophils is treated with ionophore (1 micromolar), several metabolites can be detected by thin-layer chromatography (TLC) and high performance liquid chromatography (HPLC). One is 12-HETE, derived from the stimulated platelets, and the others include 5S,12S-

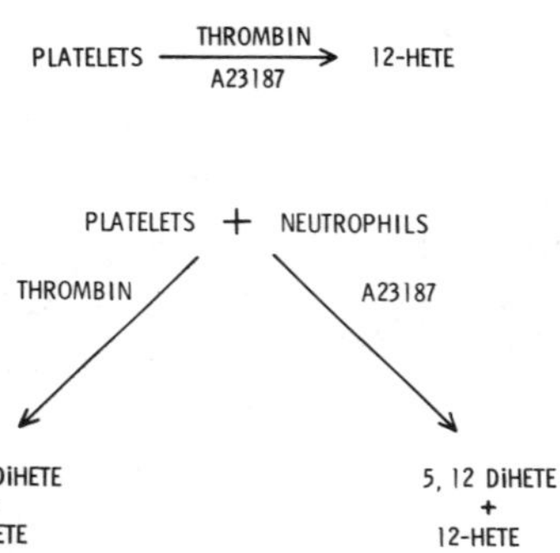

FIGURE 2. Specificity of thrombin stimulation in platelet-neutrophil interactions. The upper panel depicts a reaction sequence that occurs when aspirin-treated platelets are stimulated with either thrombin or ionophore A23187. The major product released from these stimulated platelets is 12-HETE. Also released is free arachidonic acid (not shown). If the platelets were not treated with aspirin thromboxane, HHT and MDA would also form in addition to 12-HETE. In a platelet-neutrophil mixture, product formation is stimulus-specific. Shown on the right is the effect of stimulation of platelets and neutrophils by ionophore A23187. Both components are activated by this agonist, and therefore 5,12-DiHETE and 12-HETE are detectable in the supernatant. Also formed is LTB_4 and 5-HETE. In sharp contrast, stimulation of this platelet-neutrophil mixture by thrombin results in formation of 12,20-DiHETE and 12-HETE. This is because thrombin has no effect on the neutrophil, but the unstimulated neutrophil processes released 12-HETE from the platelet to 12,20-DiHETE by way of an omega-hydroxylation mechanism.[11]

DiHETE that was metabolized by the ionophore-stimulated neutrophil from platelet 12-HETE.[7,12] In addition, released platelet arachidonate served as precursor for stimulated neutrophil-derived leukotriene B_4 and 5-HETE.[12]

The above results are in sharp contrast to those obtained when thrombin was used as antagonist for a platelet-neutrophil mixture.[7] In control studies, thrombin did not initiate eicosanoid metabolism in neutrophils, as evidenced by a lack of production of radiolabeled 5-HETE or leukotriene B_4 (LTB_4), when such neutrophils were exposed to thrombin. Thus, thrombin-stimulation of cell suspensions containing radiolabeled platelets and unlabeled neutrophils resulted in production of a labeled compound subsequently identified as 12,20-dihydroxy-5,8,10,14-eicosatetraenoic acid (12,20-DiHETE).[7] Pretreatment of the platelet-neutrophil donors with aspirin did not inhibit synthesis of 12,20-DiHETE and indicated that this platelet lipoxygenase product, released by thrombin stimulation had been omega-hydroxylated by the unstimulated neutrophil. It was then directly ascertained that 12-HETE was the precursor of 12,20-DiHETE by addition of radiolabeled 12-HETE to unlabeled, unstimulated neutrophil suspensions.[7]

These results (summarized in FIGURE 2) were of interest because they demonstrated the discriminatory nature of thrombin stimulation. When the ionophore was the stimulus, and eicosanoid metabolism was activated in both neutrophils and platelets, 12,20-DiHETE production by the suspensions was markedly decreased. This may have been due to ionophore-induced activation of the neutrophil 5-lipoxygenase, which then diverted 12-HETE released from platelets to 5,12-DiHETE synthesis. In addition, it is possible that the 5,12-DiHETE and LTB_4 produced by ionophore stimulation may compete with 12-HETE for a C-20 hydroxylating enzyme in the neutrophil. Thrombin has no such stimulatory effect on the neutrophil.

It therefore appears that unstimulated neutrophils omega-hydroxylate 12-HETE released from stimulated platelets. The reaction is unusual because most neutrophil eicosanoid activities require strong stimuli such as the ionophore, opsonized bacteria, or formylated peptides.[4]

Implications of cell-cell interactions as induced by stimuli such as thrombin have yet to be fully appreciated. Platelets from patients who have ingested aspirin can still release free arachidonate and 12-HETE upon stimulation. This arachidonate and 12-HETE may interact with other cell types for production of products in the lipoxygenase pathway that have biological activities yet to be described.

REFERENCES

1. MARCUS, A. J. 1985. Hemorrhagic disorders: Abnormalities of platelet and vascular function. *In* Cecil Textbook of Medicine. J. B. Wyngaarden & L. H. Smith Jr., Eds.: **17:** 1028-1040. W. B. Saunders. Philadelphia, PA.
2. HIRSH, J. & E. A. BRAIN, Eds. 1983. Hemostasis & Thrombosis: A Conceptual Approach. 2nd edit. Churchill Livingstone. New York.
3. MARCUS, A. J., L. B. SAFIER, H. L. ULLMAN, M. J. BROEKMAN, N. ISLAM, T. D. OGLESBY, R. R. GORMAN & J. W. WARD. 1985. Circulation **72**(4): 698-701.
4. MARCUS, A. J., L. B. SAFIER, H. L. ULLMAN, M. J. BROEKMAN, N. ISLAM, T. D. OGLESBY, R. R. GORMAN & C. VON SCHACKY. 1986. Platelet-neutrophil interactions in the eicosanoid pathway. *In* Leukocytes and Host Defense. J. J. Oppenheim & D. M. Jacobs, Eds.: **5:** 365-371. Alan R. Liss, Inc. New York.
5. PACKHAM, M. A. & J. F. MUSTARD. 1986. Semin. Hematol. **23**(1): 8-26.
6. MARCUS, A. J. 1987. Transcellular metabolism of arachidonic acid metabolites. *In* Progress in Hemostasis and Thrombosis. B. S. Coller, Ed.: Vol. 8. Grune & Stratton. New York. In press.
7. MARCUS, A. J., L. B. SAFIER, H. L. ULLMAN, M. J. BROEKMAN, N. ISLAM, T. D. OGLESBY & R. R. GORMAN. 1984. Proc. Nat. Acad. Sci. USA **81:** 903-907.
8. MARCUS, A. J. 1978. J. Lipid Res. **19**(7): 793-826.
9. DOUGLAS, W. W. 1985. Autacoids. *In* Goodman and Gilman's: The Pharmacological Basis of Therapeutics. A. G. Gilman, L. S. Goodman, T. W. Rall & F. Murad, Eds.: 7th edit: 604-673. Macmillan Publishing Company. New York.
10. MARCUS, A. J. 1984. J. Lipid Res. **25:** 1511-1516.
11. A. J. MARCUS *et al.* 1987. J. Clin. Invest. **79.**
12. MARCUS, A. J., M. J. BROEKMAN, L. B. SAFIER, H. L. ULLMAN & N. ISLAM. 1982. Biochem. Biophysics Res. Comm. **109**(1): 130-137.

Thrombin Interactions with Platelet Membrane Proteins[a]

M. C. BERNDT,[b] C. GREGORY, G. DOWDEN, AND P. A. CASTALDI

Department of Medicine
University of Sydney
Westmead Hospital
Westmead, N.S.W. 2145, Australia

INTRODUCTION

Thrombin is among the most potent of the physiological stimuli for platelets. In response to thrombin, platelets change shape from discoid to spherical, secrete the contents of their storage organelles, and providing extracellular calcium ions are present, aggregate. Despite intensive efforts during the past 10-20 years, the mechanism by which α-thrombin stimulates platelets is an essentially unresolved problem in hemostasis. One difficulty in understanding the mechanism of thrombin interaction with platelets is that the reaction contains elements consistent with both a catalytic event (receptor processing) and a more classical receptor-agonist equilibrium.[1] In addition, there is evidence to suggest that there may be more than one type of thrombin receptor on platelets. The potent thrombin inhibitor, hirudin, rapidly dissociates bound thrombin from platelets.[2] If hirudin is added during the lag period between thrombin addition and the onset of dense body secretion, no secretion occurs.[3] If hirudin is added after this lag, the subsequent platelet secretion and aggregation responses are unaffected.[3,4] By contrast, hirudin added at this point blocks lysosomal secretion and the mobilization of arachidonic acid, indicating a difference in the requirement for receptor occupancy with these reactions. A similar conclusion can be derived from the analysis of the interaction between the dysthrombin, thrombin quick I, and platelets.[5]

There is considerable evidence that the activation of platelets by thrombin involves the interaction of platelets with the thrombin active site. First, the catalytic active site of α-thrombin is essential for the physiological platelet response inasmuch as active-site-blocked α-thrombin does not stimulate platelets.[6-8] Second, proteases whose cleavage specificity overlaps that of α-thrombin, trypsin,[6,9] papain,[9] thrombocytin,[10] and α-clostripain,[11] activate platelets, but only when catalytically active, whereas proteases with dissimilar specificity such as plasmin and α-chymotrypsin do not.[9] Third, a competitive inhibitor of α-thrombin, *p*-(*p*-nitrophenoxypropoxy)-benzamidine benzenesulfonate inhibits platelet stimulation with a K_i essentially identical to that

[a]This work was supported by Grants 6K14277 and 6K14443 from the National Health and Medical Research Council of Australia.

[b]Michael C. Berndt is the recipient of a Wellcome Australian Senior Research Fellowship.

obtained with synthetic substrates.[9] Further, the rate of stimulation of platelets has the same pH dependence as the rate of hydrolysis of synthetic substrates.[9] Finally, Shuman and coworkers have demonstrated that washed platelets after pretreatment with prostacyclin and thrombin (0.1-2 nM) become refractory to a subsequent addition of thrombin (2 nM) but respond normally with other stimuli.[12] Active-site-blocked thrombin did not induce refractoriness. Treatment of platelets with higher concentrations of thrombin (>2 nM) overcame the refractoriness. The degree of refractoriness was proportional to the concentration of thrombin in the initial incubation but was independent of the time of preincubation with thrombin. By contrast, McGowan and Detwiler found that the degree of refractoriness was time-dependent and interpreted their results as favoring the catalytic modification of a receptor.[13]

Other studies indicate that the interaction of α-thrombin with platelets has characteristics similar to that of an agonist-receptor equilibrium reaction. For example, Detwiler and Feinman showed that the extent of dense body secretion was a function of thrombin concentration.[3,14] In another example, Martin *et al.* found that unstimulated platelets remain in the presence of catalytically active thrombin.[15] It can be argued that neither of these reactions is consistent with a normal enzymatic reaction; that is, catalysis predicts that a reaction would proceed to completion. Binding studies with α-thrombin indicate that there are $\simeq$500 high affinity binding sites with a K_d of $\simeq$1 nM and $\simeq$5,000-50,000 low-affinity binding sites with a K_d of $\simeq$100 nM.[7,8,15–17] The measured binding sites appear to be specific for α-thrombin; platelets do not bind prothrombin or the prothrombin activation intermediates.[18] The binding of α-thrombin to the high-affinity binding site is closely correlated with the extent of the platelet response as determined by dense body secretion. The concentration of α-thrombin that causes half-maximal saturation of the high-affinity binding sites is essentially identical to what causes half-maximal dense body release.[15] Perturbation of the binding of α-thrombin by anions,[19] or in the rate of binding of α-thrombin,[15] is directly reflected in the functional response of the platelets.

In apparent contradiction with these results, other evidence would appear to be inconsistent with the measured binding sites playing a role in the functional response of platelets. Despite the requirement of a free thrombin active site for platelet response, binding studies using active-site-blocked α-thrombin yield the same number of high- and low-affinity binding sites and, within experimental error, identical dissociation constants.[7,8] In addition, blocked thrombin directly competes for the same binding sites as native thrombin.[7,20] This competition for binding, however, is not reflected in the functional response of platelets because platelets equilibrated even with a thousandfold excess of blocked thrombin show an identical or slightly enhanced time course and extent of platelet activation.[7,9]

Tam, Fenton, and Detwiler have investigated thrombin-platelet interaction by analysis of the effect of brief chymotrypsin treatment of the platelet membrane surface.[21] Brief treatment of platelets with a low concentration of chymotrypsin (1 μM) did not alter thrombin binding to the platelets nor the extent of release of aggregation. In contrast to normal platelets, however, release and aggregation occurred only after a prolonged lag. Addition of hirudin during the prolonged lag period completely inhibited the subsequent platelet response. The prolonged lag period was specific for the interaction of the chymotrypsin-modified platelets with α-thrombin. The prolonged lag was qualitatively similar to that seen with normal platelets when stimulated by γ-thrombin or trypsin. The combined results indicate that binding of thrombin and signal generation are separate processes and that a component very sensitive to chymotrypsin is involved in the signal generation step. Thus "while the high affinity binding [site] is not essential for reaction with the signal-generating site, it greatly facilitates the reaction, leading to the much greater specificity of α-thrombin compared to γ-thrombin (or trypsin). Chymotrypsin appears to disconnect these two aspects of the receptor, abolishing the advantage of α-thrombin."[21] In this paper, recent evidence is discussed that suggests that the high-affinity binding site is probably located on glycoprotein Ib and that binding of α-thrombin to this site modulates the rate of stimulation of platelets by α-thrombin. The sole apparent thrombin substrate on the platelet membrane surface, glycoprotein V, although fulfilling some of the requirements expected of the functional thrombin receptor, probably does not represent the signal generation site on platelets.

THE GLYCOPROTEIN Ib COMPLEX

The glycoprotein Ib complex is an intrinsic membrane protein that has been identified as the platelet receptor mediating the factor VIII/von Willebrand factor-dependent adhesion of platelets to exposed vascular subendothelium (for a review, see reference 22). Recent evidence suggests that this complex also plays an important but not critical role in the response of platelets to α-thrombin. The glycoprotein Ib complex is a heterodimer complex and contains both glycoprotein Ib (M_r = 170,000) and glycoprotein IX (M_r = 22,000) (FIGURE 1).[23] There are 20,000-25,000 copies of the complex per platelet. Glycoprotein Ib consists of two disulfide-linked subunits, glycoprotein Ib_α (M_r = 135,000) and glycoprotein Ib_β (M_r = 25,000). The human platelet calcium-dependent protease cleaves the α-chain on the plasma side of this disulfide to yield the water-soluble derivative, glycocalicin, and a 30,000 molecular weight fragment that remains membrane-bound and disulfide-linked to the β-subunit.[24] Tryptic digestion of glycocalicin yields a macroglycopeptide of molecular weight 118,000, which contains the bulk of the carbohydrate (O-linked oligosaccharide), and a poorly glycosylated peptide of molecular weight 45,000.[25] Purified glycocalicin is a competitive inhibitor of α-thrombin binding to platelets (K_i = 30 nM), the inhibitory activity residing with the 45,000 molecular weight tryptic peptide.[26] Treatment of platelets with human leukocyte elastase releases a 35,000 molecular weight poorly

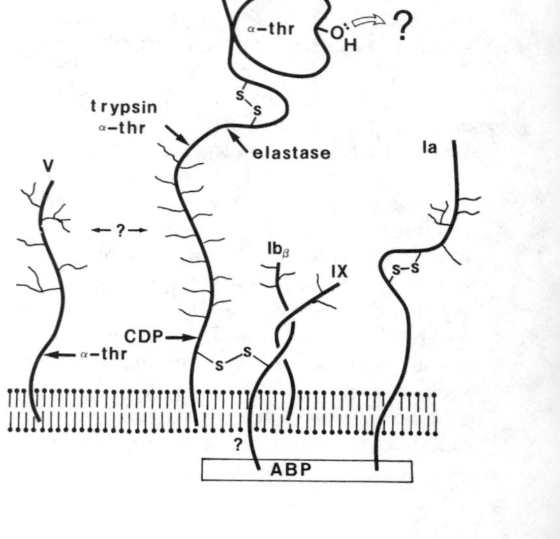

FIGURE 1. Structure of the human platelet membrane glycoprotein Ib complex, glycoprotein Ia, and glycoprotein V.

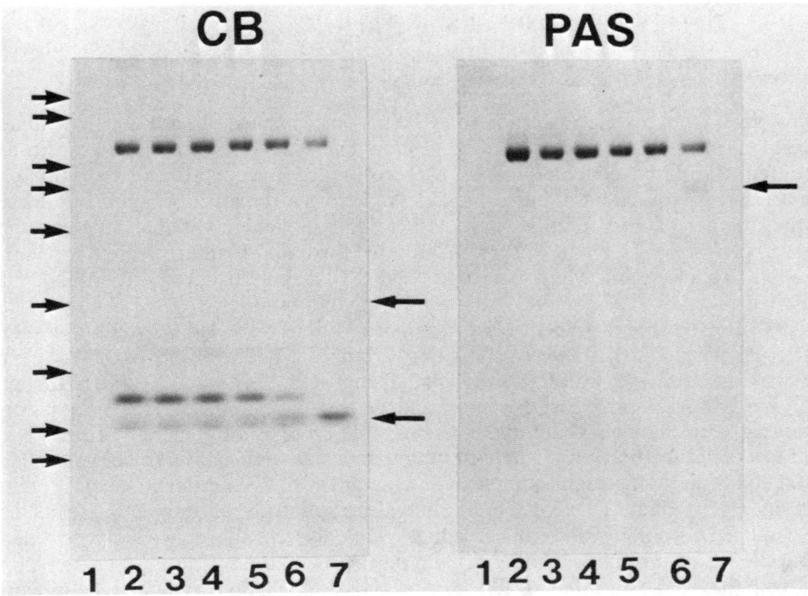

FIGURE 2. Time course for the hydrolysis of the human platelet glycoprotein Ib complex (200 μg/ml) by α-thrombin (10 U/ml). The proteolysis experiment was performed at 25°C. At the indicated times, samples were removed, quenched with 2% sodium dodecyl sulfate (SDS), and analyzed by electrophoresis on 5-20% exponential gradient SDS-polyacrylamide gels under reducing conditions. The gel was stained either for protein with Coomassie brilliant blue (CB) or for carbohydrate using Schiff's reagent (PAS). Hydrolytic fragments are indicated by the arrows on the right hand sides of the gels. Lane 1: thrombin alone; lanes 2-7: proteolysis products at time 0, 10 min, 30 min, 1 hr, 4 hr, and 24 hr, respectively. Molecular weight markers indicated by the arrows in the left-hand margin of the figure in decreasing order of molecular weight: myosin (200,000), α-2 macroglobulin (170,000), α-galactosidase (130,000), phosphorylase b (94,000), bovine serum albumin (68,000), ovalbumin (43,000), carbonic anhydrase (29,000), soybean trypsin inhibitor (21,000), and lysozyme (14,000).

glycosylated peptide from the α-chain of glycoprotein Ib, leaving a 102,000 highly glycosylated α-chain remnant that remains membrane-associated.[27] This places the tryptic peptide and hence the thrombin-binding domain at the plasma end of the α-chain of glycoprotein Ib. At least one subunit of the glycoprotein Ib complex spans the platelet membrane and is bound to actin-binding protein in the platelet endoskeleton.[28,29] Although glycocalicin has been reported not to be a substrate for α-thrombin,[26] studies in our laboratory indicate that the purified glycoprotein Ib complex is slowly hydrolyzed by α-thrombin (FIGURE 2). There is a cleavage site in the α-chain that yields an ≃95,000 molecular weight highly glycosylated fragment and an ≃43,000 molecular weight poorly glycosylated peptide. There is also a cleavage point in the β-subunit that decreases the apparent size of this subunit by ≃2,500 molecular weight. Glycoprotein IX is thrombin-resistant. These hydrolytic products in the α- and β-subunits of glycoprotein Ib appear to be identical to those generated with trypsin. On a mole basis, however, thrombin is approximately 250-fold less efficient than trypsin in generating these fragments.

There is considerable evidence that the thrombin binding site on glycoprotein Ib probably represents the high-affinity binding site on human platelets. Bernard-Soulier syndrome platelets, which apparently genetically lack the components of the glycoprotein Ib complex and glycoprotein V,[30,31] display markedly defective binding of α-thrombin.[32,33] Treatment of human platelets with calcium-dependent protease appears to be selective for the proteolysis of glycoprotein Ib and the removal of glycoprotein V from platelets (Berndt and Phillips, unpublished observations).[34] Calcium-dependent protease-treated platelets also show markedly decreased levels of thrombin binding.[34] Similarly, concomitant with hydrolysis of glycoprotein Ib by human leukocyte elastase treatment of human platelets, there is a statistically significant decrease in the number of high-affinity binding sites for α-thrombin.[27] Other studies suggest that glycoprotein Ib is the major membrane thrombin-binding protein on human platelets. Tollefsen and Majerus cross-linked ^{125}I-labeled diisopropylfluorophosphate-inhibited thrombin to intact platelets using 1 mM glutaraldehyde.[35] SDS-polyacrylamide gel electrophoresis under nonreducing conditions revealed a single complex of molecular weight 200,000 over a range of thrombin concentrations (0.02-1.5 U/ml), a result consistent with the cross-linking of glycoprotein Ib (M_r = 170,000) to thrombin (M_r = 36,000). More recently, Jung and Moroi have analyzed the interaction of thrombin with platelets using disulfide-cleavable cross-linking agents.[36] Cross-linking with low concentrations of ^{125}I-labeled inhibited or native thrombin (6 nM) also yielded a 200,000 molecular weight complex. This complex had a similar isoelectric point to that of glycoprotein Ib. Crossed immunoelectrophoresis of human platelets using immobilized thrombin in the intermediate gel is also consistent with glycoprotein Ib being the major thrombin-binding protein on the membrane surface.[37] Similarly, probing with blocked thrombin of Western blots of SDS-polyacrylamide gel-separated human platelet proteins detects only glycoprotein Ib.[38] In addition, Moroi and coworkers have used affinity chromatography on thrombin-sepharose for the purification of glycocalicin.[39] Glycocalicin bound equally well to sepharose columns coupled either with native or blocked thrombin and could be specifically eluted with heparin. The combined evidence therefore indicates that binding of α-thrombin to glycoprotein Ib does not involve the active site but involves the macromolecular binding domain on α-thrombin. Binding of α-thrombin to glycoprotein Ib is therefore similar to the known binding characteristics of α-thrombin towards the high-affinity binding sites on platelets, because this binding is also not dependent on the integrity of the α-thrombin active site. Workman and coworkers have shown that modification of a single tryptophan in the macromolecular binding site of α-thrombin coincides with the loss of binding to the high-affinity binding sites and with a shift in the dose-response curves for dense body secretion to higher thrombin concentrations.[8] Modification of lysine residues in the heparin binding domain of α-thrombin yields similar findings.[40] In addition, nitro-α-thrombin and γ-thrombin have essentially no fibrinogen-clotting activity and are much weaker platelet stimuli as compared to α-thrombin. Consistent with the importance of the macromolecular binding site of thrombin in the binding of thrombin to the high-affinity binding sites of platelets, α-thrombin has no effect on the binding of either nitro-α-thrombin or γ-thrombin to platelets.[20]

There are three principal lines of evidence that the thrombin binding site on glycoprotein Ib serves the modulator function in thrombin activation of platelets suggested by the chymotrypsin experiments of Tam, Fenton, and Detwiler.[21]

Antiglycoprotein Ib Antibodies as Inhibitors of Thrombin-Platelet Interaction

In 1983, Jenkins *et al.* reported that the response of washed platelets to 0.05 U/ml of α-thrombin was blocked by Fab fragments of rabbit antiglycoprotein Ia/Ib and antiglycocalicin antibodies.[41] Similarly, McGregor *et al.* observed that P_1, a monoclonal antibody against glycoprotein Ib, was a potent inhibitor of platelet aggregation induced by low levels of α-thrombin, but was without effect on collagen-induced platelet aggregation.[42] We have observed similar effects in our laboratory using the Fab fragments of an affinity-purified rabbit antiglycoprotein Ib_α antibody (FIGURE 3). Inhibition of thrombin-induced platelet aggregation was marked at low (0.1 U/ml) but not high concentrations of α-thrombin (>0.5 U/ml). The major effect of the Fab fragments was a marked prolongation of the lag period between thrombin addition and the onset of platelet aggregation.

Effect of Selective Proteolytic Modification of Glycoprotein Ib on Thrombin-Platelet Aggregation

In 1983, Yoshida, Weksler, and Nachman found that proteolytic removal of glycocalicin, which contains the glycoprotein Ib/thrombin binding site, by purified human

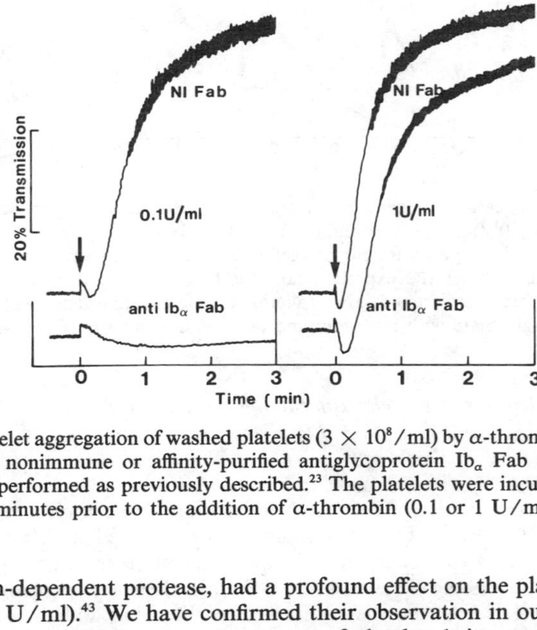

FIGURE 3. Platelet aggregation of washed platelets (3×10^8/ml) by α-thrombin in the presence of 20 μg/ml of nonimmune or affinity-purified antiglycoprotein Ib_α Fab fragments. Platelet aggregation was performed as previously described.[23] The platelets were incubated with the Fab fragments for 3 minutes prior to the addition of α-thrombin (0.1 or 1 U/ml).

platelet calcium-dependent protease, had a profound effect on the platelet response to thrombin (0.12 U/ml).[43] We have confirmed their observation in our laboratory, the effect of calcium-dependent protease treatment of platelets being more pronounced at low concentrations of α-thrombin (FIGURE 4). McGowan, Yeo, and Detwiler have examined the effects of calcium-dependent protease treatment of platelets on platelet-thrombin response in much greater detail.[34] Although treatment of platelets with calcium-dependent protease produced a prolonged lag in the rate of response of platelets to α-thrombin, protease treatment had no effect on the extent of the thrombin response as measured by dense body secretion. Protease treatment was without effect on the response of platelets to γ-thrombin. Somewhat surprisingly, they observed prolongation of the lag in response to α-thrombin at low concentrations of protease with no apparent membrane protein hydrolysis. Although the cause of this phenomenon is unclear, one possible explanation is that this effect is due to the presence of β-mercaptoethanol during the protease treatment. There appears to be at least one intramolecular disulfide in the tryptic peptide that contains the α-thrombin binding domain.[22,44] *Serratia marcescens* metalloprotease appears to be more specific than the calcium-dependent protease and apparently hydrolyzes only glycoprotein Ib on intact platelets.[45,46] Metalloprotease-treated platelets also show the pronounced lag before α-thrombin-induced dense body secretion and aggregation.[45,46] Again, protease treatment had little effect on the extent of dense body secretion in response to α-thrombin.[45] Treatment of platelets with human leukocyte elastase also abolishes the aggregation response to low concentrations of α-thrombin (0.1 U/ml).[27] In contrast to the above studies, however, elastase treatment shifts the thrombin dose-response curve for dense body secretion to high thrombin concentrations, suggesting that elastase may also modify the thrombin receptor responsible for signal generation.

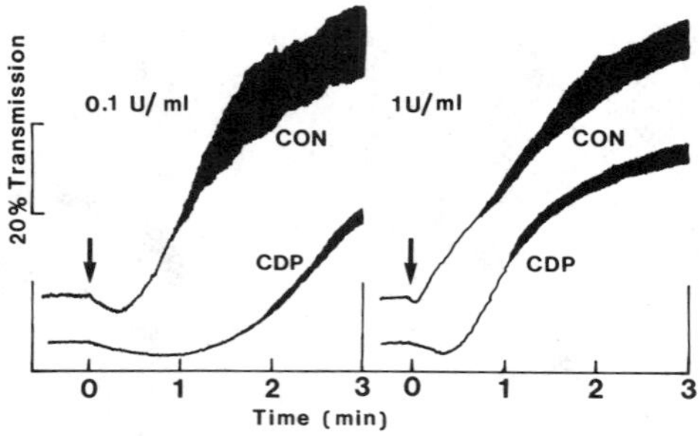

FIGURE 4. Effect of calcium-dependent protease treatment on the aggregation response of washed platelets (3×10^8/ml) to α-thrombin (0.1 or 1 U/ml). Platelet aggregation was performed as previously described.[23] The treatment of platelets with calcium-dependent protease was as previously described.[24] Under the experimental conditions, >90% of the platelet membrane glycoprotein Ib had been converted to glycocalicin, and the calcium-dependent protease-treated platelets failed to agglutinate with ristocetin and purified human von Willebrand factor.

Analysis of Thrombin-Platelet Interaction with Bernard-Soulier Syndrome Platelets

The aggregation responses of Bernard-Soulier syndrome platelets toward α-thrombin are shown in FIGURE 5. This experiment was performed with a Bernard-Soulier syndrome patient (L.S.) who completely lacks detectable levels of the glycoprotein Ib complex.[31] At low levels of α-thrombin (0.1 U/ml), there is a prolonged lag relative to the control platelets between the addition of α-thrombin and the onset of platelet aggregation. This effect is much less marked at higher concentrations of α-thrombin (1 U/ml). The aggregation responses are similar to those reported by Jamieson and Okumura in two other patients with the Bernard-Soulier syndrome.[33] Despite the marked differences in the rate of the thrombin response between the control and Bernard-Soulier syndrome platelets, the control and Bernard-Soulier syndrome platelets had an essentially identical thrombin dose-response curve for dense body secretion (FIGURE 6), suggesting that the Bernard-Soulier syndrome platelets, although lacking glycoprotein Ib, have normal levels of the thrombin receptor responsible for signal generation.

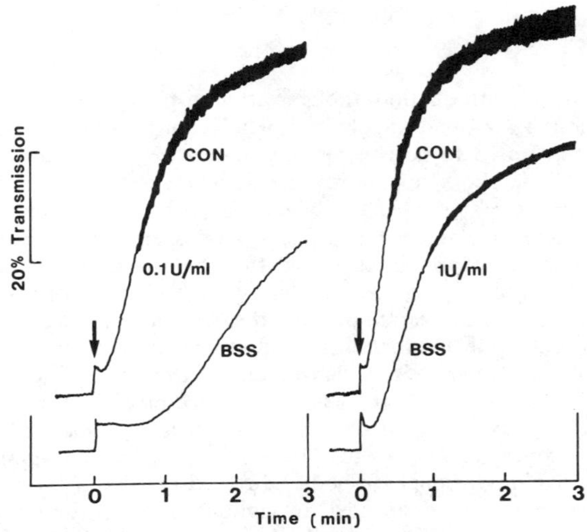

FIGURE 5. Platelet aggregation of washed normal and Bernard-Soulier syndrome platelets (3×10^8/ml and 1.5×10^8/ml, respectively; equivalent optical density) by α-thrombin (0.1 or 1 U/ml). Platelet aggregation was performed as previously described.[23]

The combined evidence therefore suggests that glycoprotein Ib plays an important but not critical role in the response of platelets to α-thrombin. Binding of α-thrombin to glycoprotein Ib accelerates the rate of platelet-thrombin response but has no effect on the extent of this response. In the absence of glycoprotein Ib, α-thrombin loses this kinetic advantage and the response of the platelets becomes qualitatively similar to that observed with γ-thrombin or trypsin.[20]

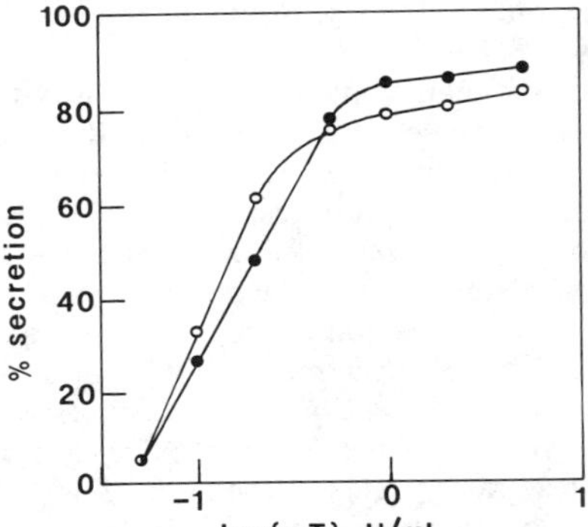

FIGURE 6. Dose-response curves for [^{14}C]serotonin secretion versus the log of the α-thrombin concentration. The experimental conditions were equivalent to those in FIGURE 5. The percent secretion was measured 3 minutes after the addition of α-thrombin by quenching with an equal volume of 1% formaldehyde. Closed circles: control platelets; open circles: Bernard-Soulier syndrome platelets.

GLYCOPROTEIN V

As discussed in the introduction, the activation of platelets by thrombin is dependent on the thrombin active site. Only one platelet membrane protein, glycoprotein V, has been demonstrated to be a thrombin substrate.[47–49] Because glycoprotein Ib and glycoprotein V are both apparently genetically absent in the Bernard-Soulier syndrome,[30,31] it has been suggested that glycoprotein Ib and glycoprotein V may be associated in the normal platelet membrane.[30] This is an attractive proposition, for α-thrombin bound to glycoprotein Ib would then be localized for the hydrolysis of glycoprotein V, hydrolysis of glycoprotein V providing the signal for platelet response.[30] McGowan and Detwiler, however, found that the *Serratia marcescens* metalloprotease hydrolyzed glycoprotein Ib without loss of glycoprotein V from the platelet membrane.[46] Inasmuch as glycoprotein V can be eluted from the platelet membrane by variations in the ionic strength of the suspending medium,[49] it seems unlikely that it would remain membrane-associated after metalloprotease treatment if it were strongly associated with glycoprotein Ib. FIGURE 7 shows the result of an immunoprecipitation experiment using five monoclonal antibodies directed against distinct epitopes on the glycoprotein Ib complex and performed throughout either in the presence of 1 mM EDTA or 1 mM calcium ions. All fives antibodies immunoprecipitated the glycoprotein Ib complex. Glycoprotein Ia was also immunoprecipitated presumably because of its mutual association with actin-binding protein (FIGURE 1).[28,29] None of the five antibodies immunoprecipitated glycoprotein V either in the absence or presence of calcium ions. It would therefore appear that if glycoprotein V is associated with the glycoprotein Ib complex that this association must be weak.

Glycoprotein V contains $\simeq$48% carbohydrate and has an apparent molecular weight of 82,000.[49] It is the most basic of the surface membrane glycoproteins on human platelets.[30] Glycoprotein V is directly cleaved by α-thrombin, because purified glycoprotein V is a thrombin substrate, and on hydrolysis yields a major fragment, glycoprotein V_{fl} (M_r = 69,500), identical in molecular weight to that observed in the supernatant of thrombin-treated, periodate-labeled platelets. Glycoprotein V fulfills several of the requirements expected of the functional thrombin receptor (signal generation site) on platelets. Glycoprotein V is the only detectable membrane surface protein hydrolyzed by thrombin.[47–49] Hydrolysis occurs at all physiologically active thrombin concentrations.[11] Further, proteases of widely divergent evolutionary origin whose cleavage specificity is similar to that of α-thrombin, γ-thrombin, thrombocytin, and α-clostripain, aggregate platelets and all catalyze the hydrolysis of glycoprotein V to glycoprotein V_{fl} as the sole or major hydrolytic event on the platelet membrane surface.[11] Other evidence, however, is inconsistent with glycoprotein V playing a functional role in the physiological response of platelets to thrombin. First, the rate of thrombin hydrolysis of platelet-bound glycoprotein V as measured by the rate of appearance of glycoprotein V_{fl} in the platelet supernatant is slow.[50] Maximum platelet activation occurred with thrombin treatments resulting in hydrolysis of as little as 4% of glycoprotein V per minute. One proviso in this type of experiment that has not been addressed, however, is whether the rate of release of glycoprotein V_{fl} from the platelet membrane accurately reflects the rate of glycoprotein V cleavage by α-thrombin. Second, both chymotrypsin and calcium-dependent protease release essentially all the glycoprotein V from platelets in apparently intact form[50] without affecting the thrombin dose-response curves for platelet dense body secretion.[21,34] Third, platelets that are refractory to thrombin by prior treatment with thrombin and prostacyclin (see introduction), show an essentially unaltered rate of glycoprotein V hydrolysis by thrombin as measured by the rate of appearance of glycoprotein V_{fl} in the supernatant.[50] Finally, Bernard-Soulier syndrome platelets apparently deficient in glycoprotein V[30,31] have an essentially normal thrombin dose-response curve for platelet dense body secretion (FIGURE 6). The available evidence therefore suggests that hydrolysis of glycoprotein V by thrombin is unlikely to represent the mechanism by which signal generation occurs when platelets are exposed to thrombin.

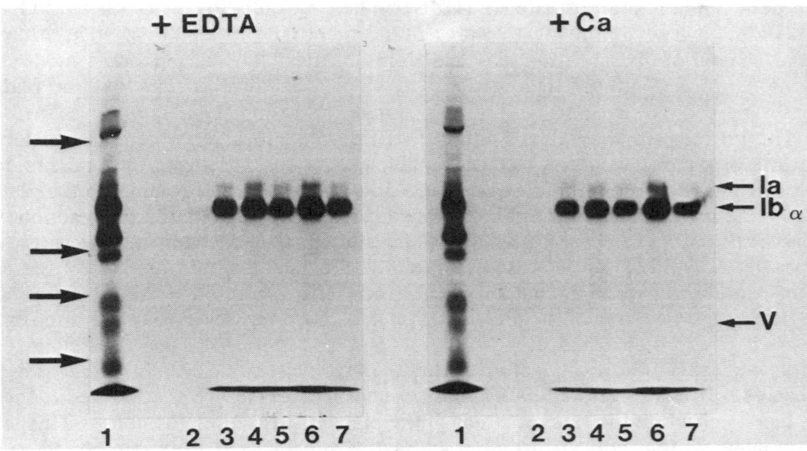

FIGURE 7. Fluorography of a 5% SDS-polyacrylamide gel run under reduced conditions of the antiglycoprotein Ib complex immunoprecipitates derived from the Triton X-100 lysate of periodate-labeled platelets. Platelets were lysed in the presence of 100 μg/ml of leupeptin and either 1 mM EDTA or 1 mM calcium chloride. Platelet labeling, lysis, and immunoprecipitation with fixed *S. aureus* cells was performed as previously described[31] except that the *S. aureus* cells were only washed once before solubilization with SDS. Lane 1: Triton X-100 lysate of periodate-labeled platelets; lane 2: immunoprecipitate, negative control using WM 21 (anti-CALLa); lanes 3-7: immunoprecipitates using the antiglycoprotein Ib complex monoclonal antibodies, WM 23, AN 51, SZ 2, AP 1, and FMC 25, respectively. SZ 2 and AP 1 were the generous gifts of Dr. Changgeng Ruan and Dr. Tom Kunicki, respectively. Molecular weight markers indicated by the arrows in the left-hand margin of the figure in decreasing order of molecular weight: myosin (200,000), β-galactosidase (130,000), phosphorylase b (94,000), and bovine serum albumin (68,000). None of the five monoclonal antibodies coimmunoprecipitated glycoprotein V under either set of conditions.

CONCLUSIONS

Two platelet membrane proteins, glycoprotein V and the glycoprotein Ib complex, have been shown to interact with α-thrombin. As discussed above, however, glycoprotein V is unlikely to play an important functional role in thrombin-platelet interaction at least with respect to thrombin activation of platelets. By contrast, there is good evidence that glycoprotein Ib plays an important but not critical role in the α-thrombin activation of platelets. The binding of α-thrombin to glycoprotein Ib increases the rate but not the extent of the platelet response to α-thrombin. There is a precedent for the binding of a ligand (asialo von Willebrand factor) to glycoprotein Ib causing platelet activation.[51,52] Bernard-Soulier syndrome platelets, however, which lack the glycoprotein Ib complex, have a normal thrombin dose-response curve for dense body secretion, suggesting that glycoprotein Ib is not the platelet thrombin receptor involved in signal generation. In unstimulated platelets, the glycoprotein Ib complex forms part of a larger transmembrane complex that includes actin-binding protein, glycoprotein Ia, and possibly a minor glycoprotein with a molecular weight of 250,000.[28,29] The combined molecular weight of these components ($\simeq$820,000) is in good agreement with the apparent molecular size ($\simeq$900,000) of the high-affinity thrombin binding site on platelets as determined by radiation inactivation.[53] Glycoprotein Ia, however, is unlikely to represent the membrane protein involved in thrombin signal generation, because the platelets from a patient lacking glycoprotein Ia show normal thrombin-induced aggregation.[54] It would therefore appear that the platelet membrane protein involved in thrombin signal generation remains to be defined.

The mechanism by which binding of α-thrombin to glycoprotein Ib accelerates the rate of platelet response to α-thrombin has yet to be defined. One possibility is that binding of α-thrombin to glycoprotein Ib localizes the α-thrombin on the platelet membrane such that the thrombin active site is sterically orientated for reaction with adjacent thrombin receptor (signal generation site). Such a mechanism, however, would appear to be unlikely on at least two grounds. First, one would predict on the basis of an equilibrium reaction that the localization of α-thrombin would be reflected in the dose-response curve of the platelets. Platelets, however, respond to the same extent whether glycoprotein Ib is present or not. Second, one would also predict in terms of this mechanism the prolongation of the lag in response to α-thrombin in the presence of excess active-site-blocked α-thrombin, whereas excess active-site-blocked α-thrombin has no effect on the rate or extent of the platelet α-thrombin response.[7] This latter result suggests that both α-thrombin and active-site-blocked thrombin bound to glycoprotein Ib can specifically facilitate the response of platelets to α-thrombin. Studies on collagen-platelet interaction provide an interesting parallel to this conclusion. Nieuwenhuis and coworkers have recently provided convincing evidence that platelet membrane glycoprotein Ia probably represents the collagen receptor on human platelets.[54] In another recent study, Sinigaglia *et al.* reported that low levels of α-thrombin (0.66 U/ml) stimulated the adhesion of washed platelets to fibrillar collagen.[55] This phenomenon was not apparently dependent on platelet stimulation and occurred equally well with active-site-blocked α-thrombin. Detachment of thrombin from thrombin-treated platelets with hirudin restored normal platelet adhesiveness to collagen. These results suggest that active-site-blocked thrombin can modulate platelet response even though it cannot itself cause platelet activation; in the case of collagen, thrombin binding to the α-chain of glycoprotein Ib is presumably affecting the binding of collagen to glycoprotein Ia, possibly by way of mutual association with actin-binding protein.[28,29] Future studies should define whether a similar mechanism applies in the glycoprotein-Ib-dependent modulation of α-thrombin-platelet response.

ACKNOWLEDGMENTS

We thank Mrs. A. Webster for the typing of the manuscript and Mr. P. J. Woods for his assistance in the preparation of the figures.

REFERENCES

1. BERNDT, M. C. & D. R. PHILLIPS. 1981. *In* Platelets in Biology and Pathology 2. J. L. Gordon, Ed.: 43-75. Elsevier. Amsterdam.
2. TAM, S. W., J. W. FENTON & T. C. DETWILER. 1979. J. Biol. Chem. **254:** 8723-8725.
3. DETWILER, T. C. & R. D. FEINMAN. 1973. Biochemistry **12:** 282-289.
4. HOLMSEN, H., C. A. DANGELMAIER & H.-K. HOLMSEN. 1981. J. Biol. Chem. **256:** 9393-9396.
5. HENRIKSEN, R. A. & A. F. ADAMS BROTHERTON. 1983. J. Biol. Chem. **258:** 13717-13721.
6. DAVEY, M. G. & E. F. LUSCHER. 1967. Nature (London) **216:** 857-858.
7. TOLLEFSEN, D. M., J. R. FEAGLER & P. W. MAJERUS. 1974. J. Biol. Chem. **249:** 2646-2651.
8. WORKMAN, E. F., G. C. WHITE & R. L. LUNDBLAD. 1977. J. Biol. Chem. **252:** 7118-7123.
9. MARTIN, B. M., R. D. FEINMAN & T. C. DETWILER. 1975. Biochemistry **14:** 1308-1314.
10. NIEWIAROWSKI, S., E. P. KIRBY, T. M. BRUDZYNSKI & K. STOCKER. 1979. Biochemistry **18:** 3570-3577.
11. BERNDT, M. C. & D. R. PHILLIPS. 1981. Ann. N.Y. Acad. Sci. **370:** 87-95.
12. SHUMAN, M. A., M. BOTNEY & J. W. FENTON. 1979. J. Clin. Invest. **63:** 1211-1218.
13. MCGOWAN, E. B. & T. C. DETWILER. 1983. Thromb. Res. **31:** 297-304.
14. DETWILER, T. C. & R. D. FEINMAN. 1973. Biochemistry **12:** 2462-2468.
15. MARTIN, B. M., W. W. WASIEWSKI, J. W. FENTON & T. C. DETWILER. 1976. Biochemistry **15:** 4886-4893.
16. SHUMAN, M. A., D. M. TOLLEFSEN & P. W. MAJERUS. 1976. Blood **47:** 43-54.
17. TAM, S. W. & T. C. DETWILER. 1978. Biochim. Biophys. Acta **543:** 194-201.
18. TOLLEFSEN, D. M., C. M. JACKSON & P. W. MAJERUS. 1975. J. Clin. Invest. **56:** 241-245.
19. SHUMAN, M. A. & P. W. MAJERUS. 1975. J. Clin. Invest. **56:** 945-950.
20. ALEXANDER, R. J., J. W. FENTON & T. C. DETWILER. 1983. Arch. Biochem. Biophys. **222:** 266-275.
21. TAM, S. W., J. W. FENTON & T. C. DETWILER. 1980. J. Biol. Chem. **255:** 6626-6632.
22. BERNDT, M. C. & J. P. CAEN. 1984. *In* Progress in Hemostasis and Thrombosis. T. H. Spaet, Ed. Vol. 7: 111-150. Grune and Stratton. Orlando, FL.
23. BERNDT, M. C., C. GREGORY, A. KABRAL, H. ZOLA, D. FOURNIER & P. A. CASTALDI. 1985. Eur. J. Biochem. **151:** 637-649.
24. BERNDT, M. C., B. H. CHONG, H. A. BULL, H. ZOLA & P. A. CASTALDI. 1985. Blood **66:** 1292-1301.
25. OKUMURA, T., C. LOMBARD & G. A. JAMIESON. 1976. J. Biol. Chem. **251:** 5950-5955.
26. OKUMURA, T., M. HASITZ & G. A. JAMIESON. 1978. J. Biol. Chem. **253:** 3435-3443.
27. BROWER, M. S., R. I. LEVIN & K. GARRY. 1985. J. Clin. Invest. **75:** 657-666.
28. FOX, J. E. B. 1985. J. Clin. Invest. **76:** 1673-1683.
29. FOX, J. E. B. 1985. J. Biol. Chem. **260:** 11970-11977.
30. CLEMETSON, K. J., J. L. MCGREGOR, E. JAMES, M. DECHAVANNE & E. F. LUSCHER. 1982. J. Clin. Invest. **70:** 304-311.
31. BERNDT, M. C., C. GREGORY, B. H. CHONG, H. ZOLA & P. A. CASTALDI. 1983. Blood **62:** 800-807.
32. GANGULY, P. 1977. Br. J. Haematol. **37:** 47-51.
33. JAMIESON, G. A. & T. OKUMURA. 1978. J. Clin. Invest. **61:** 861-864.
34. MCGOWAN, E. B., K.-T. YEO & T. C. DETWILER. 1983. Arch. Biochem. Biophys. **227:** 287-301.
35. TOLLEFSEN, D. M. & P. W. MAJERUS. 1976. Biochemistry **15:** 2144-2149.
36. JUNG, S. M. & M. MOROI. 1983. Biochim. Biophys. Acta **761:** 152-162.
37. HAGEN, I., F. BROSSTAD, N. O. SOLUM & R. KORSMO. 1981. J. Lab. Clin. Med. **97:** 213-220.
38. MOROI, M., S. M. JUNG & N. YOSHIDA. 1984. Blood **64:** 622-629.
39. MOROI, M., A. GOETZE, E. DUBAY, C. WU, M. HASITZ & G. A. JAMIESON. 1982. Thromb. Res. **28:** 103-114.
40. WHITE, G. C., R. L. LUNDBLAD & M. J. GRIFFITH. 1981. J. Biol. Chem. **256:** 1763-1766.

41. JENKINS, C. S. P., K. J. CLEMETSON & E. F. ALI-BRIGGS. 1983. Br. J. Haematol. **53:** 491-501.
42. MCGREGOR, J. L., J. BROCHIER, F. WILD, G. FOLLEA, M.-C. TRZECIAK, E. JAMES, M. DECHAVANNE, L. MCGREGOR & K. J. CLEMETSON. 1983. Eur. J. Biochem. **131:** 427-436.
43. YOSHIDA, N., B. WEKSLER & R. NACHMAN. 1983. J. Biol. Chem. **258:** 7168-7174.
44. CLEMETSON, K. J., H. Y. NAIM & E. F. LUSCHER. 1981. Proc. Nat. Acad. Sci. USA **78:** 2712-2716.
45. COOPER, H. A., W. P. BENNETT, G. C. WHITE & R. H. WAGNER. 1982. Proc. Nat. Acad. Sci. USA **79:** 1433-1437.
46. MCGOWAN, E. B. & T. C. DETWILER. 1985. Blood **65:** 1033-1035.
47. PHILLIPS, D. R. & P. P. AGIN. 1977. Biochem. Biophysics Res. Commun. **75:** 940-947.
48. MOSHER, D. F., A. VAHERI, J. J. CHOATE & C. G. GAHMBERG. 1979. Blood **53:** 437-445.
49. BERNDT, M. C. & D. R. PHILLIPS. 1981. J. Biol. Chem. **256:** 59-65.
50. MCGOWAN, E. B., A. DING & T. C. DETWILER. 1983. J. Biol. Chem. **258:** 11243-11248.
51. GRALNICK, H. R., S. B. WILLIAMS & B. S. COLLER. 1985. J. Clin. Invest. **75:** 19-25.
52. DE MARCO, L., A. GIROLAMI, S. RUSSELL & Z. M. RUGGERI. 1985. J. Clin. Invest. **75:** 1198-1203.
53. HARMON, J. T. & G. A. JAMIESON. 1985. Biochemistry **24:** 58-64.
54. NIEUWENHUIS, H. K., J. W. N. AKKERMAN, W. P. M. HOUDIJK & J. J. SIXMA. 1985. Nature (London) **318:** 470-472.
55. SINIGAGLIA, F., C. L. BALDUINI, A. BISIO & C. BALDUINI. 1985. Br. J. Haematol. **59:** 587-592.

Platelet Activation by α-Thrombin Is a Receptor-Mediated Event[a]

JOAN T. HARMON AND G. A. JAMIESON

American Red Cross
Biomedical Research Laboratories
Bethesda, Maryland 20814

BACKGROUND

Thrombin is one of the most potent and physiologically significant activators of platelet function and can cause platelet activation and secretion at concentrations below 1 nM. Despite its importance, the mechanism by which thrombin activates platelets is not known, specifically the question of whether or not it is a receptor-mediated event.

Extensive studies have been carried out in several laboratories on the binding of α-thrombin to platelets [1–4] and platelet membranes.[5] Graphical analysis of the data has supported a two-site model with high nonspecific binding: about 300 binding sites of high affinity (K_d 1 nM) and about 30 000 sites of lower affinity (K_d 30 nM).

We have recently reexamined the binding of α-thrombin to platelets using computer-assisted analysis (LIGAND)[6] and have found that the binding data is best represented by a three-site model: about 50 high-affinity sites (K_d 0.3 nM), about 1700 moderate-affinity sites (K_d 10 nM), and 600 000 low-affinity sites (K_d 3 μM).

In these studies the functional sizes of the binding sites for thrombin on both human platelets and isolated membranes were determined by the technique of radiation inactivation. Independent studies using different radiation doses (0, 3, and 48 Mrad) and different thrombin concentrations (10^{-10} M, 10^{-8} M, and 10^{-6} M) established the presence of three binding sites with functional sizes of 900 000, 30 000, and 4000. Upon examination of the equilibrium parameters, the lowest affinity site (M_r 4000) appears to represent what would generally be considered nonspecific binding, that is, the dissociation constant of approximately 3 μM is well outside the probable range of thrombin concentrations occurring under physiological concentrations. The presence of a very low-affinity site, however, does explain the difficulty of other investigators, as well as ourselves, in being able to demonstrate complete competition of labeled α-thrombin (10^{-10} M) with 10^{-6} M unlabeled thrombin. To compete for a site with a dissociation constant of 3 μM, one should be using an α-thrombin concentration of approximately 30 μM. Under the conditions of the binding assay, for example, ionic strength, α-thrombin is not soluble at these concentrations.

The binding site with moderate affinity has a dissociation constant (K_d 10 nM) that is also beyond the minimum thrombin concentration required to induce platelet activation, but is within the probable range of physiological thrombin concentrations.

[a] This work was supported, in part, by USPHS Grants HL34364 and RR05737.

The site with the highest affinity has a dissociation constant (K_d 0.3 nM) in the range of thrombin concentrations required for platelet activation. The functional size calculated for this component (900 000) suggests that it may represent a complex of several individual molecules whose mutual interaction is required for the effective binding of thrombin to platelets.

The binding of thrombin and stimulation of platelets by thrombin have some unusual features. Studies of calcium secretion in response to thrombin,[1] or heat production during stimulation,[8] have shown that thrombin concentration affects the extent of the reaction but not its rate. Thus, although proteolytically active thrombin is required, there is apparently no catalytic turnover of thrombin, suggesting that the interaction of thrombin with platelets has the characteristics both of an enzyme-catalyzed reaction and of an agonist-receptor equilibrium.[9]

From studies on changes in the stimulus-response relationship in chymotrypsinized platelets, we have proposed that there is first a receptor step involving the binding of thrombin to platelets, and then an effector step leading to signal generation.[10] Thus, the role of the receptor could be to ensure the correct orientation of the thrombin to induce platelet stimulation in the subsequent effector step (FIGURE 1). Similar models have been subsequently proposed by others[11] and could also explain similar changes in platelet stimulation seen in platelets treated with *Serratia marcescens* protease[12] and with the platelet calcium dependent protease.[13] Following the initial interaction with thrombin, there is evidence of receptor processing to forms that are more slowly dissociating and possibly covalently linked.[14]

The question of the membrane structures involved in these interactions has not been satisfactorily answered. Glycoprotein I (GPIb: M_r 185 000) has been suggested as being a receptor because its proteolytic product glycocalicin can effect the reversible inhibition of platelet activation by thrombin[10] and by the antithrombin activity of GPI itself.[15] The possible role for GPI in thrombin binding and activation has been supported by the correlation between decreased GPI and the reduction of thrombin reactivity in the Bernard-Soulier syndrome,[16] in myeloproliferative disorders,[17,18] and in polymorphic variants.[19]

Cross-linking of bound thrombin to the platelet surface with glutaraldehyde suggested a molecular weight of ca 200 000 for the high-affinity binding site,[20] which would be compatible with GPI, whereas the use of a photoactivatable cross-linking derivative of thrombin has also suggested M_r 200 000 for the high-affinity sites and values of 400 000 and 46 000 as possible low-affinity thrombin binding sites (K_d 30 nM).[21] Other studies have proposed binding sites of M_r 74 000[22] as part of a multi-molecular complex containing other components of M_r 55 000, 27 000, and 20 000.[23] In addition, three complexes stable in sodium dodecyl sulfate (SDS) and dithiothreitol of M_r 58 000, 75 000, 77 000 have been identified.[24,25] As noted above, however, these covalently linked complexes may arise from receptor processing. Immunological techniques have been used to identify other thrombin-binding proteins of unknown function.[26]

A major question has been the relevance of this bound thrombin to the process of platelet activation. Half saturation of high-affinity sites corresponds to 50% of maximal platelet activation,[27] and binding affinity and platelet stimulation are affected in parallel by changes in buffer composition.[28] Moreover, the number of high-affinity receptors and sensitivity of platelets to thrombin also move in parallel as membrane microviscosity is changed.[29] Lectins, particularly wheat germ agglutinin, can also have synergistic effects on both thrombin binding and platelet activation.[30,31]

Even though these changes suggest a relationship between thrombin binding and response, they have by no means established it. A major problem in determining whether thrombin activation is a receptor-mediated event has been the observation that thrombins blocked at the active site, such as Nα-tosyl-L-lysine chloromethyl ketone-treated (TLCK)-thrombin and diisopropyl fluorophosphate-treated (DFP)-thrombin, do not inhibit the activation of platelets by α-thrombin, but do compete with α-thrombin in the binding studies at high and moderate affinity sites as determined using graphical methods of analysis.[1-3] This has led to the suggestion that the measurable binding of thrombin to platelets is not involved in platelet activation.

Because proteolytically active α-thrombin is required for platelet activation, glycoprotein V (GPV; M_r 75 000) has also been proposed as a modulator of platelet function, because it is a substrate for thrombin in the platelet membrane[32,33] and in its purified form.[34] The kinetics of hydrolysis for GPV, however, do not parallel those of platelet activation by thrombin,[12,35] and it appears that its hydrolysis during thrombin-induced platelet activation may be an epiphenomenon.

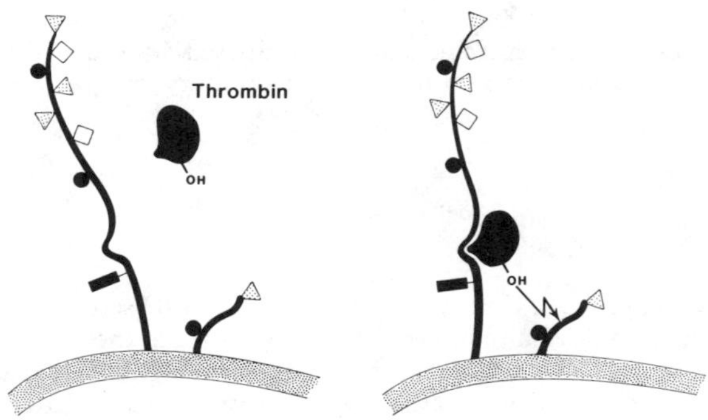

FIGURE 1. Schematic representation of the mechanism proposed for the activation of platelets by thrombin.[10,38] In this model, α-thrombin binds to a specific site on GPIb in the receptor complex and is oriented to interact with another component of the complex. (G. A. Jamieson.[38] With permission from *Plasma Therapy and Transfusion Technology*.)

EXPERIMENT

Binding Studies

Our standard binding assay was used as described.[29] In brief, thrombin was purified by the procedure of Fenton *et al.*[36] All thrombin preparations (total of 6 to date) have had specific clotting activities of > 2700 US U/mg protein and were at least 98% pure by Coomassie blue staining of SDS-polyacrylamide gels or by autoradiography of [^{125}I]thrombin. The [^{125}I]thrombin was prepared by use of an iodogen-bead procedure[29] to a radio-specific activity of 20-30 μCi/μg (< 0.6 moles radioiodine per thrombin molecule). The [^{125}I]thrombin retained 100% of the clotting activity and was identical to unlabeled thrombin in the radioreceptor assay.

For the binding assay, platelets were removed from platelet-rich plasma (pH adjusted to 6.5) by centrifugation, washed with citrate wash buffer (pH 6.5), and resuspended to a concentration of 1×10^9 platelets/ml in a modified Tyrode's buffer ($Ca^{++}-Mg^{++}$ free, 10 mM HEPES pH 7.4).[29] In a total volume of 0.1 ml, the final concentration of reactants was 0.09-0.2 nM [^{125}I]thrombin, 10 mg/ml bovine serum albumin, and 4×10^8 platelets/ml. A thrombin-binding isotherm was obtained by adding increasing concentrations up to 1000 nM of unlabeled thrombin. The bound thrombin was rapidly separated from the free thrombin by centrifugation. The supernatant (free thrombin) was removed by aspiration, and [^{125}I]thrombin, associated with the platelet pellet, was quantitated by gamma counting. Steady-state binding was achieved after 10 minutes at 22°C. Binding was constant with pH from 7.4 to 8.0, but it decreased at lower pH. Binding was not affected by Ca^{++} concentrations of up to 1 mM, but higher concentrations were inhibitory, with 10 mM causing a ~60% reduction. The degradation of thrombin was less than 4% during the course of the binding assay as followed by the amount of ^{125}I soluble in 5% trichloroacetic acid. Thrombin binding (B/F) was linear with the platelet number over the range of 1-7 $\times 10^8$/ml. Thrombin binding studies and data analysis by the LIGAND program were performed as routinely carried out in our laboratory.[7,29]

Serotonin Release

Washed platelets (1×10^9/ml) were incubated with [^{14}C]serotonin (0.25 μCi/ml, 1.6 μM) for 1 hour at 37°C. Imipramine (2 μM) was added at the end of the incubation to prevent reuptake of serotonin. The release assay was conducted using 4×10^8 platelets/ml in the absence and presence of increasing concentrations of thrombin and in the absence and presence of increasing concentrations of thrombin analogues for 10 minutes at 22°C. After 10 minutes, further release was inhibited by the addition of a mixture of EGTA, imipramine, and formaldehyde, and the platelets removed by centrifugation. An aliquot of the supernatant was counted in a beta-scintillation counter

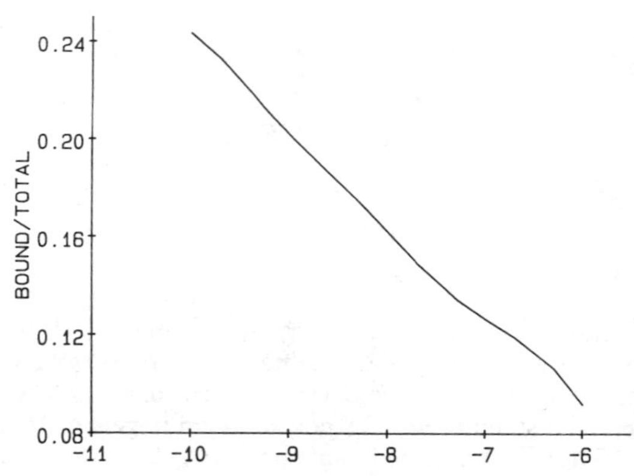

FIGURE 2. Binding isotherm for the interaction of α-thrombin with human platelets.

TABLE 1. Binding Parameters for α- , TLCK-, and PPACK-Thrombins with Washed Human Platelets

	Number of Sites (nM)					Dissociation Constant (nM)				
	B1	B2	B3	B-TLCK	B-PPACK	K1	K2	K3	K-TLCK	K-PPACK
α-Thrombin	0.02	2	66			0.1	16	740		
TLCK-Thombin	—	0.6	67	0.01		—	2	950	0.03	
PPACK-Thrombin	0.02	1	56		0.01	7	3	510		0.4

to quantitate the serotonin released. The serotonin released in the absence of thrombin was considered background and was subtracted.

RESULTS

Thrombin Binding Studies

The binding isotherm for α-thrombin on human platelets is shown in FIGURE 2. Alpha-thrombin bound to high, moderate, and low affinity sites as previously shown,[7] and the binding parameters are shown in TABLE 1.

To ascertain whether the high-affinity binding site is a receptor necessary for biological activity, competition binding studies were carried out to evaluate the antagonism of the proteolytically inhibited thrombin analogues, TLCK-thrombin and D-phenylalanyl-L-prolyl-L-arginine chloromethyl ketone-treated (PPACK)-thrombin, with α-thrombin, using computer-assisted analysis of the binding isotherms (LIGAND).

The best fit for the TLCK-thrombin/α-thrombin binding isotherms indicated TLCK-thrombin bound with similar affinity to α-thrombin at the moderate and low-affinity sites but did not bind to the high-affinity site accessible to α-thrombin: instead TLCK-thrombin bound with high affinity to another site (B-TLCK), which was not accessible to α-thrombin. By contrast, PPACK-thrombin bound to all three sites accessible to α-thrombin and, with high affinity, to a fourth site (B-PPACK) inaccessible to α-thrombin. The binding parameters for TLCK-thrombin and PPACK-thrombin at these sites are given in TABLE 1.

Studies on serotonin secretion in the presence of TLCK- and PPACK-thrombins following challenge with α-thrombin (2 nM, 200 mU/ml) were carried out as described in MATERIALS AND METHODS. As expected, TLCK-thrombin had no effect on secretion at concentrations as high as 0.5 uM. On the other hand PPACK-thrombin showed about 10% inhibition of secretion at 0.1 μM concentrations and complete inhibition by 0.5 μM (TABLE 2).

The protease from *Serratia marcescens* specifically cleaves GPIb.[12,37,39] Examination of the thrombin-binding isotherms before and after digestion demonstrated a complete loss of high-affinity thrombin binding. The platelets were still responsive, however, to α-thrombin albeit with a rightward shift in the dose-response curve for serotonin secretion. That is, an α-thrombin concentration of 1 nM was necessary to elicit a

50% secretion response in *Serratia* protease-treated platelets as compared with about 0.25 nM in control platelets. When these protease-treated platelets were challenged with thrombin (2 nM), TLCK-thrombin showed a 50% inhibition of secretion at 1 μM, whereas secretion was totally inhibited by PPACK-thrombin at the same concentration (TABLE 2).

DISCUSSION

Our previous studies[7] have demonstrated that α-thrombin binds to intact platelets at three sites with high, moderate, and low affinities: these binding sites may be termed B1, B2, and B3. In the present studies, the best fit, as determined by F-test comparison of the sum of squares, for the binding of PPACK-thrombin to intact platelets, was a model in which the modified thrombin bound to all of the three sites but, in addition, bound to a fourth site (B-PPACK) with high affinity (0.4 nM). The binding affinity (K_d) at the high-affinity site accessible to α-thrombin was reduced to 7 nM as compared

TABLE 2. Inhibition by TLCK- and PPACK-Thrombins of Serotonin Secretion Induced by α-Thrombin[a]

	Intact Platelets	Serratia Protease-Treated
TLCK-Thrombin	No inhibition (1 μM)	1 μM
PPACK-Thrombin	0.2 μM	0.3 μM

[a] Values given are the concentration of blocked thrombins giving 50% inhibition of serotonin secretion from the challenge of intact platelets and *Serratia* protease-treated platelets with α-thrombin at 2 nM.

to a value of 0.1 nM with α-thrombin itself. From this it could be inferred that PPACK-thrombin should compete with α-thrombin for platelet activation. This was found to be the case, and the degree of inhibition was roughly proportional to the differences in the binding affinities of α-thrombin and PPACK-thrombin at this site.

By contrast, the best fit for the binding data of TLCK-thrombin was a three-site model in which the modified thrombin bound to the moderate- and low-affinity sites but also with high affinity (0.03 nM) to another site (B-TLCK) that was not accessible to α-thrombin. TLCK-thrombin was not found to bind to the high-affinity site accessible to α-thrombin (B1) and therefore would not be expected to compete with it for platelet activation at low thrombin concentrations, as found in the present work and, previously, by others. These results demonstrate that the high-affinity binding site for α-thrombin on human platelets is a classical receptor, occupancy of which is necessary for platelet activation by low concentrations of thrombin; and that TLCK-thrombin does not occupy this high-affinity site and hence cannot inhibit platelet activation by α-thrombin. Whether the high-affinity binding sites for TLCK-thrombin (B-TLCK) and PPACK-thrombin (B-PPACK) are related is not known.

The binding studies indicate that only PPACK-thrombin binds to the high-affinity α-thrombin receptor, but that both TLCK-and PPACK-thrombins bind to the moderate-affinity binding site. Hence the model predicts that both TLCK-thrombin and

PPACK-thrombin should compete with moderate concentrations of α-thrombin in platelet activation under conditions in which the high-affinity binding site was not functional: this was achieved by treating the platelets with *Serratia marcescens* protease that cleaves GPIb and causes a rightward shift in stimulus-response coupling with α-thrombin. With these protease-treated platelets, we found, as predicted, that platelet activation was inhibited by both of the blocked thrombins. These results demonstrate that the moderate affinity-binding site for α-thrombin on human platelets is also a classical receptor, occupancy of which is necessary for platelet activation by moderate concentrations of α-thrombin; and that PPACK-thrombin and TLCK-thrombin both compete for the moderate-affinity binding site. Both inhibit α-thrombin response mediated by way of this receptor.

These results resolve the paradox regarding the relative interactions of platelets with blocked thrombins, particularly TLCK-thrombin, and demonstrate conclusively that platelet activation by α-thrombin is a receptor-mediated event. The mechanism by which this interaction with the receptor is transduced to the platelet interior remains to be elucidated.

SUMMARY

Computer-assisted data analysis of binding isotherms (LIGAND) has shown that human platelets have binding sites for α-thrombin of high (K_d 0.3 nM), moderate (K_d 10 nM), and low affinities (K_d 3 μM).[7] Application of similar techniques has shown that TLCK-thrombin does not, whereas PPACK-thrombin does, bind to the high-affinity binding site accessible to α-thrombin, but that both bind to the moderate and low-affinity sites. Treatment of platelets with *Serratia marcescens* protease destroys the high-affinity site but does not affect moderate-affinity binding. In accordance with this model, both modified thrombins compete with α-thrombin for platelet activation at the moderate-affinity site, but only PPACK-thrombin competes at the high-affinity site. These results establish that platelet activation by either low or moderate concentrations of thrombin are receptor-mediated events and explain the paradox of the differential effects of TLCK-thrombin on the binding and activation of platelets by α-thrombin.

REFERENCES

1. Detwiler, T. C. & R. D. Feinman. 1973. Kinetics of the thrombin-induced release of calcium (II) by platelets. Biochemistry **12:** 282.
2. Tollefson, D. M. , J. R. Feagler & P. W. Majerus. 1974. The binding of thrombin to the surface of human platelets. J. Biol. Chem. **249:** 2646.
3. Ganguly, P. 1974. Binding of thrombin to human platelets. Nature (London) **247:** 306.
4. Ganguly, P. & W. J. Sonnichsen. 1976. Binding of thrombin to human platelets and its possible significance. Br. J. Haematol. **34:** 291.
5. Tam, S. W. & T. C. Detwiler. 1978. Binding of thrombin to human platelet plasma membranes. Biochim. Biophys. Acta **543:** 194.
6. Munson, P. J. & D. Rodbard. 1980. LIGAND: A versatile computerized approach for characterization of ligand-binding systems. Anal. Biochem. **107:** 220.

7. HARMON, J. T. & G. A. JAMIESON. 1985. Thrombin binds to a high affinity $\approx$ 900,000 dalton site on human platelets. Biochemistry **24:** 58.
8. ROSS, P. D., A. P. FLETCHER & G. A. JAMIESON. 1973. Microcalorimetric study of isolated blood platelets in the presence of thrombin and other aggregating agents. Biochim. Biophys. Acta **313:** 105.
9. MARTIN, B. M., R. D. FEINMAN & T. C. DETWILER. 1975. Platelet stimulation by thrombin and other proteases. Biochemistry **14:** 108.
10. OKUMURA, T., M. HASITZ & G. A. JAMIESON. 1978. Platelet glycocalicin: interaction with thrombin and role as thrombin receptor of the platelet surface. J. Biol. Chem. **253:** 3435.
11. TAM, S. W., J. W. FENTON II & T. C. DETWILER. 1980. Platelet thrombin receptors: binding of α-thrombin is coupled to signal generation by a chymotrypsin-sensitive mechanism. J. Biol. Chem. **255:** 6626.
12. COOPER, H. A., W. P. BENNETT, G. C. WHITE II & R. H. WAGNER. 1982. Hydrolysis of human platelet membrane glycoproteins with a *Serratia marcescens* protease: effect on response to thrombin and von Willebrand factor. Proc. Natl. Acad. Sci. USA **79:** 1433.
13. MCGOWAN, E. B., K-T. YEO & T. C. DETWILER. 1983. The action of calcium-dependent protease on platelet surface glycoproteins. Arch. Biochem. Biophys. **227:** 287.
14. TAM, S. W., J. W. FENTON II & T. C. DETWILER. 1979. Dissociation of thrombin from platelets by hirudin: evidence for receptor processing. J. Biol. Chem. **254:** 8723.
15. GANGULY, P. & N. L. GOULD. 1979. Thrombin receptors of human platelets: thrombin binding and antithrombin properties of glycoprotein I. Br. J. Haematol. **42:** 137.
16. JAMIESON, G. A. & T. OKUMURA. 1978. Reduced thrombin binding and aggregation in Bernard-Soulier platelets. J. Clin. Invest. **61:** 861.
17. BOLIN, R. B., T. OKUMURA & G. A. JAMIESON. 1977. Changes in distribution of platelet membrane glycoproteins in patients with myeloproliferative disorders. Am. J. Hematol. **3:** 63.
18. GANGULY, P., S. B. SUTHERLAND & H. B. BRADFORD. 1978. Defective binding of thrombin to platelets in myeloid leukemia. Br. J. Haematol. **39:** 599.
19. BOLIN, R. B., T. OKUMURA & G. A. JAMIESON. 1977. A new polymorphism of platelet membrane glycoproteins. Nature (London) **269:** 69.
20. TOLLEFSON, D. M. & P. W. MAJERUS. 1976. Evidence for a single class of thrombin binding sites on human platelets. Biochemistry **15:** 2144.
21. LARSEN, N. E. & E. R. SIMONS. 1981. Preparation and application of a photoreactive thrombin analogue: binding to human platelets. Biochemistry **20:** 4141.
22. GANGULY, P. & N. G. FOSSETT. 1981. Inhibition of thrombin-induced platelet aggregation by a derivative of wheat germ agglutinin. Evidence for a physiologic receptor of thrombin in human platelets. Blood **57:** 343.
23. CHELLADURAI, M., N. G. FOSSETT & P. GANGULY. 1983. A novel thrombin-reactive protein complex in human platelets. J. Biol. Chem. **258:** 1407.
24. SHUMAN, M. A., M. BOTNEY & L. K. JOHNSON. 1981. Identification of a specific binding site for thrombin on platelets. Ann. N. Y. Acad. Sci. **370:** 57.
25. BENNETT, W. F. & K. C. GLENN. 1978. Hypersensitivity of platelets to thrombin: Formation of stable thrombin receptor complexes and the role of shape change. Cell **22:** 621.
26. HAGEN, I., G. O. GOGSTAD, F. BROSSTAD & N-O. SOLUM. 1983. Demonstration of ^{125}I-labelled thrombin-binding platelet proteins by use of crossed immunoelectrophoresis and autoradiography. Biochim. Biophys. Acta **732:** 600.
27. MARTIN, B. M., W. W. WASIEWSKI, J. W. FENTON II & T. C. DETWILER. 1976. Equilibrium binding of thrombin to platelets. Biochemistry **15:** 4886.
28. SHUMAN, M. A. & P. W. MAJERUS. 1975. The perturbation of thrombin binding to human platelets by anions. J. Clin. Invest. **56:** 945.
29. TANDON, N. N., J. T. HARMON, D. RODBARD & G. A. JAMIESON. 1983. Thrombin receptors define responsiveness of cholesterol-modified platelets. J. Biol. Chem. **258:** 11840.
30. JUNG, S. M., A. ORDINAS & G. A. JAMIESON. 1981. Synergistic effects of lectins in the interaction of thrombin with human platelets. Biochim. Biophys. Acta **673:** 312.

31. TANDON, N. N., A. ORDINAS & G. A. JAMIESON. 1982. Effects of *N*-acetylglucosamine and platelet inhibitors on the synergistic interaction of platelets and aggregating agents in the presence of wheat germ agglutinin. Biochim. Biophys. Acta **719:** 388.
32. PHILLIPS, D. R. & P. P. AGIN. 1977. Platelet membrane glycoproteins. Identification of a proteolytic substrate for thrombin. Biochem. Biophysics Res. Commun. **75:** 940.
33. MOSHER, D. F., A. VAHERI, J. J. CHOATE & C. G. GAHMBERG. 1979. Action of thrombin on surface glycoproteins of human platelets. Blood **53:** 437.
34. BERNDT, M. C. & D. R. PHILLIPS. 1981. Purification and preliminary physicochemical characterization of human platelet membrane glycoprotein V. J. Biol. Chem. **256:** 59.
35. MCGOWAN, E. B., A-H. DING & T. C. DETWILER. 1983. Correlation of thrombin-induced glycoprotein V hydrolysis and platelet activation. J. Biol. Chem. **258:** 11243.
36. FENTON II, J. W., M. J. FASCO, A. B. STACKROW, D. L. ARONSON, A. M. YOUNG & J. S. FINLAYSON. 1977. Human thrombins. Production, evaluation, and properties of α-thrombin. J. Biol. Chem. **252:** 3587.
37. COOPER, H. A., W. P. BENNETT, A. KREGER, D. LYERLY & R. H. WAGNER. 1981. The effect of extracellular proteases from gram-negative bacteria on the interaction of von Willebrand factor with human platelets. J. Lab. Clin. Med. **97:** 379.
38. JAMIESON, G. A. 1982. Biochemical and ultrastructural relationships in platelet function. Plasma Ther. Transfus. Technol. **3:** 239.
39. MCGOWAN, E. B. & T. C. DETWILER. 1985. Differential effect of Serratia protease on platelet surface glycoproteins Ib and V. Blood **65:** 1035.

Thrombin-Induced Fibronectin Binding to Rat Platelets: Relationship to Other Inducing Agents[a]

R. E. CIAGLOWSKI, D. G. MOON, L. K. WESTON, AND J. E. KAPLAN[b]

Department of Physiology
Albany Medical College
Union University
Albany, New York 12208

Thrombin stimulates human platelets to express specific, saturable receptors for plasma fibronectin (Fn).[1] Scatchard analysis of [^{125}I]Fn binding indicated a single class of receptors with an apparent dissociation constant of 3×10^{-7} M and approximately 120 000 Fn binding sites per platelet. Human platelets have also been demonstrated to contain Fn (3 μg Fn/10^9 platelets) within their alpha granules, which is secreted with other granular proteins during stimulation by thrombin and collagen.[2,3] *In vitro* assay systems have indicated that whereas Fn enhances adhesion and spreading of platelets on collagen,[4,5] it can inhibit platelet aggregation.[6,7] Observations such as the above have led to considerable speculation as to the actual role of Fn in platelet function. We have hypothesized that Fn exerts an antithrombotic effect *in vivo* by modulating collagen-induced platelet deposition at sites of vascular injury.[7,8] We have been investigating this hypothesis using both *in vitro* and *in vivo* rat model systems. The present study was undertaken to determine whether rat platelets also express Fn receptors and whether other platelet activators or proteases induce platelet binding of Fn.

Rat Fn was purified from fresh plasma by gelatin-sepharose affinity chromatography as previously described[7] and labeled with ^{125}I using the lactoperoxidase method. Highly purified human thrombins (alpha, gamma, and diisopropyl phosphate [DIP]) were the generous gift of Dr. John Fenton II of the New York State Department of Health, Albany, NY. Bovine factor X_a was graciously provided by Dr. Daniel Walz (Wayne State University, Detroit, MI). All other reagents were obtained commercially.

Platelets were isolated from 300 g male Sprague-Dawley rats (Taconic Farms, Germantown, NY). Isolation was accomplished by isopycnic centrifugation of rat platelet-rich plasma into a Stractan II step gradient (details may be found in reference 7). Fn binding assays were performed in a manner similar to that of Plow and

[a]This work was supported in part by HHS Grants GM-25946, HL-32418, and GM-07033.

[b]To whom correspondence should be addressed.

Ginsberg.[1] Isolated platelets (1-5 × 10^7/mL) were incubated with [^{125}I]Fn at 37°C in Tyrodes solution containing 1% bovine serum albumin with the desired concentration of inducers and/or inhibitors. Aliquots (100 μL) were removed and quickly layered over 500 μL of 20% sucrose (in Tyrodes/BSA) and centrifuged for 3 min at 10 000 g in a microfuge (Beckman Instruments). Then the supernatants were aspirated; the tips containing the cell pellets were amputated and counted for bound [^{125}I]Fn.

Binding of [^{125}I]Fn to alpha and gamma thrombin-stimulated rat platelets was time-dependent. Both thrombins induced maximum binding after 20-25 minutes of incubation. This is very similar to the time course reported for binding of Fn by human platelets.[1] [^{125}I]Fn binding was also dependent upon the form and dose of thrombin added. Alpha thrombin at concentrations of 1.0 μg/mL (2.7 × 10^{-8} M) induced near maximal binding of [^{125}I]Fn (10 ng/10^7 platelets), whereas gamma thrombin only induced half as much Fn binding even at a concentration of 60 μg/mL. Concentrations of gamma thrombin less than 0.2 μg/mL failed to induce any Fn binding. DIP-thrombin, (the enzymatically inactive form of thrombin), failed to induce [^{125}I]Fn binding by platelets at any concentration and it did not competitively inhibit the action of alpha thrombin. DIP-thrombin also did not augment the effect of gamma thrombin.

Other proteases were compared to thrombin with regard to their ability to stimulate [^{125}I]Fn binding to rat platelets. At the concentrations tested (nM-μM), bovine chymotrypsin, bovine factor X_a, porcine elastase, bovine cathepsin, human plasmin, and human urokinase all failed to induce any Fn binding. Bovine trypsin (0.1 μM) induced approximately half the binding of Fn observed with alpha-thrombin. These findings indicate that the proteolytic activity of thrombin is necessary to induce Fn binding, and this action is relatively specific to alpha-thrombin.

Adenosine diphosphate (ADP) at concentrations of 1-40 μM, induced only a slight amount of [^{125}I]Fn binding (< 10% of that induced by thrombin). Platelet-activating factor (PAF) failed to induce any Fn binding, but PAF does not stimulate rat platelets to aggregate as it does human platelets, so this finding may be species specific. Two other platelet activators, arachidonic acid (AA) and the calcium ionophore A-23187, both induced about 60% of the Fn binding that alpha-thrombin induced. Preliminary studies suggest that phospholipase c (*Clostridium perfringens*) also induces Fn binding. Thus, other platelet stimulatory agents can induce at least partial expression of the Fn receptor on platelets. It is somewhat surprising that ADP did not significantly enhance the amount of Fn bound, because ADP is an excellent inducer of the fibrinogen receptor on platelets.[9] Recent evidence indicates that both Fn and fibrinogen bind to the GPIIb-IIIa complex on the platelet surface.[10] How then can ADP induce expression of the fibrinogen receptor but not the Fn receptor? Perhaps the binding sites for fibrinogen and Fn are close together on the GPIIb-IIIa complex but not identical, as suggested by recent monoclonal antibody studies.[11]

The effect of various inhibitors of platelet activation was investigated using three inducers of Fn binding: alpha-thrombin, arachidonic acid, and A-23187. The amount of [^{125}I]Fn bound to platelets in the absence of any inhibitor was considered to 100% binding for each inducing agent. The effect of each inhibitor was then expressed in terms of relative percent Fn bound. The results are shown in FIGURE 1. As can be seen, the tripeptide Phe-Pro-Arg-Ch_2Cl or PPACK (a potent active-site inhibitor of thrombin) specifically inhibited the thrombin-induced Fn binding. In turn, aspirin (an inhibitor of the cyclooxygenase enzyme) primarily inhibited the arachidonic acid-induced Fn binding. Although the A-23187-induced binding is somewhat attenuated by aspirin, the thrombin response is essentially unaffected. This would suggest the existence of at least two pathways leading to expression of Fn receptors on rat platelets. Addition of the divalent cation chelators, EGTA and EDTA, inhibited all Fn binding.

These data indicate that much like fibrinogen binding to platelets, Fn binding is calcium-dependent.

In summary, rat platelets do express FN receptors upon stimulation by alpha thrombin. Gamma thrombin, arachidonic acid, and A-23187 can also induce [^{125}I]Fn binding but only about half as much as alpha-thrombin. Induction of Fn receptors appears to be able to proceed by at least two pathways, and Fn binding seems to be calcium- (or divalent cation) dependent.

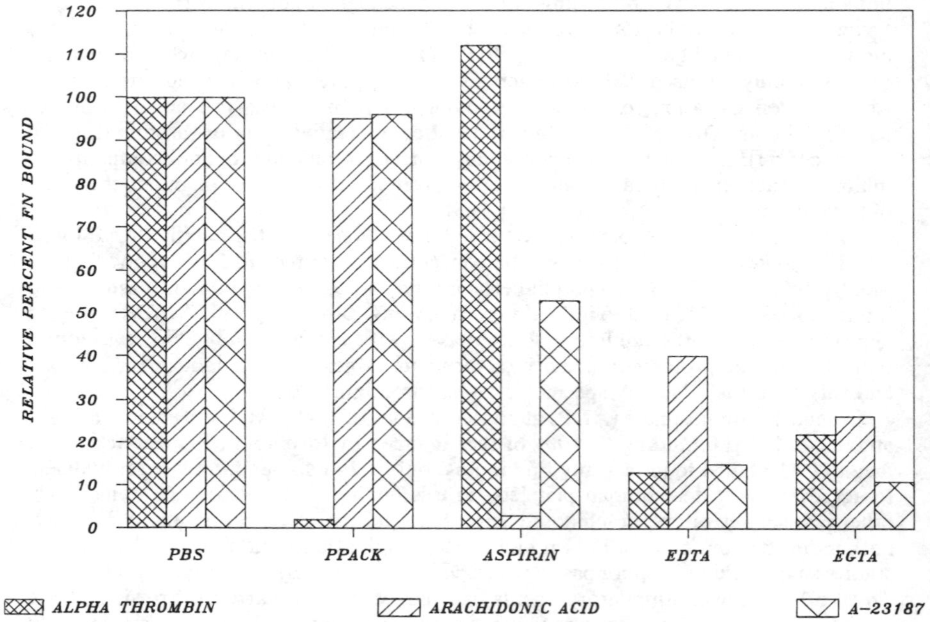

FIGURE 1.

REFERENCES

1. PLOW, E. F. & M. H. GINSBERG. 1981. Specific and saturable binding of plasma fibronectin to thrombin-stimulated human platelets. J. Biol. Chem. **256:** 9477.
2. ZUCKER, M. B., M. W. MOSESSON, M. J. BROEKMAN & K. L. KAPLAN. 1979. Release of platelet fibronectin from alpha granules induced by thrombin or collagen; lack of requirement for plasma fibronectin in ADP-induced platelet aggregation. Blood **54:** 8.
3. GINSBERG, M. H. & E. F. PLOW. 1981. Fibronectin expression on the platelet surface occurs in concert with secretion. J. Supramol. Struct. Cell. Biochem. **17:** 91.
4. HOFFMAN, R. P. & R. O. HYNES. 1980. Hemostasis: The role of fibronectin in the adhesion of platelets to collagen. Clin. Res. **28:** 297.
5. KOTELIANSKY, V. E., V. L. LEYTIN, D. D. SVIRIDOV, V. S. REPIN & V. N. SMIRNOV. 1981. Human plasma fibronectin promotes the adhesion and spreading of platelets on surfaces coated with fibrillar collagen. FEBS Lett. **123:** 59.

6. SANTORO, S. A. 1983. Inhibition of platelet aggregation by plasma fibronectin. Biochem. Biophysics Res. Commun. **116:** 135.
7. MOON, D. G., J. E. KAPLAN & J. E. MAZURKEWICZ. 1986. The inhibitory effect of plasma fibronectin on collagen-induced platelet aggregation. Blood **67:** 450.
8. KAPLAN, J. E., P. W. SNEDEKER, S. H. BAUM, D. G. MOON & F. L. MINNEAR. 1983. Influence of plasma fibronectin on the response to infusion of thrombin and adenosine diphosphate. Thromb. Haemostasis **49:** 217.
9. BENNETT, J. S. & G. VILAIRE. 1979. Exposure of platelet fibrinogen receptors by ADP and epinephrine. J. Clin. Invest. **64:** 1393-1401.
10. PLOW, E. F., A. H. SROUJI, D. MEYER, G. MARGUERIE & M. H. GINSBERG. 1984. Evidence that three adhesive proteins interact with a common recognition site on activated platelets. J. Biol. Chem. **259:** 5388.
11. RUGGERI, Z. M. 1985. Distinct epitopes on the platelet membrane glycoprotein IIb/IIIa complex are relevant for interaction with von Willebrand Factor and fibrinogen. (abstr.) Thromb. Haemostasis **54:** 225.

Concluding Remarks

WALTER H. SEEGERS[a]

Department of Physiology
Wayne State University School of Medicine
Detroit, Michigan 48201

INTRODUCTION

Ten of the contributors to this conference have made a career of experimental work involving some aspect of the function of thrombin; others have built on past advances. Furthermore, all inherit the theory and technology supplied by persons specialized in diverse disciplines. During the midcentury period it was first realized that thrombin had multiple functions. This conference covers recently recognized ones, mostly bioregulatory. The presentations stand on their own merits; the purpose of this paper is to correlate some of the facts presented from the past to the present.

PURIFICATION OF THROMBIN

From the beginning, it was self-evident that to purify prothrombin and thrombin was of utmost importance. The real question was how and whether it could be done with the technology available. I began purification work on bovine prothrombin and thrombin in 1937. The publications that appeared from time to time are listed in reference 1, the first report appearing in 1938 and the last in 1980. Consider some of the working conditions of the early years: It was the decade in which threonine was discovered. There was no glass electrode for measuring pH, no freeze-drying apparatus, and no accepted way to assess purity. There were no conferences on hemostasis and thrombosis, nor scheduled air flights. Just as today, however, use was made of the latest technology. Intellectual capacity was not lacking, and in 1939 John Northrop published his book on crystalline enzymes. With rapid progress, industrial production of thrombin began in 1943. The product was of limited use in research. Purified bovine prothrombin,[2] suitable for research work, was first obtained in 1953; purified bovine thrombin[3,4] was available in 1958, and crystals of thrombin[5] in 1972.

About 18 years ago, in association with one of my publications, a referee made a comment that I will remember for a long time. One of the remarks was: "Thrombin is a most intriguing enzyme. However, either because of its inherent complexity or more likely because of the tradition of the blood clotting field, the advances in our

[a]Present address: 2857 Ptarmigan #5, Walnut Creek, CA 94595.

chemical understanding of thrombin are minute compared to the advances in the understanding of many other enzymes. Thus, a dichotomy of standards occurs—judged by 'thrombin standards,' this paper is a milestone pushing our understanding a great deal; on the other hand, judged by normal biochemical standards, it is woefully incomplete. When either standard is applied, it should be published." The referee was right about complexity, and there is a tradition in the blood clotting field. This tradition is characterized by diversity, modesty, enthusiasm, a pioneering spirit, and freedom.

Knowing how to isolate thrombin did not make it easily available for research. To proceed implied a means to obtain plasma, equipment, and reagents. John Fenton saw his opportunity to prepare human thrombin and make it available to many laboratories. His own account[6] of the history is as follows: "Procoagulant α-thrombin is not only the central bioregulatory enzyme in hemostasis but is also the most extensively studied regulatory protease to date. Methods originating from those of Dr. Kent D. Miller while in Albany, New York, and dating back to his graduate studies under Dr. Seegers in Detroit, Michigan, have enabled the preparation of gram amounts of the human enzyme and have permitted numerous investigations over the past decade."

RECOGNITION OF NONFIBRINOGEN-RELATED FUNCTIONS OF THROMBIN

A break with the restricted view that thrombin clots fibrinogen was first made when it was discovered that other factors of the clotting mechanisms were modified by thrombin. A second break came when still other functions such as those considered in this volume were found. One of the first nonfibrinogen-related functions of thrombin involved factor V (Ac-globulin).[7] Shortly after this factor was discovered, it was shown that thrombin increased its activity and, in larger quantities than needed for activation, destroyed the activity.[8] A similar scenario applied to factor VIII:C (antihemophilic factor, platelet cofactor I). Special emphasis was placed on failure to find the activity in natural serum or anticoagulated plasma treated with thrombin.[9,10] These early reports on factors V and VIII:C are now in the background, and inactivation by active protein C (factor XIV_a) is featured.[11,12] Activation of plasma factor XIII by thrombin was recorded in 1962, and a detailed paper appeared in 1964.[13] Stimulation of platelets by thrombin[14] was reported in 1953. Production of factor XIV_a was demonstrated in 1960.

How are the above functions of thrombin possible despite plasma antithrombin III? The answer is all the more remarkable when it is realized that the antithrombin III concentration of plasma is sufficient to neutralize twice the thrombin potential of plasma. Thrombin, factor X_a, and other enzymes neutralize some antithrombin III, but still much antithrombin III remains in serum. Antithrombin III does block thrombin formation and activity if heparin is present.

Ordinarily, during the clotting of blood in test tubes, the thrombin concentration rises to about one hundreth the potential plasma concentration, and antithrombin III does not readily neutralize low concentrations of thrombin. Antithrombin III is characterized by high capacity but low-grade fine-tuning when functioning as inhibitor of thrombin. The fraction of thrombin and/or other enzymes not diverted to antithrombin III can function and be potentiated by a plasma, platelet, or tissue protein. These proteins have variously been called cofactors, accelerators, or modifiers. The respective meaning in each case is (1) together with, (2) accelerating enzyme activity, as will accelerator globulin (factor V), or (3) modification of enzyme specificity.

MODIFIED ENZYME SPECIFICITY

The concept of modified enzyme specificity had its experimental roots in work reported by Landaburu and myself in 1957.[15,16] We observed that storage of purified bovine thrombin preparations was associated with loss of fibrinogen clotting activity. By contrast, large amounts of esterase activity remained. I believe this observation was the first one to bring attention to functional changes in enzyme specificity due to intrinsic modification of structure. The spontaneously modified enzyme was called esterase thrombin or thrombin E. Like fibrinogen, factor V was also refractory to thrombin E. Eventually it could be shown that autolysis of bovine thrombin broke the B-1 polypeptide from the heavy chain and that the fragment remained noncovalently bound to the modified enzyme.[17] Today bovine thrombin E corresponds to beta-thrombin.

Modifications in enzyme specificity occur spontaneously in the presence of proteins with special properties, and by enzymes as well as by chemicals. The latter way is artificial and not within the purview of the present discussion. Modified enzyme catalysis permeates the blood-clotting mechanisms and is one of the important concepts introduced in this century. Some illustrations of cofactor, accelerator, or modifier function follow:

(1) Accelerator globulin (factor V) is essential in the prothrombinase complex for generating thrombin by factor X_a.

(2) Factor VIII:C is needed in the tenase complex for generating factor X_a by factor IX_a.

(3) As a predicting adventure, a protein might be found for the generation of factor IX_a by factor XI_a.

(4) Thrombomodulin is important in the generation of protein Ca (autoprothrombin II-A, factor XIV_a). Thrombomodulin modifies thrombin specificity. In the thrombin-thrombomodulin complex only esterase activity remains, but it can be neutralized by antithrombin III.

(5) Protein S has a place in the inactivation of factor V_a by active protein C.

(6) Possibly, platelet factor 2 modifies thrombin for acceleration of the thrombin-fibrinogen reaction.

(7) Fibrin accelerates the activation of factor XIII with thrombin.

(8) Prothrombin fragment 2 enhances the esterase activity of thrombin. This is an example of a molecular fragment functioning by itself, independent of parent molecule.

(9) Prothrombin fragment 2 accelerates the conversion of prethrombin 2 to thrombin by ecarin.

(10) Prothrombin fragment 2 retards the thrombin-fibrinogen reaction.

(11) Prothrombin fragment 2, covalently bound to thrombin A chain (meizothrombin 1), is thrombin with esterase activity 14.5 times that of activity on fibrinogen.

It seems to me that the above illustrations are sufficient for demonstrating that modified enzyme specificity occurs as a result of variously called cofactors, accelerators, or modifiers. Small quantities from a proenzyme source become effective at locations where needed. In the case of thrombin and factor X_a, functioning occurs in the presence of antithrombin III, which is a high-capacity inhibitor. It is a weak inhibitor at low concentrations of thrombin and/or factor X_a. With heparin, antithrombin III prevails over all.

ZYMOGEN ACTIVITY IN 25% SODIUM CITRATE SOLUTIONS

The generation of thrombin and/or factor X_a in certain concentrated salt solutions represents a discovery[18] used as a base for strong inferences in blood coagulation studies. Enzyme and zymogen function more effectively in 25% sodium citrate than in low salt concentration such as physiological saline solution. Much is known about reactions that occur. No studies, however, are recorded regarding likely conformational changes, nor are there extensive kinetic studies. Experiments to date are characterized by simplicity. They help with considerations taken into account with the complicated prothrombinase and tenase systems for thrombin and factor X_a production. A review can indicate the nature of recorded studies.[19] (1) Thrombin activates purified factor X (FIGURE 1). (2) Prethrombin 1 activates factor X. (3) Prethrombin 2 activates factor X. (4) Prothrombin activates factor X. (5) Factor X activation is accelerated by factor X_a. (6) Factor X plus prothrombin mixtures generate both active enzymes. (7) Prethrombin 1 activation with factor X_a is inhibited with protein Ca (autoprothrombin II-A). (8) Degradation of synthetic substrates with factor X_a or thrombin is accelerated.

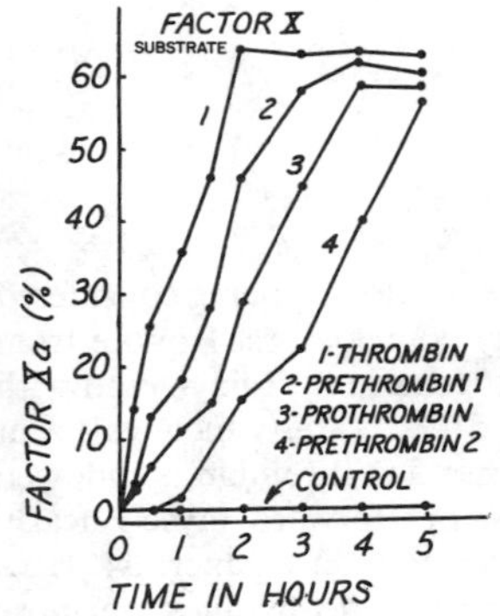

FIGURE 1. Activation of purified bovine factor X in 25% sodium citrate solution at 27°C with thrombin. Purified zymogens were also active in the given order: prethrombin 1, prothrombin, and prethrombin 2. With thrombin activation as activator, no factor X remained as determined by polyacrylamide electrophoresis. Beta factor X_a was the form of the active enzyme.

THROMBIN AND FIBRINOLYSIS

Much current interest centers on the induction of fibrinolysis with active protein C. As soon as active bovine factor XIV_a was obtained as pure protein, it was infused intravenously in dogs.[20] Fibrinolysis was observed shortly after the infusion and for hours thereafter. From further experiments, the initial observation on fibrinolysis was confirmed. Direct activation of purified plasminogen was found to be minimal. Inhibitors of fibrinolysis were depressed. Marlar[12] has reviewed papers on fibrinolysis induced with protein Ca, and the main direction of evidence favors the conclusion that there is a release of tissue fibrinogen activator. An inhibitor of factor XIV_a must also be taken into account, and might be depressed. There are now self-evident questions that imply avenues for further work.

Thrombin does not activate purified plasminogen.

In 1979, Ouyang and I completed a review on snake venoms and blood coagulation.[21] One feature of this survey was the attention to thrombin-like enzymes in venoms and the induction of fibrinolysis *in vivo.* Ancrod has been used to defibrinogenate the blood of patients. By reducing fibrinogen concentration and inducing fibrinolysis, by unknown mechanisms, it was/is possible to deal with undesired thrombosis. The fact that factor XIII was not activated by ancrod may have enhanced the effectiveness of the fibrinolytic process.

Good therapeutic results were at one time obtained with thrombin infusion.[22] The procedure was abandoned, probably because thrombin is presumed to be dangerous under all conditions. Testifying to that can easily be imagined.

In the dog as an animal model, the infusion of acetylated thrombin produced fibrin deposits that disappeared due to fibrinolysis.[23] Although acetylated thrombin preparations produced only esterase activity, some residual thrombin may have made a difference, even though experiments apparently ruled that out. To elicit the thrombolytic effect with thrombin, acetylated thrombin, or thromboserpentin enzymes, they must be infused intravenously. Just adding the enzyme to blood in a test tube is not sufficient. As discussed in the review with Ouyang, factor XIV is the most likely pathway to account for the induction of fibrinolysis with thrombin. By postulating *in vivo* augmented effectiveness of thrombin due to thrombomodulin[24] and/or some other accelerator, one could account for enzyme effectiveness. That thrombin has a role in fibrinolysis is well established as one of the pathways for promoting fibrinolysis.

CONCLUSION

Thrombin and fibrinolysis are not new subjects. They were already being considered before my birth. P. Nolf in Brussels was one of the early contributors. I quote from a letter he sent me in 1951, when he was probably an octogenarian. "I have read with great interest the paper of M. Mason Guest and Arnold G. Ware, which you sent me recently. One of the conclusions of the authors is that purified thrombin is endowed with fibrinolytic activities, an opinion which I have first put forward myself nearly fifty years ago. In 1908, I devoted to the defense of this conception a paper, 54 pages long, of which I send you a copy by separate mail. I considered this question more from the point of view of biology and am glad to see that there are now new arguments in favour of it which are of a chemical nature."

REFERENCES

1. Seegers, W. H. 1981. A personal perspective on hemostasis and thrombosis (1937-1981). Semin. Thromb. Hemostasis **7:** 177-307.
2. Seegers, W. H. & N. Alkjaersig. 1953. Comparative properties of human and bovine prothrombin. Am. J. Physiol. **172:** 731-736.

3. SEEGERS, W. H., W. G. LEVINE & R. S. SHEPARD. 1958. Further studies on the purification of thrombin. Can. J. Biochem. Physiol. **36:** 603-611.
4. SEEGERS, W. H., G. CASILLAS, R. S. SHEPARD, W. R. THOMAS & P. HALICK. 1959. Some properties of thrombin preparations. Can. J. Biochem. Physiol. **37:** 775-785.
5. TSERNOGLOU, D., D. A. WALZ, L. E. MCCOY & W. H. SEEGERS. 1972. A new thrombin: purification, amino acid composition, and crystallization. Thromb. Res. **1:** 533-537.
6. FENTON II, J. W. 1981. Thrombin specificity. *In* Contributions to Hemostasis. D. A. Walz & L. E. McCoy, Eds. Ann. N.Y. Acad. Sci. **370:** 468-495.
7. WARE, A. G. & W. H. SEEGERS. 1948. Serum Ac-globulin: formation from plasma Ac-globulin, role in blood coagulation, partial purification, properties, and quantitative determination. Am. J. Physiol. **152:** 567-576.
8. WARE, A. G., J. L. FAHEY & W. H. SEEGERS. 1948. Platelet extracts, fibrin formation and interaction of purified prothrombin and thromboplastin. Am. J. Physiol. **154:** 140-147.
9. GRAHAM, J. B., G. D. PENICK & K. M. BRINKHOUS. 1951. Utilization of antihemophilic factor during clotting of canine blood and plasma. Am. J. Physiol. **164:** 710-717.
10. JOHNSON, S. A. & W. H. SEEGERS. 1954. Studies on the plasma defect in hemophilia. Rev. Hematol. **9:** 529-535.
11. SEEGERS, W. H. & O. N. ULUTIN. 1961. Autoprothrombin-II anticoagulant (autoprothrombin-IIA). Thromb. Diath. Haemorrh. **6:** 270-281.
12. MARLAR, R. A. 1986. Protein C: activation, anticoagulant and fibrinolytic action. *In* Prothrombin and Other Vitamin K Proteins. W. H. Seegers & D. A. Walz, Eds.: 69-80. C.R.C. Press. Boca Raton, FL.
13. LORAND, L. & K. KONICHI. 1964. Activation of the fibrin stabilizing factor of plasma by thrombin. Arch. Biochem. Biophys. **105:** 58-67.
14. DEROBERTIS, E., P. PASEYRO & M. REISSIG. 1953. Electron microscopic studies of the action of thrombin on blood platelets. Blood **8:** 587-595.
15. LANDABURU, R. H. & W. H. SEEGERS. 1957. Further studies of prothrombin derivatives. Proc. Soc. Exp. Biol. Med. **94:** 708-710.
16. SEEGERS, W. H. & R. H. LANDABURU. 1957. Esterase and clotting activity derived from purified prothrombin. Am. J. Physiol. **191:** 167-173.
17. SEEGERS, W. H., J. REUTERBY, G. MURANO, L. E. MCCOY & B. B. L. AGRAWAL. 1971. Studies on the nature of thrombin. Thromb. Diath. Haemorrh. (Suppl.) **47:** 325-337.
18. SEEGERS, W. H. 1949. Activation of purified prothrombin. Proc. Soc. Exp. Biol. Med. **72:** 677-680.
19. TENG, C. M. & W. H. SEEGERS. 1981. Activation of factor X and thrombin zymogens in 25% sodium citrate solution. Thromb. Res. **22:** 203-212.
20. SEEGERS, W. H., L. E. MCCOY, H. D. GROBEN, N. SAKURAGAWA & B. B. L. AGRAWAL. 1972. Purification and some properties of autoprothrombin II-A: an anticoagulant perhaps also related to fibrinolysis. Thromb. Res. **1:** 443-460.
21. SEEGERS, W. H. & C. OUYANG. 1979. Snake venoms and blood coagulation. *In* Handbook of Experimental Pharmacology. C. Y. Lee, Ed. **52:** 685-750. Springer Verlag. Berlin, Heidelberg, New York.
22. BRAMBEL, C. E. 1957. Proteases in the clotting mechanism. Ann. N.Y. Acad. Sci. **68:** 67-69.
23. BROERSMA, R. J., L. E. MCCOY & W. H. SEEGERS. 1971. Production of microvascular thrombosis and lysis with acetylated thrombin. Thromb. Diath. Haemorrh. **47:** 353-360.
24. OWEN, W. G. & C. T. ESMON. 1981. Functional properties of an endothelial co-factor for thrombin catalyzed activation of protein C. J. Biol. Chem. **256:** 5532-5535.

Proteolysis of Human α-Thrombin by Human Neutrophil Elastase Results in Decreased Fibrinogen Clotting and Platelet-Stimulatory Activity

MARK S. BROWER,[a] KIMBERLY E. GARRY,[a] AND JOHN W. FENTON II[b]

[a]*Specialized Center for Research in Thrombosis*
Division of Hematology-Oncology
Department of Medicine
The New York Hospital-Cornell Medical Center
New York, New York 10021

[b]*Wadsworth Center for Laboratories and Research*
New York State Department of Health
Albany, New York 12201

As blood clots, elastase, the major polymorphonuclear leukocyte (PMN) neutral protease, is released in amounts that can exceed 4 μg/ml.[1,2] Elastase is also released in a variety of other inflammatory conditions.[3,4] We therefore studied the interaction between human PMN elastase and human α-thrombin.

Highly purified elastase (specific activity 95% by active site titration) cleaved human α-thrombin, resulting in two fragments that could not be separated under nondenaturing conditions. As analyzed by sodium dodecyl sulfate-polyacrylamide gel electrophoresis (SDS-PAGE), the larger fragment ($M_r \sim 22{,}000$) was disulfide-linked to the thrombin A chain. The smaller fragment ($M_r \sim 13{,}000$) contained the active-site serine as indicated by the recovery of a covalent bond between this fragment and antithrombin III on SDS-PAGE. These findings suggested that elastase cleaved the α-thrombin B chain near the thrombin γ-cleavage site. Heparin accelerated the proteolysis of α-thrombin by elastase.

Elastase-modified α-thrombin retained amidolytic activity. It was approximately 14% as potent as α-thrombin, however, in stimulating platelet aggregation and release, and it was approximately 32% as potent as α-thrombin in clotting fibrinogen.

We conclude that the limited digestion of α-thrombin by elastase could be an important physiologic mechanism for regulation of thrombin-substrate and thrombin-membrane interactions. Additionally, elastase-modified thrombin, and its two halves, FI, containing the chemotactic site, and FII, containing the active-site serine, can serve as useful probes for investigating the interactions of thrombin with fluid phase substrates and with membrane receptors.

REFERENCES

1. BROWER, M. S. & P. C. HARPEL. 1983. α_1-Antitrypsin-human leukocyte elastase complexes in blood: Quantification by an enzyme-linked differential antibody immunosorbent assay and comparison and α_2-plasmin inhibitor-plasmin complexes. Blood **61:** 842-849.
2. PLOW, E. F. 1981. Leukocyte elastase release during blood coagulation: A potential mechanism for activation of the alternate pathway. J. Clin. Invest. **69:** 564-572.
3. OHLSSON, K. & I. OLSSON. 1977. The extracellular release of granulocyte collagenase and elastase during phagocytosis and inflammatory processes. Scand. J. Haematol. **19:** 145-152.
4. EGBRING, R., W. SCHMIDT, G. FUCHS & K. HAVEMANN. 1977. Demonstration of granulocytic proteases in plasma of patients with acute leukemia and septicemia with coagulation defects. Blood **49:** 219-231.

Effect of Terbium on Thrombin and Antithrombin-Thrombin Interaction

D. DEL PRINCIPE, A. MENICHELLI,
A.M. FIORENTINO, C. COLISTRA, P.M. STRAPPINI,
AND A. FINAZZI-AGRO[a]

Department of Pediatrics
[a]Department of Experimental Medicine, II
University of Rome
Rome, Italy

Interactions between thrombin and antithrombin are influenced by calcium ions.[1] In fact, it has been reported that $CaCl_2$ potentiates the heparin-modulated antithrombin III inhibition of thrombin. A similar potentiation of calcium on thrombin inactivation by antithrombin may occur in the absence of heparin. Thus, calcium appears to play a complex role in the interactions involving thrombin, heparin, antithrombin, and fibrinogen. The mechanisms of these effects are poorly understood. Because lanthanide ions show chemical properties that make them suitable probes for the interactions of Ca^{2+} with biological systems, we investigated the effect of one of them, namely Tb^{3+}, on thrombin and on thrombin-antithrombin interactions.

MATERIAL AND METHODS

Commercial bovine thrombin was purified by Amberlite chromatography. Human plasma was freed from fibrinogen, heating citrated plasma at 56°C for 5 min, followed by centrifugation. Partially purified fibrinogen was obtained from Sigma Chemical Company. All other chemicals were at least reagent grade and used without further purification. The thrombin clotting activity was determined at 37°C, using fibrinogen as substrate.[1] Amidase activity was determined by the TAME-esterase activity. Isotachophoresis was performed as previously reported.[2] Fluorescence measurements were made on a FICA-L55 spectrofluorometer.

RESULTS

The addition of Tb^{3+} (1 mM) to thrombin was accompanied by a 20% quenching in intrinsic protein fluorescence (FIGURE 1A). We were unable to detect any Tb^{3+}

binding, however, by protein-sensitized luminescence of the lanthanide.[3] Calcium ions quenched the thrombin fluorescence in the same way (FIGURE 1B), ruling out any specific effect of the lanthanide. This effect was concomitant with a drop in coagulant and esterase activity of thrombin, as reported in a previous report.[4] Moreover, the metals enhanced the inhibitory effect of the fibrinogen-free plasma. Ca^{2+} and Tb^{3+} modified the isotachophoretic pattern of thrombin, in that the peak of high mobility decreased, whereas the low-mobility peak increased.[2]

DISCUSSION

Our results show that Tb^{3+} and Ca^{2+} affect some properties of thrombin, such as the intrinsic fluorescence and the isotachophoretic mobility. Moreover, the metals

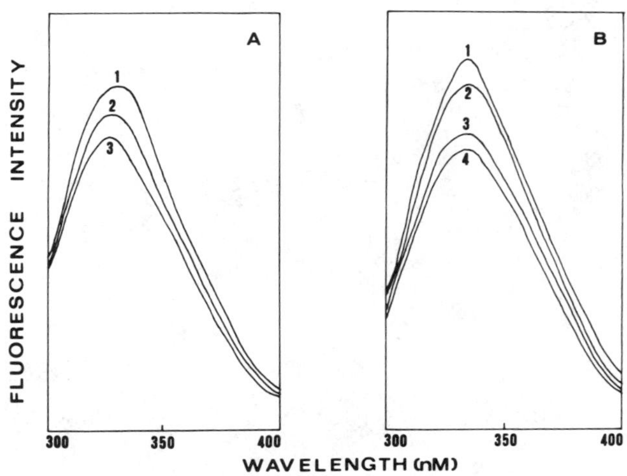

FIGURE 1. A: Emission spectra of 5 μM thrombin (1), thrombin plus 10^{-3} M Tb^{3+} (2), thrombin plus 5 × 10^{-3} M Tb^{3+} (3). **B**: Emission spectra of thrombin (1), thrombin plus 10^{-3}M (2), 5 × 10^{-3}M (3), or 7 × 10^{-3}M (4) Ca^{2+}.

reduce the functional activity of the enzyme and enhance the rate of the inactivation of thrombin by antithrombin III. Martin and Richardson[3] have pointed out that the Ln^{3+} substitution for Ca^{2+} in proteins is important for evaluating the role of the latter. They speculated that if Ln^{3+}-substitute protein still retains activity, Ca^{2+} may play a structural role. Even though binding of Tb^{3+} to thrombin was not directly demonstrated by fluorescence studies, our results may suggest that both Ca^{2+} and Tb^{3+} affect thrombin, possibly by a weak binding. This binding may cause a conformational change or a proteolytic cleavage of the protein, which favors the inactivation brought about by antithrombin.

REFERENCES

1. LUNDBLAD, R. L., J. C. ROBERTS, D. K. JOHNSTON, G. L. FEATHERSTONE & M. J. GRIFFITH. 1981. Thromb. Res. **22:** 135-146.
2. DEL PRINCIPE, D., G. MANCUSO, C. D'ARCANGELO, A. MENICHELLI, P. M. STRAPPINI, S. DEL VECCHIO. 1980. Thromb. Res. **20:** 137-142.
3. MARTIN, R. B. & F. S. Q. RICHARDSON. 1979. Rev. Biophys. **12:** 181-209.
4. LONG, W. F. & F. B. WILLIAMSON. 1982. Biochem. Biophysics. Res. Commum. **104:** 363-368.

A New Form of Proteolyzed Bovine Thrombin[a]

BRIAN F. P. EDWARDS, VINOD KUMAR, BARBARA A. BEDFORD, PHILIP D. MARTIN, AND RAJU D. KUNJUMMEN

Department of Biochemistry
Wayne State University
Detroit, Michigan 48201

Three forms of proteolyzed bovine alpha-thrombin are known.[1] If the polypeptide structure of alpha-thrombin is represented as [A:1-49, B:1-259] where the 49 residue A chain is linked to the 259 residue B-chain by a disulfide bond between A:22 and B:119, then beta-thrombin has the structure [A:14-30, B:1-65, B:74-259], and gamma-thrombin has an additional cut near residue B:180 that has not been defined precisely due to lack of material. A similar but not identical pattern exists for human alpha-thrombin.[2]

As part of a project to determine the crystallographic structure of bovine thrombin, we have investigated the proteolysis of bovine thrombin under conditions that are close to those used in crystallization. As shown in lane A of FIGURE 1, the dominant species after incubation at 24°C without ammonium sulfate is beta-thrombin, which has a B:1-65 chain of 14 kDa and a B:74-259 chain of 24 kDa. These identifications were made by comparison with a sample of beta-thrombin supplied by R. Lundblad. The band at 33 kDa is the B:1-259 chain of alpha-thrombin; the molecular weights of the B:1-259 band and its derivatives that contain asparagine-53 are anomalously high due to the polysaccharide chain that is attached to that residue. Lanes B and C show that a different species is produced in 35% ammonium sulfate; the process is much slower at 4°C (lane B) than at 22°C (lane C). Electroelution and Edman sequencing indicated that the new bands were B:1-150 at 21 kDa, B:151-259 at 13 kDa, and B:74-150 at 10 kDa. The carboxyl termini of these peptides might be shorter than what is shown. FIGURE 2 shows the production of the chains over time. Our interpretation of these data, summarized in the insert, is that a new form, which we have labeled beta-2-thrombin, is produced that has B:1-150 and B:151-259 chains. The presence of an A-chain attached to the 21 kDa species has been shown by electrophoresis on nonreducing gels. A subsequent cut at arg-73 produces a species similar to gamma-thrombin that contains the 10 kDa chain. The model predicts that the concentrations of the 14 kDa and 13 kDa chains should be the sum of the concentration of the 10 kDa and, respectively, the 24 kDa or 21 kDa chains. The data for the 13 kDa chain agrees with this prediction, but the data for the 14 kDa chain does not, probably because it breaks down further to chains below 10 kDa. Comparison with

[a] This work was supported by NIH Grant GM33192 and a Grant-in-aid from the American Heart Association of Michigan.

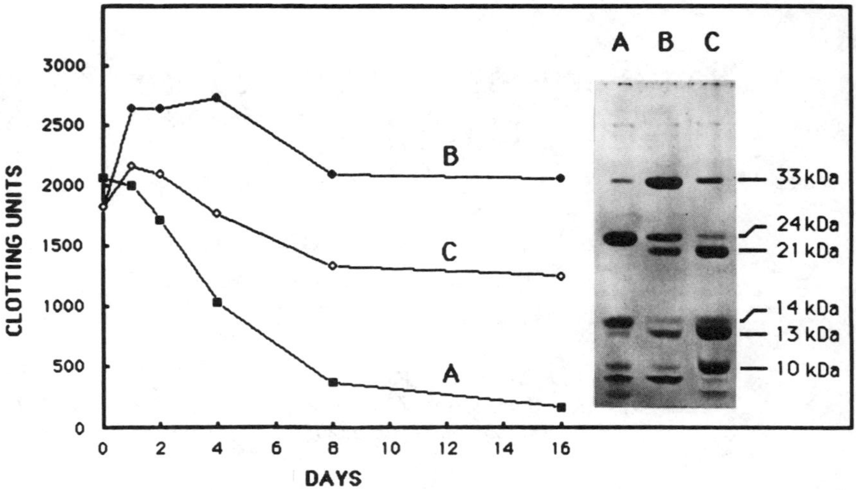

FIGURE 1. Concentrated solutions of bovine alpha-thrombin (23 mg/ml) were incubated for 16 days in 0.05 M phosphate buffer, pH 7.0: (A) 24°C; (B) 4°C with 35% saturated ammonium sulfate; (C) 24°C with 35% saturated ammonium sulfate. Samples were electrophoresed in 1% sodium dodecyl sulfate on a 17% polyacrylamide Laemmli gel under reducing conditions.

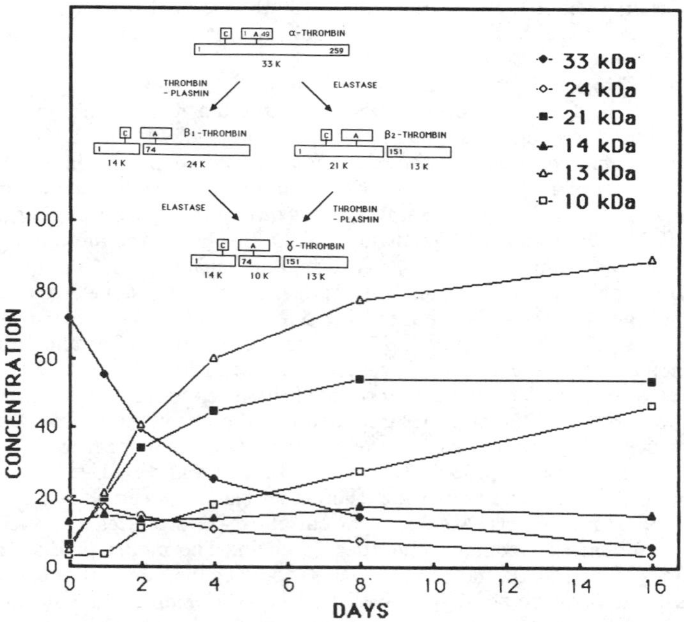

FIGURE 2. The relative concentrations, in arbitrary units, of the different polypeptide chains that were generated as a function of time in experiment C of FIGURE 1 were determined by integrating spectrophotometric scans of the polyacrylamide gel. The integrated area for each band, expressed as a fraction of the total area for the lane, was converted to relative moles and then scaled by a factor that made the total thrombin, that is, the sum of the concentrations of the 33 kDa, 24 kDa, 21 kDa, and 10 kDa bands, at zero time equal to 100 units. The insert shows the model used to explain the data and identifies the various chains.

the data of FIGURE 1 indicates that beta-2-thrombin has significantly more clotting activity than beta-thrombin. Apparently, separation of thr-150 and ser-151 does not disturb the active site as severely as does separation of arg-73 and lys-74. Recently, elastase has been reported to cut human alpha-thrombin at the same position, but between ala-150 and asn-151.[3] We have confirmed that porcine elastase will rapidly cleave bovine thrombin into the 21 kDa and 13 kDa fragments. Consequently, it is very likely that beta-2-thrombin is generated by an elastase-like protease that copurifies with it. In contrast to the porcine enzyme, however, this contaminating enzyme must be activated by ammonium sulfate, or perhaps requires thrombin to be potentiated as a substrate by a salt-induced conformational change.

REFERENCES

1. KINGDON, H. S., C. M. NOYES & R. L. LUNDBLAD. 1977. *In* Chemistry and Biology of Thrombin. R. L. Lundblad, J. W. Fenton II & K. G. Mann, Eds.: 91-96. Ann Arbor Sci. Publ. Inc., Ann Arbor, MI.
2. BOISSEL, J. P., B. LE BONNIEC, M. J. RABIET, D. LABIE & J. ELION. 1984. J. Biol. Chem. **259:** 5691-5697.
3. KAWABATA, S, R. MORITA, S. IWANAGA & H. IGARASHI. 1985. J. Biochem. (Tokyo) **97:** 325-331.

Inhibition of Tissue Plasminogen Activator by Protein or Synthetic Thrombin Inhibitors[a]

N. GILBOA AND J. W. FENTON II

Wadsworth Center for Laboratories and Research
New York State Department of Health
Albany, New York 12201

and

Albany Medical College
Department of Pediatrics
Albany, New York 12208

INTRODUCTION

Selective inhibition of active thrombin in clots and following fibrinolysis[1] is required when the amidolytic activity of tissue plasminogen activator (TPA) has to be determined. This is due to the fact that the K_m of thrombin's reaction with the chromogenic substrate Leu-Pro-Arg-pNa (S2288), which is commonly used to determine the amidolytic activity of TPA, is much lower (3×10^{-6}M) than with the two-chain TPA (3×10^{-4}M).

METHODS

The effects of four thrombin inhibitors on human thrombin purified as described previously[2] and on TPA (a gift from Dr. Collen) were compared. The studies were performed using S2288 (Leu-Pro-Arg-pNa), as the chromogenic substrate for thrombin, and TPA in the presence or absence of antithrombin III (ATIII), hirudin, PPACK (D-Phe-Pro-Arg-CH_2-C1), and Thromstop [*N*-20-naphthylsulfonyl-glycyl)-*D,L*-amidinophenylalanin piperidine]. The rates of reactions were determined with the Biotek microplate reader set on dual wavelengths of 405 nm and 540 nm. The range of S2288 concentrations was 1×10^{-4}M to 3.25×10^{-3}M.

[a] This work has been supported in part by the New York Affiliate of the American Heart Association.

RESULTS

Hirudin inhibited the amidolytic activity of thrombin, but had no effect on TPA (FIGURE 1). With the maximum of 37.5 U/ml of thrombin used in our experiments, 78% inhibition was achieved. To obtain a 50% inhibition of thrombin, 0.8 U/ml of hirudin were required.

ATIII, at 0.094 U/ml caused 73% inhibition in the amidolytic activity of thrombin (0.06 U/ml), with the I_{50} being approximately 0.063 U/ml. When 0.6 U/ml of thrombin were used, 3 U/ml and 0.15 U/ml of ATIII caused 93% and 50% inhibition, respectively. As was the case with hirudin, ATIII caused no inhibition of TPA. Preincubation of ATIII with heparin up to 19 U/ml had no effect on the amidolytic activities of either thrombin or TPA (not shown).

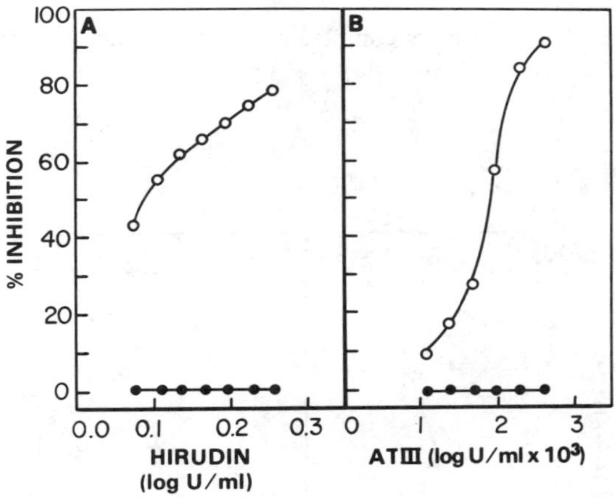

FIGURE 1. Thrombin (0.06 U/ml) (○) or TPA (●) (12.5 U/ml) in 50 μl of Tris (50 mM), NaCl (150 mM), pH 7.4 with 0.01% triton X-100 were incubated with various concentrations of hirudin or ATIII in 75 μl of the Tris NaCl-Triton buffer for 20 min at 37°. The chromogenic substrate, S2288 (0.324 mM) in H_2O, was then added to each well and the rate of the reactions determined at 25°C. **A:** Inhibition of thrombin and TPA with hirudin. **B:** Inhibition of thrombin and TPA with ATIII.

PPACK caused 100% inhibition of both thrombin (0.06 U/ml) and TPA (19 U/ml) at a concentration of 3.4×10^{-7}M (FIGURE 2). With decrease in PPACK's concentration to 1.1×10^{-8}M, however, the inhibition of TPA also decreased rapidly to 18% (I_{50}-4.4×10^{-8}M), whereas it still inhibited 96% of thrombin activity. The K_m(app) of TPA in the presence of PPACK (7.15×10^{-8}M) was 1.14×10^{-3}M, and V_{max} was 4.8×10^{-3}M/min. Without PPACK, K_m was 3.6×10^{-4}M, and V_{max} was 3.95×10^{3}M/minutes.

Thromstop caused a relatively similar inhibition of both thrombin and TPA. Thromstop (1.87×10^{-5}M) caused 93% and 57% inhibition of thrombin and TPA respectively. The I_{50} for thrombin was 9×10^{-7}M. Thrombin was inhibited 21% and

TPA 3 percent. The K_m(app) of TPA in the presence of Thromstop (9.4×10^{-6}M) was 2.4×10^{-4}M, the V_{max} was 1.8×10^{-3}M/min, and the K_i was 5.41×10^{-6}M.

DISCUSSION

Hirudin has a very high-binding affinity to thrombin (K_i 6.2×10^{-11}M),[3] but in spite of the structural similarities between thrombin and TPA, neither hirudin or ATIII inhibited TPA. Although Thromstop's affinity for thrombin is much higher (K_i 1.5×10^{-8}M)[4] than for TPA, it is apparent from FIGURE 2 that it will be difficult to achieve an adequately selective inhibition of thrombin with this competitive inhibitor. On the other hand, PPACK can be used for the selective inhibition of thrombin in the presence of TPA.

In addition, as hirudin inhibits completely thrombin's fibrin-forming activity unit for unit, it seems that it is considerably less effective in the inhibition of thrombin's amidolytic activity.

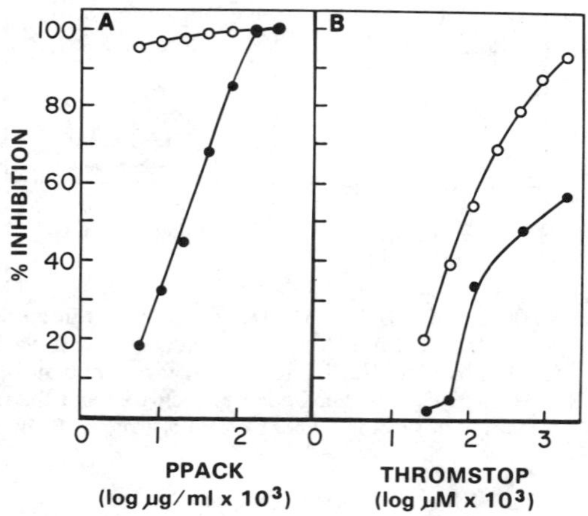

FIGURE 2. Procedure is identical to the one described in FIGURE 1, except that varying concentrations of PPACK (**A**) or Thromstop (**B**) were added to thrombin (○) or TPA (●).

ACKNOWLEDGMENT

The authors thank Mr. W. J. Collis for technical help.

REFERENCES

1. FRANCIS, C. W., R. E. MARKHAM, JR., G. H. BARLOW, T. M. FLORACK, D. M. DOBRZYNSKI & V. J. MARDER. 1983. Thrombin activity of fibrin thrombi and soluble plasmic derivatives. J. Lab. Clin. Med. **102:** 220-230.
2. FENTON II, J. W., M. J. FASCO, A. B. STACKROW, D. L. ARONSON, A. M. YOUNG & J. S. FINLAYSON. 1977. Human thrombins. Production, evaluation and properties of alpha-thrombin. J. Biol. Chem. **252:** 3587-3598.
3. LANDIS, B. H., M. P. ZAMBINSKI, G. J. M. LAFLEUR, D. H. BING & J. W. FENTON II. 1978. Human alpha-thrombin differential inhibition with hirudin. Fed. Proc. **37:** 1445.
4. SVENDSEN, L., M. BROGLI, G. LINDEBERG & K. STOCKER. 1984. Differentiation of thrombin and factor Xa amidolytic activity in plasma by means of a synthetic proteinase inhibitor. Thromb. Res. **34:** 457-462.

Hematin-Derived Anticoagulant Retards Fibrin Formation and Is Inhibited by Iron Chelators

ROBERT L. JONES

Rockefeller University
New York, New York 10021

In clinical trials for the treatment of acute intermittent porphyria, hematin infusions were found to produce prolongation of coagulation times.[1] Addition of hematin solutions to plasma *in vitro* has also been found to produce this phenomenon.[2] We have shown that the prolongation of APTT, thrombin time and prothrombin times, is due to an oxidative degradation product of hematin rather than the parent compound. We have designated this product hematin-derived anticoagulant (HDA).[3] To examine the mechanism of HDA, we have studied the effect on fibrin formation as assessed by fibrinopeptide A generation. We have also found that the activity of HDA is inhibited by imidazole and by the iron chelator desferrioxamine.

HDA was prepared by allowing hematin to stand in carbonate buffer (pH = 7.4) for four weeks. The resultant HDA prolonged thrombin clotting times by at least 200 percent. FPA generation was studied by mixing fibrinogen (2.5 mg/ml) and thrombin (.25 U/ml) in .05 M Hepes buffer, pH 7.5, and measuring resultant FPA by radioimmunoassay. Inhibition of FPA generation was studied after incubating HDA (0.006 mg/ml) with thrombin for 15 minutes before mixing with fibrinogen. At 60 seconds of thrombin-fibrinogen reaction, HDA showed a 100-fold suppression of FPA generation (2.45 ng/mg fibrinogen with HDA versus 240 ng/mg fibrinogen without HDA). HDA also showed a marked suppression of the rate of FPA generation in this system (FIGURE 1).

HDA prolongation of thrombin clotting times was examined and found to be blocked or reversed by iron chelating compounds. Thrombin times were performed with human fibrinogen with the addition of imidazole (0-50 mM) or desferrioxamine (0-.6 mM) before or after the addition of HDA. Both imidazole and desferrioxamine showed a dose-dependent blockade (added before HDA) and reversal of HDA prolongation of thrombin times. Imidazole (30 mM) showed 100% and desferrioxamine showed 70% (.6 mM) blockade and reversal of HDA. These effects were inhibited by adding ferric citrate to the reaction mixture, indicating a role for iron in reversal and blockade of HDA by these compounds. Also, desferrioxamine, converted to ferrioxamine with ferric chloride, showed no effect on HDA when added at the same concentration as desferrioxamine (FIGURE 2).

Inasmuch as imidazole and desferrioxamine are both capable of chelating iron, and because blockade and reversal of HDA activity are both reversed by adding iron, we propose that the mechanism of HDA involves iron or another chelatable metal. Reversal of HDA activity by these agents also suggests that HDA does not produce covalent modification or destruction of the coagulation proteins involved in the mech-

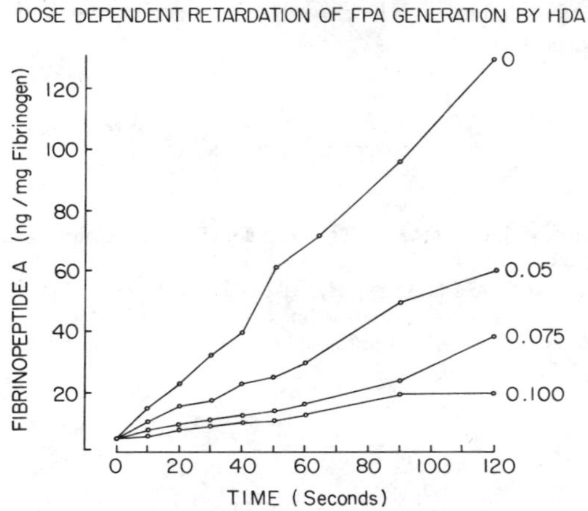

FIGURE 1. Dose dependent blockade of HDA by desferal. Thrombin times were performed with human fibrinogen (2.5 mg/ml) in veronal buffer and thrombin. Prior to the clotting time, either desferrioxamine of ferrioxamine was added to the fibrinogen solution. After 5 minutes, HDA (0.06 mg/ml) was added and the thrombin time performed 2 minutes later.

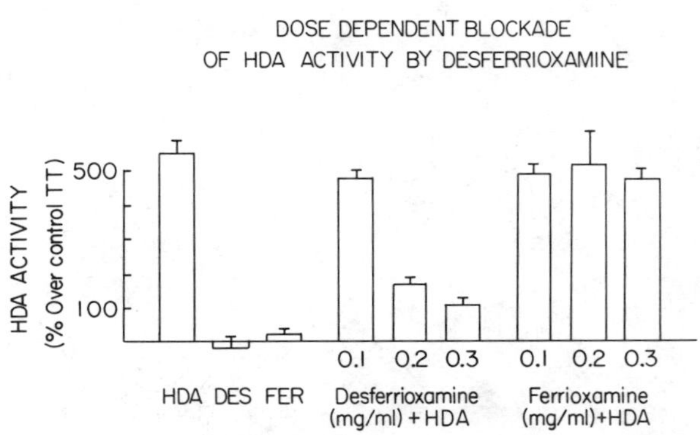

FIGURE 2. Suppression of the rate of FPA generation with HDA. Fibrinogen 1 mg/ml was reacted with thrombin (.1 U/ml) at 37°C. The reaction was terminated by the addition of 100 μl of FPA anticoagulant solution. HDA was added at various concentrations (0-.10 mg/ml). Each point represents the mean of duplicate determinations. HDA produces a dose-dependent suppression of the rate of FPA generation.

anism. Imidazole inhibition of HDA might also be explained by displacement of HDA from a histidine residue on a coagulation protein such as thrombin. Histidine residues are important in the proteolytic mechanism of thrombin and other coagulation proteases. The precise mechanism of HDA awaits the purification and definition of the structure of this compound.

REFERENCES

1. GLUECK, R., D. GREEN, I. COHEN & C. TS'AO. 1983. Hematin: Unique effects on hemostasis. Blood **61:** 243-248.
2. GREEN, D., N. REYNOLDS, J. KLEIN, H. KOHL & C. TS'AO. 1983. The inactivation of hemostatic factors by hematin. J. Lab. Clin. Med. **102:** 361-369.
3. JONES, R. L. 1986. Hematin derived anticoagulant: Generation *in vitro* and *in vivo.* J. Exp. Med. **163:** 724-739.

Modulation of Thrombin Activity by Zinc

GERARD MARX

Department of Hematology
Beilinson Medical Center
Petah Tikva, Israel

DISCUSSION

Initial interest in the role of zinc in hemostasis was based on the observations that Zn^{2+} accelerates the formation of thrombin-induced fibrin clots (FIGURE 1).[1] Altered thermal stability and decreased intrinsic fluorescence of human thrombin in the presence of zinc (FIGURE 2) attest to the formation of a Zn^{2+}-thrombin complex. Moreover, the proteolytic effectiveness of thrombin toward fibrinogen and synthetic substrate is severely reduced by physiologic levels of Zn^{2+} (FIGURE 2A and B).[2–4] This is similar to Zn^{2+} inhibition of other serine proteases, notably nerve growth factor and trypsin.[5,6] Apparently, the net procoagulant effect observed with Zn^{2+} (FIGURE 1) is due an increased rate of fibrin polymerization, which actually masks the inhibitory influence of zinc on thrombin proteolytic activity.

A noteworthy aspect of this is that the thrombin complexed by Zn^{2+} becomes less susceptible to the inhibitory effect of antithrombin III (AT-III) (FIGURE 1B, middle and upper curve).[1] In the presence of Ca^{2+}, preincubation of thrombin with Zn^{2+} precludes inhibition by AT-III. These experiments demonstrate that the effective activities of thrombin and AT-III can be modified by zinc in a concentration-dependent manner. How this impinges on the anticoagulant activity of heparin, which operates as a cofactor of AT-III, remains to be explored.

Studies with bone marrow-derived mast cells (BMMC) reveal that Zn^{2+} significantly inhibits BMMC activation by thrombin. Flow cytometry with FITC-thrombin indicates that zinc does not alter the binding of thrombin to the cells and that catalytically active thrombin is required for BMMC activation.[3,5] Apparently, the inhibitory effect of Zn^{2+} on thrombin activation of mast cells is due to either interference with the proteolysis of BMMC thrombin receptor or blockage of the calcium channel associated with the Ca^{2+} influx of thrombin-stimulated cells.

Modulation of thrombin activities by zinc may have physiological implications. The nutritional requirement of zinc for normal coagulation and immune response has been documented.[12–16] Platelets and mast cells accumulate zinc,[6–11] activated platelets secrete zinc,[10] and one might expect activated mast cells to release stored zinc, although this has not been examined. In the context of the above-described experiments and the cited literature, it seems that a measure of physiologic control over coagulation processes and immune response could be exercised by the timely secretion of Zn^{2+} from activated cells.

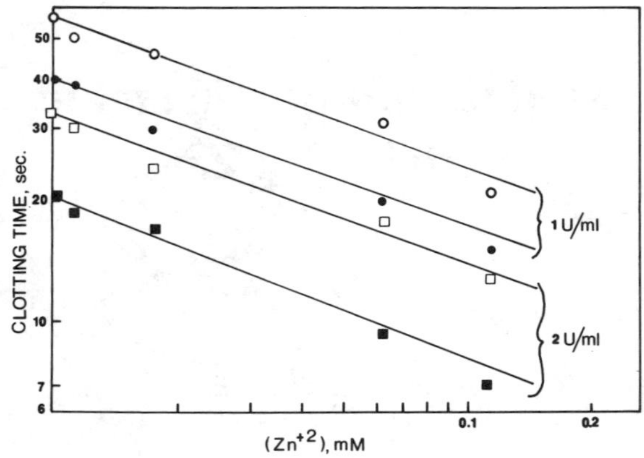

FIGURE 1A. Thrombin-induced (1 and 2 U/ml) clotting time of fibrinogen at increasing Zn^{2+} (0.□) with 2.5 mM Ca (●,■). (G. Marx & A. Eldor.[1] With permission from the *American Journal of Hematology*.)

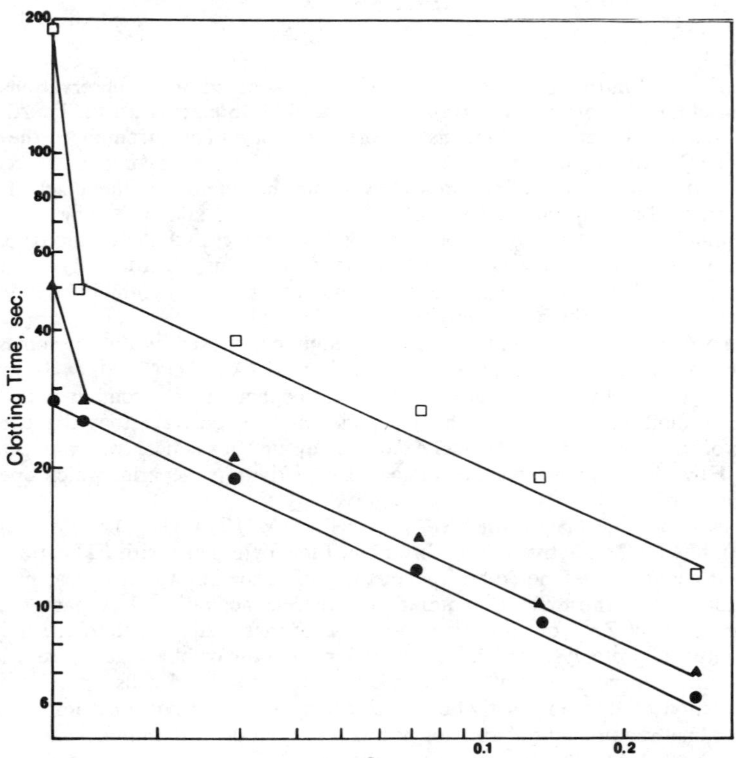

FIGURE 1B. Log clotting time of thrombin-induced fibrin clot formation (●), preincubated with 0.1 U/ml AT-III (□), with 2 mM calcium (▲).[1] Based purely on clotting time, it would be difficult to specify thrombin activity. (G. Marx & A. Eldor.[1] With permission from the *American Journal of Hematology*.)

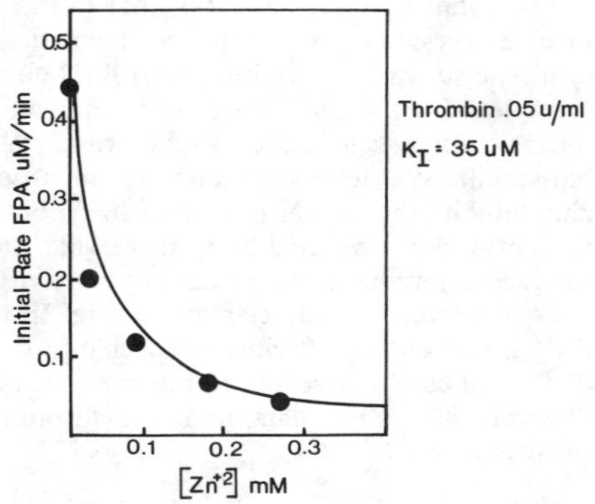

FIGURE 2A. Decreased thrombin-induced release of FPA (0.05 U/ml) at increasing Zn^{2+} (by radioimmunoassay). (G. Marx & P. Hopmeier.[2] With permission from the *American Journal of Hematology.*)

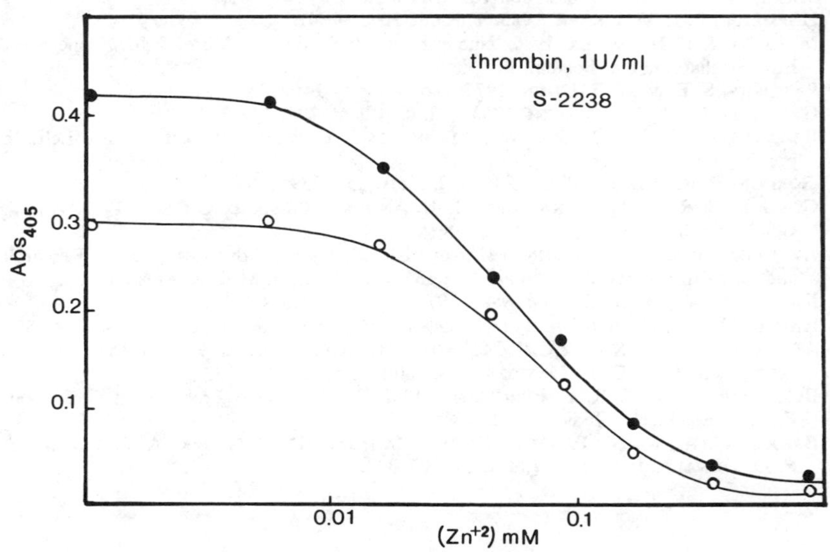

FIGURE 2B. Decreased rate of amidolysis of S-2238 by thrombin (1 U/ml) with increasing Zn^{2+}.[4] Both assays (2A and B) indicate that the proteolytic (amidolytic) activity of thrombin decreases in the presence of Zn^{2+}.

SUMMARY

The ability of Zn^{2+} (< 100 μM) to modify thrombin activity has been examined in a few systems, including transformation of fibrinogen into fibrin, amidolysis of synthetic substrate, inhibition by AT-III, and activation of cultured murine mast cells. Complexation of Zn^{2+} by purified human thrombin is accompanied by decreased intrinsic fluorescence, decreased thermal stability, and decreased amidolysis of thrombin-specific synthetic substrates. In the absence of chelating agents (citrate, EDTA), zinc inhibits the rate of release of FPA, but nevertheless accelerates the formation of the fibrin clot, presumably by increasing the rate of fibrin polymerization. Zinc also significantly reduces the proimmune activity of thrombin to mast cells, but does not alter its binding to the cell membrane. In all of the above systems, the influence of Zn^{2+} on thrombin activities is specific in that it is not mimicked by Mg^{2+}, Mn^{2+}, or Cu^{2+}, and can be observed in the presence of millimolar levels of Ca^{2+}. These findings illustrate how Zn^{2+} can modulate thrombin activity towards plasma and cellular substrates.

REFERENCES

1. Marx, G. & A. Eldor. 1985. Am. J. Hematol. **19:** 151-159.
2. Marx, G. & P. Hopmeier. 1986. Am. J. Hematol. **22:** 347-353.
3. Hopmeier, P. & M. Fisher. 1985. Thromb. Res. **54:** 41.
4. Marx, G. & P. Hopmeier. 1986. Zinc enzymes. I. Bertini, W. Maret & M. Zeppezaver, Eds. Birkhäuser, Inc. Boston.
5. Pattison, S. E. & M. F. Dunn. 1975. Biochemistry **14:** 2733-2739.
6. Green, N. M. & H. Neurath. 1953. J. Biol. Chem. **204:** 379-390.
7. Baranes, D., F. T. Liu, G. Marx, M. Shalit & E. Razin. 1986. Immunol. Lett. In press.
8. Gordon, P. R. & B. L. O'Dell. 1983. J. Nutr. **113:** 239-245.
9. Gordon, P. R., C. W. Woodruff, H. L. Anderson & B. L. O'Dell. 1982. Am. J. Clin. Nutr. **35:** 113-120.
10. Aktulga, A. & O. N. Ulutin. 1975. *In* Platelets: Recent Advances In Basic Research and Clinical Aspects. A. Aktulga, Ed.: 185-191. Excerpta Medica. Amsterdam.
11. Kazimierczak, W. & C. Maslinski. 1974. Agents Actions **4:** 1-6.
12. Hansen, M. A., G. Fernandes & R. Good. 1982. Ann. Rev. Nutr. **2:** 151-177.
13. Allen, J. L., N. E. Kay & C. J. McLain. 1981. Ann. Int. Med. **95:** 154-157.
14. Chandra, R. K. & D. H. Dayton. 1982. Nutr. Res. **2:** 721-733.
15. Bergmann, K. E. & R. L. Bergmann. 1982. *In* Nutritional Problems in Childhood. F. Balli, Ed. Piccin Medical Books.
16. Briggs, W. A., M. M. Pedersen, S. K. Mahajan, D. H. Sillik, A. S. Prasad & F. D. Donald. 1982. Kidney Int. **21:** 827-832.

Proimmune Activity of Thrombin

GERARD MARX

Department of Hematology
Beilinson Medical Center
Petah Tikva, Israel

DISCUSSION

It has been demonstrated that bone marrow-derived mast cells (BMMC) can be activated by thrombin.[1–5] Their stimulation, which results in degranulation, the parallel release of histamine and β-hexosaminidase, is calcium dependent, and is associated with calcium uptake and a transient rise in cAMP (FIGURES 1-3). A major distinction between BMMC activation by IgE-Ag complexes and thrombin is that the former leads to the release of leukotrienes and the latter does not.[1] Unlike monocytes, which can be stimulated by catalytically inactive thrombin or by thrombin-AT-III complexes,[6,7] mast cells require proteolytically effective thrombin.

One could hypothesize that mast cells and platelets are functionally interactive. The responses associated with exposure of BMMC and platelets to stimuli, and their sensitivity to drugs, appear to overlap remarkably (TABLES 1 and 2). Metabolites released by one cell type seem to be particularly suited to the activation of the other. This is exemplified by the generation of thrombin on the platelet membrane, and the release of relatively large amounts of PAF (platelet aggregating factor) by mast cells. Depending on the specific stimulant, both cell types release arachidonic acid derivatives (prostaglandins or leukotrienes), serotonin, and histamine, all of which have wide-ranging physiologic impact. Concomitantly, both cells release metabolites that are capable of modulating the activity of thrombin, notably heparinoids and zinc.[8,9]

Platelets circulate in the blood, and mast cells are usually located in subendothelial regions. Exposure of platelets to the collagen-rich environment in which mast cells abound stimulates platelets and leads to the generation of thrombin on their surface, which induces the release of metabolites from mast cells, including histamine and PAF. An explosive and mutually instigative paroxysm of release occurs among platelets and mast cells.

Functional complementarity between mast cells and platelets accords with the physiologic overview that the activation of the coagulation system triggers a cascade of responses, exemplified by the mutual mobilization of platelets and mast cells through the vehicle of thrombin.

SUMMARY

Exposure of cultured BMMC to thrombin induces the release of histamine, β-hexosaminidase, and degranulation, but does not generate leukotrienes. By contrast,

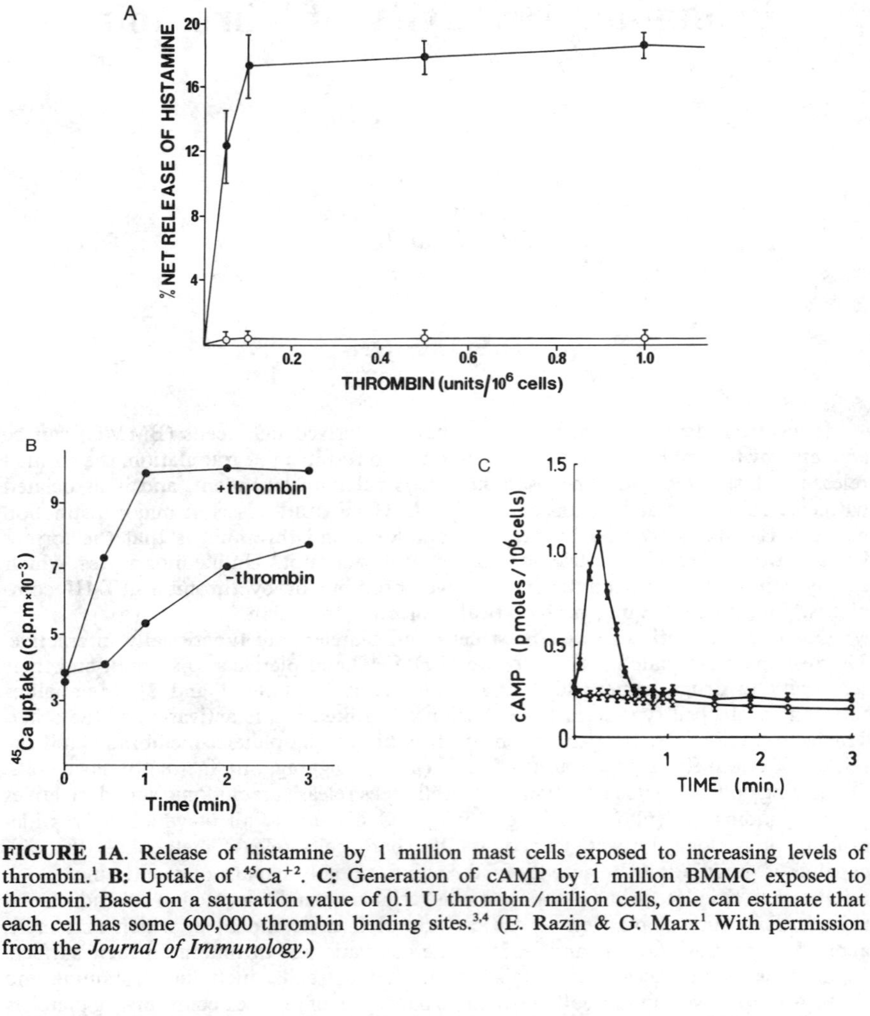

FIGURE 1A. Release of histamine by 1 million mast cells exposed to increasing levels of thrombin.[1] **B:** Uptake of $^{45}Ca^{+2}$. **C:** Generation of cAMP by 1 million BMMC exposed to thrombin. Based on a saturation value of 0.1 U thrombin/million cells, one can estimate that each cell has some 600,000 thrombin binding sites.[3,4] (E. Razin & G. Marx[1] With permission from the *Journal of Immunology*.)

TABLE 1. Comparison of Mast Cell and Platelet Response to Stimuli[8–18]

Stimulant	Platelet Aggregation	Mast Cell Secretion
IgE-Ag	+	+
Thrombin	+	+
Histamine	+ [a]	−
Serotonin	−	+
Collagen	+	−
Complement	+	+
PAF	+	−
Zinc	+ [a]	+ [a]

[a] Inhibited

TABLE 2. Comparison of Metabolites Released by Mast Cells and Platelets

Metabolite Released	From/On Platelet	From Mast Cell
Thrombin[a]	+	−
Lytic enzymes	+[a]	+[b]
Histamine	+/−	+
Serotonin	+	+
Arachidonic acid derivatives	+	+
Heparinoids	+	+
PAF	+	+
Zinc	+	?

[a] Coagulant factors II_a, IX_a, X_a (serine proteases) are generated from their zymogens on the platelet membrane.

[b] Preformed β-hexosaminidase and glycosidases are released from granules.

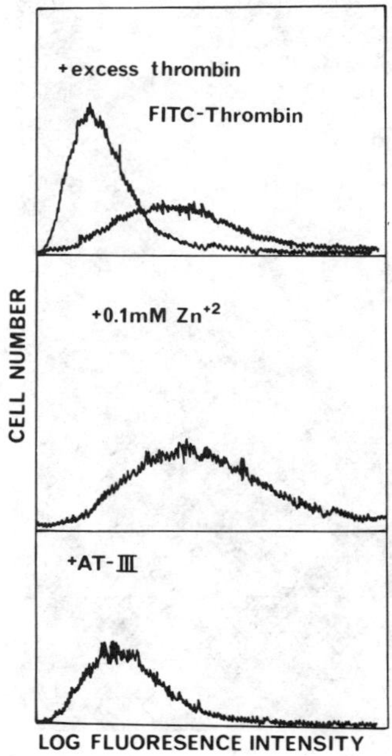

FIGURE 2. Flow cytometry of mast cells exposed to FITC-thrombin. Top panel: with excess thrombin. Middle: with 0.1 mM Zn.[2] Bottom: with AT-III.[3,5] (G. Razin *et al.* With permission from *Experimental Cell Research.*)

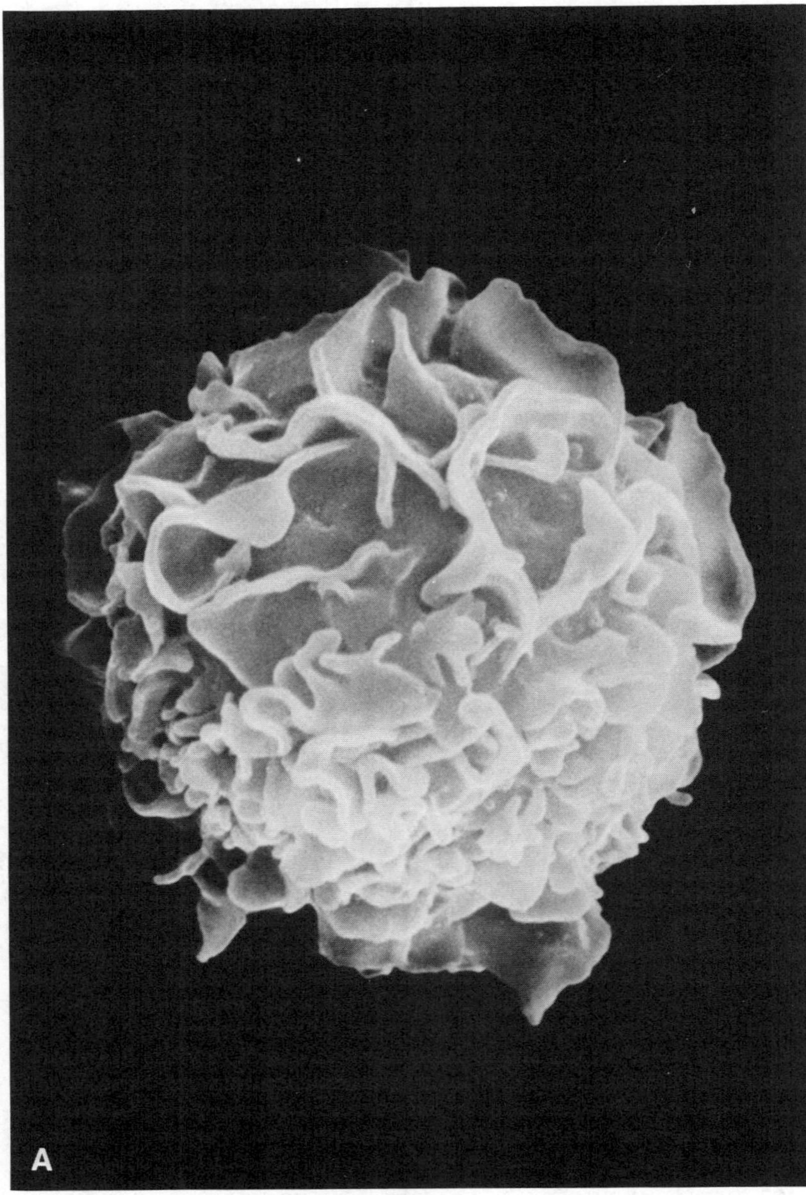

FIGURES 3A and B. Before (A) and after (B) exposure to 0.5 U/ml thrombin in Tyrode's buffer with 1 mM Ca. The activated cells do not aggregate, but the broad-based ruffled membranes appear to have become less anchored to the cell surface. SEM (×6000) of mast cells (BMMC).

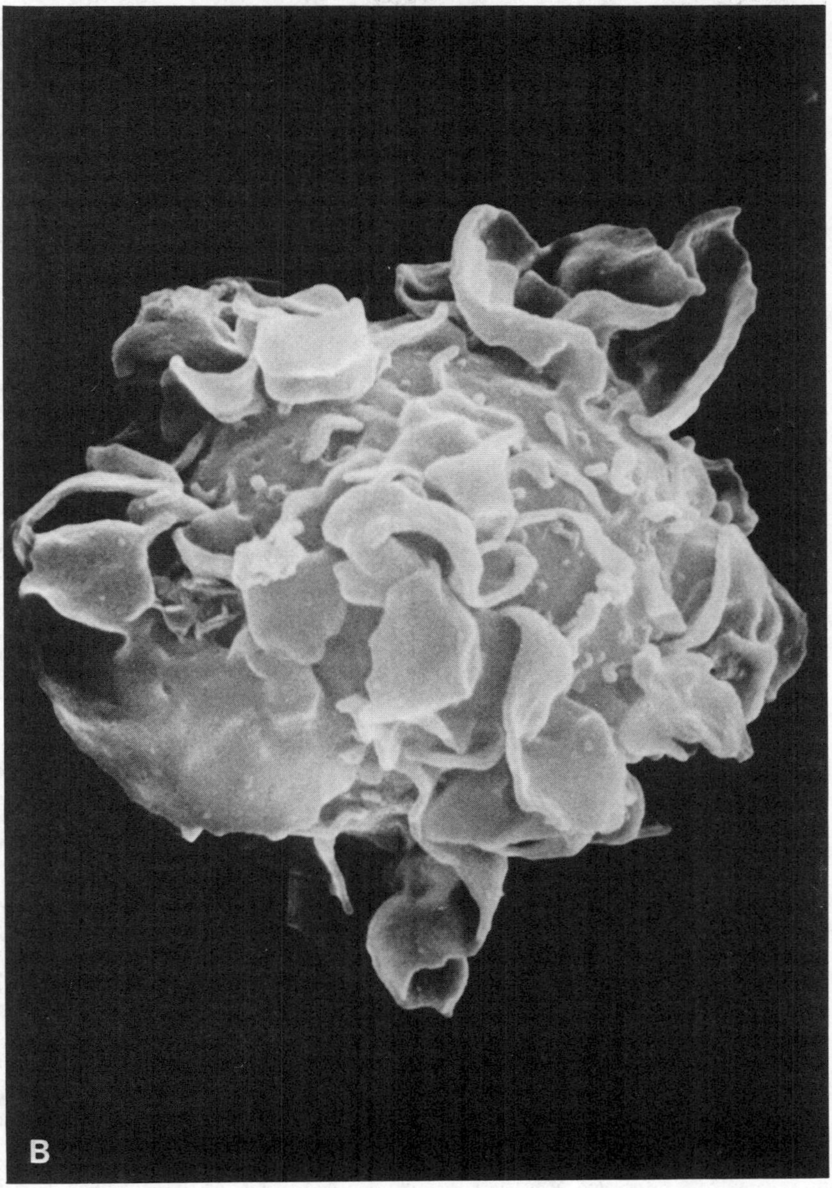
B

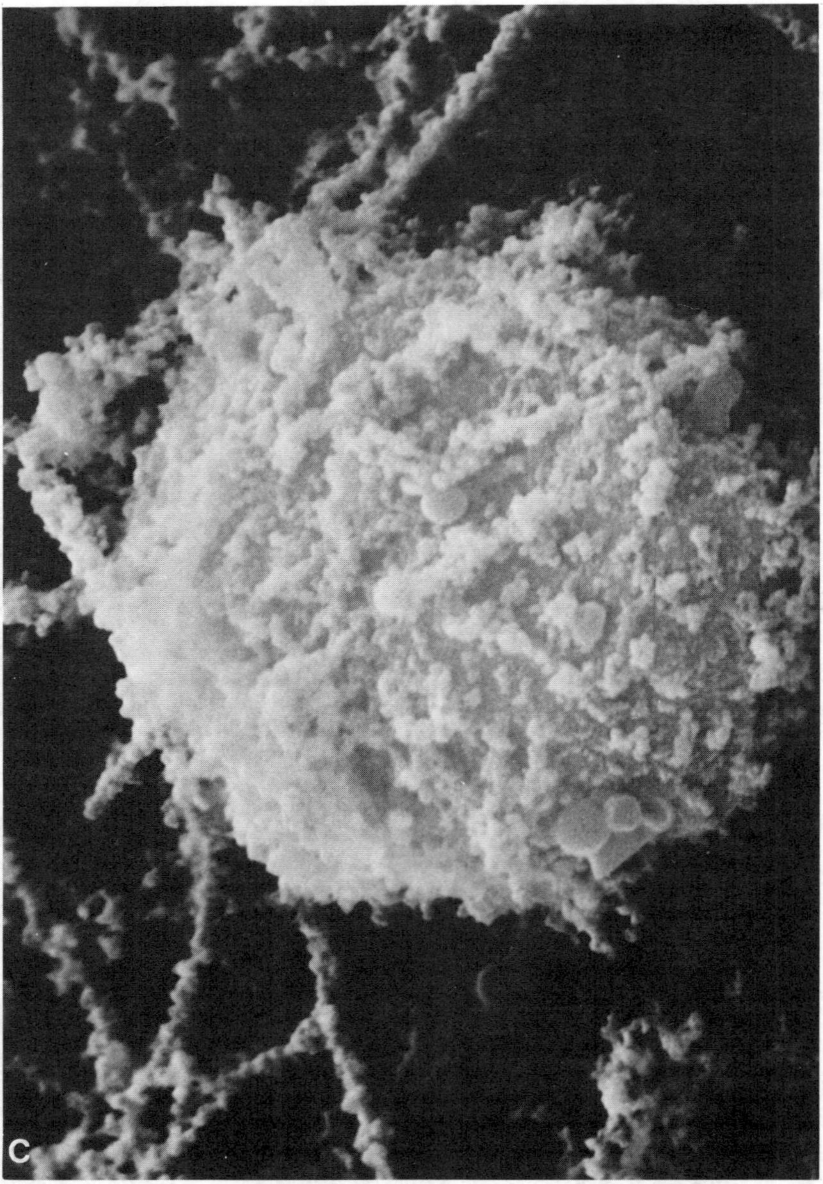

FIGURE 3C. Mast cells entrapped in fibrin, instigated by the addition of cephalin (Merz-Dade) and calcium to a suspension of mast cells in citrated human plasma (essentially an activated partial thromboplastin (APTT) assay mixture). SEM (×6000) of mast cells (BMMC).

rat peritoneal mast cells (RMP) are not stimulated by thrombin, though both types of mast cells are activated by IgE-Ag complexes. Thrombin stimulation of BMMC, which coincides with a transient rise in intracellular cAMP and a rapid influx of Ca(II), can be inhibited by AT-III and hirudin. Studies with fluorescein-labeled thrombin indicate that both binding and catalytic activity are required for full expression of cell-stimulating activity. The locus of thrombin action on the surface of BMMC seems to be distinct from that of IgE-Ag. In a physiologic context, these findings indicate that the generation of thrombin by the clotting system can activate cellular components of the immune response.

REFERENCES

1. RAZIN, E. & G. MARX. 1984. Thrombin-induced degranulation of cultured bone marrow derived mast cells. J. Immunol. **133:** 3282-3285.
2. MARX, G., D. BARANES & E. RAZIN. 1985. Thrombin selective activation of mast cells. Fed. Proc. Fed. Am. Soc. Exp. Biol. **44:** 1324.
3. RAZIN, G., D. BARANES & G. MARX. 1985. Thrombin-mast cell interactions: Binding and cell activation. Exp. Cell Res. **160:** 380-386.
4. PERVIN, R., B. I. KANNER, G. MARX & E. RAZIN. 1986. Immunology **56:** 667-672.
5. BARANES, D., F. T. LIU, G. MARX, M. SHALIT & E. RAZIN. 1986. Immunology Letters. **12:** 95-99.
6. BAR-SHAVIT, R., A. KAHN, G. D. WILNER & J. W. FENTON II. 1983. Science **220:** 728-730.
7. BAR-SHAVIT, R., A. KAHN, M. S. MUDD, C. WILNER, K. G. MANN & J. W. FENTON II. 1984. Biochemistry **23:** 397-400.
8. HEYNS, A. DUP., A. ELDOR, R. YAROM & G. MARX. 1985. Blood **66:** 213-219.
9. MARX, G. & A. ELDOR. 1985. Am. J. Hematol. **19:** 151-159.
10. KAZIMIERCZAK, W. & C. MASLINSKI. 1974. Agents Actions **4:** 1-6.
11. HALLBERG, T., M. DOHLSTEN & B. BALDETORP. 1984. Scand. J Haematol. **32:** 113-118.
12. LAPETINA, E. G. & F. L. SIEGEL. 1983. J. Biol. Chem. **258:** 7241-7244.
13. KIEM, J. *et al.* 1979. Clin. Chem. **25:** 705-710.
14. MUSTARD, J. F. & M. A. PACKHAM. 1970. Pharmacol. Rev. **22:** 97-186.
15. WIEDMER, T. & P. J. SIMS. 1985. J. Biol. Chem. **260:** 8014-8019.
16. SCHREIBER, A. D., D. B. CINES, C. ZMIJEWSKI & R. W. COLMAN. 1979. Blood **53:** 578-587.
17. WATHEWR, J. L., H. SONDON, K. B. REID, A. P. PETTIER & J. P. CAEN. 1977. Immunochemistry **14:** 763-766.
18. VOELKEL, N. F., S. WORTHEN, J. T. REEVES, P. M. HENSON & R. C. MURPHY. 1982. Science **218:** 286-288.

Thrombin-Induced Increase in Pulmonary Endothelial Permeability *in Vitro*: Protective Effect of Isoproterenol[a]

FRED L. MINNEAR, DUDLEY G. MOON, AND LORI A. HILL

Department of Physiology
Albany Medical College of Union University
Albany, New York 12208

Activation of β-adrenergic receptors by isoproterenol or terbutaline reduces the edema produced by histamine and bradykinin in the hindlimb and hamster cheek-pouch preparations.[1–4] Studies in the lung have shown that β-agonists attenuate pulmonary edema as produced by histamine, hydrochloric acid, and *Pseudomonas* bacteremia.[5–7] We recently observed that preinfusion of isoproterenol protected against the increased pulmonary transvascular fluid and protein fluxes produced by thrombin-induced intravascular coagulation in sheep.[8]

Two mechanisms have been proposed to explain this protective effect of β-agonists. β-agonists may relax endothelial cells and thereby reduce the width between endothelial cells[1–4] that may be initially widened by permeability-increasing substances such as histamine, bradykinin, and thrombin.[9,10] Secondly, β-agonists, by virtue of their vasodilatory properties, may also reduce the pulmonary capillary pressure and subsequently decrease transvascular fluid filtration and protein flux.[5] Because it is difficult to differentiate between changes in vascular permeability and hemodynamics *in vivo,* we used an *in vitro* model to control for hemodynamic changes and to determine if isoproterenol could reduce the thrombin-induced increase in endothelial permeability.

METHODS

Alterations in endothelial permeability were tested by measurement of the clearance rate of [^{125}I]albumin across a monolayer of bovine pulmonary artery endothelial cells. The cell line (CCL-209) of Del Vecchio and coworkers[11] was obtained at the 16th passage from the American Type Culture Collection (Rockville, MD). At the 22d passage, the cells were seeded onto gelatinized polycarbonate micropore membranes

[a]This work was supported by HL-27016, HL-32418, and in part, by BRSG Grant S07RR05394-4.

(13 mm diameter, 0.8 μm pore size; Nucleopore) that were mounted on the base of plastic cylinders (11 mm inner diameter; Adaps, Inc.). The experimental apparatus used to study transendothelial transport consisted of a 700 μl luminal compartment that communicated with a 25 ml albuminal compartment solely by the polycarbonate membrane lined with the endothelial cell monolayer. Both compartments contained Dulbecco's Modified Eagle Medium (DMEM) and 1% BSA. Since the luminal chamber floated in the abluminal chamber, there was no hydrostatic pressure between the two chambers.

A concentration gradient of [^{125}I]albumin was established across the endothelial monolayer by placement of DMEM containing tracer albumin in the luminal compartment. The [^{125}I]albumin was prepared from ^{251}NaI and purified bovine albumin using the chloramine-T procedure.[12] The [^{125}I]albumin was separated from free iodine by dialysis against phosphate buffered saline at 4°C and was maintained in dialysis until used. Baseline clearance rates were measured for an initial 30 min with the cells incubated at 37°C in DMEM. At 30 min, 70 μl of either DMEM, human α-thrombin (final concentration of 10^{-6} M), α-thrombin and isoproterenol (10^{-6}M), or isoproterenol alone was added to the luminal chamber (total volume = 700 μl). Experimental clearance rates were determined at 30-60 min in each group (n = 15) and normalized to the baseline clearance rates of each cell monolayer. The change in clearance of albumin (Cl_{alb}) over time was determined by least squares regression and was calculated from the equation

$$Cl_{alb} = \frac{V_A [A]_t}{[L]}$$

where V_A is the volume in the abluminal side at each 5-min time point (corrected for changes in volume due to sampling), $[A]_t$ is the concentration of tracer in the abluminal side at each time point, and [L] is the concentration of tracer in the luminal side at each time point (corrected for dilution from volume of fluid added to effect an intervention).

RESULTS

The baseline and experimental clearance rates and the experimental/baseline values are shown in TABLE 1. α-Thrombin increased ($p < 0.05$, by analysis of variance) the clearance rate from the control DMEM value, and isoproterenol reduced ($p < 0.05$) this response to thrombin. Isoproterenol also decreased ($p < 0.05$) the clearance rate below the control DMEM value.

DISCUSSION

This study was designed to examine the permeability-decreasing effect of the β-agonist, isoproterenol, independent of its vasodilatory properties. Isoproterenol

(10^{-6}M) significantly attenuated the thrombin-induced increase in the clearance rate of [^{125}I]albumin across a monolayer of bovine pulmonary artery endothelial cells. Furthermore, isoproterenol decreased endothelial permeability below control values. The findings indicate that isoproterenol can prevent increases in endothelial permeability and can possibly decrease normal endothelial permeability.

The possible mechanisms for the permeability-decreasing effect of isoproterenol may be related to a direct action of isoproterenol on endothelial cells and/or on the thrombin molecule itself. Thrombin acts directly on endothelial cells to produce gaps between endothelial cells and thus increase the transendothelial clearance rate of albumin (reference 9 and personal observation). It has been hypothesized that this effect is due to contraction of actin fibrils within the endothelial cytoplasm that results in increased gap formation between endothelial cells.[4,9,10] Isoproterenol may counteract the contraction of endothelial cells by relaxing the endothelial cells and reducing the width between the cells. Preliminary data suggest that a direct action of isoproterenol on the thrombin molecule is unlikely in that isoproterenol does not alter the fibrinogen-clotting activity of thrombin.

TABLE 1. The Effect of Isoproterenol on the Clearance Rate of [^{125}I]Albumin across Pulmonary Artery Endothelial Cell Monolayers[a]

	Control (DMEM)	Thrombin (10^{-6}M)	Thrombin and Isoproterenol (10^{-6}M)	Isoproterenol (10^{-6}M)
Baseline clearance rate, μl/min	0.36 ± 0.03	0.29 ± 0.02	0.32 ± 0.03	0.30 ± 0.03
Experimental clearance rate, μl/min	0.33 ± 0.03	0.57 ± 0.03	0.45 ± 0.05	0.22 ± 0.04
Experimental to baseline ratio	0.91 ± 0.05	1.96 ± 0.09[b]	1.39 ± 0.07[c]	0.68 ± 0.08[b]

[a] Values are means ± 1 SE.
[b] $p < 0.05$ from DMEM.
[c] $p < 0.05$ from thrombin.

ACKNOWLEDGMENT

Human α-thrombin was generously supplied by Dr. John Fenton II, New York State Department of Health.

REFERENCES

1. ARFORS, K. E., G. RUTILI & E. SVENSJO. 1979. Microvascular transport of macromolecules in normal and inflammatory conditions. Acta Physiol. Scand. Suppl. **463:** 93-103.

2. GREGA, G. J., J. J. MACIEJKO, R. M. RAYMOND & D. P. SAK. 1980. The interrelationship among histamine, various vasoactive substances, and macromolecular permeability in the canine forelimb. Circ. Res. **46:** 264-275.
3. MARCINIAK, D. L., D. E. DOBBINS, J. J. MACIEJKO, J. B. SCOTT, F. J. HADDY & G. J. GREGA. 1978. Antagonism of histamine edema formation by catecholamines. Am. J. Physiol. **234:** H180-H185.
4. SVENSJO, E., C. G. A. PERSSON & G. RUTILI. 1976. Inhibition of bradykinin-induced macromolecular leakage from postcapillary venules by a β_2-adrenotropic stimulant, terbutaline. Acta Physiol. Scand. **101:** 504-506.
5. FOY, T., J. MARION, K. L. BRIGHAM & T. R. HARRIS. 1979. Isoproterenol and aminophylline reduce lung capillary filtration during high permeability. J. Appl. Physiol.: Respir. Environ. Exercise Physiol. **46:** 146-151.
6. MIZUS, I., W. SUMMER, I. FARRUKH, J. R. MICHAEL & G. H. GURTNER. 1985. Isoproterenol or aminophylline attenuate pulmonary edema after acid lung injury. Am. Rev. Respir. Dis. **131:** 256-259.
7. PERSSON, C. G. A., M. EKMAN & I. ERJEFALT. 1979. Vascular anti-permeability effects of β-receptor agonists and theophylline in the lung. Acta Pharmacol. Toxicol. **44:** 216-220.
8. MINNEAR, F. L., A. JOHNSON & A. B. MALIK. 1986. β-Adrenergic modulation of pulmonary transvascular fluid and protein exchange. J. Appl. Physiol. **60:** 266-274.
9. GALDAL, K. S., S. A. EVENSEN & F. BROSSTAD. 1982. Effects of thrombin on the integrity of monolayers of cultured human endothelial cells. Thromb. Res. **27:** 575-584.
10. MAJNO, G., S. M. SHEA & M. LEVENTHAL. 1969. Endothelial contraction induced by histamine-type mediators: An electron microscopic study. J. Cell Biol. **42:** 647-672.
11. DEL VECCHIO, P. J. & J. R. SMITH. 1981. Expression of angiotensin converting enzyme in cultured pulmonary artery endothelial cells. J. Cell Physiol. **108:** 337-345.
12. BOCCI, V. 1964. Efficient labelling of serum proteins with ^{131}I using chloramine-T. Int. J. Appl. Radiat. Isot. **15:** 449-456.

S-Protein Modulates the Inactivation of Thrombin by Antithrombin III-Heparin[a]

KLAUS T. PREISSNER AND G. MÜLLER-BERGHAUS

Clinical Research Unit for Blood Coagulation and Thrombosis
Max Planck Gesellschaft at the Justus-Liebig-Universität
Gaffkystr. 11, D-6300 Giessen
Federal Republic of Germany

The direct inhibition of thrombin by antithrombin III in the fluid phase results in the formation of an inactive, equimolar complex between the enzyme and the inhibitor.[1] The slow rate of inactivation of thrombin is accelerated several fold in the presence of heparin due to an interaction of antithrombin III with the mucopolysaccharide.[2,3] Besides antithrombin III, other plasma proteins such as histidine-rich glycoprotein[4] or platelet factor 4[5] show high affinity to heparin, which results in the neutralization of heparin activity in the inhibition reaction.[6] In this respect, the plasma protein S-protein, known as an inhibitor of the assembly of the membrane attack complex of complement,[7,8] has been shown to express similar antiheparin activity[9] and appears to be identical to the serum spreading factor, vitronectin.[10]

The interference of human S-protein, a glycoprotein with an approximate M_r of 78 000, with thrombin inactivation by antithrombin III-heparin mixtures, was studied in a purified system. While under pseudo first-order conditions, thrombin amidolytic activity was totally inhibited by antithrombin III in the presence of 0.05 U/ml heparin in less than one minute; the addition of S-protein induced a concentration-dependent reduction of the inhibition rate and thereby counteracted the accelerative effect of heparin (TABLE 1). Control experiments revealed no influence of S-protein on the thrombin-antithrombin III reaction in the absence of heparin. The same effect of S-protein on the thrombin inhibition by antithrombin III in the presence of 0.05 U/ml heparin was demonstrated in a clotting assay system. The addition of increasing concentrations of S-protein progressively reduced the clotting times in this system. At a molar ratio of S-protein to antithrombin III of 2:1, the heparin effect was almost abolished.

The influence of various heparin concentrations on the inhibition of thrombin (30 nM) by antithrombin III (1 μM) was studied in an amidolytic assay system at 37°C. In the absence of S-protein, thrombin activity was progressively inhibited due to the presence of increasing concentrations of heparin, and complete inhibition was observed at 0.1 U/ml heparin. By contrast, the presence of 4 μM S-protein shifted the point of complete inhibition of thrombin to 1 U/ml heparin. The heparin-neutralizing activity of S-protein was mainly expressed within the range of 0.01-0.2 U/ml.

[a]This work was supported by the Stiftung Volkswagenwerk, Hannover, West Germany.

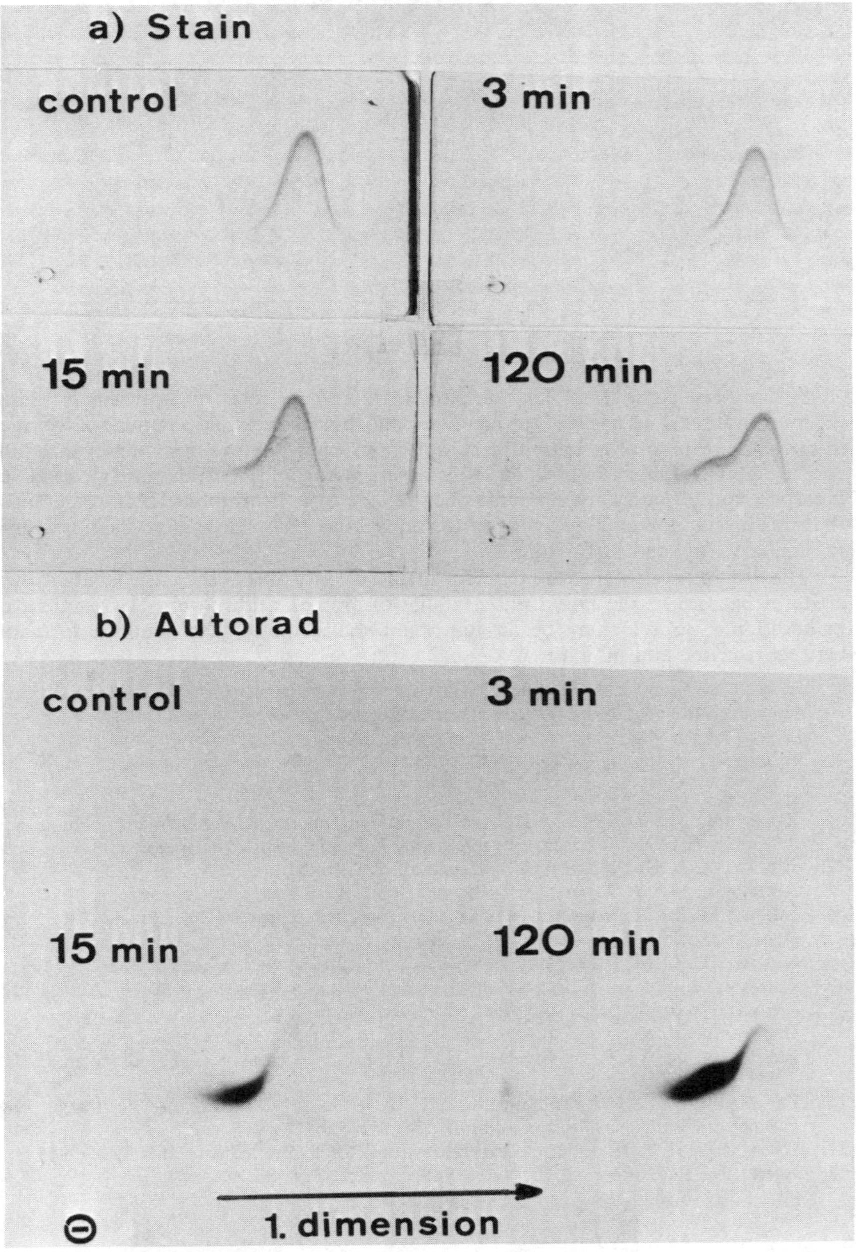

FIGURE 1. Formation of the thrombin-antithrombin III-S-protein complex. Native whole blood was substituted with radiolabeled antithrombin III and kept at 37°C for various time intervals as indicated. The samples were made 2 mM in diisopropyl fluorophosphate and centrifuged, and the supernatants were subjected to crossed immunoelectrophoresis. The second dimension into agarose gel contained anti-(human S-protein). The control sample was kept at 37°C for 2 hr in the presence of 10 mM EDTA. Upper panel: Stain of the immunoprecipitates. Note the development of the two peaks in the serum samples with time. Lower panel: Autoradiographs of the same plates. Note the precipitation of increasing amounts of radiolabeled antithrombin III by anti-(human S-protein).

S-protein (μM)	S-protein/AT III (mol/mol)	Apparent first-order rate constant k (min^{-1})
0	0	8.5
0.9	0.45	4.2
1.8	0.9	2.5
2.7	1.35	1.9
4.1	2.05	1.3

It had been recognized that the electrophoretic mobility of S-protein in plasma differs from that in serum.[11,12] The characteristic immunoprecipitin pattern of S-protein in serum appears to be due to formation of a ternary complex consisting of thrombin, antithrombin III, and S-protein. During serum formation from native blood, the incorporation of increasing amounts of radiolabeled antithrombin III into a complex that was immunoprecipitated with antiserum against S-protein was verified by crossed immunoelectrophoresis (FIGURE 1).

These findings demonstrate that S-protein not only affects the anticoagulant properties of heparin in the initial phase of the thrombin-antithrombin III reaction, but in addition, S-protein may be an important modulator of the complex formation between enzyme and inhibitor.

REFERENCES

1. ROSENBERG, R. D. 1982. *In* Hemostasis and Thrombosis. R. W. Colman, J. Hirsh, V. J. Marder & E. W. Salzman, Eds.: 962-985. J. P. Lippincott, Philadelphia.
2. ABILDGAARD, U. 1968. Scand. J. Haematol. **5:** 440-453.
3. JORNVALL, H., W. W. FISH & I. BJÖRK. 1979. FEBS Lett. **106:** 358-362.
4. LIJNEN, H. R., M. HOYLAERTS & D. COLLEN. 1973. Thromb. Res. **29:** 443-446.
5. HANDIN, R. I. & J. H. COHEN. 1976. J. Biol. Chem. **251:** 4273-4282.
6. LIJNEN, H. R., M. HOYLAERTS & D. COLLEN. 1983. J. Biol. Chem. **258:** 3803-3808.
7. PODACK, E. R., K. T. PREISSNER & H. J. MÜLLER-EBERHARD. 1984. Acta Pathol. Microbiol. Immunol. Scand. Sect. C. 92 (Suppl. 284): 89-96.
8. DAHLBÄCK, B. & E. R. PODACK. 1985. Biochemistry **24:** 2368-2374.
9. PREISSNER, K. T., R. WASSMUTH & G. MÜLLER-BERGHAUS. 1985. Biochem. J. **231:** 349-355.
10. PREISSNER, K. T., N. HEIMBURGER, E. ANDERS & G. MÜLLER-BERGHAUS. 1986. Biochem. Biophysics Res. Commun. **134:** 951-956.
11. PODACK, E. R. & H. J. MÜLLER-EBERHARD. 1979. J. Biol. Chem. **254:** 9908-9914.
12. JENNE, D., F. HUGO & S. BHADKI. 1985. Thromb. Res. **38:** 401-412.

Identification of a Tripeptide Analogue (SC-40476) That Acts as a Selective Partial Agonist-Antagonist at the Human Platelet Thrombin Receptor

E. M. RUDA,[a] M. C. SCRUTTON,[a] AND D. P. TUFFIN[b]

[a] *Department of Biochemistry*
King's College
Strand, London WC2R 2LS
United Kingdom

[b] *Searle Research and Development*
High Wycombe HP12 4HL
United Kingdom

High-affinity receptors for thrombin have been detected on human platelets,[1] but many aspects of the mechanism(s) by which this proteolytic enzyme induces aggregation of, and secretion from, this cell remain unclear. In common with platelet excitatory agonists, which do not exhibit proteolytic activity, for example, platelet-activating factor, thrombin increases phosphoinositide breakdown[2,3] and elevates the levels of 1,2-diacylglycerol[4,5] and cytosolic [Ca^{2+}],[6,7] suggesting that it acts by way of a classical receptor occupancy mechanism. A proteolytic event, however, has been proposed as an integral feature of the signal transduction mechanism used by thrombin inasmuch as derivatives of this enzyme selectively inactivated at the catalytic site are ineffective as platelet excitatory agonists[1] and because a surface membrane substrate (glycoprotein V) has been identified that is cleaved by thrombin.[8]

Many compounds have been described that inhibit the catalytic activity of thrombin. Similar attention has not, however, been given to the identification of synthetic agonists or antagonists for cellular thrombin receptors, despite the potential of such compounds to provide insight into the mechanisms by which thrombin stimulates cells. We have identified a novel tripeptide analogue (SC40476) (FIGURE 1) as a selective partial agonist-antagonist for the platelet thrombin receptor. SC40476, when added at mM concentrations, has no significant effect on thrombin-induced catalytic activity monitored either as hydrolysis of a small model substrate (S2238), or as conversion of fibrinogen to fibrin. Over this concentration range, however, SC40476 induces a parallel shift to the right in the dose/response curve describing the relationship between the extent of aggregation and thrombin concentration. The pA_2 calculated from these data is 2.4. Inhibition by SC40476 of adenosine triphosphate

(ATP) secretion induced by thrombin occurs over a similar concentration range (IC_{50} = 0.5 mM at 2 nM thrombin). Inhibition is selective, for over this concentration range, SC40476 causes no inhibition of aggregatory responses induced by addition of saturating concentrations of adenosine diphosphate (ADP), vasopressin, collagen, or 11,9-epoxymethano prostaglandin H_2 (U-46619). Instead, SC40476 tends to enhance the responses induced by a nonsaturating concentration of these latter agonists. Furthermore inhibition by SC40476 of aggregatory and secretory responses induced by thrombin is incomplete, with a maximum of 60-70% inhibition being obtained in the presence of saturating concentrations. These findings, which suggest additional efficacy as a weak partial agonist for the platelet thrombin receptor, accord with observation in platelet-rich plasma of a weak aggregatory response induced when SC40476 is added alone. This response can, however, only be observed when aggregation is measured as a decrease in the number of single platelets because no change in the light transmittance of a platelet suspension results from addition of SC40476.

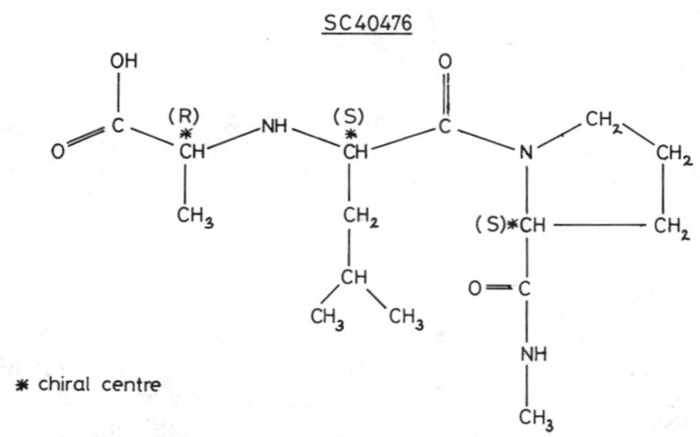

FIGURE 1. Structure of SC40476.

No change in cytosolic Ca^{2+} concentration (as measured using Quin 2) occurs as a consequence of stimulation by SC40476, although addition of this compound inhibits the increase induced by thrombin. In platelets prelabeled with [^{32}P]phosphate, however, addition of SC40476 causes increased ^{32}P incorporation into phosphatidate (FIGURE 2). No significant change occurs in the levels of ^{32}P in phosphatidylserine, phosphatidylethanolamine, or phosphatidylcholine under these conditions (FIGURE 2), suggesting that the phosphatidate formed derives from breakdown of phosphoinositides. The agonist activity observed for SC40476 may therefore result from its production of an enhanced level of 1,2-diacylglycerol, although more recent studies cast doubt on this postulate.

No detectable cleavage of glycoprotein V occurs as a consequence of stimulation of platelets with SC40476, and this compound causes only weak inhibition of cleavage induced by thrombin. Hence, proteolytic cleavage of glycoprotein V is not an absolute requirement for transmembrane signaling from the thrombin receptor, although our data do not exclude a facilitative role for proteolysis in this process (but see reference 9).

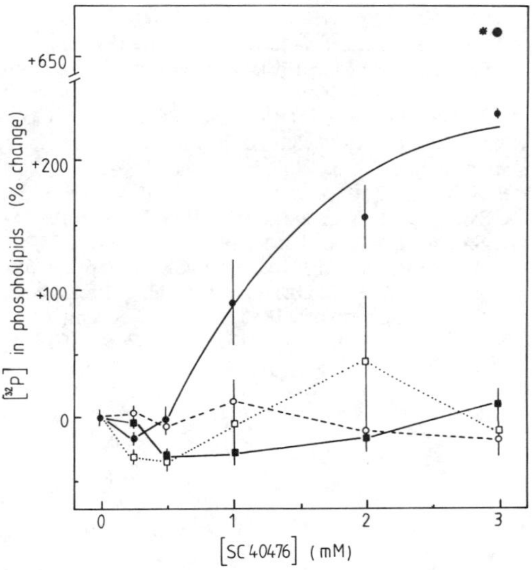

FIGURE 2. Pattern of incorporation of ^{32}P into platelet phospholipids following stimulation with SC40476. A washed platelet suspension (2×10^9 platelets/ml) in modified phosphate-free Tyrode's medium was prepared essentially as described previously.[10] The suspending medium also contained 0.2% (w/v) bovine serum albumin, 0.05 units/ml hirudin, and 1 μM prostacyclin. This suspension was incubated for 90 mins at 37°C with 30 μCi/ml carrier-free [^{32}P]phosphate, and the platelets were then collected by centrifugation at $350 \times g$ for 25 mins (20°C). The platelet pellet was resuspended in the modified phosphate-free Tyrode's medium without additions to give a cell count of 4×10^8 platelets/ml. Ca^{2+} (1 mM) and fibrinogen (1 mg/ml) were added to aliquots (0.4 ml) of this suspension after warming to 37°C. SC40476 at the concentration indicated, or thrombin (25 nM), was then added, and after 2 mins at 37°C, the reaction was terminated by addition of 3.75 volumes $CHC1_3$:CH_3OH (1:2 (v/v)). Phospholipids were extracted as described by Bligh and Dyer[11] and the solvent removed by drying under N_2. The phospholipid residues were redissolved in $CHC1_3$ at a ratio of 0.025 ml/10^8 platelets extracted, and phospholipids were separated by one-dimensional thin layer chromatography on aluminum silica gel sheets (Merck Kieselgel 60) using $CHC1_3$;$CH_3 \cdot CH_2 \cdot COOH$; $CH_3 \cdot CH_2 \cdot CH_2OH$; H_2O (50:75:50:20 (v/v) as developing solvent. The phospholipid spots were located under a U.V. lamp after spraying with rhodamine 6G and identified by comparison to the extent of migration of phospholipid standards. Areas corresponding to these spots were cut out and the ^{32}P content was estimated by liquid scintillation counting. In the figure, the symbols indicate the ^{32}P content after 2 mins stimulation in phosphatidic acid (●), phosphatidylethanolamine (○), phosphatidylcholine (■), and phosphatidylserine (□). The filled circle (●) indicated beside a star (*) shows the extent of increase in the ^{32}P content of phosphatidic acid caused by addition of 25 nM thrombin. For convenience, the data are presented as percentage increases in ^{32}P content as compared to the ^{32}P content of unstimulated controls. The actual level of ^{32}P incorporation observed for such controls was phosphatidic acid (138 ± 10 cpm), phosphatidylserine (152 ± 30 cpm), phosphatidylcholine (95 ± 5 cpm), and phosphatidylethanolamine (2044 ± 145 cpm). Phosphatidylinositol is not well stained by rhodamine and hence cannot routinely be located in this system. Thus, data for this phospholipid are not included.

REFERENCES

1. Majerus, P. W., D. M. Tollefsen & M. A. Shuman. 1976. *In* Platelets in Biology and Pathology. J. L. Gordon, Ed.: 2-260. Elsevier/North Holland Biomedical Press. Amsterdam.
2. Agranoff, B. W., P. Murphy & E. B. Seguin. 1983. J. Biol. Chem. **258:** 2076-2078.
3. Shukla, S. D. & D. J. Hanahan. 1983. Arch. Biochem. Biophys. **227:** 626-629.
4. Rittenhouse-Simmons, S. 1979. J. Clin. Invest. **63:** 580-587.
5. Macintyre, D. E. & W. K. Pollock. 1984. Biochem. J. **219:** 833-842.
6. Rink, T. J., S. W. Smith & R. Y. Tsien. 1982. FEBS Lett. **148:** 21-26.
7. Hallam, T. J., A. Sanchez & T. J. Rink. 1984. Biochem. J. **218:** 819-827.
8. Berndt, M. C. & D. R. Phillips. 1981. J. Biol. Chem. **256:** 59-65.
9. McGowan, E. B., A. Ding & T. C. Detwiler. 1983. J. Biol. Chem. **258:** 11243-11248.
10. Thompson, N. T. & M. C. Scrutton. 1985. Eur. J. Biochem. **147:** 421-427.
11. Bligh, E. G. & W. J. Dyer. 1959. Can. J. Biochem. **37:** 911-917.

Determination of Antithrombin III (AT III) Using the Coatest® Antithrombin Kit and a Microplate System

CHERYL F. SCOTT

Temple University Thrombosis Research Center
Philadelphia, Pennsylvania 19140
and
Helena Laboratories
Beaumont, Texas 77704

INTRODUCTION

AT III (heparin cofactor), the major regulatory inhibitor of plasma coagulation proteases, can be congenitally decreased, or decreased in kidney and liver disease, in disseminated intravascular coagulation, in pregnancy, in women taking oral contraceptives, or in patients following surgery, with resultant predisposition to thromboembolic disease. At present, AT III is either assayed antigenically or functionally by means of coagulant or chromogenic determinations. The preferred assay, however, is the functional chromogenic determination because coagulation assays, in general, have a high coefficient of variation, and antigenic assays may detect inactive AT III. The chromogenic assays employ synthetic, tripeptide paranitroanilide substrates that measure residual thrombin activity, spectrophotometrically, either by initial rate or acid-stopped (fixed hydrolysis time) measurements. In this report, a chromogenic assay for AT III, performed at room temperature in microplates using the Coatest® Antithrombin[a] kit, will be described (TABLES 1-4).

TABLE 1. Principle of the Assay

1. AT III + heparin (excess) → (AT III − heparin)
2. (AT III − heparin) + thrombin (excess) → (AT III − heparin + thrombin + residual thrombin)
3. Substrate $\xrightarrow{\text{thrombin}}$ peptide + pNA (yellow)

TABLE 2. Predilution of Samples

Buffer working solution	1.50 ml
Plasma (reference or patient)	50 μl

[a] The Coatest® Antithrombin kit is available from KabiVitrum or Helena Laboratories (USA).

TABLE 3. Preparation of Standard Curve (FIGURE 1)

Buffer Working Solution (μl)	Diluted Plasma (μl)	Percent of Normal AT III Obtained
400	0	0
300	100	25
200	200	50
100	300	75
0	400	100

TABLE 4. Microassay Procedure 23°C[a]

Diluted standard or sample		100 μl
Thombin		20 μl
	incubate 7 min	
S-2238		60 μl
	incubate 1.5 min	
50% acetic acid		70 μl

[a] Read in microplate reader at 405 nm; (blank = all reagents minus thrombin).

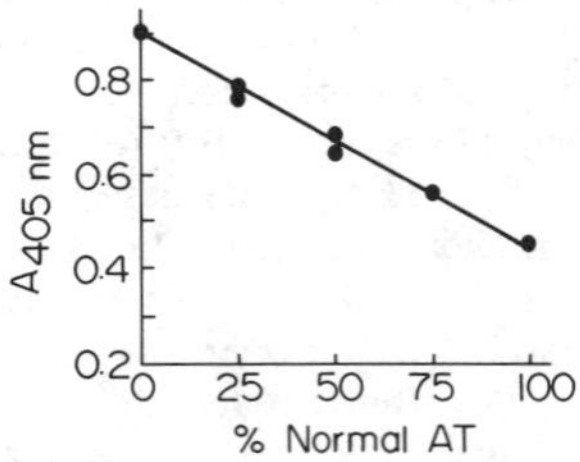

FIGURE 1. Standard curve.

The chromogenic microassay is an easy, accurate, and inexpensive way to assay AT III. It is approximately 5 times less expensive than the spectrophotometric determinations, is five to ten times faster, does not require a thermostated chamber, and requires only minimal bench space. These features make the microplate assay attractive for even the smallest clinical laboratory.

Careful and accurate monitoring of AT III levels, coupled with replacement therapy when levels fall below 80% of normal, may lead to a decreased risk of thrombosis.

Effect of Deuterium Oxide on Thrombin-Activated Fibrinogen Clotting

CHARLES R. SPILLERT, KATE R. SPILLERT, JOHN C. KERR, AND ERIC J. LAZARO

Department of Surgery
UMDNJ-New Jersey Medical School
Newark, New Jersey 07103

The kinetics of fibrin clot formation have usually been determined by measuring increased turbidity by changes in optical density.[1] These optical changes, however, are not related to the mechanical properties of the resultant clot. Other authors have successfully used mechanical impedance measurements to study dysfibrinogens in a clinical setting.[2] The purpose of this study was to use changes in viscous drag (clot impedance) to evaluate the effect of thrombin and deuterium oxide (D_2O) concentrations on thrombin-induced fibrinogen gelation. The Sonoclot Coagulation Analyzer (Scienco Inc., Morrison, CO) with an attached strip recorder was used to monitor the clot formation. This instrument produces a continuous readout of clot impedance as a function of time. The greater the slope, the more rapid the clot formation.

Lyophilized normal human citrated plasma and bovine thrombin were dissolved in water or in varying D_2O water compositions. The plasmas were mixed with thrombin at 37°C, and the clotting process was monitored for seven minutes. The curves asymptotically approach their maximum values in this seven-minute period of time. The results are shown in TABLE 1.

The results obtained in this study indicate that (1) at low concentrations of thrombin (0.5 U/cc), mean clot impedance is significantly lower in the D_2O-containing solution than in the solution without D_2O; (2) at higher concentrations of thrombin (2.0 U/cc), there is no significant difference in clot impedance between the solutions with and without D_2O); (3) when comparing the same solvent compositions, but varying the thrombin concentrations, there are significant differences in the samples containing D_2O, but not in samples containing only water.

Conclusions

D_2O markedly affects fibrin formation. The exact mechanism by which this occurs remains to be determined. The Sonoclot Coagulation Analyzer offers a new approach to the study of mechanical aspects of clot formation.

TABLE 1. Effects of D_2O and Thrombin Concentrations on Thrombin-Induced Fibrinogen Gelation as Measured by Clot Impedance

	Maximum Mean Clot Impedance (CM) Percent D_2O			
Thrombin Concentrations	0	30	60	90
0.5U/cc	(A) 3.7	(B) 3.1	(C) 1.6	(D) 1.0
2.0U/cc	(E) 4.6	(F) 5.0	(G) 3.9	(H) 3.5

Significance: B,C,D < .02 vs A; F,G,H NS vs E;
A vs E NS; B vs F < .005; C vs G < .001; D vs H < .03

REFERENCES

1. REGANON, E., V. VILA & J. AZNAR. 1984. Haemostasis **14:** 170-178.
2. SCHREIBER, W E. & G. SCHMER. 1984. J. Lab. Clin. Med. **104:** 494-500.

Structured Base of Thrombin-Regulating Functions in Hemostasis

S. M. STRUKOVA, B. A. UMAROVA, E. G. KIREEVA,
E. F. LUKYANENKO, AND B. A. KUDRYASHOV

Department of Physiology
Moscow State University
Moscow, USSR

Thrombin, the central regulatory enzyme in hemostasis, is capable of facilitating or inhibiting the clotting process. Many of its reactions require the catalytically active enzyme, whereas thrombin stimulation of monocyte chemotaxis[1] and excitation of the anticoagulating system[2] does not, suggesting that thrombin may have both enzymic and hormonal functions. The latter functions are the result of the high-affinity binding of the thrombin recognition center with cellular receptors. The loss of the important functions—the clotting of fibrinogen, the induction of platelet aggregation, the anticoagulating system activation—in β/γ-thrombin, which retains the original conformation of the active site, is likely due to destruction of the recognition center.[2,3] In the present work we provide evidence that blockade of the thrombin-recognition center by thrombomodulin (TM) or heparin results in loss of the same functions.

TM was prepared from rabbit lungs by the modified method.[4] Incubation of bovine α-thrombin, obtained by the method in reference 2, with TM, resulted in a dose-dependent decrease in clotting activity (FIGURE 1).

The treatment of α-thrombin by TM was shown to reduce thrombin-induced aggregation of platelets obtained through Lukyanenko.[3] The degree of inhibition depended on the concentration of TM (FIGURE 2). TM was shown not to alter adenosine diphosphate (ADP)-induced platelet aggregation. These data are in agreement with the results of Esmon *et al.*[6]

The binding of heparin with the cationic site of the thrombin-recognition center results in an essential decrease in its clotting and aggregating activity. Thus, the binding of the thrombin-recognition center with either TM or heparin causes loss in thrombin high substrate specificity, but hydrolysis of nonspecific substrates (TAME, BAME) does not cause such a loss.

At the same time, catalytically nonactive DIP-α-thrombin conserved the ability to bind and caused the activation of cellular receptors.[2,3] But the formation of heparin-DIP-α-thrombin complex resulted in loss of this ability. This complex did not cause the excitation of the anticoagulating system upon perfusion of the humorally isolated carotid sinus of the rabbit, but DIP-α-thrombin alone initiated the rise in fibrinolytic activity to 152.4% ($p < 001$).

We suggest that thrombin functions could be modulated by ligands either to the active site or to the thrombin-recognition center.

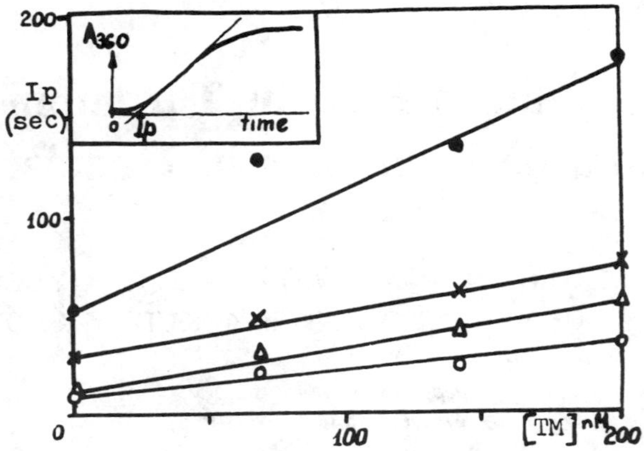

FIGURE 1. The effect of increasing concentrations of TM (nM) on the clotting activity of α-thrombin, determined as Ip (sec) by Sato and Nakajima.[5] α-Thrombin (●, 3.75 nM; ×, 7.5 nM; △, 11.2 nM; ○, 15.0 nM) was incubated with TM for 2 minutes. The induction period, Ip, of a system was obtained by extrapolating along the maximum slope of a turbity-time curve (Hitachi spectrophotometer model EPS-3T).

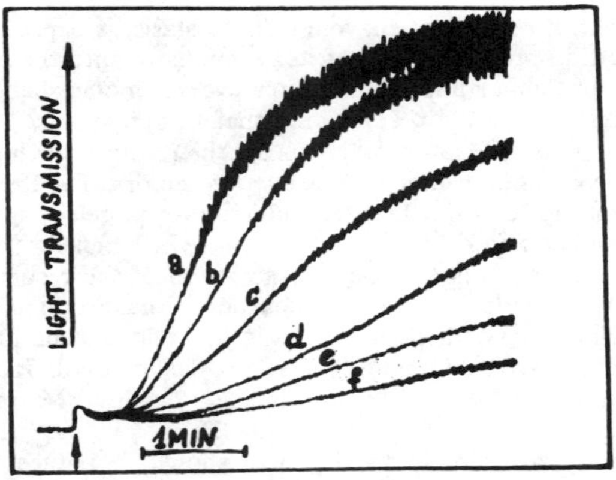

FIGURE 2. Inhibition of α-thrombin-induced platelet aggregation by increasing concentrations of TM. α-Thrombin (1.5 nM) with different concentrations of TM was added into platelets at the arrow. a is the control, b is the addition of 20 nM TM, c of 50 nM TM, d of 70 nM TM, e of 90 nM TM, and f of 100 nM TM.

REFERENCES

1. BAR-SHAVIT, R., A. KAHN, G. D. WILNER & J. W. FENTON II. 1983. Science **220:** 728-731.
2. STRUKOVA, S. M., B. A. UMAROVA, T. N. MITROSHINA, O. A. SEMIONOVA & B. A. KUDRYASHOV. 1982. Thromb. Res. **26:** 259-266.
3. LUKYANENKO, E. F., S. M. STRUKOVA, E. G. KIREEVA, T. A. BALAKINA & N. A. GORBUNOVA. 1985. Biokhimia USSR **50:** 1433-1439.
4. ESMON, N. L., W. J. OWEN & C. T. ESMON. 1982. J. Biol. Chem. **257:** 859-864.
5. SATO, H. & A. NAKAJIMA. 1984. Thromb. Res. **33:** 645-651.
6. ESMON, N. L., R. C. CARROLL & C. T. ESMON. 1983. J. Biol. Chem. **258:** 12238-12242.

Index of Contributors